OSTEOPOROSIS: ETIOLOGY, DIAGNOSIS AND TREATMENT

OSTEOPOROSIS: ETIOLOGY, DIAGNOSIS AND TREATMENT

BILAR E. MATTINGLY
AND
ALBERT C. PILLARE
EDITORS

Nova Biomedical Books
New York

For permission to use material from this book please contact us:
Telephone 631-231-7269; Fax 631-231-8175
Web Site: http://www.novapublishers.com

LIBRARY OF CONGRESS CATALOGING-IN-PUBLICATION DATA

Osteoporosis : etiology, diagnosis, and treatment / editors, Bilar E. Mattingly and Albert C. Pillare.
p. ; cm.
Includes bibliographical references and index.
ISBN 978-1-60692-397-9 (hardcover)
1. Osteoporosis. I. Mattingly, Bilar E. II. Pillare, Albert C.
[DNLM: 1. Osteoporosis--diagnosis. 2. Osteoporosis--etiology. 3. Osteoporosis--therapy. 4. Risk Assessment. WE 250 O851245 2009]
RC931.O73O715 2009
616.7'16--dc22

2008055493

Published by Nova Science Publishers, Inc. ✝ New York

CONTENTS

PREFACE

Osteoporosis is a disease of bone that leads to an increased risk of fracture. In osteoporosis the bone mineral density (BMD) is reduced, bone microarchitecture is disrupted, and the amount and variety of non-collagenous proteins in bone is altered. Osteoporosis is defined by the World Health Organization (WHO) in women as a bone mineral density 2.5 standard deviations below peak bone mass (20-year-old healthy female average) as measured by DXA; the term "established osteoporosis" includes the presence of a fragility fracture.[1] Osteoporosis is most common in women after menopause, when it is called postmenopausal osteoporosis, but may also develop in men, and may occur in anyone in the presence of particular hormonal disorders and other chronic diseases or as a result of medications, specifically glucocorticoids, when the disease is called steroid- or glucocorticoid-induced osteoporosis (SIOP or GIOP). Given its influence on the risk of fragility fracture, osteoporosis may significantly affect life expectancy and quality of life. This new book presents the latest research results in the field.

Chapter 1 - Osteoporosis currently poses a major public health problem and vertebral fractures are considered one of the hallmarks of this condition. Bone mineral density (BMD) testing using dual energy x-ray absorptiometry (DXA) is the most efficient, safe and economical tool to assess skeletal integrity and fracture risk in the clinical environment. However, conventional DXA has limited ability to discriminate between individuals with and without vertebral fractures. Recent histological and *ex vivo* research has identified differences in BMD distribution and bone structural properties within the vertebral body. This intra-vertebral (subregional) heterogeneity may be a defining characteristic between individuals with and without vertebral fractures. The aim of the studies described in this Chapter was to determine whether individuals with and without vertebral fracture(s) differed in areal subregional BMD (srBMD) profiles. Individuals with primary osteoporotic, vertebral fracture (n=7) or without vertebral fracture (n=15), and comparable controls with normal BMD (n=9) were recruited. Fractures were diagnosed from lateral thoracolumbar radiographs. Areal BMD was measured from a lateral projection DXA scan of the L3 vertebral body and in 6 manually-selected subregions (Hologic 4500A densitometer, Waltham, MA, USA). A two-way repeated measures ANOVA revealed a main effect for region ($p<0.001$) but not group. Trends demonstrated greater deficits in areal BMD when comparing srBMD profiles with standard DXA parameters between fracture and non-fracture cases. Differences in BMD between the groups across the subregions ranged from 13.1-16.3%, while for standard DXA parameters the differences were smaller in the range of 0.7-5.4%. The inability to detect statistically-significant differences between groups was attributed to low power in the study. Irrespective of group, significantly lower areal BMD was observed in the anterior and central subregion of the L3 vertebral body ($p<0.05$), consistent with previous data. Mean srBMD and standard DXA output values of the fracture group were also expressed as the number of standard deviations (SDs) from the corresponding non-fracture group means. Greater deviation below the non-fracture mean was observed with srBMD data (0.60-1.04 SDs) compared to standard DXA values (0.04-0.51 SDs). Subregional BMD measures were also found to be stronger predictors of vertebral morphology compared to standard DXA parameters ($r^2=0.18$-0.28, $p\leq0.05$; $r^2=0.06$-0.08, $p>0.05$). The subregional BMD method was considered accurate with preliminary concurrent validity established against histomorphometry methods (r=0.52-0.78). These findings suggest that subregional analysis may be superior to current standard DXA analyses in discriminating fracture from non-fracture cases. The predictive value of lateral subregional DXA for incident vertebral fractures warrants evaluation. Moreover, this method may be applied to other clinical situations, such as the monitoring of bone responses to medications, glucocorticoid-induced osteoporosis, and in disabling conditions such as chronic back pain.

Chapter 2 - Osteoporosis is a systemic skeletal syndrome characterized by low bone mass and microarchitectural deterioration of bone tissue, with a consequent increase in bone fragility and susceptibility to fracture [1]. It is a “silent” and progressive disease that may be undiagnosed until a fragility fracture occurs. Postmenopausal osteoporosis is the most common metabolic disease in the developed countries.

Non-invasive measurements of bone mineral density and estimation of fracture risk are crucial to the diagnosis and management of osteoporosis [2].

Dual Energy X-ray Absorptiometry (DXA) is the most widely employed method for estimation of bone mineral density (BMD). It is accepted as the “gold standard”, carries a low radiation exposure, and has the ability to measure BMD in spine, hip, forearm, other peripheral sites and throughout the entire skeleton. It uses two X-ray beams of different energy levels to scan the region of interest and measure the attenuation as the beam passes through the bone.

DXA estimates the average concentration of bone mineral in the area that is being scanned and allows calculation of BMD in g/cm^2 and bone mineral content (BMC) in grams. In 1994, the World Health Organization (WHO) selected the T-score as the standard for defining BMD [3]. The WHO criteria intend to provide a reasonable standard for evaluation of individual BMD values in comparison to existing databases. Comparisons are stated as standard deviation (SD) from normal BMD values obtained from young, healthy persons of the same sex, race, and age. These young normal scores, or T-scores, can then be used to decide whether a patient has a reduced BMD consistent with osteoporosis or osteopenia. The Z-score compares one patient's BMD, in standard deviations, with the mean BMD people of similar age and gender.

Osteoporosis is defined as a BMD of 2.5 SD or more below the young average value, whereas established osteoporosis uses the same threshold, but in the presence of fragility fractures [4]. In case of osteoporosis fracture risk increases continuously with decreasing

BMD, but there is no biological break-point to characterize absolutely an individual who will fracture from one who will not.

According to the International Society of Clinical Densitometry (ISCD) measurement of BMD is recommended for women 65 years and older, postmenopausal women under 65 years with risk factors, men 70 years and older, adults with a fragility fracture, adults with a disease or condition associated with low bone mass or bone loss, adults taking medications associated with low bone mass or bone loss, anyone being considered for pharmacological therapy, anyone being treated, to monitor treatment effect, and anyone not receiving therapy in whom evidence of bone loss would lead to treatment [5,6,7,8].

Chapter 3 - This chapter discusses the steps in the nutritional assessment of osteoporotic patients. It focuses on the nutritional clinical history, but anthropometry and diagnostic tests are also described. Within the former, familiar and personal health history important in bone metabolism are described. In addition, different nutritional questionnaires are discussed in assessing diet in osteoporotic patients. This chapter also emphasizes on the nutritional requirements for bone health and osteoporosis, focuzing on the key bone nutrients such as protein, calcium, phosphorus, magnesium, fluoride and vitamin D. Other nutrients important to bone are also discussed, such as zinc, copper, boron, manganese, potassium, vitamins A, K, C and the B vitamins. Nutritional recommendations on how to reach these requirements through diet are given, as well as the use of nutritional supplements for osteoporotic patients. The substances and the nutrients that interfere with calcium metabolism, as well as in the metabolism of other important bone nutrients are also described, along with nutritional recommendations to avoid these interactions. In conclusion, this review paper gives insights to the nutritional management of osteoporosis, a very important complement to medical and technology therapies.

Chapter 4 - In this chapter the authors discuss the epidemiology, pathogenesis and management of glucocorticoid-induced osteoporosis. One third to almost half of patients with endogenous or exogenous hypercortisolemia (particularly patients affected by rheumatoid arthritis and treated with synthetic glucocorticoids) presents bone loss. Trabecular bones (such as the ribs and vertebral bodies) are more affected but corical bones (such as the upper femur) are not spared. Bone turnover markers and assessments of bone mineral density (BMD) assist in the evaluation of bone loss. Glucocorticoids stimulate bone resorption and suppress bone formation. Even during the first few months after glucocorticoid administration bone loss is rapid. Nevertheless, only few patients on steroids receive prophylaxis or treatment for glucocorticoid-induced bone loss,which is required even when BMD measurements point to osteopenia (a milder form of bone loss) rather than osteoporosis. Lifestyle changes, calcium and vitamin D, bisphosphonates, are currently standard therapy for most cases of glucocorticoid-induced osteoporosis. Recent studies indicate that parathyroid hormone (PTH) might also offer a valid therapeutic option.

Chapter 5 - Individuals with stroke sustain a much higher risk of fragility fractures than the reference population. Secondary bone loss is a common phenomenon following a stroke and is a major contributing factor to the exaggerated rate of bone fractures. The pattern of bone loss in stroke survivors follows a distinct pattern, with the paretic (weaker) side sustaining a much higher degree of bone loss than the non-paretic side. In addition to progressive decline in bone mass, stroke-induced alterations in bone geometry may also compromise bone strength. Various demographic and physiological factors have been associated with bone status in individuals with stroke. There is also some evidence that certain pharmacological and non-pharmacological interventions may improve bone health and decrease the incidence of fractures in stroke patients. This chapter will review the research findings on the specific bone changes after stroke, the determinants of bone status post-stroke, as well as the current evidence on the use of different pharmacological and non-pharmacological treatments to improve bone health in stroke patients.

Chapter 6 - During the last years, several medications have been used for the management of osteoporosis. Bisphosphonates are the most prescribed drugs: daily or weekly alendronate and risedronate have demonstrated their ability to reduce fracture rates at the spine and hip; ibandronate has demonstrated spine antifracture efficacy with intervals between dosings greater than weekly. New developments in this class include intravenous administration of ibandronate or zoledronate, once every three months or once yearly. Raloxifene, a selective estrogen-receptor modulator, reduces spine fractures and, in post-hoc analyses, non-spine fractures in high-risk subjects. New selective estrogen-receptor modulators, including lasofoxifene, bazedoxifene and arzoxifene, are expected to demonstrate antifracture efficacy at the hip level, whilst retaining the extra-skeletal benefits (such as in the breast). The peptides from the parathyroid hormone family are potent stimulators of bone formation: teriparatide reduces spine and non-spine fractures for up to 30 months after the withdrawal of treatment. Strontium ranelate is suggested to be the first medication to uncouple bone formation from bone resorption. New developments include: inhibitors of cathepsin K, a cysteine protease that is involved in the cleavage of collagen, and, mainly, denosumab, a monoclonal antibody against a cytokine responsible for osteoclastogenesis.

This last perspective is born from the discovery of OPG/RANK/RANKL system. Osteoprotegerin (OPG) is a protein expressed by osteoblasts that, linking the receptor activator of nuclear factor κB (RANK) ligand (RANKL), produced by osteoblasts, blocks the process of osteoclastic differentiation and modulates osteoclastic apoptosis. The importance of OPG in bone metabolism is suggested by the positive correlation between the gene production of OPG and the bone mass increase in animal models. In humans, OPG is implicated in the pathogenesis of postmenopausal osteoporosis and of other metabolic diseases, characterized by bone loss. Estrogens and other drugs used in the treatment of osteoporosis stimulate the production of OPG from osteoblasts carrying out their antiresorption activity, at least in part, as means of the OPG/RANK/RANKL system. In vitro and in vivo data demonstrate that these drugs could improve osteoporosis, also through an increase of OPG production by osteoblasts, opening further therapeutic use of OPG or anti-RANKL drugs. The fully human monoclonal antibody denosumab (formerly known as AMG 162) binds RANKL with high affinity and specificity and inhibits RANKL action. In postmenopausal women with low bone mass, subcutaneously administered denosumab increased bone mineral density and decreased bone resorption. These preliminary data suggest that denosumab might be an effective treatment for osteoporosis.

Chapter 7 - Calcitonin (CT), through its action via a specific receptor, is a powerful inhibitor of osteoclast activity. Unlike the bisphosphonates, CT has only a transitory action and is quickly eliminated from the skeleton. Calcitriol (Vt.D_3; 1α,25-$(OH)_2D_3$) has been reported to increase lumbar BMD in postmenopausal and senile osteoporoses, but its clinical use is limited due to considerable calcemic activity, particularly after higher doses or prolonged use. Recent data showing that another calciotropic hormone, PTH, when used intermittently reduces fracture risk through considerable bone forming activity, led us to investigate the action of a combination treatment paradigm using Vt.D_3 and CT. Utilization of Vt.D_3 and calcitonin treatment in combination intuitively makes sense from a therapeutic perspective since these two hormones act on different cellular targets and could potentially create an additive beneficial effect on bone structure and strength.

Experiments were carried out in Ovx female S-D rats that had surgery at 8 weeks. Four weeks post surgery the rats were allocated to one of the following groups: 1. Sham vehicle; 2. Ovx vehicle; 3. Ovx + CT; 4. Ovx + Vt.D_3; 5. Ovx+Vt.D_3 + CT and 6. Ovx+Vt.D_3 + CT. Both CT (2μg/kg, sc) and Vt.D_3 (2μg/kg, PO) were administered once per day, 5 days/week. Rats in group 3 received calcitonin every week throughout the study. Rats in group 4 received Vt.D_3 only one week every month. Rats in group 5 received Vt.D_3 during the first week, followed by 3 weeks of calcitonin, while rats in group 6 received simultaneous dosing with Vt.D_3 and calcitonin during the first week, followed by 3 weeks of calcitonin treatment. The 4-week dosing cycle was repeated 3 times with a monthly evaluation of bone metabolism and structure.

In vivo m-CT revealed that ovariectomy resulted in deterioration in bone mass, reduced trabecular number and thickness and impaired connectivity of cancellous bone. *Ex vivo* m-CT data paralleled *in vivo* findings at the tibial metaphysis. Unlike metaphisis, epiphyseal cancellous bone was only moderately affected by ovariectomy. Intermittent dosing with calcitriol and calcitonin improved bone mass and structure at both epiphysis and metaphysis, with group 5 being particularly effective. Cortical bone was more affected with calcitonin treatment due to low endocortical resoprtion and periosteal modeling due to ovariectomy. Our data demonstrate that uncoupling of bone resorption and formation can be achieved by intermittent treatment with two calciotropic hormones that separately target bone formation (Vt.D_3) and bone resorption (calcitonin).

Chapter 8 - It has been accepted for decades that osteoclasts, the cells responsible for bone breakdown, are derived from precursors that circulate among the monocyte/macrophage population, cells more commonly associated with immune surveillance and defense. However, it is only relatively recently that the depth of integration and interaction between components of the immune and skeletal systems has begun to be appreciated. A large body of evidence has begun to accumulate implicating T cells in the bone destruction commonly associated with inflammatory and autoimmune conditions such as rheumatoid arthritis, periodontitis, Crohn's disease, and infection. Compelling data from animal models, [1] supported by recent human studies [2,3] now suggest that T cells may also play a critical role in exacerbating bone destruction in postmenopausal osteoporosis, the archetypal osteoporotic condition.

In contrast to T cells, the role of B cells in physiological and pathological bone turnover is more obscure. However, recent animal studies demonstrate that B cells may be a critical component of the mechanism by which peak bone mass is achieved and maintained. Bone homeostasis is regulated by a delicate balance between bone formation by osteoblasts and bone resorption by osteoclasts. Physiological osteoclast renewal is controlled primarily by the ratio of the key osteoclastogenic cytokine, Receptor Activator of NF-kappaB Ligand (RANKL), relative to that of its physiological inhibitor, osteoprotegerin (OPG), a RANKL decoy receptor. Historically, the predominant source of both RANKL and OPG under physiological conditions has been attributed to osteoblasts and their precursors, the bone marrow stromal cells. Human B cells have long been known to make OPG especially in response to CD40 costimulation in vitro [4]. Recently, studies from our laboratory have found that in mice, B cell precursors, immature and mature B cells, and plasma cells together account for up to 64% of total bone marrow OPG production, with 45% derived from mature B cells alone [5]. Consequently B cells are essential to the attainment and maintenance of peak bone mineral density (BMD) and bone structure in the mouse. Interestingly, B cell OPG production is regulated, in part, through interactions with T cells, via the costimulatory molecule CD40 ligand (CD40L), suggesting a critical role of lymphocytes in the regulation of basal bone mass.

This chapter will review the current knowledge base concerning the potential role of B cells and their precursors in the regulation of physiological and pathological bone turnover.

Chapter 9 - Since the mid-eighties, several medications, aiming at the inhibition of bone resorption, have consistently shown their ability to reduce fracture rates, at various skeletal locations, in osteoporotic post-menopausal women. Unfortunately, the diagnosis of osteoporosis is frequently made after the first fracture occurs. At this stage, bone strength has significantly decreased, as a result of low bone mineral density and disrupted bone micro architecture. Medications have now been developed to specifically stimulate bone formation, with the ultimate goal to restore the affected skeleton and to bring back bone biomechanical resistance to a normal level. The peptides from the parathyroid hormone family (1-34 human recombinant fragment or teriparatide and the 1-84 full length hormone) are potent stimulators of bone formation. They both have shown their ability to dramatically reduce vertebral fractures, whereas teriparatide alone has, so far, confirmed this effect on non-spinal events. These peptides were shown to have a carry-over effect, with their anti-fracture efficacy (teriparatide) maintained up to 30 months after treatment has been interrupted. However, the prescription of an anti-resorptive agent after withdrawal of teriparatide prevents further bone loss. Strontium ranelate is characterized by a dual mechanism of action, combining an inhibition of bone resorption and a simulation of bone formation. This new chemical entity has been tested in long-term studies which have shown, after 5 years, a reduction of fracture rates at the spine, at non vertebral locations and at the hip (in patients above 74 years old with prevalent low bone density at the femoral neck). Strontium ranelate reduces fractures in patients with or without prevalent vertebral fractures, in osteoporotic patients, in osteopenia and in subjects above the age of 80 years. Development of medications aiming at the restoration of normal bone strength and resistance is one of the most exciting perspectives in the management of post-menopausal osteoporosis.

Chapter 10 - *Background:* Osteoporosis is a skeletal disorder characterized by reduced bone mass and deterioration of bone microarchitecture, predisposing it to an increased risk of fracture (NIH Consensus, 2001). There are many strategies to prevent osteoporosis and maintain (or gain) bone mineral density, and physical exercises are among the most important ones. Bone is constantly built and rebuilt through remodeling, which is controlled by endogenous hormones and external mechanical forces which result from physical activity, for example.

Purposes: To update the specific physical exercise and rehabilitation protocols that show significant effects on the treatment and prevention of osteoporosis and to review the mechanisms through which exercise can maintain (or augment) bone mass and strength.

Methods: Research studies published until March 2008 were identified through a review of the literature available on the NLM PubMed and Elsevier-Science Direct databases.

Results: Most of the physical exercise and rehabilitation programs elaborated for osteoporotic patients showed that weight-bearing exercises, high-impact activities and strength training were able to maintain or increase bone mineral density. Balance and coordination exercises could decrease the fall risk, and aerobic exercises could also benefit osteoporotic patients, since they provide them more disposition to perform their activities of daily living, leading to a more active life style.

Conclusion: Recent evidences confirm that certain physical exercises are not only important to maintain or increase bone mass, but also to reduce fall risk and to improve the quality of life of osteoporotic patients.

Chapter 11 - Most current studies on the pathogenesis of osteoporosis emphasize the bone metabolic activities occurring on endosteal surfaces, whereas the periosteal aspect is somewhat neglected. In terms of bone physiology, periosteum plays a determining role in *de novo* cortical bone formation and cortical bone expansion through periosteum is the most efficient way of increasing bone strength against fractures. Despite the important role of periosteum in the pathogenesis and treatment of osteoporosis, little is known about the structural and cellular features of periosteum in osteoporosis. This chapter will focus on the major changes occurring in the periosteum of osteoporosis and the possible implications of these changes in the pathogenesis of osteoporosis. The changes identified in the periosteum of osteoporosis are mainly located in the metaphyseal compartment, which include: (a) much thicker and more cellular cambial layer; (b) increased number of $TRAP^{+}$ (tartrate resistant acid phosphatase), $VEGF^{+}$ (vascular endothelial growth factor) cells and the degree of vascularization; and (c) enhanced expression of sympathetic nerve fibers. The structural and cellular changes of osteoporotic periosteum indicate that periosteum plays an important role in the cortical bone resorption in metaphyseal areas and this pathological process may be regulated by the sympathetic nervous system.

Chapter 12 - Osteoporosis is known as the 'silent epidemic' due to the asymptomatic nature of the disease, prior to fracture. It is estimated that by 2020, half of all US citizens over the age of 50 will be at risk of fracture from osteoporosis if no immediate action is taken by individuals at risk, healthcare professionals, health systems and policy makers. In the US, caring for individuals with osteoporotic bone fractures costs $18 billion per annum in direct medical costs. With the global population aging rapidly, these costs will affect increasing numbers of people. Early diagnosis has the potential to substantially reduce the social and economic costs associated with this disease.

The current clinical gold standard in non-invasive bone evaluation is dual energy X-ray absorptiometry (DEXA) scanning. This technique measures areal bone mineral density (aBMD) which is a 2D parameter, whereas in reality BMD is a 3D phenomenon. This, obviously, leads to limitations in the usefulness of this measurement with respect to fracture prediction. Some have gone so far as to say that DEXA-measured in vivo BMD methodologies are intrinsically flawed and represent a misleading indicator of bone mineral status and is an erroneous gauge of relative fracture risk (Bolotin, 2007).

The mechanical properties of bone are in fact determined not only by bone mass but also by bone quality, the parameters of which include the overall shape, internal microarchitecture, mineralization and microdamage within the tissue. Bone turnover is the metabolic process which underlies all of these parameters and is important in several ways to the understanding of osteoporosis. It mediates the effects of all of the skeletal stimuli; endocrine, nutritional and mechanical. Although turnover is a key aspect of bone physiology, very little is known about it, particularly in terms of how site-specific variations can affect local mechanical properties and overall fracture risk.

This paper addresses some of the issues relating to parameters of bone quality, specifically bone turnover and microdamage and their relationship to local mechanical properties. The clinical relevance of these issues is also addressed, particularly in relation to the use of bisphosphonates in osteoporosis therapy.

Chapter 13 - Osteoporosis is a major health concern for our growing elderly population. It represents one major health condition accounting for significant morbidity and mortality in postmenopausal women and an emerging health problem even in aging men.

Screening of the population at risk for bone demineralization and treatment of patients to prevent consequent fractures would be useful tools to increase quality of life in the elderly and to lighten the related socio-economic impact.

The most common approach to osteoporosis diagnosis in clinical practice is the estimate of bone mineral content (BMD) by means of dual-energy X-ray absorptiometry (DEXA). However, BMD alone is not a good predictor for fracture risk. From a clinical point of view, bone microarchitecture is an interesting aspect to study and to define patterns of bone alterations with aging and pathology. In fact, microarchitecture seems to be a determinant of bone fragility independent of bone density, and as a result is important to understand the mechanisms of bone fragility as well as the action of the drugs used to prevent osteoporotic fractures.

The rapid diffusion of medical imaging techniques in clinical practice as well as the surprising development of information technologies with an increased power calculation capacity has allowed proliferation of new methods to assess trabecular bone architecture changes with aging and osteoporosis. Recently, magnetic resonance imaging (MRI) has emerged as a means of measuring trabecular bone structure in vivo. Developments in high-resolution MRI techniques have opened up new perspectives for the characterization of trabecular bone architecture by non-invasive non-ionizing methods. However, texture analysis is not frequently used as the interpretation of the large number of calculated parameters is difficult.

A proper combination of medical imaging technique, texture analysis procedure, and mathematical approach to the study of trabecular bone architecture allows the development of computerized methods that, by providing a limited number of parameters sensitive to pathology onset and progression, would speed up their application into clinical practice.

The introduction in the biomedical field of paradigms, such as theory of complexity, chaos, and fractals, suggests new approaches and provides innovative tools to the study of aging phenomena. Taking into account the complexity of living beings and fractal properties of many anatomic and physiologic structures, it is possible to quantify morpho-functional changes with aging and pathology by means of fractal analysis. In this particular context, fractal lacunarity appears the most suitable tool to characterize trabecular bone texture as it is able to describe discontinuity of the bone network as well as sizes of bone marrow spaces, changes of which are an index of increased fracture risk.

Chapter 14 - Osteoporosis is a world wide problem and its incidence is rising as life expectancy increases. A common complication of osteoporosis is that of wedge compression fractures of the vertebrae. Traditionally, wedge compression fractures have been treated conservatively with analgesia, bed rest and subsequently back physiotherapy when the pain has subsided to an acceptable level.

Following its introduction in the 1980s, vertebroplasty has gained popularity in the management of osteoporotic compression fractures and is fast becoming the standard of care for painful compression fractures. Performance of the procedure is quick and simple yet affords rapid and efficacious pain relief, while maintaining an excellent safety profile. Despite its excellent safety profile, complications have been reported post vertebroplasty, some of which are potentially devastating. As such, one must practice careful patient selection in order to maximize benefits from the procedure while minimizing complications.

Chapter 15 - Drugs may affect bone turnover and density in many ways. However, the disease for which the drugs are administered may also contribute to bone loss. Drugs against epilepsy may be associated with a limited increase in the risk of fractures. However, much of the increase may be linked to the underlying disease. Sedatives and anxiolytics may be associated with a limited increase in the risk of fractures, especially among the drugs with long half-lives. Among the antidepressants, especially those which inhibit serotonin reuptake (SSRI) are associated with an increase in the risk of fractures, possibly linked to the effect of serotonin on the bone cells, but also through an increased risk of falls. Neuroleptics may be associated with a limited increase in the risk of fractures. In contrast to mosh other psychotropic drugs, lithium seems associated with a decrease in the risk of fractures, possibly mediated through a bone anabolic effect via the Wnt signalling system. Type 1 diabetes is associated with a decrease in bone mineral, while type 2 diabetes is associated with an increase. The new class of thiazolidinediones (glitazones) has been associated with an increased loss of bone mineral. Most cardiovascular drugs (thiazide diuretics, nitrates, digoxin, antihypertensive drugs, and statins) are associated with a decrease in the risk of fractures, possibly though an amelioration of the negative effects of the underlying cardiovascular system on the skeleton. A few exceptions are amiodarone, which is associated with an increased risk of fractures, and vitamin K antagonists, which do not seem to affect the risk of fractures much. Infection with human immunodeficiency virus leads to a loss of bone mineral, while treatment with highly active antiretroviral therapy does not seem to contribute to further bone loss. Proton pump inhibitors may lead to decreased calcium absorption and thus a decreased bone mineral and an increased risk of fractures. In breast cancer treatment tamoxifen is associated with an increased bone mineral, while the newer class of aromatase inhibitors through a decrease in serum estradiol are associated with an increased loss of bone mineral. Strong analgesics (opioids) may decrease bone mineral density through inhibition of gonadotrophins while weak analgesics such as the non-steroidal anti-inflammatory drugs may increase bone mineral through an effect on the prostaglandin system. However, possibly through an increased risk of falls, the weak analgesics are associated with an increased risk of fractures.

By analysing these differences much can be learned about signalling pathways in the skeleton much in the same way as through screening of the human genome.

Chapter 16 - In recent years, it has been suggested that not only thyroid hormone excess but also thyroid stimulating hormone (TSH) deficiency may be the cause of bone loss in patients with hyperthyroidism.

The excess of thyroid hormone (T3) leads to increased bone remodeling, characterized by an imbalance between bone resorption and formation which results in net bone loss and an increased risk of fragile fractures. A brief overview of the molecular actions of thyroid hormone in adult bone is provided as well as a review of the clinical effects of excess levels of thyroid hormones and the long-term effects of the treated manifest hyperthyroidism on the skeleton.

Since thyrotropin receptors have been demonstrated in several extrathyroidal tissues and cells, including human and rat osteosarcoma cell lines and primary cultures of human osteoblast-like (hOB) cells, its role in bone metabolism has been discussed. In this article, the authors will evaluate the results of different research concerning molecular actions of TSH on bone and estimate its input in comparison to thyroid hormones.

With the development of sensitive thyrotropin assays, subclinical hyperthyroidism has become a commonly diagnosed endocrine disorder especially in the elderly population in iodine deficient areas. Whereas manifest thyrotoxicosis is usually diagnosed and treated at a very early stage, subclinical thyroid dysfunction has often remained undiagnosed and even artificially maintained with suppressive thyroid hormone therapy in patients after surgical treatment for differentiated thyroid cancer. The clinical significance of subclinical hyperthyroidism on bone mineral density and fracture risk and the first experience in the antiosteoporotic treatment of these patients will be discussed.

Chapter 17 - Osteoporosis is the most frequent metabolic bone disorder. Defined as a reduction of bone tissue compared to the anatomic volume of the bone with a preserved ratio between the mineral content and the organic matrix, this pathology leads to an enhanced bone fragility and a consequent increased susceptibility to spontaneous fractures even in the case of low energy traumas; the most frequent sites of these fractures are skeletal portions with a high trabecular content such as the spine, hip and wrist.

Up till now, the quantitative evaluation of osteoporosis and the assessment of fracture risk have been essentially based on the measurement of bone mineral density (BMD) that can be obtained with radiological techniques such as Dual X-Ray Absorpiometry (DEXA) and Quantitative Computed Tomography (QCT). The main limit of this kind of evaluation is that it exclusively considers the amount of mineral content without assessing the structure of the bone. The structure of the trabecular bone is in fact an important parameter to determine bone strength. For this reason the use of Magnetic Resonance imaging has been proposed since, by means of different techniques, it provides important morfological and structural information on the bone as well as on the presence and evolution of contingent fractures.

Besides 3 Tesla high field MR, which is a direct imaging method of the bone structure that can provide a quantitative evaluation, the trabecular bone network may be assessed with

Diffusion Tensor Imaging (DTI) and spectroscopic analysis. These techniques identify early changes in the microarchitecture of cancellate bone before such phenomenon can be detected with DEXA.

It has been demonstrated that an increased marrow fat content with a decreased unsaturated lipidic component and a reduced Apparent Diffusion Coefficient (ADC) correlate to a reduction of trabecular bone, typical of this disease. The aforementioned MR techniques, by evaluating these biological characteristics through which important structural information is provided, may therefore be useful not only in fracture risk assessment, but in pre- and post- operative diagnostics for joint prosthesis placement as well. In pre-collapse osteoporotic vertebrae there is a narrowing and a rarefaction of the bone trabeculae, with a growth of inter-trabeculary spaces that are then filled by fat and liquids. Anisotropy calculation and colorimetric vectorial evaluation provide a new intuitive non-invasive instrument for the evaluation of osteoporotic levels to be treated with vertebroplasty before any difference is grossly assessable with conventional imaging.

Chapter 18 - Young females have a high incidence of menstrual irregularities, and one of the most common forms of menstrual dysfunction is oligomenorrhea and amenorrhea as a result of prolonged anovulation. The common underlying causes include idiopathic hypothalamic amenorrhea, polycystic ovarian syndrome, exercise induced hypothalamic dysfunction, eating disorders, and other rarer congenital anomalies such as gonadal dysgenesis. Each of these conditions would have specific implications on bone mineral density (BMD) changes in affected women. While those with idiopathic hypothalamic amenorrhea are at risk of osteoporosis because of prolonged hypo-oestrogenism, the high androgen states in those with polycystic ovarian syndrome would compensate for the estrogen deficiency, so that BMD is preserved or better than eumenorrhoeic women. In exercise-induced amenorrhea, the positive stimulating effects of weight-bearing exercises would stimulate bone accrual and again off-set the negative effects of anovulation on BMD. Those with eating disorders suffer not only from the effects of amenorrhea, but also from the associated low energy intake and malnutrition. Women affected with gonadal dysgenesis, such as Turner's syndrome, would require long term hormonal therapy to maintain bone accretion and BMD, as well for induction of pubertal development. While genuine osteoporosis and its sequalae would only be expected in later life in these young women, the implications of menstrual dysfunction at this early reproductive age would need to be explored.

Chapter 19 - Postmenopausal osteoporosis is one of the most common diseases to confront elderly women. The disease is characterized by low bone mass and micro-architectural deterioration, hence resulting in increased fracture risk. In fact, this risk is greater than breast, cervical and endometrial cancer combined. Unfortunately, the exact causes of osteoporosis are not very clear although multifactorial pathology is recognized as contributors to development of the disease. Iron is ubiquitous in the human body and its homeostasis strictly relates to human health and wellbeing. What is observable in postmenopausal women, however, is the moderate, but significant, increase in stored body iron. This increase has been suggested as a risk factor of several chronic diseases such as atherosclerosis albeit with controversy. While the relationship between the moderate elevations of stored body iron and postmenopausal osteoporosis has been rarely explored, in this chapter the authors have provided evidence that iron concentrations increase in osteoporotic and osteopenic bones of postmenopausal women and estrogen-deficient animals, respectively. Importantly, the authors have also shown that iron reduction in bone through chelation therapy mitigates the osteopenic development in estrogen-deficient rats. These strongly suggest that iron buildup plays a causal role in the development of postmenopausal osteoporosis, thus providing novel preventive and therapeutic strategies. Moreover, the evidence may further help raise awareness about iron nutrition, iron supplements and Western diets that may be associated with excessive iron accumulation, and thereby increase the risks of postmenopausal and senile osteoporosis.

Short Communication 1 - Osteoporosis, the most prevalent metabolic bone disease, is characterized by compromised bone strength predisposing to an increased risk of fracture in response to mild trauma. The social and economic burden of osteoporosis is rapidly growing due to the aging of the world population. This disease, therefore, is a severe problem for current public health systems. Postmenopausal women and patients under glucocorticoid treatment are the two main groups of individuals who suffer from osteoporosis. The latter group is of particular relevance, because glucocorticoids are widely used to treat various conditions such as allergic and inflammatory disorders as well as asthma. Currently, physiological actions of glucocorticoids with potential implications in osteoporosis include decreased calcium absorption in the gastrointestinal tract and its increased urinary excretion, thus causing resistance to vitamin D and subsequent loss of bone mineral density. Despite several studies that have focused on the physiological actions of glucocorticoids, the authors still lack a clear picture of the ultimate molecular mechanism(s) underlying osteoporosis onset and progression in humans.

Osteoclasts are multinucleated cells originated from the fusion of macrophages, which play essential roles in bone development and remodeling. They possess a unique capacity for bone resorption, and are thus important mediators of the bone loss that leads to osteoporosis. Recently, the cellular and molecular bases of osteoclast involvement in osteoporosis have been analyzed in several independent investigations. It has been shown that increases in osteoclast number and/or activity lead to several diseases associated with both general and localized bone loss such as osteoporosis and rheumatoid arthritis, respectively. Here the authors discuss molecular mechanisms that underlie glucocorticoid-induced osteoporosis, focusing on newly identified regulators of osteoclatogenesis and osteoclast activation such as IRAK-M. Indeed, this pseudokinase not only acts as a negative modulator of innate immune responses mediated by Toll-like receptors (TLRs) and interleukin-1 receptor (IL-1R), but also participates in the control of macrophage differentiation into osteoclasts. IRAK-M knockout mice develop a strong osteoporosis phenotype, suggesting that the down-regulation of this molecule activates osteoclast-mediated bone resorption. Data from human studies indicate that blood monocytes differentiated into osteoclasts express high levels of IRAK-M at both mRNA and protein level. Glucorticoids down-regulate IRAK-M expression, which correlates with an increased activation of bone resorption.

Short Communication 1a - The vertebral fractures are generated when the combination of the axial and rotational charges on the spine exceed the resistance offered by vertebral body.

Reduction in the individual vertebral body strength may result from infiltrative processes created by benign or malignant tumors or, more commonly, from bone mineral loss precipitated by osteoporosis.

Osteoporosis, which may be age-related (primary) or due to steroid use (secondary), is the most common cause of VCF in Europe and United States. The frequency of radiographic evidence of VCF increases from 500/100,000 person years (py) in women aged 50 to 54 years to 2960/100,000 py in women more than 85 years old. Radiographic changes may be present without the patient experiencing pain.

Patients with VCFs may experience severe and prolonged pain that can markedly alter activities of daily living. Complications include progressive kyphosis of the spine and reduction of volumes of the thoracic and abdominal cavities, with consequent reduction of vital capacity (VC) and "forced expiratory volume to 1 second" (FEV1), as well as gastrointestinal dysfunction.

In osteoporotic vertebral collapses a conservative therapy is generally achieved with bed rest, bracing, analgesics, and physical therapy.

Instead for patients with painful bone metastases current conventional treatments are primarily palliative and include localized therapies (fractionated external beam radiation therapy and surgery), systemic therapies (chemotherapy, hormonal therapy, radiopharmaceuticals, and bisphosphonates), and analgesics (opioids and non-steroidal anti-inflammatory drugs).

These conventional therapies with their well known drawbacks and side effects provide reasonable pain relief obtaining variable success rates.

All painful vertebral collapses are adequately treated through percutaneous injection of polymethylmethacrylate (PMMA) bone cement into the vertebral body, described for the first time by Galibert et al. in 1984 as " Vertebroplasty ", and successfully applied to the treatment of C2 aggressive hemangiomas, and subsequently used on VCF secondary to osteoporosis and osteolytic tumors.

Vertebroplasty is a technique utilized in the field of VCF, based on Osteoporosis or neoplasms.

It is extremely useful in the treatment of aggressive vertebral hemangiomas, bone osteolytic metastases and destructive multiple myeloma, which is associated with VCF in 55-70% of the cases.

New tendencies are essentially directed, according to Medline, toward developments of a new generation of injectable bone cements.

Short Communication 2 - Osteoporosis is associated with a considerable degree of mortality and morbidity in elderly patients. Back pain, disfigurement and fractures of the hip and spine are well known consequences of the end stage disease. Hip fracture causes a reduction in life expectancy of almost 6 years in both men and women [1] and often has a devastating effect on the quality of life, with a severe curtailment of independent living. The challenge is to detect fracture-prone patients in the early stages when effective treatment can be instituted.

Short Communication 3 - Osteoporosis is a multifactorial, age-related metabolic bone disease characterized by low bone mineral density (BMD), deterioration of the microarchitecure of cancellous bone, and changes in the material properties of bone, leading to enhanced bone fragility and to a consequent increase in the risk of fracture.

Those factures do not seem to occur in the jaws. Studies investigating the effect of osteoporosis on the jaws have generally relied on relating changes in bone mass in different skeletal sites to changes in a range of mandibular variables measured in different ways, including height of residual ridge, altered trabecular and cortical pattern, and reduced bone density.

Oral signs of the bone loss in elderly patients are manifested by excessive alveolar ridge resorption and tooth loss. Reduction of the residual alveolar ridges could be described as a resorptive athrophy, a fundamental and physiologic reaction to loss of function and inactivity that presumably is influenced and modulated by individually varying factors, such as condition of the bone, period of edentulousness, denture-wearing habits, and unfavorable loading patterns.

Radiographic intraoral microdensitometry, next to the clinical examination, is definitely one of the most often used bone-mass measuring techniques in assessing the quantity of the mandibular bone loss caused by osteoporosis. It has been developed to increase the precision of bone mass assessment on conventional radiographs, including panoramic radiographs and periapical radiographs. This tool has been proved in several clinical studies to be accurate enough in detecting patients with low bone mineral density.

In the recent study, determing the relative usefulness of BMD measurements on dental panoramic radiographs in the diagnosis of patients with postmenopausal osteoporosis it was found that the mandibular BMD values, measured on panoramic radiographs, are a significant factor in predicting postmenopausal osteoporosis ($p<0.05$).

Partially and completely edentulous patients, with the diagnosed osteporosis, require special prosthodontic treatment.

Short Communication 4 - This article brings the biomechanical analysis of sport – Nordic walking – for patients with osteoporotic fractured vertebrae and shows that it is suitable for them.

Based on the biomechanical model of skeletal load the authors have developed a method of walking movement for patients, different from the method of walking movement for healthy people. And so came into being the "first sport"for patients with osteoporotic fractures. They can go for regular walks in easy terrains outdoors with friends and family, and so be liberated from social isolation. It requires only one-off financial costs of buying the poles and special footwear.

Short Communication 5 - *Patients and methods*. The authors analysed 498 ($n = 498$) densitometric findings from the area of proximal femur: Neck (ROI_1), Ward ´s area (ROI_2), great trochanter (ROI_3) (DXA - dual energy X–ray absorptiometry, from the population of Bratislava women of the average age of 59.71 years ⟨58.63; 60.80⟩. Measured values of T and Z– score were categorized as follows: 1 – increased fracture risk (T – score < - 2.5 SD/ T = 1, Z–score ≤ - 1.0 SD/ Z = 1), 0 – without increased fracture risk (T – score > - 2.5 SD/ T = 0, Z – score > - 1.0 SD / Z = 0).

The objective of the study. The authors aimed to prove that the relative risk of fractures (RR) is higher in women whose T and Z–score values come under the category of increased risk than in the women whose T–score only falls within the category of increased risk.

Statistical analysis: 1. Contingency tables, measurement of the intensity of the association of categorized variables 2. Determination of probability (P) and relative risk (RR)

Results: RR for development of fracture was higher for all measurement sites (ROI_1 – 29.87; ROI_2 – 15.3; ROI_3 – 5.5) for women having T – score < - 2.5 SD and simultaneously Z – score ≤ - 1.0 SD than for the women having T – score < - 2.5 SD and simultaneously Z – score > - 1.0 SD. When the women were divided according to age into two groups: a) women< 65 years, b) women ≥ 65 years, it was found that the RR of fracture for women < 65 years having T – score < - 2.5 SD and also Z – score ≤ - 1.0 SD is very high (RR = ∞), old women (≥ 65 years) had the RR for ROI_1 – 32.61, for ROI_2 – 7.72, and for ROI_3 – 6.9. Probability (P) of the presence of women with T – score values < - 2.5 SD and Z – score ≤ - 1.0 SD in the group under 65 years is for ROI_1 – 12.5%; ROI_2 – 34.4%; ROI_3 – 20.5%, and the probability for women ≥ 65 years is for ROI_1 – 75%; ROI_2 – 98%; and ROI_3 – 100%.

Conclusions: The study's contribution lies in the finding that the relative fracture risk in proximal femur in women increases, if T-core < - 2.5 SD and, simultaneously, Z-score ≤ - 1.0 SD, and this risk is especially high for women under the age of 65.

In assessing the individual fracture risk by questionnaires in female patients the authors recommend to add also Z – score values in the measured area to T –score values and to other anamnestic and biochemical risk factors.

Short Communication 6 - The article presents an analysis of statistical methods used for estimating fracture risk in patients with osteoporosis. Mathematical relations of different methods are explained (risk – R, risk ratio - RR, RD – risk difference, odds - O, odds ratio - OR, Yule's Q, Yule's Y, logistic model). What is important to keep in mind is that: 1) relative risk and odds ratio are statistics that only describe an association, not causation; 2) relative risk and odds ratio refer to a population, not to an individual patient; 3) the studies of small groups are more likely to find an association that might actually just be due to chance, the larger the groups, the less likely the association between a risk factor and an outcome (fracture); 4) when the incidence of an outcome of interest in the study population is low (< 10%), the OR is close to the RR, the more frequent the outcome becomes, the more the OR will overestimate the RR when it is more than 1 or underestimate the RR when it is less than 1.

Sophisticated statistical packages are available which can calculate many of the tests of association but the problem is that the investigator must know which the desirable is. The incorrect option of statistical analysis, the incorrect interpretation of risk ratio or odds ratio and overestimation of the importance of a risk factor may lead to unintentional errors in the economic analysis of potential programs or treatments in osteoporosis. This article could be a contribution for investigators, who are concerned with assessment of fracture risk.

Short Communication 7 - The article brings a biomechanical analysis of the determination of the position of gravity centre of a trainee in the plane, both graphically and by calculation.

The importance of determining the position of the gravity centre in different postures of a trainee should not be underestimated, as it belongs to the basic principles in the development of methodology of kinesitherapy for both healthy and ill people.

An erudite methodology of kinesitherapy for osteoporotic patients can be developed only on the basis of biomechanical analysis of each exercise element, i.e., the knowledge of the position of the gravity centre, the knowledge of the support area and the distance of the gravity centre projection from the stability limit, the knowledge of the magnitude of the stability angle, and the knowledge of the regularity of mechanical stress of weakened osteoporotic vertebrae. A correctly chosen methodology of kinesitherapy for osteoporotic patients prevents the development of microfractures in the vertebrae, prevents patient's fall during the exercise, and stimulates the bone neoformation with increasing the bone mineral density and periosteal apposition of bone, followed by the enlargement of the bone cross sectional area as well as of the cross sectional moment of inertia.. The resulting effect is an improvement of the bone quality and its mechanical resistance.

Short Communication 8 - The article presents a biomechanical model of articulatio and mm. coxae with the characteristics of the vectors of reaction forces generated in flexors and extensors 1) in muscular balance; 2) in muscular dysbalance; 2a) with permanent load of the model of a hip by the body weight; 2b) with simulated live load during a fall or an impact. In case of muscular dysbalance the application of action force on a hip during a fall results in a sharp increase of the reaction compressive force in flexors and the tensile force in extensors. Muscular dysbalance of external (extensors) and internal (flexors) muscles of mm. coxae facilitates in this way complicated splintered fractures in the collum femoris area, and in the pertrochanteric and subtrochanteric areas.

Muscular balance achieved by balancing exercises and mechanical protection of the joint reduce the risk of splintered and complicated fractures in the described area.

Short Communication 9 - *Patients and methods:* In a prospective study the authors observed which female patients developed depression following an acute and painful vertebral fracture. On the day of diagnosing the vertebral fracture the patients filled the questionnaires 1 and 2. The depression developed in some patients was diagnosed by means of the DSM – IV questionnaire. For the statistical evaluation of questionnaires the authors chose randomly 32 patients with depression (out of 33 patients) aged 51-73, and 32 patients without depression (out of 44 patients) aged 52-70.

The aim of the study: To verify the hypothesis that the patients with more traumatic experience in the anamnesis (Questionnaire No. 1) are more depression prone following the osteoporotic vertebrae fractures and their character features are typical for subjects with higher emotional vulnerability (Questionnaire No. 2).

Statistical analysis: 1. Questionnaires 1 and 2 were evaluated by two statistical methods:

automatization of mathematical and statistical estimates and tests based on binomial distribution;

ADALINE Programme. 2. Assessment of relative risk for developing depression.

Results: 1. Questionnaire No. 1 completed by depressed patients contained statistically significant higher number of positive answers to questions defining experienced stress situations (differences in values of weights of questionnaire parameters expressed in percentages within linear combination of the whole group). 2. Questionnaire No. 2 completed by depressed patients contained statistically significant higher number of positive answers by more depression prone subjects in comparison with non-depressed patients (differences in values of weights of questionnaire parameters. 3. Patients lapsed into depression most often on the 32nd day following the vertebra fracture. 4. Proposed questionnaires are according to validity criteria (sensitivity, specificity, prediction value of positive test, prediction values of negative test, test effectiveness) indicated for identification of persons risking the onset of depression following the osteoporotic fracture of vertebrae. 5. Relative risk (RR) for developing depression in patients with osteoporotic fracture, which answered in Questionnaire No. 1 eight and more questions positive is *7,0 time* higher than in patiens with osteoporotic fracture, which answered in Questionnaire No. 1 less than eight guestions positive. For Questionnaire No. 2 it is *8,5 time* higher.

Conclusion: The authors recommend to use questionnaires No. 1 and 2 in female patients with acute painful vertebrae fractures to select patients with the risk of depression development. These patients should be followed more frequently as outpatients and in case of first clinical symptoms of depression should be recommended for special psychiatric care. Early therapy of depression enables to accelerate the mobilisation, rehabilitation and resocialisation of patients, to improve the quality of their lives and to reduce the costs of analgetic treatment of pain, sedatives and rehabilitation.

Short Communication 10 - *Patients and methods.* The authors analysed 498 women (n = 498) in Bratislava (BA) population aged 21 to 90. The authors measured bone mineral density (BMD) in the area of proximal femur with one densitometric instrument DXA (dual energy X–ray absorptiometry), applying BMD and T-score values in three standard regions of interest: Neck (ROI_1), Ward ´s area (ROI_2), great trochanter (ROI_3).

Statistical analysis: 1. Chi-square goodness-of-fit statistics (χ^2 - test). 2. Analysis of variance (ANOVA).

Results: Measured values of T–score in ROI_1 , ROI_2 have normal distribution and a lognormal distribution of frequency in ROI_3. Using χ^2 - test (chi-square goodness-of-fit statistics), the authors determined the distribution of frequency of T-score values and the percentage of osteoporosis incidence in Bratislava female population. The osteoporosis incidence in Bratislava female population, according to T-score values measured in ROI_1 is 2.40%, in ROI_2 16.34% and in ROI_3 3.83% . Following the division of women into ten-year intervals, the statistically significant sample averages of T-score values were decreasing in relation to age only for ROI_2. The osteoporosis incidence in age intervals was rising with age for ROI_2, for ROI_1 the number of osteoporotic patients in the 61 to 70-year interval was lower than in the 41 to 50-year interval, and for ROI_3 the number of osteoporotic patients in the 51 to 60-year interval was lower than in the 41 to 50-year interval. Expect of the above mentioned intervals, T-score values decreased in relation to age also in ROI_1 and ROI_3 . According to the analysis of variance, the age category explains 9.6% of the overall variability of T-score values for ROI_1, 24.7% for ROI_2 and 11.70% for ROI_3.

Conclusion: As in ROI_2 (Ward's area) greater fraction of the trabecular bone is measured in comparison with ROI_1 and ROI_3, the ROI_2 reflects best the age-related BMD changes. It is due to the fact that the trabecular bone is eight times more active metabolically than the cortical bone, and so it is more sensitive than the cortical bone for the determination of BMD changes. In ROI_1 and ROI_3 the relation was distorted by a greater fraction of cortical bone in comparison with ROI_2 and by an accidental selection of a higher number of osteoarthrotic patients in the 61 to 70-year interval for ROI_1 , and in the 51 to 60-year interval for ROI_3 . The age of patients is a significant risk factor. Bone mass decreases with age independently of the period of other risk factors activities, and also independently of the fact whether the patient suffers from primary or secondary osteoporosis (osteopenia). The development and application of densitometric methods measuring separately the trabecular and cortical bone excludes the distorting factor of osteoarthrosis and should be preferred in densitometric examination methods for a continuous observation of BMD changes.

Short Communication 11 - According to the instruction manual of the producer of kits for determining the levels of aminoterminal telopeptide of type I collagen of organic bone matrix (NTx), the time of the collection of second morning urine is arbitrary, i.e., that a patient can urinate anytime within the period from about 6 to 8.30 a.m. This time interval is within the period of the change in circadian rhythm of the NTx excretion (maximum excretion with the transition into the fast decrease of excretion). That is the reason why the authors considered appropriate to standardise conditions for the collection of second morning urine and the authors suggested to apply the so-called two-hour morning diuresis NTx2 (from 6 to 8.00 a.m. after an overnight fast). The authors examined 48 women patients aged 33-65 with a primary or secondary osteopenia or osteoporosis (all patients had normal renal functions). In these patients the authors determined NTx (Osteomark, OSTEX, USA) in a standardly used 24-hour diuresis (NTx24) and in the suggested two-hour morning diuresis (NTx2).

Aim of the study: To find a mathematical character of the dependence of values of dependent variable NTx2 from an independent variable NTx24 and to evaluate the statistic significance of this dependence. To compare the ratio of the widths of 95% confidence intervals (C.I.) for NTx2 and NTx24 in patients (index: IO) with the ratio of the widths of reference limits for NTx in arbitrary second morning urine ($NTx2_{ostex}$) and in 24-hour diuresis ($NTx24_{ostex}$) in healthy women (index: IR). To evaluate the suggested two-hour diuresis for the determination of NTx.

Statistical analysis: Stochastic and deterministic linear regressive analysis. Index of 95% C.I., index of reference limits.

Results: Statistically significant ($p < 0.01$) regressive dependence ($r^2 = 0.781$) was found between the values of NTx24 and NTx2. The index of the widths of reference limits (IR) is 1.5 times bigger that the index for osteopenic and osteoporotic patients (IO), meaning that the scatter of the $NTx2_{ostex}$ values is bigger than NTx2 in the suggested two-hour diuresis.

Conclusion: Based on statistically significant linear regressive dependence between NTx24 and NTx2 values it is possible to use the suggested two-hour morning diuresis to determine the NTx levels in women. The introduction of two-hour morning diuresis NTx2 will decrease the fluctuation range of NTx values in its repeated examination and will make the conclusiveness of its values more accurate in comparison with the determination of $NTx2_{ostex}$ in any second morning urine in compliance with the instructions of the producer of kits OSTEX, USA.

Research and Review Studies

In: Osteoporosis: Etiology, Diagnosis and Treatment
Editors: Bilar E. Mattingly and Albert C. Pillare
ISBN 978-1-60692-397-9

Chapter 1

SUBREGIONAL BONE MINERAL DENSITY MEASUREMENT IN THE LUMBAR SPINE USING DXA: POTENTIAL FOR THE APPLICATION TO OSTEOPOROSIS AND VERTEBRAL FRACTURES

Andrew M. Briggs[1,2]***, John D. Wark***[2]***, Alison M. Greig***[3]***,***
Nicola L. Fazzalari[4]***, Susan Kantor***[2] ***and Kim L. Bennell***[5]
[1]Curtin University of Technology, Western Australia, Australia;
[2]University of Melbourne, Royal Melbourne Hospital, Victoria, Australia;
[3]University of British Columbia, BC, Canada;
[4]Institute for Medical and Veterinary Sciences and Hanson Institute, South Australia, Australia.
[5]Univerity of Melbourne, Victoria, Australia.

ABSTRACT

Osteoporosis currently poses a major public health problem and vertebral fractures are considered one of the hallmarks of this condition. Bone mineral density (BMD) testing using dual energy x-ray absorptiometry (DXA) is the most efficient, safe and economical tool to assess skeletal integrity and fracture risk in the clinical environment. However, conventional DXA has limited ability to discriminate between individuals with and without vertebral fractures. Recent histological and *ex vivo* research has identified differences in BMD distribution and bone structural properties within the vertebral body. This intra-vertebral (subregional) heterogeneity may be a defining characteristic between individuals with and without vertebral fractures. The aim of the studies described in this Chapter was to determine whether individuals with and without vertebral fracture(s) differed in areal subregional BMD (srBMD) profiles. Individuals with primary osteoporotic, vertebral fracture (n=7) or without vertebral fracture (n=15), and comparable controls with normal BMD (n=9) were recruited. Fractures were diagnosed from lateral thoracolumbar radiographs. Areal BMD was measured from a lateral projection DXA scan of the L3 vertebral body and in 6 manually-selected subregions (Hologic 4500A densitometer, Waltham, MA, USA). A two-way repeated measures ANOVA revealed a main effect for region ($p<0.001$) but not group. Trends demonstrated greater deficits in areal BMD when comparing srBMD profiles with standard DXA parameters between fracture and non-fracture cases. Differences in BMD between the groups across the subregions ranged from 13.1-16.3%, while for standard DXA parameters the differences were smaller in the range of 0.7-5.4%. The inability to detect statistically-significant differences between groups was attributed to low power in the study. Irrespective of group, significantly lower areal BMD was observed in the anterior and central subregion of the L3 vertebral body ($p<0.05$), consistent with previous data. Mean srBMD and standard DXA output values of the fracture group were also expressed as the number of standard deviations (SDs) from the corresponding non-fracture group means. Greater deviation below the non-fracture mean was observed with srBMD data (0.60-1.04 SDs) compared to standard DXA values (0.04-0.51 SDs). Subregional BMD measures were also found to be stronger predictors of vertebral morphology compared to standard DXA parameters (r^2=0.18-0.28, $p\leq0.05$; r^2=0.06-0.08, $p>0.05$). The subregional BMD method was considered accurate with preliminary concurrent validity established against histomorphometry methods (r=0.52-0.78). These findings suggest that subregional analysis may be superior to current standard DXA analyses in discriminating fracture from non-fracture cases. The predictive value of lateral subregional DXA for incident vertebral fractures warrants evaluation. Moreover, this method may be applied to other clinical situations, such as the monitoring of bone responses to medications, glucocorticoid-induced osteoporosis, and in disabling conditions such as chronic back pain.

1. INTRODUCTION

1.1. Why is Osteoporosis Important?

Osteoporosis affects 30% of postmenopausal women and 8% of men aged over 50 in Western societies [1,2]. As the global population ages and expands these percentages are expected to increase. Clinically, osteoporosis is recognised by the occurrence of characteristic, pathologic fractures presenting most commonly in the thoracic spine, thoracolumbar junction, hip and wrist; and to a lesser extent in the proximal humerus and ribs [3,4]. Osteoporosis-related fractures have been associated with significant morbidity, decreased quality of life, psychological effects and loss of independence, and place a significant burden on the health system. The residual lifetime risk of fracture for men and women aged 60 years and over is estimated to be 25% and 44% respectively, while in the context of osteoporosis these risks increase to 42% and 65% respectively [5]. The estimated annual direct health care expenditure for osteoporosis in the United States is $US 14 billion, in the United Kingdom £UK1 billion and in Australia $AU 7.4 billion [1,3,6]. These estimates are based on health care audits from several years ago; therefore current costs are likely to be even greater. In Australia, health care expenditure for osteoporosis is now in excess of other diseases such as diabetes and asthma, both of which are National Health

Priority Area conditions as determined by the Australian Federal Government [7]. In recognition of the worldwide problem of osteoporosis and other musculoskeletal diseases, many nations have joined the World Health Organization (WHO) and United Nations in designating the first decade of the 21st century as the Decade of Bone and Joint Disease.

1.2. The Significance of Vertebral Fractures

Vertebral fractures account for 46% of all osteoporotic fracture presentations [8]. However, this figure may underestimate the true prevalence of these fractures considering that only 1 in 4 comes to clinical attention, either due to lack of radiographic attention or absence of recognised classical symptoms [9]. However, estimates of vertebral fracture prevalence are influenced by the radiographic method used to diagnose fracture. The mortality rate in individuals who have sustained a vertebral fracture is greater than in those individuals with no history of vertebral fracture, and is comparable to that of one year post hip fracture [10]. Deaths are likely attributable to the physical and psychosocial sequelae of vertebral fractures, rather than the fracture *per se*. For example, Jalava et al. [11] reported that although vertebral fractures were associated with a 4-fold increase in mortality, other known predictors of mortality, such as medication intake, gender, serum albumin, renal function, body mass and age, could explain a significant proportion of the increased risk..

Vertebral fractures impose a significant burden on the health system. A recent study by Delmas et al. [8] found that the global rate of false-negative reporting ranged from 29.5-46.5%. Therefore, estimates of financial, physical and psychological costs likely underestimate the true burden of these fractures. The majority of health care expenditure estimates related to disease report the direct costs only. For osteoporosis-related expenditure, direct costs have been estimated to account for only 25-34% of the total costs [3,12]. A recent report examined the annual health care utilisation and expenditures for patients with osteoporosis who sustained a new vertebral fragility fracture from 1997-2001 [13]. The authors found that direct medical costs in the fracture group were more than ten times higher than those without vertebral fractures. This may have been related to higher incidence of co-morbidities in the vertebral fracture group to which health care costs were attributable, for example myalgia, back pain and chest pain. Notably, patients who had sustained a vertebral fracture within the study period incurred more than twice the overall health care expenditure compared to non-fracture cases ($US15,942 *vs*. $6,476) and nearly three times those of a control group ($US15,942 *vs*. $4,658). Similarly, Lindsay et al. [14] and Gabriel et al. [15] estimated that the cost of subsequent fracture after an initial fracture was much higher compared to individuals who did not re-fracture. Therefore, identification of individuals at risk of vertebral fracture or re-fracture is of great importance in terms of public health expenditure and individual quality of life.

The issue of identifying individuals at risk of fracture becomes more critical when considering that the risk of subsequent fracture rises exponentially after an initial fracture is sustained, with a concurrent rise in the associated sequelae. Within the first year after sustaining an initial vertebral fracture, the risk of sustaining a second vertebral fracture is reported to be 20% [16,17], while other studies report the risk of sustaining a subsequent vertebral fracture to increase by 4-7 fold, and then exponentially with greater numbers of prior vertebral fractures [4,18-20]. Although bone mineral density (BMD) derived from dual energy X-ray absorptiometry (DXA) is the most widely used method to assess skeletal integrity and infer fracture risk, it cannot be used reliably to determine who will sustain a fracture and who will not [21,22]. For example, in the prospective, population-based Rotterdam Study only 44% and 21% of all non-vertebral fractures in women and men, respectively, with a T-score below -2.5 [23]. Analogously, although the risk of stroke can be inferred from blood pressure, and the risk of myocardial infarction from serum cholesterol levels, these parameters cannot identify who will sustain a stroke or myocardial infarction. Minimal trauma failure of one vertebral body is indicative of critical weakness at multiple other vertebral levels, unless bone strength is improved with treatment. Currently, clinicians are faced with the dilemma of how to prevent subsequent fractures, and more importantly how to predict with confidence which patients are at increased risk of incident and prevalent fractures. Improvement in this area would allow more efficient use of health care resources.

1.3. The Vertebral Fracture Cascade

The *vertebral fracture cascade* refers to the increased risk of sustaining subsequent vertebral fractures (prevalent fractures) after an initial vertebral fracture (incident fracture). The exponential increase in fracture rate is coupled with more pronounced physical, psychosocial and public health sequelae [14,15,24,25]. The aetiopathogenesis of the vertebral fracture cascade has been comprehensively reviewed elsewhere [26]. The vertebral fracture cascade and indeed vertebral integrity generally can be conceptualised with a dynamic systems approach, where properties of several domains are considered as well as their interactions [26,27]. Domains relevant to vertebral fractures include bone properties, spinal properties (local and global), and neurophysiologic properties [26,27]. In this chapter, only bone properties are discussed.

1.4. Bone Properties Relevant to Vertebral Integrity and the Fracture Cascade

1.4.1. Bone Mineral Density (BMD)

Areal BMD refers to the amount of bone mineral (hydroxyapatite) per unit of projected area in which the bone mineral is measured. In individual patients, BMD is primarily determined by their peak bone mass and bone loss since the time peak bone mass was achieved [28]. Measurement of BMD holds important clinical value, since low BMD measured at the spine and hip is a recognised risk factor for osteoporotic fracture [29]. BMD is also used to monitor responses to pharmacotherapy in patients at higher risk of fracture. Measurement of BMD has been used in many large clinical trials as a primary outcome measure to evaluate the effect of anti-resorptive medications in reducing vertebral fracture risk [30-32]. These studies highlight the importance of BMD in clinical decision-making.

Bone mineral density can be measured with several tools including DXA and quantitative computed tomography (QCT), and research is now being directed towards the application of magnetic resonance imaging (MRI) for this purpose. Both QCT and MRI have been applied to the lumbar spine previously *in vivo* for densitometric purposes [33,34]. Application of MRI technology in the field of bone densitometry is relatively new, with the majority of *in vivo* studies directed towards examining bone structure in the appendicular skeleton [35,36]. However, some studies point to the utility of this technology for axial structures [37,38]. Utilisation of QCT and high-resolution MRI may present some advantages over DXA since measures of volumetric density and multidimensional geometry can be accurately collected with these technologies. QCT scanning provides information on densitometric and geometric characteristics of both cortical and trabecular bone independently, while MRI has the potential to make measurements of bone geometry and bone quality without ionising radiation [39-42]. In addition, vertebral deformities may be quantified with greater precision and accuracy using conventional MRI since projection errors such as scoliosis and sagittal obliquity are overcome with tomographic features of MRI [43].

Although all non-invasive measurement tools for BMD perform well [44], DXA is the most common method of BMD assessment. DXA functions by using two photon energy beams, each of a different energy level, to distinguish between bone and non-bone structures within the beam fields. The relative areal composition of the bone and non-bone structures is then calculated according to how much of the photon energy is absorbed from each beam [28,45]. The clinical utility of DXA is attributed to its economic, efficient, practical and precise measuring capabilities compared to other technologies. In addition, the radiation dose delivered to the patient with DXA is much less than QCT [46].

Although DXA is the most widely-used tool to measure BMD, and in combination with other clinical variables is used to diagnose osteoporosis and estimate fracture risk, it does carry several limitations. The most significant limitation of DXA is that it cannot measure true BMD (volumetric: g/cm^3), but rather only apparent or two-dimensional BMD (areal: g/cm^2). Studies indicate that areal BMD is strongly correlated with age, while volumetric density is not [47,48]. This highlights the confounding effect of bone (or body) size on BMD. Larger bones will have greater bone mineral content (BMC) and to some extent greater apparent BMD. The BMD expression (BMC/area) was originally introduced as a normalising factor to minimise the effect of bone size on BMC results. However, individuals with larger bones still demonstrate greater BMD. A problematic consequence of body or bone size is that small-framed individuals are more likely to be misdiagnosed with osteoporosis by virtue of their smaller bones when compared to a reference (normative) population. Normative data are derived from the averages of both large and small people. Therefore, calculated T and Z scores do not consider bone size [49]. In some circumstances areal BMD derived from DXA can be transformed to apparent volumetric BMD using simple engineering principles.

Variation in results between densitometer instruments, which can reach up to 20%, is also a major problem and is attributable to variation in calibration procedures, edge detection algorithms, and assumptions regarding fat distribution [50,51]. Differences also exist between machines of the same manufacturer [52,53]. However, even with these limitations, DXA has remained the most easily used and efficient way of determining skeletal status in patients since its introduction in 1987. Table 1 summarises the advantages and disadvantages of DXA technology described in the literature.

In vivo scanning of the lumbar spine can be performed with X-ray projections orientated in either the postero-anterior [PA] (or antero-posterior [AP]) or lateral directions. Lateral scanning has been used less frequently in the past due to the high precision errors associated with difficulties in positioning patients in the decubitus position [54,55]. This difficulty has been largely overcome with development of the matched supine-lateral scan sequence, which eliminates the need to change the position of the patient. Instead, the radiation source moves around the patient. Lateral scanning has the advantage of eliminating cortical bone of the vertebral posterior elements from the analysis. Consequently, lateral scanning allows preferential calculation of BMD in the trabecular bone-rich vertebral centrum, where the pathologic effects of osteoporosis are most significant. This explains why the diagnostic sensitivity of lateral scanning is superior to that of AP scanning [56-59]. Blake et al. [59] demonstrated that the treatment effects of a pharmacologic intervention were larger when evaluating lateral BMD data compared to AP data. However, in that study, greater sensitivity of the lateral data was offset by larger precision errors.

Table 1. Advantages and disadvantages of using DXA for the measurement of BMD

Advantages	Disadvantages
Low radiation dose	Cannot measure volumetric BMD (g/cm^3) directly
Short scanning time	Affected by bone/body size
High accuracy	Cannot separate trabecular and cortical components
High short-term precision	T and Z scores do not consider body size
High long-term stability	Cannot compare results between densitometers or sites
Lower public health cost	Cannot differentiate well individuals with and without fracture
Simple to use technology	Cannot assess bone quality
Less sensitive to bone marrow fat	Affected by calcified tissues and vertebral fractures
Can measure at a range of sites	Affected by bone sclerosis (e.g. degenerative spondylosis)
Can measure lean and fat mass	
Can measure vertebral morphometry	

Lateral scan images are less affected by aortic calcification and degenerative spinal conditions compared to AP DXA [57]. In addition to superior diagnostic sensitivity, lateral DXA has also been shown to possess greater predictive validity for bone strength. As a result, many centres now choose not to scan the lumbar spine in an AP projection for patients aged over 60-65 years [49,60]. Although the diagnostic advantages offered by lateral DXA may be superior to AP scanning, concern still exists regarding the precision of this scan mode, as it tends to be poorer than AP projection. This limitation was clearly a concern before the introduction of supine-lateral scanning capabilities, now available on newer densitometers. Lateral-projection DXA may also be more affected by signal to noise ratio than AP-projection DXA owing to the greater volume of soft tissue content required for the X-ray beam to pass through in lateral projection. Precision of BMD measures is important since thresholds of BMD are often used as criteria for prescribing medications and assessing fracture risk. Generally, DXA has the advantage of producing precise results. For *in vivo* spine scanning, the precision errors depend greatly on the projection mode used. AP/PA scans possess greater precision, in the range of 0.6-3.2% (% coefficient of variation [CV]), depending on the age and health status of the cohort (see Table 2). Lateral scanning is generally associated with greater precision errors, in the range of 1.6-7.1% for decubitus lateral and 0.9-4.9% for supine-lateral modes (Table 2). The higher precision costs of lateral scanning are offset by the greater clinical value of the data collected. Table 2 summarises the precision errors reported in the literature for spine scanning using DXA. Importantly, data provided in Table 2 show minimal difference in precision errors between AP and supine-lateral scanning, suggesting that this mode of lateral scanning is appropriate for clinical and research use.

Table 2. Summary of precision errors reported in the literature for *in vivo* measures of lumbar spine BMD. All studies involved patient repositioning. Errors are expressed %CV

Study	AP (PA)	Decubitus lateral	Matched supine-lateral
Mazess et al [61]		2.00%	
Slosman et al [62]		2.80%	
Steiger et al[63]			0.90%
Lilley et al [64]		3.60%	
Banks et al [65]		3.80%	
Larnach et al [66]		3.80%	
Pye et al [67]		5.20%	
Slosman et al [68]			1.00%
Economou et al [69]		5.90%	
Devogelaer et al [70]		6.90%	
Devogelaer et al [71]			1.20%
Blake et al [54]	0.8-1.66%		1.2-2.11%
Duboeuf et al [72]	1.15%		2.31%
Peel and Eastell [73]	0.80%	6.40%	
Jergas et al [74]			3.3-4.9%
Del Rio et al [75]		1.6-2.0%	
Engelke et al [76]	0.90%	7.10%	
Grey et al [77]	1.20%		
Nguyen et al [78]	0.8-3.2%		
Nanjo et al [79]	0.60%		2.40%

1.4.2. Bone Mineral Density and Bone Strength

The ability of bone to resist failure (fracture) is dependent on bone strength. However, bone strength cannot be measured directly *in vivo* and therefore must be inferred from other parameters, such as BMD and bone geometry (e.g. cross sectional area). Research suggests that BMD accounts for 70-90% of the variance observed in bone strength, with the remaining 10-30% attributable to bone quality parameters [6,80,81]. Bone quality refers to micro-architecture, cumulative micro-damage, bone turnover and mineralization. BMD alone cannot provide a complete picture of bone strength, highlighting the drawback of relying solely on

BMD as a predictor of fracture risk and the need to also consider bone quality [26]. The relationship between BMD and bone quality is uncertain. For example, studies examining pharmacologic interventions demonstrate reductions in fracture risk before increases in BMD are apparent [30,82]. These findings may suggest that standard measurement tools do not detect BMD responses with enough sensitivity or that changes in bone quality parameters also account for the increased bone strength. Histological studies highlight aspects of independence between BMD and bone quality. A comprehensive study by Fazzalari et al. [83] reported no relationship between bone micro-damage and BMD. In addition, an *in vivo* study examining iliac trabecular architecture among women with and without vertebral fracture determined differences in three-dimensional architecture between the groups, independent of BMD [84]. However, Feldkamp et al. [85] reported a moderate correlation between the number of trabecular connections in a three-dimensional lattice and trabecular bone volume, suggesting that some aspects of architecture can be captured with bone densitometry. BMD assessment is the focus of this Chapter; therefore bone quality will not be addressed further, though its role in determining bone strength is acknowledged.

Table 3. Synthesis of the literature examining the relationship between DXA-derived areal BMD (g/cm^2) and vertebral bone strength tested *ex situ*. The strength of correspondence between variables is expressed as Pearson's correlation co-efficient (*r*)

Study	Gender (Mean age)	Specimen	Correlation (*r*) AP-DXA *vs.* load		Correlation (*r*) Lateral-DXA *vs.* load	
			Failure*	Stress^	Failure*	Stress^
Edmondston et al [87]	10M / 6F (65yrs)	250 isolated vertebrae T1-L5, posterior elements excised	-	-	0.82-0.86	0.73-0.78
Yang et al [92]	swine model	51 isolated vertebrae T1-L5, posterior elements excised	0.89-0.91	0.75-0.79	-	-
Cheng et al [99]	34M (66yrs) / 28F (72 yrs)	62 L3 vertebrae, posterior elements excised	0.80	0.66	-	-
Cheng et al [100]	38M (72yrs) / 32F (67yrs)	70 L3 vertebrae, posterior elements excised	0.80	-	-	-
Ebbensen et al [93]	50M (55.1yrs) / 51F (59yrs)	101 central sections of L3 vertebrae (trabecular bone)	-	-	0.91-0.93	0.84-0.86
Myers et al [55]	16M / 6F (52-75yrs)	61 isolated vertebrae L2-L4, posterior elements excised	0.67	0.54	0.78	0.58
Singer et al [80]	10M (58yrs) / 8F (77yrs)	287 isolated vertebrae T1-L5, posterior elements excised	-	-	0.78-0.93	0.73-0.89
Lochmuller et al [95]	32M (82.1yrs) / 17F (83.1yrs)	49 L4 vertebrae, posterior elements excised	0.53-0.55	-	-	-
Moro et al [101]	3M / 8F (72yrs)	11 L1/2-L2/4 motion segments, posterior elements excised	0.72	-	0.89	-
Edmondston et al [86]	5M (65.2yrs) / 7F (78.6yrs)	58 motion segments T2-4 - T12-L2 with posterior elements	-	-	0.62-0.84	0.40
Bürklein et al [97]	43M (77yrs) / 76F (82yrs)	68 L2-4 motion segments, posterior elements excised	0.69-0.77	-	0.83	-

Bjarnason et al [96]	14 cadavers (61yrs)	32 isolated vertebrae L2-L4 with posterior elements	0.48-0.51	-	0.45-0.71	-
Renau et al [94]	15M / 7F (63yrs)	42 vertebrae (L2 and L3), posterior elements excised	0.57	0.74		

* Failure: compression force to point of vertebral failure identified on a force-displacement curve (measured in Newtons [N]);
^ Stress: defined as failure load (N) / vertebral cross sectional area (m^2).

The relevance of bone mass, specifically BMD in vertebral bone strength has been established unequivocally in *ex vivo* studies. Table 3 provides a synthesis of the published studies examining the relationship between BMD and ultimate vertebral compressive force and compressive stress. The Table describes only studies in which BMD was derived from DXA. Many other studies have examined the relationships between bone strength and bone mass parameters derived from QCT, MRI, ultrasound and histology; however, these are not the focus of this Chapter.

Results presented in Table 3 demonstrate that BMD correlates strongly with compressive strength of bone tissue, independent of gender. Specifically, up to 86% of the variance in ultimate vertebral compressive force could be accounted for by DXA-derived BMD. Importantly, vertebral compressive strength is also influenced by vertebral size, for example cross sectional area (CSA), as evidenced in biomechanical studies [80,86,87]. Whereas areal BMD measured by DXA captures vertebral size to a degree, vertebral trabecular density (VTD) as measured by QCT does not. It is not surprising therefore, that the relationship between areal BMD and compressive strength is stronger than VTD and compressive strength [80,87], and that the latter relationship is improved when vertebral CSA is added to a regression model [80]. Generally, the studies contained in Table 3 indicate that the relationship between vertebral BMC and mechanical strength is weaker than BMD and mechanical strength, therefore in this Chapter, BMD is the primary variable of interest. Data also indicate that the relationship between vertebral bone strength and BMD is stronger when BMD is measured with lateral-projection DXA. Lateral DXA therefore appears to be a more valid predictor of vertebral strength than conventional AP-DXA. Indeed, epidemiologic studies indicate that lateral DXA has significantly greater discriminant validity compared to AP-DXA for distinguishing between individuals with and without osteoporotic vertebral fractures [88,89], while a trend to this effect was reported in another study [44]. Considering the superior diagnostic ability of lateral-projection DXA, applications of this scanning mode are explored in this Chapter.

A recently published study reported that when scanning the thoracic spine with lateral DXA, the most accurate representation of thoracic bone mineral is achieved when BMC is used rather than BMD [90]. This finding is not surprising considering that the concurrent validity was established against ash weighting of the T6 vertebral bodies. A stronger association will exist between BMC and ash weight since both variables are independent of bone area. However, the implications of these data are uncertain for the clinical context given that BMD of thoracic vertebrae cannot be measured with DXA *in vivo*, interpretation of bone mineral properties are predominantly based on BMD in the clinical environment, and measurement of BMC is grossly affected by bone size (or region of interest size). Several studies have also reported a stronger association between BMD and mechanical strength of vertebrae compared to BMC and mechanical strength [55,80,87,91-95].

The *ex vivo* studies described in Table 3 support epidemiologic data that a decrease in BMD as measured with DXA (lateral DXA in particular) is a risk factor for osteoporotic vertebral fracture [21]. However, *ex vivo* designs cannot be regarded as representative of *in vivo* loading conditions, and therefore the findings should be interpreted with some caution. For example, *in vivo* load distributions are dependent on the integrity of the intervertebral disc, while *ex vivo* load applications tend to be axial and symmetrical [87]. Studies that use vertebral motion segments in mechanical tests may be more representative of *in vivo* physiologic loading conditions compared to studies that test isolated vertebrae with posterior elements removed. In addition, correlations between DXA data and failure loads tend to be greater when DXA is performed *ex situ* compared to *in situ* [96-98].

The strong relationship between BMD and bone strength underlines the rationale for the use of densitometry in assessing fracture risk and skeletal status. However, evidence from epidemiologic studies suggests a lack of discriminant power of standard BMD measures, derived from DXA. For example, compared to DXA-derived BMD data acquired from AP scans of the lumbar spine, BMD data acquired from the hip is better able to identify individuals with prevalent vertebral fractures and the predictability of hip data is not enhanced with lumbar spine BMD data [102]. Further, studies indicate marked differences in the prevalence rate of vertebral fracture among individuals with comparable BMD, measured predominantly with AP DXA [74,77,103-112] and a poor sensitivity of areal BMD T-scores in identifying fracture cases [102,113]. Certainly, this may reflect differences between cohorts in factors other than BMD, but it is also likely that BMD differences exist given the strong relationship between BMD and compressive strength of bone (Table 3). Ciarelli et al. [114] used back-scattered electron microscopy to examine mineralization profiles in the cancellous bone of the iliac crest in individuals with and without osteoporotic vertebral fractures. The authors found that although the fracture group had the same mean value of mineralization, the distribution of mineralization differed markedly between groups, supporting the hypothesis that vertebral fracture aetiology is also influenced by the *distribution of bone mineral*. The inability to accurately identify BMD differences between fracture and non-fracture groups may be attributable, in part, to limitations in the measurement approach (AP-DXA) and failure to consider the distribution of bone mass within vertebrae.

1.4.3. Subregional Bone Mineral Density (srBMD)

Standard *in vivo* densitometry testing at the lumbar spine using AP or lateral-projection DXA measures BMC within the whole vertebral area to derive a whole vertebral BMD value from which total spine BMD is usually calculated and interpreted. This approach precludes assessment of the distribution of bone mineral within the vertebral body. Any regional variations in BMD are undetected since whole vertebral BMD remains unaffected. However, previous *ex vivo* (and *ex situ*) research using histomorphometry, QCT, quantitative radiography and DXA has established that bone mineral distribution within the vertebral centrum is not homogenous. In general, histomorphometry studies indicate greater trabecular separation and lower bone volume, trabecular thickness and trabecular number in the central and anterior zones of vertebrae compared to other zones [115-119]. Similarly, studies utilising QCT report lower volumetric bone density in central and anterior regions of vertebral bodies [120-123], while studies using computed quantitative radiography and DXA report lower BMD anteriorly and centrally [124-127]. Moreover, observed differences in srBMD measured by DXA are independent of measurement error [128].

1.4.4. Subregional BMD (srBMD) and Bone Strength

Alterations in regional trabecular architecture, as evidenced by histomorphometric and finite element modelling studies, significantly affect the mechanical integrity of the vertebral body [129,130]. Given the heterogeneity in BMD and trabecular architecture present within the vertebral body, it is likely that mechanical strength of vertebral bone varies according to the area upon which load is applied. Indeed, differences have been reported in static and fatigue failure properties of vertebral bone according to the region at which mechanical loads were imposed [131-135]. Considering the heterogeneity in bone mineral distribution and consequently mechanical strength within the vertebral body, it is likely that the nature of the distribution of bone mineral will influence vertebral fragility and therefore the risk of vertebral fracture. It follows that individuals who have sustained vertebral fractures may display different subregional BMD profiles compared to those without vertebral fractures even when global BMD measures remain comparable, as is commonly demonstrated in epidemiology studies (see section 1.4.2). It is also likely that subregional bone mass will have a stronger association with vertebral morphometry than a gross or average measure of vertebral bone mass. Both these issues are explored in this Chapter.

The majority of research examining intra-vertebral BMD distribution has been conducted with *ex vivo* models using methods that cannot be applied *in vivo* (e.g. histomorphometry), or are less commonly applied in a clinical context *in vivo* (QCT). Therefore, there is a lack of information in the literature describing BMD distribution patterns measured *in vivo,* in a clinical population and using clinical tools. Two previous *in vivo* studies reported that the use of a subregion in lateral DXA analysis of lumbar spine BMD increased diagnostic sensitivity compared to standard DXA analysis of the entire vertebral body [74,126]. Jergas et al. [74] found that the greatest percentage difference in BMD between 331 postmenopausal women with and without vertebral fractures was obtained when using a subregion in a lateral DXA scan. Mazess et al. [136] reported a trend to the same effect. Similarly, Sandor et al. [137] reported that subregional analysis of lumbar BMD using QCT could discriminate between fracture and non-fracture cases with 90% accuracy, while conventional BMD analysis resulted in complete overlap of BMD values between the groups. It would seem plausible that consideration of vertebral subregions in DXA-derived measurements may help to resolve the issue of poor discriminant power of standard DXA assessment between individuals with and without vertebral fractures. In addition, analysis of vertebral subregions may improve insight into vertebral fragility rather than relying on gross vertebral BMD and criteria established by the World Health Organisation (WHO). Indeed, Sandor et al. [138] argue that a significant limitation of current bone mineral densitometry is the overlap in BMD among individuals with and without vertebral fractures, bringing into question the accuracy of standard DXA for assessing vertebral fragility, and the over-simplistic nature of the classification criteria for osteoporosis established by the WHO. Those authors argued that intra-vertebral BMD distributions should be assessed as part of routine densitometric tests, and proposed that evaluation of subregional volumetric BMD using QCT should form the basis of standard clinical practice due to the scanning and analysis limitations of standard DXA. However, studies in this Chapter challenge that suggestion by specifically examining the use of DXA to assess subregional BMD of the lumbar spine *in vivo* and *ex vivo*. By optimising precision and accuracy parameters of srBMD assessment with DXA, more sensitive information about vertebral fragility is likely to become available. This would limit reliance on tools such as QCT, where relatively high doses of ionising radiation are delivered to the patient to gain the same information.

The aims of the studies described in this Chapter were to:

1. Provide preliminary evidence for the validity of measuring srBMD in the lumbar spine using lateral-projection DXA. The correspondence between DXA-derived srBMD values and histomorphometry-derived values were examined. We hypothesised that there would be good correspondence between BMD and bone volume fraction in anatomically equivalent subregions to confirm concurrent validity of the srBMD technique using DXA (Study 1).
2. Determine whether individuals with and without osteoporotic vertebral fractures demonstrate differences in subregional BMD profiles at L3. We hypothesised that the central and anterior regions of the vertebral bodies in fracture cases would have greater deficits in areal BMD compared to other intra-vertebral areas relative to non-fracture cases and controls. We hypothesised also that the ratios of subregional BMD would differ between fracture and non-fracture cases with osteoporosis (Study 2).
3. Add to the evidence base regarding the utility of srBMD measures by examining the strength of association between vertebral morphometry and srBMD compared to vertebral morphometry and standard DXA-derived vertebral BMD parameters (Study 3).

2. Materials and Methods

Three studies are described in this Chapter which address the aims listed above. The methods of each study are described below.

2.1. Study 1: Establishing Concurrent Validity of srBMD using DXA

Although DXA is able to measure BMD in small regions of interest, as outlined in this Chapter and in previous studies [126,127,139], it is unable to characterise trabecular architectural properties. Histomorphometry is a class of histology, which can be applied to bone tissue to quantitatively describe microarchitecture and bone mass characteristics. The histomorphometric parameter most closely related to BMD is the bone volume fraction (%BV/TV), which quantifies the percentage of bone tissue within a given volume of osteoid tissue section under microscopy. Previous studies, predominantly using animal models, have compared DXA-derived subregional BMD data to bone volume fraction to establish concurrent validity of DXA techniques [140-144]. In this study, srBMD from a human specimen is compared with %BV/TV in anatomically-equivalent subregions.

2.1.1. Specimen

A single cadaver spine was harvested from a 56 year old male. The ribs and ilia were removed leaving intact vertebral bodies from T12 to sacrum. The spine was fixed in formalin using standardised embalming protocols. The intact cadaver was embalmed with 30 L of embalming fluid (55% ethanol, 5% formaldehyde, 5% phenol, 20% propylene glycol and 15% water) and stored at 4°C for 3 months prior to harvesting of the spine. An experienced medical scientist examined the spine to identify vertebral levels *ex situ*. Use of the specimen for research purposes was granted by the Human Research Ethics Committee at the Royal Adelaide Hospital, South Australia.

2.1.2. Bone Densitometry and Histomorphometry

Prior to DXA scanning the spine was placed supine in a water bath (300×500×300mm) containing 40 L of tap water to a depth of 18 cm to simulate soft tissue composition. This procedure has been used previous studies with validity and reliability established for both lumbar and thoracic vertebrae [80,97,127,145,146]. Measurements of BMD and BMC were made subregionally at L2 and L3 from the lateral DXA scan using the subregional protocol, described below. DXA scans were performed five times without repositioning, and the mean data were used for analysis.

A Hologic QDR 4500A fan beam densitometer (Hologic Inc., Waltham, MA, USA), running operating system software version 9.10D was used for scanning in this study and those described later in this Chapter. A senior technician monitored quality control of the long-term reproducibility of the densitometer by scanning an anthropomorphic Hologic spine phantom (#402, Hologic Inc.) each morning and recording these data in the machine's internal quality control database. The Hologic QDR 4500A densitometer operated in the densitometry unit at the Royal Melbourne Hospital (RMH) uses Hologic reference data to calculate BMD parameters (specifically the population norms to T and Z scores). These reference data are used for all clinical interpretations by physicians who refer patients to the RMH densitometry unit. The Hologic reference database contains 1000 lumbar spine measurements (65% women) and 1400 hip measurements. These measures were taken from volunteers at the University of California, San Diego, USA [147]. The Hologic manual outlines how this information was complied and the inclusion/exclusion criteria applied [148]. The demographic characteristics of individuals in the Hologic database are comparable to those of participants described in this Chapter.

Analysis of the AP scan was performed according to the standard protocol described by Hologic [148] and Watts [149]. This analysis was performed prior to the commencement of the lateral scan to ensure correct identification of vertebral levels and correct start position for the lateral scan. After the lateral scan was completed, areal BMD was calculated for the whole vertebral body area (defined as region of interest [ROI] 1) and in six subregions (ROI 2-7) at L2 and L3 (Figure 1). Subregions were selected manually by modifying the regions of interest during the analysis phase, using Hologic analysis software version 8.26f:3. The whole vertebral area (ROI 1) was defined by the four corners of the vertebra of interest from the lateral DXA image, including the vertebral endplate and excluding the posterior elements. Overt osteophytes were excluded from the ROIs and deleted from the bone map manually. The size and shape of this area was defined according to the morphology of the vertebral body. Generally, the endplates defined the superior and inferior margins, the anterior border of the centrum defined the anterior margin, while the posterior margin was defined by the junction between the vertebral centrum and pedicle of the posterior elements (see Figure 1). A shortcut key was used during the analysis process to progressively add subregions into the analysis screen. The size and shape of the subregions were defined manually. Subregions 2-4 formed equal thirds in the area of ROI 1, orientated vertically. Keeping the pixel width (x dimension) of these regions constant ensured consistency of areal dimensions. Subregions 5-7 formed equal thirds in area of ROI 1, orientated horizontally. To ensure consistency of areal dimensions the pixel height (y dimension) of these regions was kept constant. Once the geometry of all seven ROIs was complete, a bone map was automatically created and areal BMD calculated in each ROI. In circumstances where the automated process of bone map creation failed to detect bone tissue adequately, the map was completed manually. The final output screen for the subregional analysis is illustrated in Figure 2.

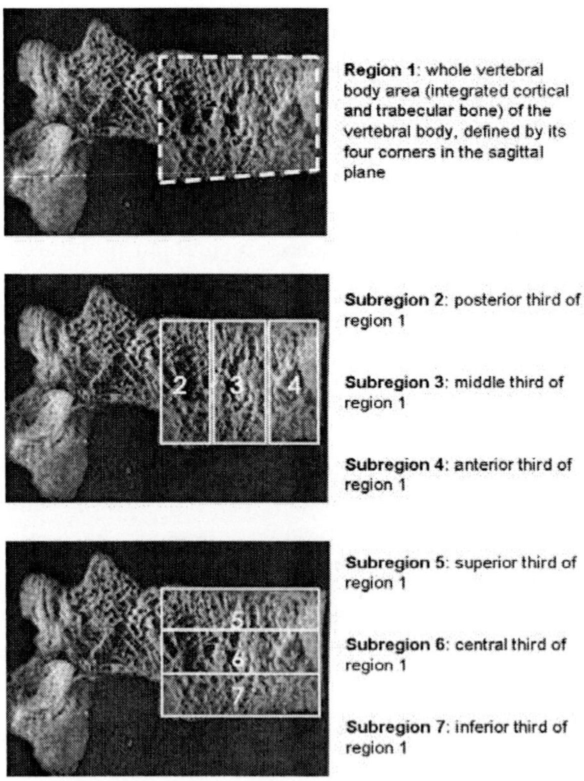

Figure 1. Whole vertebral area in the sagittal plane (ROI 1) and subregions (ROI 2-7) identified from the lateral scan.

A standard Hologic lateral analysis procedure was also performed for each scan. The standard lateral scan performed by the Hologic QDR 4500A densitometer differs to ROI 1 with respect to the completion of the bone map and the size of the region of interest. The standard Hologic analysis operates with an automatic bone map completion and does not adjust the area and shape of the region of interest according to the morphology of the vertebral body. The ROI 1 analysis used in this Chapter allows for manual completion of the bone map and adjusts the shape of the region of interest to the morphology of the individual vertebra.

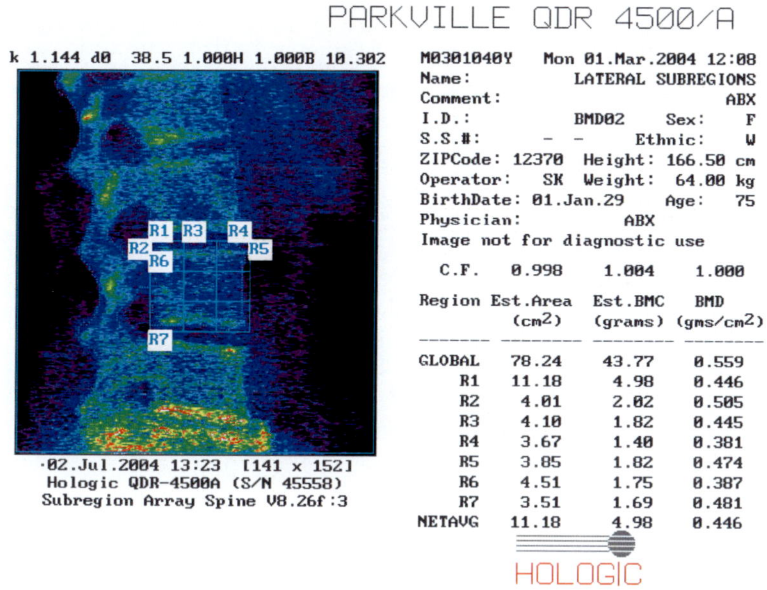

Figure 2. Screen capture of subregional analysis for L3 from a lateral scan on QDR 4500 densitometer. The Figure was not derived from a patient contained in this study and therefore the areas and BMCs have not been constructed around the morphology of the vertebral body. Instead, they show the orientation and relative positions of each subregion, relative to the whole, in a Hologic QDR 4500 output screen.

After DXA scanning, the specimen was prepared for histomorphometric analysis. Histomorphometry was performed using a pre-established protocol [115] to calculate the bone volume fraction within total volume (%BV/TV) for each region of interest, in accordance with Parfitt's formula [150]. A parasagittal slice of 5 mm width was cut close to the vertebral body midline and fixed using 10% neutral buffered formalin and decalcified with 9% nitric acid in 1% EDTA. The slice was embedded in paraffin wax and a section of 7 μm thickness was cut using a microtome. The section was then slide mounted and stained with van Gieson stain to highlight the bone matrix and imaged at 25 μm per pixel. Similar to selection of regions of interest (ROIs) for BMD and BMC measurement with DXA, the ROIs for histomorphometry were selected by dividing the vertebral body slice into equal thirds antero-posteriorly and supero-inferiorly (Figure 3).

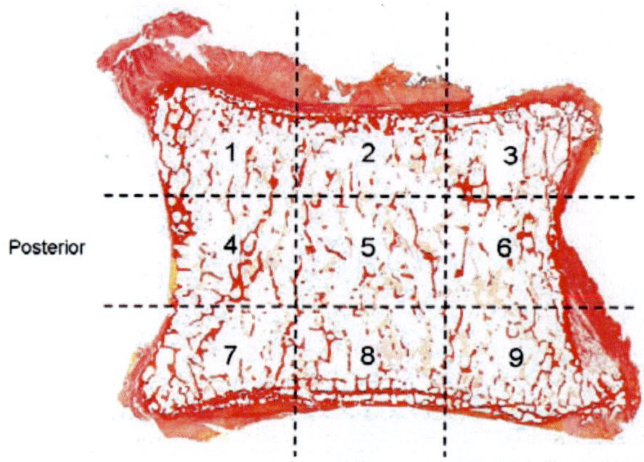

Figure 3. Slide-mounted parasagittal slice of the L3 vertebral body from a 76 year old male illustrating the staining and subregions used in this study based on the methodology reported by Simpson et al [115]. The mean bone volume fraction from combinations of histological subregions was calculated to construct anatomically equivalent subregions to those defined from the DXA analysis (mean %BV/TV regions 1-9 = DXA ROI 1; mean %BV/TV of 1,4,7 = DXA ROI 2; mean %BV/TV of 2,5,8 = DXA ROI 3; mean %BV/TV of 3,6,9 = DXA ROI 4; mean %BV/TV of 1-3 = DXA ROI 5; mean %BV/TV of 4-6 = DXA ROI 6; mean %BV/TV of 7-9 = DXA ROI 7).

2.1.3. Data Analysis

Pearson correlation was used to examine correspondence between DXA-derived BMD and BMC data and histomorphometry-derived %BV/TV data with α set at 0.05. This approach has been used for histomorphometry previously [151].

2.2. Study 2: Subregional Vertebral BMD Characteristics in Individuals with and without Osteoporotic Vertebral Fractures

2.2.1. Participants

Three groups of participants were recruited for this study (*n*=34). These were (i) individuals with primary osteoporosis who had experienced at least one thoracic vertebral fracture, (ii) individuals with primary osteoporosis who were free of vertebral fracture and (iii) comparable controls with normal BMD and no vertebral fracture. Participants had not ever taken medication known to affect BMD for a period of greater than 6 months (steroids, hormone replacement therapy, bisphosphonates, selective estrogen receptor modulator (SERM) medication, parathyroid hormone, calcitriol or vitamin D analogues) and were free of other bone diseases/conditions. Other exclusion criteria included a fracture of L2 or L3, previous spinal surgery such as laminectomy and microdiscectomy, and a period of immobilisation for greater than 1 month within the last year. Osteoporosis was diagnosed according to the WHO criteria based on T-scores from AP spine and hip DXA scans and the presence of fragility fracture(s) [152]. The level of physical activity between groups was assessed using the Physical Activity Scale for the Elderly (PASE) questionnaire [153,154].

2.2.2. Plain Film Radiography

Confirmation of vertebral fracture was made from plain film radiographs of the thoracic and lumbar spine. Participants adopted a relaxed standing posture (i.e. normal self-defined, standing posture) with their left side against an X-ray cassette. Participants were asked to pronate their forearms, placing their palms on their anterior thigh to shift the humerus slightly anterior to the vertebral column. This upper limb position was deemed necessary after pilot testing in order to minimise the structures overlying the thoracic vertebral bodies, for example the scapula, humerus and elbow joint. Previous studies have used a similar rationale, instructing participants to rest their hands on a horizontal beam positioned at the level of the pelvis [155,156]. Those researchers found that this position was necessary to remove the humeri from the X-ray volume and demonstrated that it did not significantly change spinal curvature. Radiographs were taken with a fixed film-to-focus distance (FFD) of 100cm using a General Electric Proteus XR/a General Purpose Radiographic System, model ML02F (General Electric [GE] Medical Systems, Milwaukee, WI, USA). Images were acquired using a breathing method so as to maximise bone structure clarity and minimise lung field features. AGFA (Mortsel, Belgium) imaging plates were processed with a GE Centricity SP1001 plate reader (model K2025JB). The reader scanned the exposed photo-stimulable phosphor imaging plate, converting the information to 12 bit digital data with a spatial resolution ranging from 7-10pixels/mm. The image was then transmitted electronically to a radiography workstation and labelled and viewed using GE Centricity Dicom Viewer™ software. Images were exported from the GE software into .jpeg format for further viewing and processing (Study 3) with image analysis software.

The thoracic image included vertebral bodies T1-T12, with the X-ray beam centred at T7 and acquired with energies of approximately 66 kV and 80 mA. The lumbar image included vertebral bodies T12-S1, with the beam centred at L3, with energies set at 90 kV and 100 mA. These parameters and an FFD of 100cm have been used in previous studies examining vertebral morphology [157-160]. The energy settings varied slightly at the discretion of the radiographer according to body size of the participant.

Similar to McCloskey et al. [161] a vertebral body was classified as fractured when two criteria were filled at each vertebral site to reduce the number of false positives. Vertebrae were classified as fractured if the anterior vertebral height was reduced by ≥30% compared to its posterior height *and* the posterior height of the adjacent superior or inferior vertebral body. Radiographs were also qualitatively reviewed by a radiologist, ensuring that fracture diagnosis was consistent with the semi-quantitative method described by Genant et al. [162]. Although wedge fractures are the most common osteoporotic vertebral fracture [108], qualitative review by a radiologist also ensured that compression fractures were not missed since the quantitative method used was aimed primarily at identifying wedge fractures. To account for normal anatomical wedging of thoracic vertebral bodies associating with ageing, normative wedging values of T4-L5 established by Melton et al. [163] were input into the algorithms for calculating vertebral height ratios. In that study, vertebral morphometry data were collected form 52 postmenopausal women (age >50yrs) with no history of vertebral fracture, and these data are reproduced in Table 4. In the current study mid-vertebral height was not measured due to potential imprecision introduced by indistinct vertebral margins and parallax error [164].

Table 4. Data adapted from Melton et al., 1989 [163] to describe normal vertebral height ratios expressed as a percentage and calculated adjustment factors expressed as a percentage

Vertebra	Ratio 1 Hp*i*/Hpi_{-1}	Adjust factor 1	Ratio 2 Hp*i*/Hpi_{+1}	Adjust factor 2	Ratio 3 Ha*i*/Hp*i*	Adjust factor 3
T4	-	-	95.3	4.70	96.89	3.11
T5	105.26	-5.26	96.43	3.57	95.48	4.52
T6	104.01	-4.01	97.46	2.54	93.12	6.88
T7	120.87	-20.87	97.26	2.74	92.17	7.83
T8	103.07	-3.07	96.89	3.11	93.19	6.81
T9	103.60	-3.60	95.01	4.99	94.74	5.26
T10	105.55	-5.55	90.91	9.09	96.03	3.97
T11	110.24	-10.24	93.24	6.76	93.37	6.63
T12	107.50	-7.50	96.52	3.48	94.20	5.80
L1	104.13	-4.13	98.25	1.75	97.03	2.97
L2	102.33	-2.33	98.72	1.28	101.31	-1.31
L3	101.86	-1.86	103.61	-3.61	103.41	-3.41
L4	96.82	3.18	91.85	8.15	107.13	-7.13
L5	108.87	-8.87	-	-	85.63	14.37

Hp*i* = posterior height of vertebra of interest (*i*), Ha*i* = anterior height of vertebra of interest, i_{+1} = vertebra above, i_{-1} = vertebra below.

All participants provided written informed consent and approval to conduct this study was granted by the Human Research Ethics Committees of Melbourne Health, The University of Melbourne, Northern Health, Department of Human Services Radiation Advisory Committee, Victoria.

2.2.3. Bone Densitometry

A standard right hip scan and a matched AP* and supine-lateral projection scan were performed on the lumbar spine using the same densitometer as described in Study 1. Scanning was performed according to the specifications and positioning recommendations issued by Hologic [148] and Watts [149], using the fast-array scanning mode. Analyses of the right hip, AP spine and lateral spine scans were performed according to the method recommended by the manufacturer. Areal BMD and associated T scores were calculated for the femoral neck, trochanter, intertrochanteric zone, Ward's triangle, total hip, vertebrae L1-L4 in the AP orientation, and the total AP spine (mean L1-L4). These results were used to classify the participants as normal, osteopenic or osteoporotic according to the WHO diagnostic criteria. The lateral spine scan was also used to calculate areal BMD in six intra-vertebral subregions at L3 using Hologic software version 8.26f:3, as outlined above. The

* Although the orientation of this scan is commonly referred to as antero-posterior (AP), the X-ray source for the Hologic QDR4500A densitometer lies underneath the patient so the X-ray beam travels postero-anteriorly (PA).

precision of subregional analysis has been established previously, and is reported to be best at L3. The %CV and ICC values ranged from 2.0-5.6% and 0.96-0.99 respectively in an analysis of short term *in vivo* precision [128]. For this reason, the srBMD protocol was only applied to L3 in this Study.

2.2.4. Data Analysis

To examine differences in areal subregional BMD between groups from the lateral scan at L3, two 3×4 ANOVAs with one repeated measure were performed, including mass as a covariate (see Results). 'Group' was set as the between-subject factor (k=3) and 'region of interest' (ROI) as the within-subject repeated measure. Although there were 7 regions of interest (ROIs), the ROI factor was set *a priori* to k=4 to ensure that overlapping regions were not compared *post hoc*. ANOVA 1 included the whole vertebral area (ROI 1) with regions orientated posteriorly to anteriorly (ROI 2-4), while ANOVA 2 included the ROI 1 and regions orientated superiorly to inferiorly (ROI 5-7). The critical alpha level of significance was set at 0.05 (2-tailed). Normality of the data was investigated with the Kolmogorov-Smirnov statistic and sphericity with Mauchly's W statistic for repeated measures tests. Where sphericity was violated the Greenhouse-Geisser statistic was used to calculate the F value. Homogeneity of variance was examined with the Levene statistic. Considering the small sample size in each cohort and to ensure clinical feasibility, all *post hoc* comparisons were calculated using a Bonferroni correction to reduce the risk of type 1 error.

The interpretation of differences in areal BMD between subregions was uncertain due to differences in geometry between them. It was, therefore, difficult to determine if any main effect for region was due to a difference in BMD or to geometry. Differences in bone size between participants may also confound areal BMD data (see section 1.4.1). However, a comparison of the whole L3 vertebral area (ROI 1) from the lateral scan showed no difference between groups when examined with a one-way ANOVA (Table 5), suggesting little difference in bone size between the groups. However, this analysis does not account for any potential differences in bone depth between groups. Although correction factors are available to convert DXA-derived areal BMD to volumetric BMD, such as that devised by Carter et al. [165] for the lumbar spine, correction factors have not been validated for lateral scans used without a matched AP scan or subregional BMD analyses, so no transformations to apparent volumetric BMD were applied to data in this study. To minimise the potentially confounding effect of regional geometry on BMD differences, ratios of subregional BMD were compared between groups using a one-way ANOVA, again with Bonferroni corrections for *post hoc* analyses. Comparisons of ratios between groups maximises the comparability of regional geometry between groups. Therefore, this approach can be used to identify any differences in the distribution of intra-vertebral BMD between groups (see Figure 4 for more detail). Ratios were set *a priori* and selection of ratios was made on the basis of results of previous work which suggested that ratios of posterior : anterior, whole : posterior, whole : anterior, whole : central, central : superior and central : inferior were the most relevant [127]. Data analysis was performed using SPSS version 12.1 for Windows (SPSS Inc., Chicago, IL, USA).

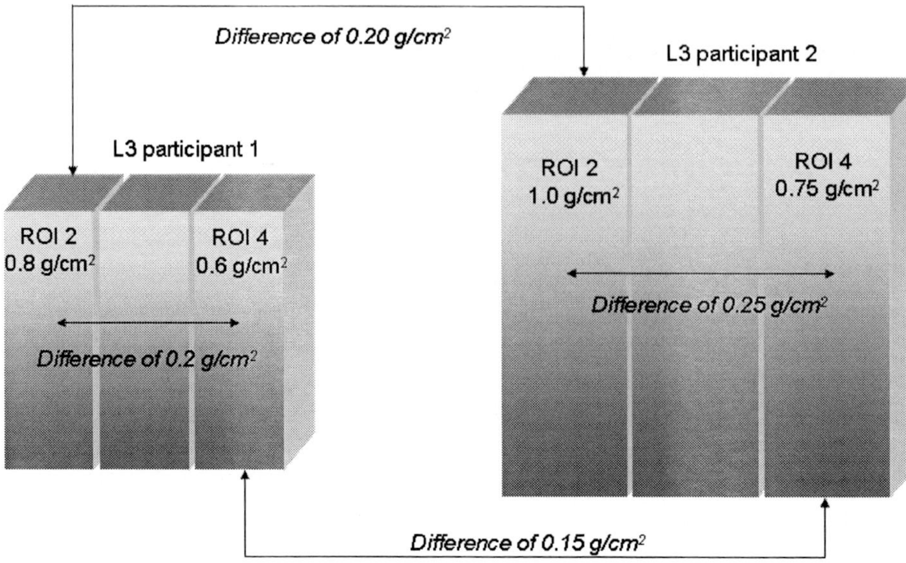

Figure 4. *i)* Comparable subregions are compared between the same vertebral body of 2 patients of different body size. There is a difference in srBMD between comparable regions. Participant 2 may have greater areal density simply due to larger vertebral size (projected area). Comparing ratios of subregional density between patients shows no difference (ROI2 : ROI4 = 1.33 for both vertebrae), suggesting the apparent differences are due to geometry. *ii)* Comparing areal density between subregions within a vertebral body may be confounded by differences in subregional geometry. This limitation may be overcome by comparing ratios of subregional BMD between participants. This keeps the geometry variable comparable and allows for any differences in BMD distribution to be identified. For example, the difference between subregions is greater in participant 2, but the relative ratios are the same between vertebral bodies, suggesting no deficit in BMD between the two participants.

2.3. Study 3: Subregional Vertebral BMD as a Predictor of Vertebral Morphology

2.3.1. Participants

Individuals with osteoporosis, described in study 2 (n=22), were included in this study.

2.3.2. Bone Densitometry

Participants were subject to the same bone densitometry procedures as described in Study 2.

2.3.3. Vertebral Morphometry

Thoracic vertebral morphometry data were acquired from digital images of the radiographs. Acquisition of radiographs is described above, in Study 2. Two-dimensional Cartesian (*x,y*) pixel co-ordinates of the corners of the vertebral bodies T1-T12 in the sagittal plane were digitised, using the 'crosshair' tool in Image J software (Image J version 1.30, National Institute of Health, Maryland, USA), using the default co-ordinate system. Image brightness, contrast and zoom were manually adjusted to achieve the optimal image clarity. Following the rationale of McCloskey et al. [161], osteophytes appearing on vertebral margins were excluded from the digitising process by visually interpolating the margins of the vertebral body to form an intersection at the vertebral corner of interest. The *x,y* pixel co-ordinate points of the vertebral corners (antero-superior, postero-superior, postero-inferior and antero-inferior) were imported into an Microsoft Excel™ spreadsheet. A formula was written to calculate the percentage reduction in anterior vertebral height for each vertebral level, based on a pixel distance. The percentage reduction of anterior vertebral height relative to posterior vertebral height was calculated for each vertebra and the maximum value for the thoracic spine recorded ($H_{A(max)}$). The mean ratio of anterior to posterior vertebral height was also recorded for T1-T12. For the current study, intra-rater reliability associated with acquiring *x,y* pixel co-ordinates of the vertebral centroids was established in a study of 10 participants . Reliability was expressed using intra-class correlation (ICC) statistics (model ICC [11]), and a percentage co-efficient of variation (%CV). Excellent intra-rater reliability was established for the upper, middle and lower thoracic spine with ICC values ranging from 0.98-0.99 and the %CV from 0.19-0.91% [166].

2.2.4. Data Analysis

Simple linear regression was used to determine the ability of standard DXA measures of areal BMD and subregional measures of areal BMD (srBMD) to predict the $H_{A(max)}$ and the mean ratio of anterior to posterior vertebral height. All data were normally distributed and the level of significance was set at $\alpha=0.05$.

3. Results

3.1. Study 1

The mean total spine areal BMD (L1-L4) from the AP scan was 0.82 ± 0.005 g/cm^2 and BMC (L1-L4) was 49.91 ± 0.84 g, with an equivalent T-score of –2.46 and Z score of –2.00. At L2 and L3, the mean areal BMD from the AP scan was 0.80 ± 0.007 g/cm^2 and 0.85 ± 0.01 g/cm^2 (T = -2.60 and –2.27 respectively; Z = -2.14 and –1.18 respectively). The mean BMC for L2 and L3 from the AP scan was 11.72 ± 0.29 g and 13.15 ± 0.28 g respectively. Correlation coefficients between areal BMD and %BV/TV across the regions were r=0.52 (p=0.23) for L2, r=0.78 (p=0.04) for L3 and r=0.59 (p=0.02) when the data sets were pooled. Weaker correlations were found for the association with BMC across the regions (p>0.05) for L2 (r=0.14), L3 (r=0.17) and pooled data (r=0.15). Figures 5A-B and 6A-B show the correspondence between the outcome measures for L2 and L3 respectively. Poorer correspondence was observed at ROI 4 at L2.

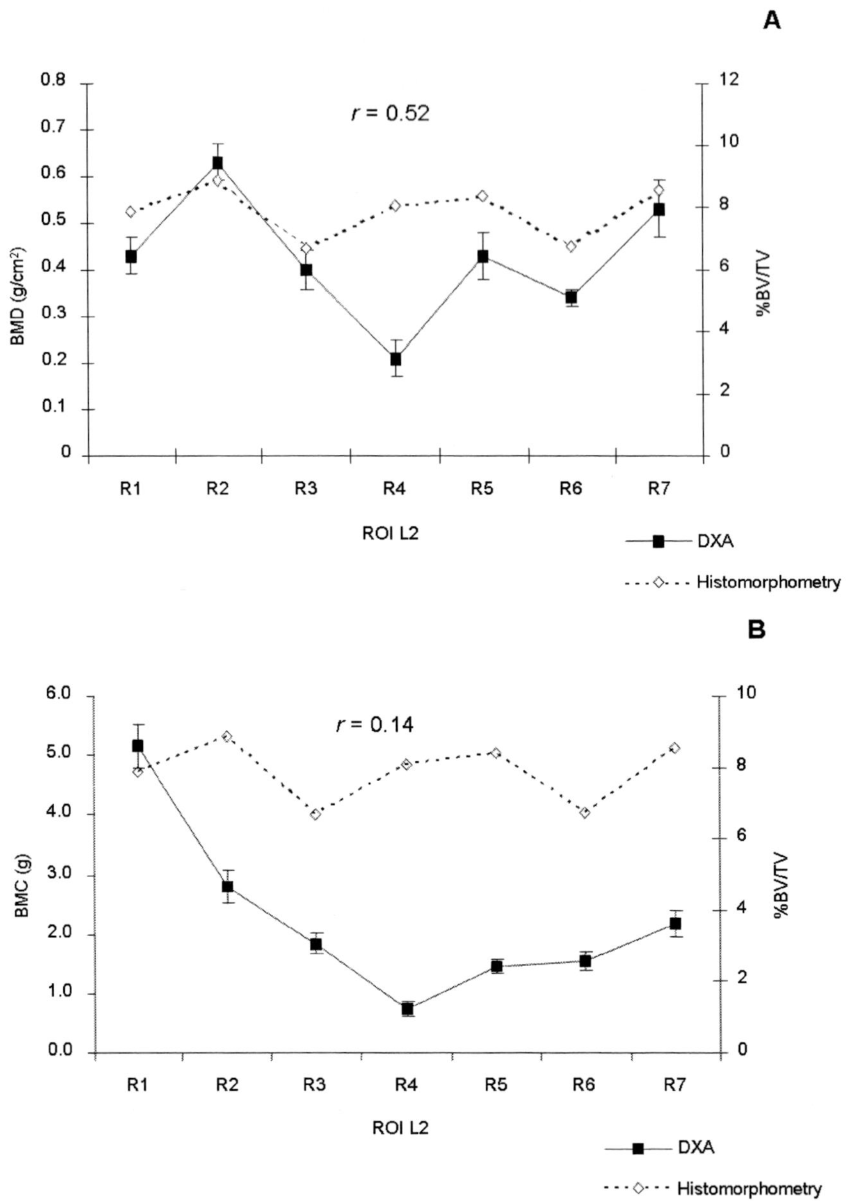

Figure 5A-B. Correspondence between DXA (mean areal BMD [A] and mean BMC [B]) and histomorphometry (%BV/TV) for L2 at each region of interest (ROI). Error bars represent 1 SD for the DXA data.

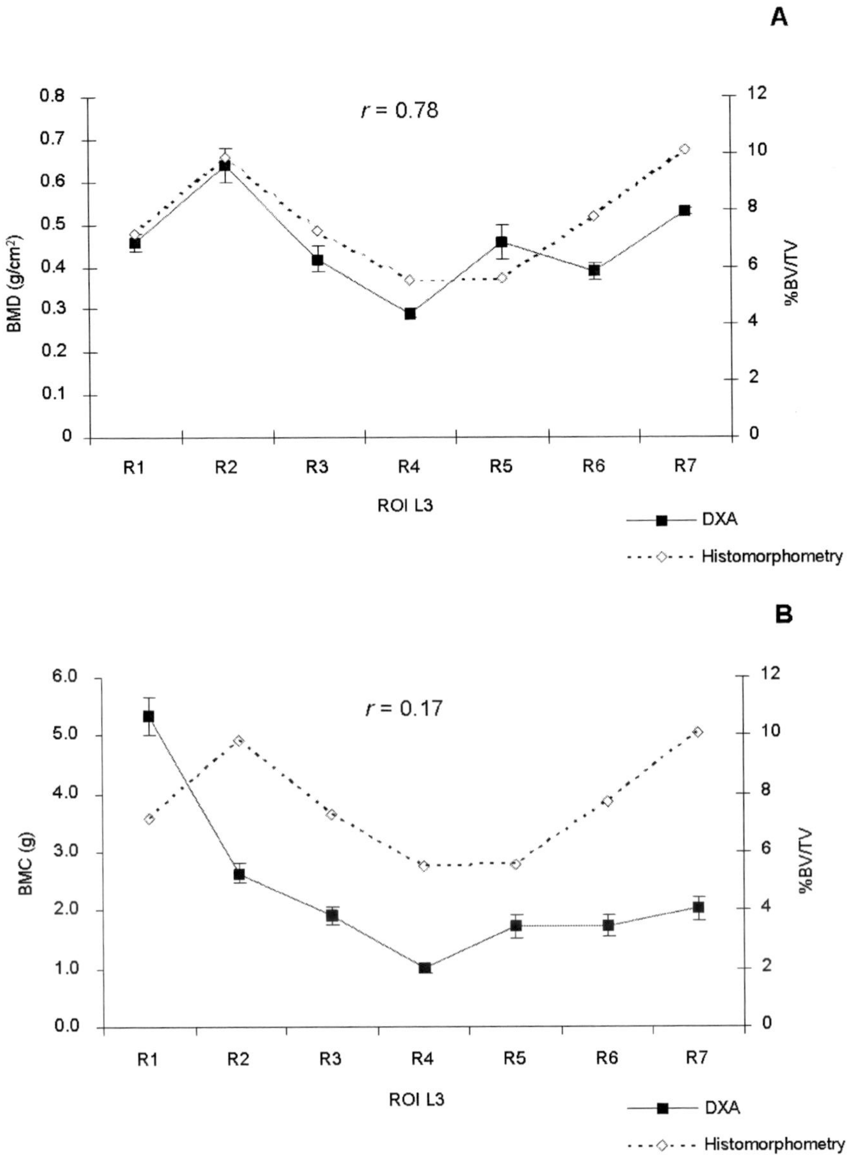

Figure 6A-B. Correspondence between DXA (mean areal BMD [A] and mean BMC [B]) and histomorphometry (%BV/TV) for L3 at each region of interest (ROI). Error bars represent 1 SD for the DXA data.

3.2. Study 2

3.2.1. Descriptive Information

Differences in physical characteristics and DXA-derived T-scores between cohorts were explored with a one-way ANOVA. Descriptive data are summarised in Table 5. There were no differences in age, height, or PASE score (physical activity index) between groups. A significant difference was found between groups based on mass, BMI and T-scores

(p<0.001). The control group had significantly greater mass and BMI compared to the fracture group, and higher T-scores than the fracture and non-fracture osteoporosis groups for AP spine, lateral spine and AP hip projections (p<0.01). Three participants from the control group were excluded since their DXA results indicated they were in the osteopenic range, based on WHO diagnostic criteria (-1>T>-2.5). The total sample size was therefore reduced to n=31. Of the 7 participants who were diagnosed with a fracture, 9 vertebral wedge fractures were identified. Wedge fractures occurred at T4 (3 fractures), T5 (1 fracture), T6 (1 fracture), T8 (3 fractures) and T9 (1 fracture).

Table 5. Summary of sample descriptive statistics for each group and pooled data, presented as the mean (SD)

Group	n	^Age (yrs)	*Mass (kg)	^Height (cm)	*BMI	^PASE†	**T-score AP spine (L1-L4)	**T-score Lateral spine (L2-L4)	**T-score Total hip	^L3 vertebral area (ROI 1) (cm²)
Fracture	7	65.6 (5.6)	65.4 (10.8)	160.2 (5.2)	25.5 (4.1)	160.1 (55.4)	-2.56 (1.81)	-2.61 (1.53)	-1.99 (1.11)	4.21 (0.98)
Non-fracture	15	63.4 (8.5)	57.0 (8.2)	157.7 (4.2)	22.8 (2.7)	154.1 (51.4)	-2.27 (0.74)	-1.70 (0.75)	-2.03 (0.84)	5.05 (0.98)
Control	9	57.2 (3.0)	74.7 (5.8)	162.3 (5.0)	28.4 (2.8)	142.1 (64.5)	0.33 (1.18)	-0.26 (1.06)	-0.23 (1.36)	5.64 (1.83)
Pooled	31	62.1 (7.3)	64.0 (11.1)	159.6 (5.1)	25.1 (3.8)	152.1 (54.8)	-1.58 (1.68)	-1.49 (1.34)	-1.50 (1.33)	5.03 (1.34)

* significant difference between control and non fracture group, p<0.01;

** significant difference between control and both osteoporotic groups (fracture and non-fracture), p<0.01;

^ no significant difference between groups;

† PASE: Physical Activity Scale for the Elderly, scored out of 400. Range in this sample was 52.5-263.1.

3.2.2. Differences in Areal Subregional BMD

For each mixed model ANOVA conducted there was neither a significant group × region interaction nor a group main effect. However, a significant difference for region was established (p<0.001). Figure 7A shows the mean areal BMD for each group for ROIs 1-4 (ANOVA 1), with areal BMD being highest at ROI 2 (posterior) and lowest at ROI 4 (anterior). Figure 7B shows mean areal BMD for ROIs 1 and 5-7 (ANOVA 2), with areal BMD being highest at ROI 7 (inferior) and lowest at ROI 6 (central).

Both Figures 7A and 7B show a trend for the fracture group to have lower areal BMD than the non-fracture group at all subregions. The percentage difference in mean areal BMD between the fracture and non-fracture groups was calculated for each region, and these results are illustrated in Figure 8. The deficit in BMD ranged from -13.1% to -16.3% with the greatest percent difference in mean BMD observed at ROI 6 (central). The percentage difference in mean areal BMD between fracture and non-fracture cases relative to controls was also calculated and these data are presented in Figure 9. The fractured cases had a much greater BMD deficit relative to the controls, compared with the non-fracture group (-10.2 to -23.5% compared to 6.1 to -10.4%). In the superior region (ROI 5) the non-fracture group had higher mean BMD than controls.

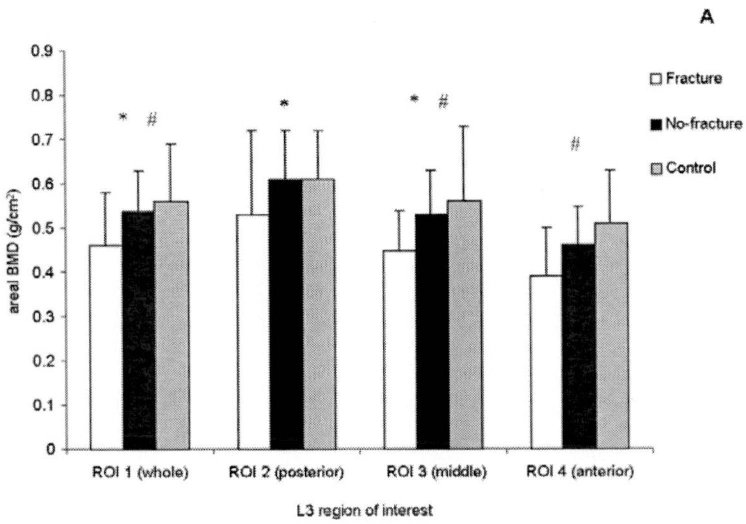

Figure 7A. Mean areal BMD for ROIs 1-4 for each group, with error bars representing 1SD. Symbols demonstrate regional differences (refer to key below).

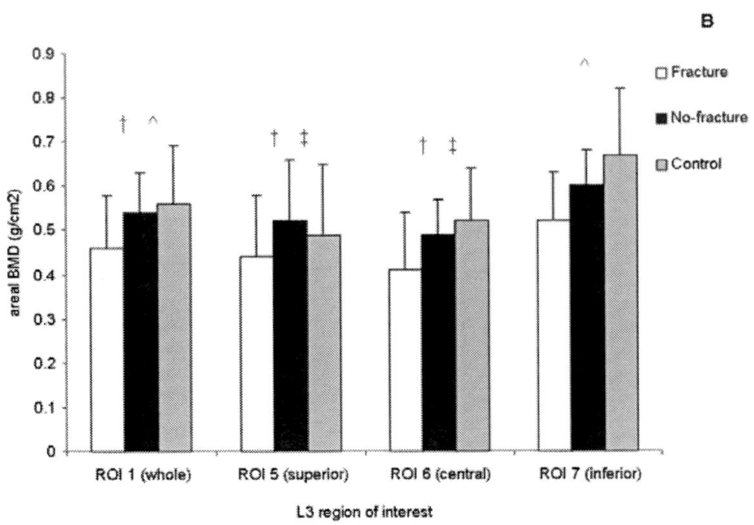

Figure 7B. Mean areal BMD for ROIs 1 and 5-7 for each group, with error bars representing 1SD. Symbols demonstrate regional differences (refer to key below).

Symbols key:

* significantly higher BMD than ROI 4, $p<0.001$; # significantly lower BMD than ROI 2, $p<0.001$; † significantly lower BMD than ROI 7, $p<0.001$; ^ significantly higher BMD than ROI 6, $p<0.001$; ‡ significantly lower BMD than ROI 1, $p<0.001$.

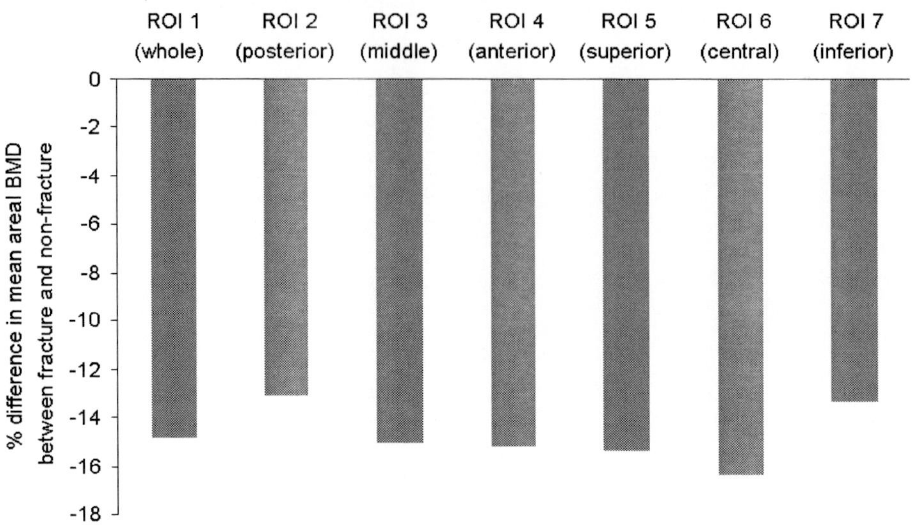

Figure 8. Percentage difference in mean areal BMD at each ROI between fracture and non-fracture groups with osteoporosis.

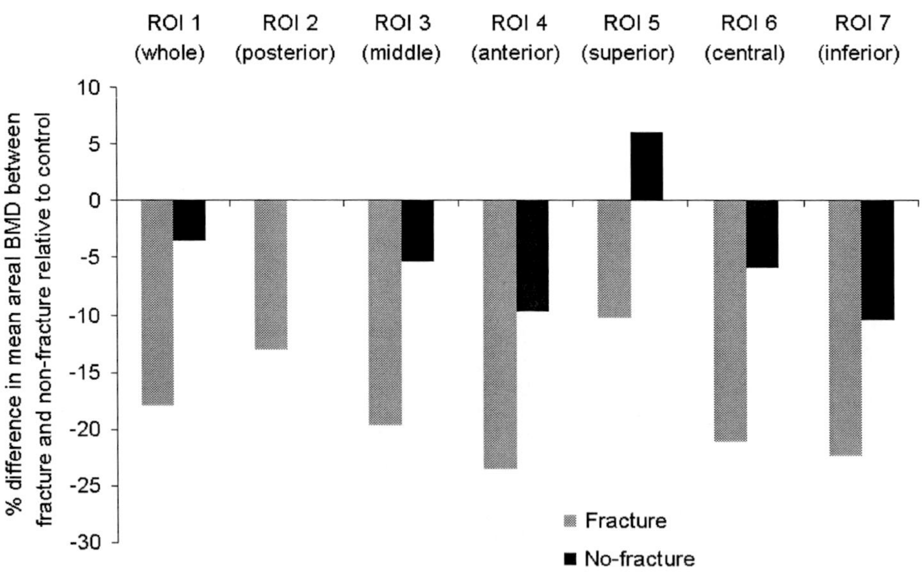

Figure 9. Percentage difference in mean areal BMD in fracture and non-fracture groups relative to controls at each ROI.

The output values for standard DXA analysis of the lumbar spine, both AP and lateral, were also compared between groups using a one-way ANOVA and these data are outlined in Table 6. The control group had significantly higher BMD than fracture and non-fracture cases ($p<0.05$) except in the L3 mid-zone calculated from the lateral scan. No differences were found between the fracture and non-fracture cases ($p>0.05$).

Table 6. Mean (SD) areal BMD for standard analysis DXA variables compared between groups. The percentage difference is calculated between fracture and non-fracture groups

	Group			
DXA variable (g/cm^2)	Fracture	Non-fracture	% Difference	Control
AP total spine (L1-L4)	0.766 (0.199)	0.797 (0.081)	3.89	1.083 (0.129)$^{\#}$
AP L3	0.785 (0.215)	0.822 (0.085)	4.50	1.145 (0.159)$^{\#}$
Standard lateral L3	0.612 (0.133)	0.647 (0.068)	5.41	0.748 (0.101)$^{\#}$
Standard lateral mid-zone L3*	0.575 (0.175)	0.579 (0.100)	0.70	0.714 (0.156)

* measured automatically from the standard lateral analysis;
# BMD of controls greater than fracture and non-fracture groups, $p<0.05$.

Mean areal srBMD and standard DXA output values of the fracture cases were then expressed as the number of standard deviations (SDs) from the non-fracture group srBMD output means and standard DXA output means. These data are presented in Figure 10. Greater deviation below the non-fracture mean was observed with srBMD data (0.60-1.04 SDs) compared to standard DXA output values (0.04-0.51 SDs). Therefore, the number of SDs below the non-fracture data means was much greater for the srBMD data compared to the standard DXA data. When srBMD SDs were expressed as a percentage increase above the standard DXA SDs, the magnitude of increase ranged from 116-2600% (Table 7).

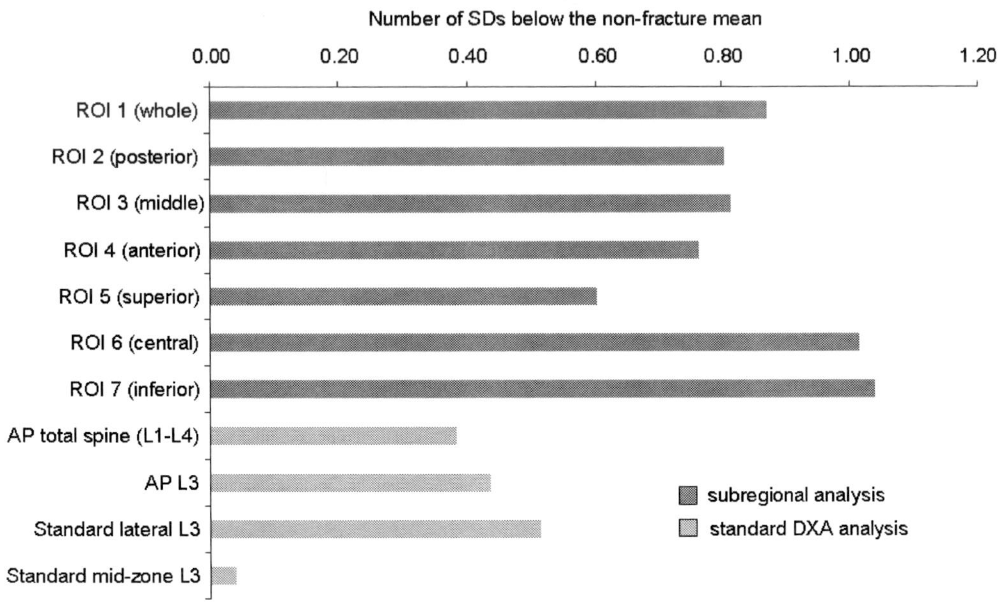

Figure 10. Mean BMD of fracture cases expressed as the number of standard deviations below the non-fracture BMD means for srBMD analysis and standard DXA analysis.

Table 7. Magnitude of increase (expressed as a percentage) of srBMD data (per region of interest [ROI]) over standard DXA analysis data. The percentage expression represents the magnitude of difference in the number of SDs below the non-fracture mean BMD data for each analysis approach between fracture and non-fracture data

	Standard DXA analysis parameter			
Region of interest	**AP spine (L1-L4)**	**AP L3**	**Lateral L3**	**Lat mid-zone L3**
ROI 1 (whole)	227.2	199.8	168.9	2173.9
ROI 2 (posterior)	209.5	184.2	155.8	2004.7
ROI 3 (middle)	212.3	186.7	157.9	2031.3
ROI 4 (anterior)	199.5	175.4	148.3	1908.6
ROI 5 (superior)	156.8	137.8	116.6	1500.0
ROI 6 (central)	264.6	232.6	196.7	2531.3
ROI 7 (inferior)	271.6	238.8	202.0	2598.7
Mean	*220.2*	*193.6*	*163.7*	*2106.9*
SD	*39.3*	*34.6*	*29.3*	*376.4*

3.2.3. Differences between Groups in Ratios of Subregional BMD

To examine differences in pre-specified srBMD ratios between groups, a one-way ANOVA was conducted. No significant difference between groups was established for any ratio compared. Table 8 shows the ratio values for each comparison.

Table 8. Mean (SD) ratio values of subregional BMD for each group

Ratio	Fracture	Non-fracture	Control	*p*-value
posterior : anterior (2:4)	1.40 (0.42)	1.36 (0.21)	1.24 (0.18)	0.432
whole : posterior (1:2)	0.89 (0.13)	0.88 (0.06)	0.91 (0.09)	0.622
whole : anterior (1:4)	1.20 (0.21)	1.18 (0.11)	1.11 (0.07)	0.396
whole : central (1:6)	1.13 (0.10)	1.10 (0.09)	1.09 (0.08)	0.644
central : superior (6:5)	0.93 (0.12)	0.97 (0.17)	1.13 (0.38)	0.205
central : inferior (6:7)	0.78 (0.11)	0.81 (0.09)	0.78 (0.13)	0.664

3.3. Study 3

3.3.1. Descriptive Information

Descriptive data for the sample are described in Study 2 results (Table 5). There were no significant differences in age, mass, height, physical activity or areal BMD measured between the fracture and non-fracture groups.

3.3.2. Vertebral Morphometry Results

The fracture group had a significantly greater $H_{A(max)}$ compared to the non-fracture group reflecting the presence of a vertebral fracture (39.2 ± 5.4% and 20.0 ± 4.0%, $p<0.0001$).

There was no difference in the mean ratio of anterior to posterior vertebral height between groups.

3.3.3. Association between BMD Data and Vertebral Morphometry

Standard measures of BMD were unable to account for a significant proportion of the variance observed in $H_{A(max)}$ (r^2=0.06-0.08, p>0.05, Table 9) other than the total lateral spine measure (L2-L4), which accounted for 19% of the observed variance in $H_{A(max)}$. However, all srBMD measures, other than ROI 5, were able to account for a significant proportion of the variance observed in $H_{A(max)}$ (r^2=0.18-0.28, $p\leq$0.05, Table 9). Neither standard DXA measures of BMD nor subregional BMD measures were able to significantly predict the mean ratios of anterior to posterior vertebral height.

Table 9. Details of simple linear regression models with BMD measures as the independent predictor variables and $H_{A(max)}$ as the dependent variable

BMD measure	Constant	Co-efficient	SE^	r^2	*p*-value
Standard BMD measure					
AP spine (L3)	42.79	-20.57	16.11	0.08	n.s
AP spine (L1-L4)	41.58	-19.64	17.46	0.06	n.s
Lateral spine L3	46.26	-31.67	23.70	0.08	n.s
Lateral spine (L2-L4)	57.08	-47.38	21.80	0.19	0.04
srBMD measure					
L3 ROI 2 (posterior)	43.92	-30.31	14.57	0.18	0.05
L3 ROI 3 (middle)	49.39	-45.95	19.98	0.21	0.03
L3 ROI 4 (anterior)	44.58	-42.10	20.36	0.18	0.05
L3 ROI 5 (superior)	40.94	-29.84	15.06	0.16	n.s
L3 ROI 6 (central)	46.98	-45.06	19.08	0.22	0.03
L3 ROI 7 (inferior)	58.93	-57.18	20.65	0.28	0.01

n.s = non significant (p>0.05);
^ SE = standard error of unstandardised co-efficient (β).

4. DISCUSSION

The studies presented in this Chapter provide robust, preliminary evidence for the potential clinical utility of vertebral srBMD measurement using DXA. With further validity testing and application to a larger prospective cohort study, it is likely that the application of this method to the clinical environment would be justified. The results demonstrate that the srBMD method using DXA is accurate and that the protocol can identify differences in BMD between vertebral subregions in vivo. The ability to identify and quantify differences in srBMD may provide very important information about vertebral fragility, as well as bone responses to therapeutic medications such as bisphosphonates, medications which deplete bone mass such as glucocorticoids and chronic conditions such as disabling back pain.

Study 1 sought to examine correspondence between subregional areal BMD measures obtained from lateral DXA scanning with bone volume fraction measured from histomorphometry in lumbar vertebral subregions. Good correspondence was found between the measures, suggesting adequate concurrent validity of the DXA protocol. The slightly poorer strength of correspondence for L2 may be explained by the relatively high bone volume fraction and low BMD measure for ROI 4. Better correspondence was observed at L3, and may reflect the higher BMD in a more caudal vertebral level and generally higher precision at L3 compared to L2 for subregional BMD measures using lateral-DXA [128]. Very high correspondence was neither achieved, nor expected, considering measurement errors associated with both tools, the inability for these errors to be diluted across a sample, and the fact that BMD does not reflect true volumetric density. Measurement errors (%CV) in histomorphometry are large, and have been reported to range from 8.5-77.0% for inter-rater analysis and 3.1-21.9% for intra-rater analysis. Specifically for %BV/TV, the %CV has been reported to be 3.8-9.4% for intra-rater and 10.2-10.3% for inter-rater precision [167,168]. Furthermore, BMD estimates were made from a combination of trabecular and cortical bone, whereas histomorphometry analyses were isolated to trabecular bone only.

Findings in this study are limited by the small sample size. However, they do suggest reasonable correspondence between areal BMD and bone volume fraction for a subregional assessment of lumbar vertebrae with low BMD. The BMD, and associated T and Z scores, in Study 1 are comparable to the samples described in Study 2, thus lending support to the suitability of the srBMD protocol for a population with osteoporosis. The results are comparable to previous studies where correlation between BMD or BMC and %BV/TV was examined in tibial metaphyses (r=0.52) [140], femoral metaphyses (r=0.77-0.88) [144] and vertebrae (r=0.75-0.79) [143] of rats. However, the association between %BV/TV and subregional BMC in the current study was poor. This may be explained by the fact that BMC is highly dependent on the size of the region in which bone is measured. The use of BMD normalises the data to minimise the confounding effect of bone or region size on the amount of bone mineral measured [169]. Furthermore, %BV/TV is a volume fraction for bone matrix, not bone mineral. It can also be transformed to an areal fraction. The areal fraction of bone matrix would therefore correlate more closely with the areal fraction of BMC (i.e. BMC/area = BMD). The use of areal BMD may therefore be a better parameter to describe the profile of subregional BMD than BMC due to the confounding effect of region size on BMC. In addition, BMD is the parameter most widely reported in the literature and the parameter most commonly used to predict fracture risk and monitor responses to pharmacotherapies. Nielsen et al. [169] also demonstrated that BMD shows less variability between individuals than BMC since body size is partially accounted for when using BMD. In addition, these authors showed that when participant Z scores were grouped into quartiles according to body surface area (an index of body size) a narrower inter-quartile range was observed for BMD compared to BMC at both the lumbar spine and femoral neck. Finally, the compressive strength of vertebral bodies has shown stronger association with vertebral BMD than BMC [55,80,86,87,92,93,95,98]. For these reasons, BMD was the primary outcome for studies in this Chapter.

Pearson correlation was applied in Study 1 to examine the correspondence between histomorphometry parameters and densitometry parameters. A parametric statistic was used given the normality of the data, as examined with the Kolmogorov-Smirnov statistic and an approach used previously [151]. Further studies with a greater number of cadaver specimens should be used to validate the srBMD protocol in order to verify the findings presented here, and consider any variability in subregional BMD between specimens of different age and gender. Measurement of srBMD using other technologies such as micro computed tomography (μCT) or QCT could also be compared against DXA [170,171]. Finally, better correspondence between bone mass and histomorphometry parameters may be found when using apparent volumetric BMD rather than areal BMD. Measuring volumetric BMD removes the potential problems that variable vertebral geometry causes with areal BMD measures, and could be acquired with QCT. Further validation may be achieved by examining the predictive validity of srBMD measured with DXA for vertebral compressive strength compared with standard DXA parameters and other imaging technologies.

Study 2 examined the utility of a using subregional analysis protocol for lateral DXA scans of the lumbar spine in a cross-sectional cohort study. Strong, although not statistically-significant, trends revealed that the fracture group had greater deficits in areal BMD across the subregional profile than the non-fracture group. The inability to detect statistically-significant differences in srBMD and ratios of srBMD between groups was likely due to low power in the study. A previous *ex vivo* study had sufficient power to detect significant differences in areal BMD of 8-43% between regions at L3 using a sample size of n=6 [127]. In this *in vivo* study, a minimum sample of n=7 in each group was selected to ensure a sufficient sample size to detect within-subject differences. It is difficult to decide what magnitude of difference in subregional BMD would be clinically relevant, since prior research has not investigated this issue and the majority of studies relate fracture risk to the per standard deviation decrease in BMD at a given site, rather than a percentage reduction. *Post hoc* sample size calculations were performed to determine whether the sample size used was also adequate to observe a 10-15% difference in areal BMD between groups with a power of 0.80. Given the findings in this study, differences in areal BMD were considered to be most important at ROI 6 (central) between fracture and non-fracture cases. Unpublished data from our group also indicate that the mean short-term precision error expressed as a percentage for ROI 6 (central) at L3 is 3.3%, while the mean across all subregions is 4.8%. Nguyen et al. [172] argue that a minimum decrease of 7.5% in BMD is required before a conclusion of significant reduction can be made. Therefore, differences of 10% to 15% in areal BMD were deemed to be to be clinically important for ROI 6 in this study. Calculations suggest a sample size per group of 82 and 37 would be required to detect changes of 10% and 15% respectively in areal BMD with a power of 0.80. To maintain power at 0.80 and detect differences of 20%, 25% and 30% between fracture and non-fracture cases at ROI 6, sample sizes of 20, 13 and 10 per group respectively would be required. However, differences in BMD of 20-30% are not clinically reasonable, as deficits of this magnitude would likely be detected with standard DXA analysis obviating the need for subregional measures. Therefore, future studies with larger sample sizes may demonstrate significant differences between groups. Moreover, in order to predict fracture risk using these data, a prospective design would be required.

In addition to the low sample size, the absence of a statistically-significant difference between the groups may also be attributable to the conservative criteria used to diagnose a vertebral fracture. The criterion of a reduction in anterior vertebral height of 30% was used to minimise the chances of false positives being classified as 'fracture' cases. Certainly, this may have increased false negative reporting. However, based on the study by McCloskey et al. [161], the false negative rate for such a criterion is low, and importantly the risk of false positives is reduced markedly. Furthermore, several anatomic studies report normal anatomic wedging of thoracic vertebrae to be as high as 20% [173-175]. Thus, epidemiologic studies which use a less stringent criterion (e.g. 20-25% reduction in anterior vertebral height) to diagnose fracture are likely to be threatened by a high false positive rate since normal anatomic wedging is not taken into account. If a less stringent criterion were used in this study, a larger proportion of participants would have been classified as 'fractured'. However, this would have increased the false positive rate, and therefore this issue was not investigated.

When examining the results of the AP DXA, there were no differences in BMD between fracture and non-fracture cases. As expected, the controls had significantly higher BMD in the AP total spine, AP L3 and standard lateral analysis. Using standard Hologic AP and lateral analyses, the percent difference in mean BMD between fracture and non-fracture cases ranged from 0.7-5.4%. This difference was much lower than the differences between fracture and non-fracture cases when comparing mean srBMD, ranging from -13.1% to -16.3%. Furthermore, there were comparably large percent differences between the fracture and non-fracture cases in BMD relative to controls across subregions. The percent differences in mean srBMD between non-fracture and controls ranged from 6% to -10.4% while differences between fracture and controls ranged from -10% to -23%. This finding was expected due to the influence of osteoporosis on BMD and the relationship between BMD and fracture [176]. The number of standard deviations below the non-fracture mean expressed the srBMD of the fracture cases relative to the distribution of srBMD in the non-fracture cases. The fracture group srBMD ranged between 0.6-1.0 SD below the non-fracture group mean across subregions and only 0-0.5 SD based on standard DXA variables (Figure 10). Therefore the sensitivity of the subregional analysis may be superior to that of current standard DXA analyses in distinguishing fracture from non-fracture cases. Previous research has established that a decrease of 1 SD in spinal areal BMD for women can increase fracture risk by 1.4-4.0 fold, which is comparable to a 17 year increase in age [113,177-180]. A 2 SD decrease in areal BMD increases subsequent fracture risk by 5.6-6 fold [19,20]. Legrand et al. [181] reported an odds ratio of 1.8 for vertebral fractures in men for each SD decrease in spinal BMD. These findings are comparable to femoral BMD, where non-vertebral fracture risk increases 1.4-1.5 times, vertebral fracture risk increases 2.7 times and hip fracture risk increases up to 2.9 times for each SD decrease in femoral neck areal BMD [23,181-184]. Collectively, these findings suggest that individuals who have sustained a vertebral fracture have greater deficits in srBMD compared to those who have not sustained a fracture and that the deficit is likely to be of clinical importance. Moreover, the nature of these differences may help to explain a mechanism for the vertebral fracture cascade.

Study 2 demonstrated that differences in intra-vertebral areal BMD can be measured *in vivo* using DXA, consistent with *ex vivo* prior work using DXA [127]. The results of areal BMD differences also agree with other *ex vivo* investigations using quantitative radiography [124]; QCT [120-123,132], histomorphometry [115,117-119,185] and an *in vivo* animal study using DXA [126]. Areal BMD was lowest in the anterior zone (ROI 4) and central zone (ROI

6) of L3. Although the interpretation of the observed differences remains uncertain since differences in subregional geometry may have a confounding effect on areal BMD values, the areal BMD data presented in this study are in agreement with volumetric BMD and bone volume fraction (%BV/TV) data presented in the previous *ex vivo* studies outlined above.

These findings may point to a potential mechanism underlying osteoporotic vertebral fracture. Vertebral fractures occur most commonly in the mid-thoracic spine and thoracolumbar junction, and this presentation is likely due to loading and geometric characteristics at these levels [186,187]. This raises the question of whether BMD profiles measured in the lumbar spine can be used to infer BMD characteristics at thoracic levels. Results of previous work suggest that the subregional profiles of areal BMD are similar for the thoracic and lumbar spine in subregions 5-7 [127]. Therefore, predictions about thoracic BMD profiles could ultimately be made from lumbar DXA data. Importantly, srBMD measured at the lumbar spine can account for a significant proportion of variance observed in thoracic vertebral morphology, while standard DXA cannot, as presented in Study 3. Technologies other than DXA have also been used to compare BMD distributions between the thoracic and lumbar spine. Both Banse et al. [121] and Singer and Breidahl [188] used QCT to compare BMD profiles between T9-L4 and T10-L1, respectively, and found no between-level differences. Similarly, Antonacci et al. [124] found no inter-level variation in bone mass profiles using quantitative radiography between T5, T12 and L4.

The low areal BMD observed in ROI 6 (central) may be explained by the predominance of trabecular bone in this region. Higher density observed in other regions could be due to the integration of cortical and trabecular bone in the srBMD measure. The greatest difference between fracture and non-fracture srBMD data was observed in ROI 6 (-16.3% difference). Vertebral compressive strength relies predominantly on trabecular bone integrity [189]. Therefore, any decrease in trabecular density, which may be most obvious at ROI 6, will affect vertebral compressive strength increasing the likelihood of fracture. Individuals with greater deficits in BMD at ROI 6 may be at increased risk of wedge or compression fracture. Future studies with larger sample sizes should therefore investigate the differences between fracture and non-fracture cases at ROI 6 and examine whether this subregion provides more useful information than other subregions or the whole vertebral body in lateral projection. In addition, studies examining responses to pharmacologic agents aimed at minimising trabecular bone loss may reveal earlier changes in bone density when examining ROI 6 with DXA. Bone quality indices may also differ between subregions; however, tools other than DXA would be required to explore this further *in vivo*, such as high resolution QCT and MRI.

A recent study reported that cortical bone thickness was strongly associated with vertebral fracture prevalence [168]. Although this association was acknowledged as a controversial issue, the authors suggested that cortical bone loss may be more important than the disruption of trabecular bone in the aetiopathogenesis of osteoporotic vertebral fracture and that this parameter could be best characterised with QCT technology. Although investigation of this parameter may be important, the clinical applicability is limited at this stage considering the health and cost issues associated with QCT imaging and its lower precision compared with DXA [190-192]. Finite element modelling studies confirm that the load-bearing role of cortical bone comprising the vertebral shell is maximal in the mid-section (ROI 6) of the vertebral body [189,193]. Although trabecular bone was confirmed as the dominant structural component in those studies, its load-bearing role was least at this mid-section. Therefore, an integrated measure of cortical and trabecular bone, as provided by a lateral DXA scan, in this region may be of significant clinical value compared to an isolated measure of each bone type as provided by QCT.

The lower areal density observed in the anterior zone (ROI 4) and higher density in the posterior zone (ROI 2) may help to explain one mechanism underlying anterior wedge fracture in the lumbar spine. However, these fractures are most common in the thoracic spine [108], owing to the larger flexion moments imposed on vertebral bodies in this area [186]. Failure of trabecular bone in the centrum may occur not only due to deficits in BMD at ROI 6 and ROI 4, but also due to endplate characteristics. Consistent with data in this study, research has found compressive strength of the inferior vertebral endplate to be greater than the superior endplate [135]. Therefore, failure of the superior endplate is likely to occur before that of the inferior endplate, which may contribute to wedge deformity. Lu et al. [123] reported a trend between L3-L5 for higher volumetric BMD at the inferior endplate. The lack of a statistically-significant difference in that study may be related to the low specimen number (n=13) and young age (mean=31yrs, range=24-36yrs). Measurement of endplate volumetric densities in an older cohort with a larger sample size may provide better clarification of this issue. Notably, in the current study participants in the non-fracture group demonstrated higher areal BMD in superior vertebral subregion (ROI 5) than controls (Figures 7B and 9). Although these data represent BMD characteristics of the lumbar spine, this finding may help to explain why individuals with higher BMD at ROI 5 did not sustain a thoracic vertebral fracture through a superior endplate failure mode.

It is well established in the literature that vertebral morphometry varies with age, gender, race and vertebral level [194]. However, vertebral morphology is also influenced by BMD as evidenced by both *in vivo* and *ex vivo* studies [86,175,195,196]. Study 3 reported the ability of both srBMD and standard DXA-derived BMD parameters to predict vertebral morphometry. A decrease in anterior vertebral height in the thoracic spine is the most common presentation of spinal osteoporosis. Reductions of up to 20% in anterior vertebral height have been reported in the thoracic spine in individuals with osteoporosis without vertebral fracture, compared to 13% for individuals with osteoarthritis and 8% in non-pathologic cases [173-175]. Furthermore, the rate of reduction in anterior vertebral height is greater in individuals with osteoporosis, reported to be 1.5% annually [175]. In combination with disc morphology, vertebral body morphology influences spinal curvature and therefore spinal loading. Therefore, the ability to predict vertebral morphology is important since increased spinal loading is likely to be a risk factor for recurrent vertebral fracture [186].

Edmondston et al. [91] examined the relationship between bone mass and vertebral shape at each vertebral level, T1-L5. The relationship between trabecular bone density measured with QCT and vertebral morphology and ratios of vertebral heights was poor (r=0.01-0.17). However, when BMD was measured by lateral DXA, the relationship was stronger (r=0.26-0.59). Nonetheless, the clinical significance of these findings remains uncertain given that BMD cannot be measured in the thoracic spine *in vivo* with DXA. Edmondston et al. [91] also reported the relationship between mean lumbar BMD, which could be measured *in vivo* with DXA, and mean vertebral height ratios to be moderate (r=0.41-0.48). Study 3 provides further evidence of a significant relationship between vertebral morphology and BMD. A reduction in anterior vertebral height is one of the most common clinical presentations among individuals with osteoporosis. Moreover, vertebral wedge fractures are routinely diagnosed based on a reduction of anterior vertebral height. Therefore, regression analyses with $H_{A(max)}$ as the dependent variable may be more clinically appropriate than using the mean of ratio of anterior to posterior vertebral height. The strength of the relationship between vertebral morphology and BMD seems to be influenced by the way BMD is measured. Study 3 provides evidence that measures of BMD derived from lateral DXA are superior to AP-projection DXA in predicting vertebral morphology. Furthermore, specific subregions defined from a lateral scan are better predictors of vertebral morphology with 28% of the variance observed in $H_{A(max)}$ accounted for by BMD in the inferior zone (ROI 7). It may be that higher density in ROI 7 is protective against reductions in anterior vertebral height, though the mechanisms explaining this observation are uncertain.

5. Conclusion

Analysis of subregional BMD is accurate and provides better discrimination between individuals with and without osteoporotic vertebral fractures than standard BMD measures derived from DXA. The largest difference in areal BMD between fracture and non-fracture cases was observed in the central subregion (ROI 6), and this difference was much larger than those observed with standard DXA parameters. Ultimately, measurement of srBMD may be used to identify patients at increased risk of sustaining an osteoporotic vertebral fracture, and assist in the long-term monitoring of vertebral fragility and efficacy of pharmaceutical treatments used to prevent fragility fractures. However, studies with larger sample sizes are required to validate these applications. Significant differences exist in intra-vertebral areal BMD, and these differences may explain, in part, mechanisms underlying vertebral fracture and helps to explain the clinically-observed vertebral fracture cascade. Considering the power limitations in Study 2, future work should be aimed at examining the clinical application of srBMD with lateral-DXA in larger scale cohort studies, both cross-sectionally and prospectively. The potentially greater predictive validity of srBMD for vertebral morphology adds to the body of evidence suggesting that srBMD measures are more informative of vertebral fragility than standard DXA-derived measures of areal BMD.

6. Acknowledgments

Funding for this work provided, in part, by the Physiotherapy Research Foundation (Australia), seeding grant #013/05. Access to bone densitometry was provided by the Bone Densitometry Unit, Royal Melbourne Hospital, Australia. The authors gratefully acknowledge Associate Professor Bev Phillips for providing statistical advice and Mr Tim Wrigley for assistance in developing the radiographic and image processing methods. Personnel from the Medical Imaging Department at St Vincent's Hospital, Melbourne, are acknowledged for their assistance in acquiring spinal radiographs. Dr Andrew Briggs is currently supported by the National Health and Medical Research Council (NHMRC) Australia.

7. REFERENCES

[1] Fraser WD. The burden of osteoporosis and the case for disease management. *Disease Management & Health Outcomes*. 2004; 12(6):409-18.

[2] Melton LJ, 3rd. Epidemiology of spinal osteoporosis. *Spine*. 1997; 22(24 Suppl):S2-S11.

[3] Harris AH, Cumming R, Watts J, Ebeling P, Crowley S. The burden of illness and the cost of osteoporosis in Australia. Technical Report. Melbourne: Centre for Health Program Evaluation; 1998 April, 1998. *Report No.: 8*.

[4] Klotzbuecher CM, Ross PD, Landsman PB, Abbott TA, Berger ML. Patients with prior fractures have an increased risk of future fractures: A summary of the literature and statistical synthesis. *Journal of Bone and Mineral Research*. 2000; 15(4):721-39.

[5] Nguyen ND, Ahlborg HG, Centre JR, Eisman JA, Nguyen TV. Residual lifetime risk of fractures in women and men. *Journal of Bone and Mineral Research*. 2007; 22(6):781-88.

[6] NIH Consensus Development Panel on Osteoporosis Prevention Diagnosis and Therapy. *Journal of the American Medical Association*. 2001; 285(6):785-95.

[7] Australian Institute of Health & Welfare. Australia's Health 2000. The seventh biennial report of the Australian Institute of Health and Welfare. Canberra: AIHW; 2000.

[8] Delmas PD, van de Langerijt L, Watts NB, Eastell R, Genant H, Grauer A, et al. Underdiagnosis of vertebral fracture is a worldwide problem: The IMPACT study. *Journal of Bone and Mineral Research*. 2005; 20(4):557-63.

[9] Ensrud KE, Nevitt MC, Palermo L, Cauley JA, Griffith JM, Genant HK, et al. What proportion of incident morphometric vertebral fractures are clinically diagnosed and vice versa. *Journal of Bone and Mineral Research*. 1999; 14:S138.

[10] Kanis JA, Oden A, Johnell O, De Laet C, Jonsson B. Excess mortality after hospitalisation for vertebral fracture. *Osteoporosis International*. 2004; 15(2):108-12.

[11] Jalava T, Sarna S, Pylkkanen L, Mawer B, Kanis JA, Selby P, et al. Association between vertebral fracture and increased mortality in osteoporotic patients. *Journal of Bone and Mineral Research*. 2003; 18(7):1254-60.

[12] Access Economics. The burden of brittle bones: costing osteoporosis in Australia. Canberra: Access Economics; 2001.

[13] Orsini LS, Rousculp MD, Long SR, Wang S. Health care utilization and expenses in the United States: a study of osteoporosis-related fractures. *Osteoporosis International*. 2005; 16:359-71.

[14] Lindsay R, Burge RT, Strauss DM. One year outcomes and costs following a vertebral fracture. *Osteoporosis International*. 2005; 16(1):78-85.

[15] Gabriel SE, Tosteson ANA, Leibson CL, Crowson CS, Pond GR, Hammond CS, et al. Direct medical costs attributable to osteoporotic fractures. *Osteoporosis International*. 2002; 13(4):323-30.

[16] Javaid MK, Cooper C. How to prevent fractures in the individual with osteoporosis. *Best Practice & Research in Clinical Rheumatology*. 2001; 15(3):497-515.

[17] Fribourg D, Tang C, Delamarter R, Bae H. Incidence of subsequent vertebral fracture after kyphoplasty. *Spine*. 2004; 29(20):2270-76.

[18] Black DM, Arden NK, Palermo L, Pearson J, Cummings SR. Prevalent vertebral deformities predict hip fractures and new vertebral deformities but not wrist fractures. Study of Osteoporotic Fractures Research Group. *Journal of Bone & Mineral Research*. 1999; 14(5):821-28.

[19] Ross PD, Genant HK, Davis JW, Miller PD, Wasnich RD. Predicting vertebral fracture incidence from prevalent fractures and bone density among non-black, osteoporotic women. *Osteoporosis International*. 1993; 3(3):120-26.

[20] Ross PD, Davis JW, Epstein RS, Wasnich RD. Pre-existing fractures and bone mass predict vertebral fracture incidence in women. *Annals of Internal Medicine*. 1991; 114(11):919-23.

[21] Marshall D, Johnell O, Wedel H. Meta-analysis of how well measures of bone mineral density predict occurrence of osteoporotic fractures. *British Medical Journal*. 1996; 312(7041):1254-59.

[22] Nguyen TV, Centre JR, Pocock NA, Eisman JA. Limited utility of clinical indices for the prediction of symptomatic fracture risk in postmenopausal women. *Osteoporosis International*. 2004; 15(1):49-55.

[23] Schuit SCE, van der Klift M, Weel A, de Laet C, Burger H, Seeman E, et al. Fracture incidence and association with bone mineral density in elderly men and women: the Rotterdam Study. *Bone*. 2004; 34(1):195-202.

[24] Ensrud KE, Black DM, Harris F, Ettinger B, Cummings SR. Correlates of kyphosis in older women. *Journal of the American Geriatrics Society*. 1997; 45(6):682-87.

[25] Pluijm SFM, Tromp AM, Smit JH, Deeg DJH, Lips P. Consequences of vertebral deformities in older men and women. *Journal of Bone and Mineral Research*. 2000; 15(8):1564-72.

[26] Briggs AM, Greig AM, Wark JD. The vertebral fracture cascade in osteoporosis. A review of aetiopathogenesis. *Osteoporosis International*. 2007; 18:575-84.

[27] Briggs AM, Greig AM, Wark JD, Fazzalari NL, Bennell KL. A review of anatomical and mechanical factors affecting vertebral body integrity. *International Journal of Medical Sciences*. 2004; 1(4):170-80.

[28] Khan K, McKay H, Kannus P, Bailey D, Wark J, Bennell K. Physical activity and bone health. Champaign, IL: Human Kinetics 2001.

[29] Cummings SR, Black DM, Nevitt MC, Browner W, Cauley J, Ensrud K, et al. Bone density at various sites for prediction of hip fractures. *Lancet*. 1993; 341(8837):72-75.

[30] Ettinger B, Black DM, Mitlak BH, Knickerbocker RK, Nickelsen T, Genant HK, et al. Reduction of vertebral fracture risk in postmenopausal women with osteoporosis treated with Raloxifene: Results from a 3-year randomized clinical trial. *Journal of the American Medical Association*. 1999; 282:637-45.

[31] Cummings SR, Black DM, Thompson DE, Applegate WB, Barrett-Connor E, Musliner TA, et al. Effect of alendronate on risk of fracture in women with low bone density but

without vertebral fractures - Results from the fracture intervention trial. *Journal of the American Medical Association*. 1998; 280(24):2077-82.

[32] Liberman UA, Weiss SR, Broll J, Minne HW, Quan H, Bell NH, et al. Effect of Oral alendronate on bone mineral density and the incidence of fractures in postmenopausal osteoporosis. *New England Journal of Medicine*. 1995; 333(22):1437-43.

[33] Link TM, Doren M, Lewing C, Meier N, Heinecke A, Rummeny E. Cross-sectional areal of lumbar vertebrae in peri and post menopausal patients with and without osteoporosis. *Osteoporosis International*. 2000; 11(4):304-09.

[34] Link TM, Koppers BB, Licht T, Bauer J, Lu Y, Rummeny EJ. In vitro and in vivo spiral CT to determine bone mineral density: Initial experience in patients at risk for osteoporosis. *Radiology*. 2004; 231(3):805-11.

[35] Arokoski MH, Arokoski JPA, Vainio P, Niemitukia LH, Kroger H, Jurvelin JS. Comparison of DXA and MRI methods for interpreting femoral neck bone mineral density. *Journal of Clinical Densitometry*. 2002; 5(3):289-96.

[36] Boutry N, Cortet B, Dubois P, Marchandise X, Cotten A. Trabecular bone structure of the calcaneus: Preliminary in vivo MR imaging assessment in men with osteoporosis. *Radiology*. 2003; 227(3):708-17.

[37] Kroger H, Vainio P, Nieminen J. Estimation of spinal bone density using conventional MRI - Comparison between MRI and DXA in 32 subjects. *Acta Orthopaedica Scandinavica*. 1995; 66(6):532-34.

[38] Maris TG, Damilakis J, Sideri L, Deimling M, Papadokostakis G, Papakonstantinou O, et al. Assessment of the skeletal status by MR relaxometry techniques of the lumbar spine: comparison with dual X-ray absorptiometry. *European Journal of Radiology*. 2004; 50(3):245-56.

[39] Faulkner KG, Pocock N. Future methods in the assessment of bone mass and structure. *Best Practice & Research in Clinical Rheumatology*. 2001; 15(3):359-83.

[40] Genant HK, Gordon C, Jiang YB, Link TM, Hans D, Majumdar S, et al. Advanced imaging of the macrostructure and microstructure of bone. *Hormone Research*. 2000; 54(1 Suppl):24-30.

[41] Link TM, Majumdar S, Grampp S, Guglielmi G, van Kuijk C, Imhof H, et al. Imaging of trabecular bone structure in osteoporosis. *European Radiology*. 1999; 9(9):1781-88.

[42] Majumdar S, Genant HK. A Review of the Recent Advances in Magnetic-Resonance-Imaging in the Assessment of Osteoporosis. *Osteoporosis International*. 1995; 5(2):79-92.

[43] Gomberg BR, Wehrli FW. Computer-assisted vertebral deformity measurement on MR spine images. 10th Annual Meeting of the International Society of Magnetic Resonance Imaging in Medicine; 2002; Honolulu, Hawaii, USA; 2002. p. 242.

[44] Grampp S, Genant HK, Mathur A, Lang P, Jergas M, Takada M, et al. Comparisons of non-invasive bone mineral measurements in assessing age-related loss, fracture discrimination, and diagnostic classification. *Journal of Bone and Mineral Research*. 1997; 12(5):697-711.

[45] Blake GM, Fogelman I. Technical principles of dual energy x-ray absorptiometry. *Seminars in Nuclear Medicine*. 1997; 27(3):210-28.

[46] Njeh CF, Fuerst T, Hans D, Blake GM, Genant HK. Radiation exposure in bone mineral density assessment. *Applied Radiation & Isotopes*. 1999; 50(1):215-36.

[47] Compston JE. BMC, BMD, or corrected BMD. *Bone*. 1995; 16:5-7.

[48] Ott SM, O'Hanlan M, Lipkin EW, Newell-Morris L. Evaluation of vertebral volumetric vs. areal bone mineral density during growth. *Bone*. 1997; 20:533-56.

[49] Nielsen SP. The fallacy of BMD: A critical review of the diagnostic use of dual energy X-ray absorptiometry. *Clinical Rheumatology*. 2000; 19:174-83.

[50] Tothill P, Avenell A, Reid DM. Precision and accuracy of measurements of whole-body bone mineral: comparisons between Hologic, Lunar and Norland dual energy X-ray absorptiometers. *British Journal of Radiology*. 1994; 67:1210-17.

[51] Fischer M, Kempers B. Phantom studies in osteoporosis. *European Journal of Nuclear Medicine*. 1993; 20:434-39.

[52] Formica CA. Standardization of BMD measurements. *Osteoporosis International*. 1998; 8:1-3.

[53] Baim S, Wilson CR, Lewiecki EM, Luckey MM, Downs RW, Lentle BC. Precision assessment and radiation safety for dual-energy X-ray absorptiometry. *Journal of Clinical Densitometry*. 2005; 8(4):371-78.

[54] Blake GM, Jagathesan T, Herd RJM, Fogelman I. Dual x-ray absorptiometry of the lumbar spine. The precision of paired anteroposterior-lateral studies. *British Journal of Radiology*. 1994; 67(799):624-30.

[55] Myers BS, Arbogast KB, Lobaugh B, Harper KD, Richardson WJ, Drezner MK. Improved assessment of lumbar vertebral body strength using supine lateral dual-energy X-ray absorptiometry. *Journal of Bone and Mineral Research*. 1994; 9(5):687-93.

[56] Sapkas GS, Papagelopoulos PJ, Stathakopoulos DP, Papadakis SA, Kiratzoulis JM, Stilianessi E. Evaluation of lumbar spine bone mineral density in the anteroposterior and lateral projections by dual-energy x-ray absorptiometry. *Orthopedics*. 2001; 24(10):959-63.

[57] Zmuda JM, Cauley JA, Glynn NW, Finkelstein JS. Posterior-anterior and lateral dual-energy x-ray absorptiometry for the assessment of vertebral osteoporosis and bone loss among older men. *Journal of Bone and Mineral Research*. 2000; 15(7):1417-24.

[58] Maricic M, Tesser J, Chen Z, Lund P, Gluck O. How often does lateral spine DXA detect low bone mass in patients with both normal PA spine and hip? *Journal of Clinical Densitometry*. 1998; 1(3):251-57.

[59] Blake GM, Herd RJM, Fogelman I. A longitudinal study of supine lateral DXA of the lumbar spine: A comparison with posteroanterior spine, hip and total-body DXA. *Osteoporosis International*. 1996; 6(6):462-70.

[60] Diez F. Guidelines for the diagnosis of osteoporosis by densitometric methods. *Journal of Manipulative and Physiological Therapeutics*. 2002; 25(6):403-15.

[61] Mazess RB, Hanson J, Gifford C. Measurement of spinal density in the lateral projection. In: Ring EFJ, ed. *Current Research in Osteoporosis and Bone Mineral Measurement*. London: British Institute of Radiology 1990:17-18.

[62] Slosman D, Rizzoli R, Donath A, Bonjour JP. Vertebral bone mineral density measured laterally by dual energy X-ray absorptiometry. *Osteoporosis International.* 1990; 1:23-29.

[63] Steiger P, von Stetten E, Weiss H, Stein JA. Paired AP and lateral supine dual X-ray absorptiometry of the spine: Initial results with a 32 detector system. *Osteoporosis International.* 1991; 1:190.

[64] Lilley J, Eyre S, Heath DA. In vivo and in vitro precision for BMD of the spine measured laterally using DEXA. In: Ring EFJ, ed. *Current Research in Osteoporosis and Bone Mineral Measurement II.* London: British Institute of Radiology 1992:27-28.

[65] Banks LM, Lees B, Stevenson JC. Comparison of bone density measurements assessed by lateral DEXA and QCT. In: Ring EFJ, ed. *Current Research in Osteoporosis and Bone Mineral Measurement II.* London: British Institute of Radiology 1992:26-27.

[66] Larnach TA, Boyd SJ, Smart RC. Reproducibility of lateral spine scans using dual energy X-ray absorptiometry. *Calcified Tissue International.* 1992; 51:255-58.

[67] Pye DW, Bassey EJ, Armstrong A. Precision in practice: Experience with a Lunar DPX-L densitometer. In: Ring EFJ, ed. *Current Research in Osteoporosis and Bone Mineral Measurement II.* London: British Institute of Radiology 1992:21-22.

[68] Slosman DO, Rizzoli R, Donath A, Bonjour JP. Bone mineral density of lumbar vertebral body determined in supine and lateral decubitus. Study of precision and sensitivity. *Journal of Bone and Mineral Research.* 1992; 7:S192.

[69] Economou G, Rushton S, Adams JE, Whitehouse RW. Precision of lateral DXA and correlation with QCT. *Calcified Tissue International.* 1993; 52:159.

[70] Devogelaer JP, Baudoux C, Nagant de Deuxchaisnes C. Lack of precision with the lumbar-BMD measurements with the QDR-1000/W when patients are lying in a lateral position. *Calcified Tissue International.* 1993; 52:163.

[71] Devogelaer JP, Baudoux C, Nagant de Deuxchaisnes C. Reproducibility of BMD measurements on the QDR-2000 Hologic, Inc. *Calcified Tissue International.* 1993; 52:164.

[72] Duboeuf F, Pommet R, Meunier PJ, Delmas PD. Dual-energy X-ray absorptiometry of the spine in anteroposterior and lateral projections. *Osteoporosis International.* 1994; 4(2):110-16.

[73] Peel NFA, Eastell R. Diagnostic-Value of Estimated Volumetric Bone-Mineral Density of the Lumbar Spine in Osteoporosis. *Journal of Bone and Mineral Research.* 1994; 9(3):317-20.

[74] Jergas M, Breitenseher M, Gluer CC, Black D, Lang P, Grampp S, et al. Which vertebrae should be assessed using lateral dual-energy X-ray absorptiometry of the lumbar spine. *Osteoporosis International.* 1995; 5(3):196-204.

[75] Del Rio L, Pons F, Huguet M, Setoain FJ, Setoain J. Anteroposterior versus lateral bone mineral density of the spine assessed by dual energy X-ray absorptiometry. *European Journal of Nuclear Medicine.* 1995; 22(5):407-12.

[76] Engelke K, Gluer CC, Genant HK. Factors influencing short-term precision of dual X-ray bone absorptiometry (DXA) of spine and femur. *Calcified Tissue International.* 1995; 56(1):19-25.

[77] Grey C, Young R, Bearcroft PWP, Compston JE. Vertebral deformity in the thoracic spine in post-menopausal women: Value of lumbar spine bone density. *British Journal of Radiology*. 1996; 69(818):137-42.

[78] Nguyen TV, Sambrook PN, Eisman JA. Sources of variability in bone mineral density measurements: Implications for study design and analysis of bone loss. *Journal of Bone and Mineral Research*. 1997; 12(1):124-35.

[79] Nanjo Y, Morio Y, Nagashima H, Hagino H, Teshima R. Correlation between bone mineral density and intervertebral disk degeneration in pre- and postmenopausal women. *Journal of Bone and Mineral Metabolism*. 2003; 21(1):22-27.

[80] Singer K, Edmondston S, Day R, Breidahl P, Price R. Prediction of thoracic and lumbar vertebral body compressive strength. Correlations with bone mineral density and vertebral region. *Bone*. 1995; 17(2):167-74.

[81] Mosekilde L. Vertebral bone quality and strength. In: Cooper C, Reeve J, eds. *Spine: Vertebral Osteoporosis*. Philadelphia: Hanley & Belfus, Inc. 1994:63-81.

[82] Black DM, Cummings SR, Karpf DB, Cauley JA, Thompson DE, Nevitt MC, et al. Randomised trial of the effect of alendronate on risk of fracture in women without existing vertebral fractures. *Lancet*. 1996; 348:1535-41.

[83] Fazzalari NL, Forwood MR, Smith K, Manthey BA, Herreen P. Assessment of cancellous bone quality in severe osteoarthrosis: Bone mineral density, mechanics, and microdamage. *Bone*. 1998; 22(4):381-88.

[84] Aaron JE, Shore PA, Shore RC, Beneton M, Kanis JA. Trabecular architecture in women and men of similar bone mass with and without vertebral fracture: II. Three-dimensional histology. *Bone*. 2000; 27(2):277-82.

[85] Feldkamp LA, Goldstein SA, Parfitt AM, Jesion G, Kleerekoper M. The direct examination of three dimensional bone architecture in vitro by computed tomography. *Journal of Bone and Mineral Research*. 1989; 4:3-11.

[86] Edmondston SJ, Singer KP, Day RE, Breidahl PD, Price RI. In-vitro relationships between vertebral body density, size, and compressive strength in the elderly thoracolumbar spine. *Clinical Biomechanics*. 1994; 9(3):180-86.

[87] Edmondston SJ, Singer KP, Day RE, Price RI, Breidahl PD. Ex vivo estimation of thoracolumbar vertebral body compressive strength: The relative contributions of bone densitometry and vertebral morphometry. *Osteoporosis International*. 1997; 7(2):142-48.

[88] Jergas M, Breitenseher M, Gluer CC, Yu W, Genant HK. Estimates of volumetric bone density from projectional measurements improve the discriminatory capability of dual X-ray absorptiometry. *Journal of Bone and Mineral Research*. 1995; 10(7):1101-10.

[89] Yu W, Gluer CC, Grampp S, Jergas M, Fuerst T, Wu CY, et al. Spinal bone mineral assessment in postmenopausal women: A comparison between dual X-ray absorptiometry and quantitative computed tomography. *Osteoporosis International*. 1995; 5(6):433-39.

[90] Sran MM, Khan KM, Keiver K, Chew JB, McKay HA, Oxland TR. Accuracy of DXA scanning of the thoracic spine: cadaveric studies comparing BMC, areal BMD and geometric estimates of volumetric BMD against ash weight and CT measures of bone volume. *European Spine Journal*. 2005; 14:971-76.

[91] Edmondston SJ, Singer KP, Price RI, Day RE, Breidahl PD. The relationship between bone mineral density, vertebral body shape and spinal curvature in the elderly thoracolumbar spine: an in vitro study. *British Journal of Radiology*. 1994; 67:969-75.

[92] Yang RS, Wang SS, Lin HJ, Liu TK, Hang YS, Tsai KS. Differential effects of bone mineral content and bone area on vertebral strength in a swine model. *Calcified Tissue International*. 1998; 63(1):86-90.

[93] Ebbesen EN, Thomsen JS, Beck-Nielsen H, Nepper-Rasmussen HJ, Mosekilde L. Lumbar vertebral body compressive strength evaluated by dual-energy X-ray absorptiometry, quantitative computed tomography, and ashing. *Bone*. 1999; 25(6):713-24.

[94] Renau A, Farrerons J, Yoldi B, Gil J, Proubasta I, Llauger J, et al. Yield point in prediction of compressive behavior of lumbar vertebral body by dual-energy X-ray absorptiometry. *Journal of Clinical Densitometry*. 2004; 7(4):382-89.

[95] Lochmuller EM, Eckstein F, Kaiser D, Zeller JB, Landgraf J, Putz R, et al. Prediction of vertebral failure loads from spinal and femoral dual-energy X-ray absorptiometry, and calcaneal ultrasound: An in situ analysis with intact soft tissues. *Bone*. 1998; 23(5):417-24.

[96] Bjarnason K, Hassager C, Svendsen OL, Christiansen C. Anteroposterior and lateral spinal DXA for the assessment of vertebral body strength: Comparison with hip and forearm measurement. *Osteoporosis International*. 1996; 6(1):37-42.

[97] Burklein D, Lochmuller EM, Kuhn V, Grimm J, Barkmann R, Muller R, et al. Correlation of thoracic and lumbar vertebral failure loads with in situ vs. ex situ dual energy X-ray absorptiometry. *Journal of Biomechanics*. 2001; 34(5):579-87.

[98] Eckstein F, Lochmuller EM, Lill CA, Kuhn V, Schneider E, Delling G, et al. Bone strength at clinically relevant sites displays substantial heterogeneity and is best predicted from site-specific bone densitometry. *Journal of Bone and Mineral Research*. 2002; 17(1):162-71.

[99] Cheng XG, Nicholson PHF, Boonen S, Lowet G, Brys P, Aerssens J, et al. Prediction of vertebral strength in vitro by spinal bone densitometry and calcaneal ultrasound. *Journal of Bone and Mineral Research*. 1997; 12(10):1721-28.

[100] Cheng XG, Lowet G, Boonen S, Nicholson PHF, van der Perre G, Dequeker J. Prediction of vertebral and femoral strength in vitro by bone mineral density measured at different skeletal sites. *Journal of Bone and Mineral Research*. 1998; 13(9):1439-43.

[101] Moro M, Hecker AT, Bouxsein ML, Myers ER. Failure load of thoracic vertebrae correlates with lumbar bone mineral density measured by DXA. *Calcified Tissue International*. 1995; 56(3):206-09.

[102] Arabi A, Baddoura R, Awada H, Khoury N, Haddad S, Ayoub G, et al. Discriminative ability of dual energy X-ray absorptiometry site selection in identifying patients with osteoporotic fractures. *Bone*. 2007; 40(4):1060-65.

[103] Mitra D, Elvins DM, Speden DJ, Collins AJ. The prevalence of vertebral fractures in mild ankylosing spondylitis and their relationship to bone mineral density. *Rheumatology*. 2000; 39(1):85-89.

[104] Bhambhani M, Crisp AJ, Compston JE. Differential involvement of the dorsal and lumbar spine in osteoporosis. *Annals of the Rheumatic Diseases*. 1992; 51(9):1069-70.

[105] Peel NFA, Moore DJ, Barrington NA, Bax DE, Eastell R. Risk of vertebral fracture and relationship to bone mineral density in steroid treated rheumatoid arthritis. *Annals of the Rheumatic Diseases*. 1995; 54(10):801-06.

[106] Spector TD, Hall GM, McCloskey EV, Kanis JA. Risk of Vertebral Fracture in Women with Rheumatoid-Arthritis. *British Medical Journal*. 1993; 306(6877):558.

[107] Spector TD, McCloskey EV, Doyle DV, Kanis JA. Prevalence of vertebral fracture in women and the relationship with bone density and symptoms - the Chingford Study. *Journal of Bone and Mineral Research*. 1993; 8(7):817-22.

[108] Eastell R, Cedel SL, Wahner HW, Riggs BL, Melton LJ, 3rd. Classification of vertebral fractures. *Journal of Bone and Mineral Research*. 1991; 6(3):207-15.

[109] Legrand E, Chappard D, Pascaretti C, Duquenne M, Krebs S, Rohmer V, et al. Trabecular bone microarchitecture, bone mineral density, and vertebral fractures in male osteoporosis. *Journal of Bone and Mineral Research*. 2000; 15(1):13-19.

[110] Stockbrugger RW, Schoon EJ, Bollani S, Mills PR, Israeli E, Landgraf L, et al. Discordance between the degree of osteopenia and the prevalence of spontaneous vertebral fractures in Crohn's disease. *Alimentary Pharmacology & Therapeutics*. 2002; 16(8):1519-27.

[111] Pors Nielsen S, Hermansen F, Barenholdt O. Interpretation of lumbar spine densitometry in women with fractures. *Osteoporosis International*. 1993; 3:276-82.

[112] Hordon LD, Raisi M, Aaron JE, Paxton SK, Beneton M, Kanis JA. Trabecular architecture in women and men of similar bone mass with and without vertebral fracture: I. Two-dimensional histology. *Bone*. 2000; 27(2):271-76.

[113] Duan YB, Duboeuf F, Munoz F, Delmas PD, Seeman E. The fracture risk index and bone mineral density as predictors of vertebral structural failure. *Osteoporosis International*. 2006; 17(1):54-60.

[114] Ciarelli TE, Fyhrie DP, Parfitt AM. Effects of vertebral bone fragility and bone formation rate on the mineralization levels of cancellous bone from white females. *Bone*. 2003; 32(3):311-15.

[115] Simpson EK, Parkinson IH, Manthey B, Fazzalari NL. Intervertebral disc disorganisation is related to trabecular bone architecture in the lumbar spine. *Journal of Bone & Mineral Research*. 2001; 16(4):681-87.

[116] Thomsen JS, Ebbesen EN, Mosekilde LI. Zone-dependent changes in human vertebral trabecular bone: Clinical implications. *Bone*. 2002; 30(5):664-69.

[117] Cvijanovic O, Bobinac D, Zoricic S, Ostojic Z, Maric I, Crncevic-Orlic Z, et al. Age and region dependent changes in human lumbar vertebral bone. A histomorphometric study. *Spine*. 2004; 24(21):2370-75.

[118] Keller TS, Moeljanto E, Main JA, Spengler DM. Distribution and orientation of bone in the human lumbar vertebral centrum. *Journal of Spinal Disorders*. 1992; 5(1):60-74.

[119] Oda K, Shibayama V, Abe M, Onomura T. Morphogenesis of vertebral deformities in involutional osteoporosis - Age-related, three-dimensional trabecular structure. *Spine*. 1998; 23(9):1050-55.

[120] Sandor TA, Felsenberg D, Kalender WA, Brown E. Global and regional variations in the spinal trabecular bone: single and dual energy examinations. *Journal of Clinical Endocrinology and Metabolism*. 1991; 72(5):1157-68.

[121] Banse X, Devogelaer JP, Munting E, Delloye C, Cornu O, Grynpas M. Inhomogeneity of human vertebral cancellous bone: Systematic density and structure patterns inside the vertebral body. *Bone*. 2001; 28(5):563-71.

[122] Nepper-Rasmussen HJ, Mosekilde L. Local differences in mineral content in vertebral trabecular bone measured by dual-energy computed tomography. *Acta Radiologica*. 1989; 4:369-71.

[123] Lu WW, Zheng YG, Holmes A, Zhu QG, Luk KDK, Zhong SZ, et al. Bone mineral density variations along the lumbosacral spine. *Clinical Orthopaedics and Related Research*. 2000; 378:255-63.

[124] Antonacci MD, Hanson DS, Leblanc A, Heggeness MH. Regional variation in vertebral bone density and trabecular architecture are influenced by osteoarthritic change and osteoporosis. *Spine*. 1997; 22(20):2393-401.

[125] Pollintine P, Tobias JH, McNally DS, Wakley GK, Dolan P, Adams MA. Intervertebral disc degeneration increases load-bearing by the neural arch and reduces BMD in the anterior vertebral body. *Journal of Bone and Mineral Research*. 2002; 17:F9.

[126] Krueger D, Todd H, Haffa A, Bruner J, Yandow D, Binkley N. Central region-of-interest analysis of lumbar spine densitometry demonstrates lower bone mass in older rhesus monkeys. *Bone*. 1999; 24(1):29-33.

[127] Briggs AM, Wark JD, Kantor S, Fazzalari NL, Greig AM, Bennell KL. Bone mineral density distribution in thoracic and lumbar vertebrae: An ex vivo study using dual energy X-ray absorptiometry. *Bone*. 2006; 38(2):286-88.

[128] Briggs AM, Wark JD, Kantor S, Teh R, Greig AM, Fazzalari NL, et al. In vivo intra-rater and inter-rater precision of measuring apparent bone mineral density in vertebral subregions using supine lateral dual- energy x-ray absorptiometry (DXA). *Journal of Clinical Densitometry*. 2005; 8(3):314-19.

[129] Polikeit A, Nolte LP, Ferguson SJ. Simulated influence of osteoporosis and disc degeneration on the load transfer in a lumbar functional spinal unit. *Journal of Biomechanics*. 2004; 37:1061-69.

[130] Snyder BD, Piazza S, Edwards WT, Hayes WC, Schaffler, Ross. Role of trabecular morphology in the etiology of age-related vertebral fractures. *Calcified Tissue International*. 1993; 53:S14-S22.

[131] Cody DD, Goldstein SA, Flynn MJ, Brown EB. Correlations between vertebral regional bone mineral density (rBMD) and whole bone fracture load. *Spine*. 1991; 16(2):146-54.

[132] McCubbery DA, Cody DD, Peterson EL, Kuhn JL, Flynn MJ, Goldstein SA. Static and fatigue failure properties of thoracic and lumbar vertebral bodies and their relation to regional density. *Journal of Biomechanics*. 1995; 28(8):891-99.

[133] Keller TS, Hansson TH, Abram AC, Spengler DM, Panjabi MM. Regional variations in the compressive properties of lumbar vertebral trabeculae. Effects of disk degeneration. *Spine*. 1989; 14(9):1012-19.

[134] Lin RM, Tsai KH, Chang GL. Distribution and regional strength of trabecular bone in the porcine lumbar spine. *Clinical Biomechanics*. 1997; 12(5):331-36.

[135] Grant JP, Oxland TR, Dvorak MF. Mapping the structural properties of the lumbosacral vertebral endplates. *Spine*. 2001; 26(8):889-96.

[136] Mazess RB, Gifford CA, Bisek JP, Barden HS, Hanson JA. DEXA measurement of spine density in the lateral projection .1. Methodology. *Calcified Tissue International.* 1991; 49(4):235-39.

[137] Sandor T, Felsenberg D, Brown E. Discriminability of fracture and non-fracture cases based on the spatial distribution of spinal bone mineral. *Journal of Computer Assisted Tomography.* 1997; 21(3):498-505.

[138] Sandor T, Felsenberg D, Brown E. Comments on the hypotheses underlying fracture risk assessment in osteoporosis as proposed by the World Health Organization. *Calcified Tissue International.* 1999; 64:267-70.

[139] Pollintine P, Garbutt SJ, Tobias JH, McNally DS, Wakely GK, Dolan P, et al. Neural arch load-bearing can weaken the anterior vertebral body and pre-dispose to osteoporotic fracture. *Journal of Bone and Mineral Research.* 2002; 17(7):P41.

[140] Libouban H, Moreau MF, Legrand E, Basle MF, Audran M, Chappard D. Comparison insight dual X-ray absorptiometry (DXA), histomorphometry, ash weight, and morphometric indices for bone evaluation in an animal model (the orchidectomized rat) of male osteoporosis. *Calcified Tissue International.* 2001; 68(1):31-37.

[141] Libouban H, Moreau MF, Legrand E, Audran M, Basle MF, Chappard D. Comparison of histomorphometric descriptors of bone architecture with dual-energy X-ray absorption for assessing bone loss in the orchidectomized rat. *Osteoporosis International.* 2002; 13(5):422-28.

[142] Pastoureau PC, Chomel AC, Bonnet J. Evidence of early subchondral bone changes in the meniscectomized guinea pig. A densitometric study using dual-energy X-ray absorptiometry subregional analysis. *Osteoarthritis and Cartilage.* 1999; 7(5):466-73.

[143] Campodarve I, Diez A, Puig J, Serrano S, Marinoso ML, Arnau MD. Correlation between densitometric and histomorphometric values in isolated vertebrae of Sprague Dawley rats. *Calcified Tissue International.* 1993; 52:470-71.

[144] Pastoureau PC, Chomel AC, Bonnet J. Specific evaluation of localised bone mass and bone loss in the rat using dual X-ray absorptiometry subregional analysis. *Osteoporosis International.* 1995; 5:143-49.

[145] Edmondston SJ, Singer KP, Price RI, Breidahl PD. Accuracy of lateral dual-energy x-ray absorptiometry for the determination of bone mineral content in the thoracic and lumbar spine: an in vitro study. *British Journal of Radiology.* 1993; 66(784):309-13.

[146] Kaymakci B, Wark JD. Precise accurate mineral measurements of excised sheep bones using X-Ray densitometry. *Bone and Mineral.* 1994; 25(3):231-46.

[147] Kelly TL. Bone mineral density reference databases for American men and women. *Journal of Bone and Mineral Research.* 1990; 5(2 Suppl):S249.

[148] Hologic Inc. QDR 4500 X-ray Bone Densitometer User's Guide. Waltham, MA: Hologic Inc.; 1996 15 October 1996. Report No.: 080-0451G.

[149] Watts NB. Fundamentals and pitfalls of bone densitometry using dual-energy X-ray absorptiometry (DXA). *Osteoporosis International.* 2004; 15:847-54.

[150] Parfitt AM. Bone histomorphometry: Proposed system for standardization of nomenclature, symbols and units. *Calcified Tissue International.* 1988; 42:284-86.

[151] Chappard D, Guggenbuhl P, Legrand E, Basle MF, Audran M. Texture analysis of X-ray radiographs is correlated with bone histomorphometry. *Journal of Bone and Mineral Metabolism*. 2005; 23(1):24-29.

[152] Alexeeva L, Burckhardt P, Christiansen C, Cooper C, Delmas P, Johnell O, et al. Report of a World Health Organization Study Group. Assessment of fracture risk and its application to screening for postmenopausal osteoporosis. Geneva: WHO; 1994. Report No.: WHO technical report series 843.

[153] Washburn RA, McAuley E, Katula J, Mihalko SL, Boileau RA. The physical activity scale for the elderly (PASE): Evidence for validity. *Journal of Clinical Epidemiology*. 1999; 52(7):643-51.

[154] Washburn RA, Smith KW, Jennet AM, Janney CA. The physical activity scale for the elderly (PASE): Development and evaluation. *Journal of Clinical Epidemiology*. 1993; 46(2):153-62.

[155] Stagnara P, Mauro JC, de Gran G, Gonon GP, Costanzo G, Dimnet J, et al. Reciprocal angulation of vertebral bodies in a sagittal plane: Approach to references for the evaluation of kyphosis and lordosis. *Spine*. 1982; 7:335–42.

[156] Berthonnaud E, Dimnet JS, Roussouly P, Labelle H. Analysis of the sagittal balance of the spine and pelvis using shape and orientation parameters. *Journal of Spinal Disorders & Techniques*. 2005; 18(1):40-47.

[157] Schneider DL, von Muhlen DG, Barrett-Connor E, Sartoris DJ. Kyphosis does not equal vertebral fractures: the Rancho Bernardo study. *Journal of Rheumatology*. 2004; 31(4):747-52.

[158] Black D, Palermo L, Nevitt M, Genant HK, Epstein RS, Valentin R, et al. Comparison of methods for defining prevalent vertebral deformities: The study of osteoporotic fractures. *Journal of Bone and Mineral Research*. 1995; 10(6):890-902.

[159] Black DM, Palermo L, Nevitt MC, Genant HK, Christensen L, Cummings SR. Defining incident vertebral deformity: a prospective comparison of several approaches. The Study of Osteoporotic Fractures Research Group. *Journal of Bone & Mineral Research*. 1999; 14(1):90-101.

[160] Mazzuoli GF, Diacinti D, Acca M, Pisani D, Rosso R, D'Erasmo E, et al. Relationship between spine bone mineral density and vertebral body heights. *Calcified Tissue International*. 1998; 62(6):486-90.

[161] McCloskey EV, Spector TD, Eyres KS, Fern ED, Orourke N, Vasikaran S, et al. The assessment of vertebral deformity: A method for use in population studies and clinical trials. *Osteoporosis International*. 1993; 3(3):138-47.

[162] Genant HK, Jergas M, Palermo L, Nevitt M, SanValentin R, Black D, et al. Comparison of semiquantitative visual and quantitative morphometric assessment of prevalent and incident vertebral fractures in osteoporosis. *Journal of Bone and Mineral Research*. 1996; 11(7):984-96.

[163] Melton LJ, 3rd, Kan SH, Frye MA, Wahner HW, O'Fallon WM, Riggs BL. Epidemiology of vertebral fractures in women. *American Journal of Epidemiology*. 1989; 129(5):1000-11.

[164] Davies KM, Recker RR, Heaney RP. Normal vertebral dimensions and normal variation in serial measurements of vertebrae. *Journal of Bone and Mineral Research*. 1989; 4:341-49.

[165] Carter DR, Bouxsein ML, Marcus R. New approaches for interpreting projected bone densitometry data. *Journal of Bone and Mineral Research*. 1992; 7(2):137-45.

[166] Briggs AM. Pathomechanics of spinal osteoporosis: Subregional bone mineral density and physiologic loading [PhD thesis]. Melbourne: The University of Melbourne; 2006.

[167] Compston JE, Vedi S, Stellon AJ. Inter-observer and intra-observer variation in bone histomorphometry. *Calcified Tissue International*. 1986; 38:67-70.

[168] Oleksik A, Ott SM, Vedi S, Bravenboer N, Compston J, Lips P. Bone structure in patients with low bone mineral density with or without vertebral fractures. *Journal of Bone and Mineral Research*. 2000; 15(7):1368-75.

[169] Nielsen SP, Kolthoff N, Barenholdt O, Kristensen B, Abrahamsen B, Hermann AP, et al. Diagnosis of osteoporosis by planar bone densitometry: can body size be disregarded? *British Journal of Radiology*. 1998; 71(849):934-43.

[170] Schmidt C, Priemel M, Kohler T, Weusten A, Muller R, Amling M, et al. Precision and accuracy of peripheral quantitative computed tomography (pQCT) in the mouse skeleton compared with histology and microcomputed tomography (μCT). *Journal of Bone and Mineral Research*. 2003; 18(8):1486-96.

[171] Horton JA, Murray GM, Spadaro JA, Margulies BS, Allen MJ, Damron TA. Precision and accuracy of DXA and pQCT for densitometry of the rat femur. *Journal of Clinical Densitometry*. 2003; 6(4):381-90.

[172] Nguyen TV, Pocock NA, Eisman JA. Interpretation of bone mineral density measurement and its change. *Journal of Clinical Densitometry*. 2000; 3(2):107-19.

[173] Goh S, Price RI, Leedman PJ, Singer KP. The relative influence of vertebral body and intervertebral disc shape on thoracic kyphosis. *Clinical Biomechanics*. 1999; 14(7):439-48.

[174] Manns RA, Haddaway MJ, McCall IW, Pullicino VC, Davie MWJ. The relative contribution of disc and vertebral morphometry to the angle of kyphosis in asymptomatic subjects. *Clinical Radiology*. 1996; 51(4):258-62.

[175] Osman AAH, Bassiouni H, Koutri R, Nijs J, Geusens P, Dequeker J. Aging of the thoracic spine. Distinction between wedging in osteoarthritis and fracture in osteoporosis: A cross-sectional and longitudinal study. *Bone*. 1994; 15(4):437-42.

[176] Ammann P, Rizzoli R. Bone strength and its determinants. *Osteoporosis International*. 2003; 14:S13-S18.

[177] Melton LJ, Atkinson EJ, Ofallon WM, Wahner HW, Riggs BL. Long-term fracture prediction by bone mineral assessed at different skeletal sites. *Journal of Bone and Mineral Research*. 1993; 8(10):1227-33.

[178] Van Staa TP, Laan RF, Barton IP, Cohen S, Reid DA, Cooper C. Bone density threshold and other predictors of vertebral fracture in patients receiving oral glucocorticoid therapy. *Arthritis and Rheumatism*. 2003; 48(11):3224-29.

[179] Nevitt MC, Ross PD, Palermo L, Musliner T, Genant HK, Thompson DE. Association of prevalent vertebral fractures, bone density, and alendronate treatment with incident

vertebral fractures: Effect of number and spinal location of fractures. *Bone*. 1999; 25(5):613-19.

[180] Gluer MG, Minne HW, Gluer CC, Lazarescu AD, Pfeifer M, Perschel FH, et al. Prospective identification of postmenopausal osteoporotic women at high vertebral fracture risk by radiography, bone densitometry, quantitative ultrasound and laboratory findings. Results from the PIOS Study. *Journal of Clinical Densitometry*. 2005; 8(4):386-95.

[181] Legrand E, Chappard D, Pascaretti C, Duquenne M, Rondeau C, Simon Y, et al. Bone mineral density and vertebral fractures in men. *Osteoporosis International*. 1999; 10(4):265-70.

[182] Papaioannou A, Joseph L, Ioannidis G, Berger C, Anastassiades T, Brown JP, et al. Risk factors associated with incident clinical vertebral and nonvertebral fractures in postmenopausal women: The Canadian Multicentre Osteoporosis Study (CaMos). *Osteoporosis International*. 2005; 16(5):568-78.

[183] Taylor BC, Schreiner PJ, Stone KL, Fink HA, Cummings SR, Nevitt MC, et al. Long-term prediction of incident hip fracture risk in elderly white women: Study of osteoporotic fractures. *Journal of the American Geriatrics Society*. 2004; 52(9):1479-86.

[184] Johnell O, Kanis JA, Oden A, Johansson H, De Laet C, Delmas P, et al. Predictive value of BMD for hip and other fractures. *Journal of Bone and Mineral Research*. 2005; 20(7):1185-94.

[185] Thomsen JS, Ebbesen EN, Mosekilde L. Predicting human vertebral bone strength by vertebral static histomorphometry. *Bone*. 2002; 30(3):502-08.

[186] Briggs AM, Wrigley TV, Dieën JHv, Phillips B, Lo SK, Greig AM, et al. The effect of osteoporotic vertebral fracture on predicted spinal loads in vivo. *European Spine Journal*. 2006; 15(12):1785-95.

[187] Lunt M, O'Neill TW, Felsenberg D, Reeve J, Kanis JA, Cooper C, et al. Characteristics of a prevalent vertebral deformity predict subsequent vertebral fracture: Results from the European Prospective Osteoporosis Study (EPOS). *Bone*. 2003; 33:505-13.

[188] Singer KP, Breidahl PD. Vertebral body trabecular density at the thoracolumbar junction using quantitative computed tomography. *Acta Radiologica*. 1990; 31:37-40.

[189] Silva MJ, Keaveny TM, Hayes WC. Load sharing between the shell and centrum in the lumbar vertebral body. *Spine*. 1997; 22(2):140-50.

[190] Ebbesen EN, Thomsen JS, Beck-Nielsen H, Nepper-Rasmussen HJ, Mosekilde LI. Vertebral bone density evaluated by DXA and QCT in vitro. *Bone*. 1998; 23:283-90.

[191] Eriksson SAV, Isberg BO, Lindgren JU. Prediction of vertebral strength by dual photon absorptiometry and quantitative computed tomography. *Calcified Tissue International*. 1989; 44(4):243-50.

[192] Johnston CC, Slemenda CW, Melton LJ. Clincal use of bone densitometry. *New England Journal of Medicine*. 1991; 324(16):1105-08.

[193] Eswaran S, Gupta A, Adams MF, Keaveny TM. Cortical and trabecular load sharing in the human vertebral body. *Journal of Bone and Mineral Research*. 2006; 21(2):307-14.

[194] O'Neill TW, Varlow J, Felsenberg D, Johnell O, Weber K, Marchant F, et al. Variation in vertebral height ratios in population studies. *Journal of Bone and Mineral Research.* 1994; 9(12):1895-907.

[195] Diacinti D, Acca M, D'Erasmo E, Tomei E, Mazzuoli GF. Aging changes in vertebral morphometry. *Calcified Tissue International.* 1995; 57:426-29.

[196] Puche RC, Morosano M, Masoni A, Perez Jimeno N, Bertoluzzo SM, Podadera JC, et al. The natural history of kyphosis in postmenopausal women. *Bone.* 1995; 17(3):239-46.

In: Osteoporosis: Etiology, Diagnosis and Treatment
Editors: Bilar E. Mattingly and Albert C. Pillare
ISBN 978-1-60692-397-9

Chapter 2

DIAGNOSIS OF OSTEOPOROSIS USING DXA TECHNIQUE

***Christos S. Baltas*[1]*, Alexia P. Balanika*[2] *and Olympia Papakonstantinou*[2]**

[1]Athens General Hospital "G.Gennimatas", Athens, Greece;
[2]Athens Medical School, University General Hospital "Attikon", Athens, Greece.

ABSTRACT

Osteoporosis is a systemic skeletal syndrome characterized by low bone mass and microarchitectural deterioration of bone tissue, with a consequent increase in bone fragility and susceptibility to fracture [1]. It is a "silent" and progressive disease that may be undiagnosed until a fragility fracture occurs. Postmenopausal osteoporosis is the most common metabolic disease in the developed countries.

Non-invasive measurements of bone mineral density and estimation of fracture risk are crucial to the diagnosis and management of osteoporosis [2].

Dual Energy X-ray Absorptiometry (DXA) is the most widely employed method for estimation of bone mineral density (BMD). It is accepted as the "gold standard", carries a low radiation exposure, and has the ability to measure BMD in spine, hip, forearm, other peripheral sites and throughout the entire skeleton. It uses two X-ray beams of different energy levels to scan the region of interest and measure the attenuation as the beam passes through the bone.

DXA estimates the average concentration of bone mineral in the area that is being scanned and allows calculation of BMD in g/cm^2 and bone mineral content (BMC) in grams. In 1994, the World Health Organization (WHO) selected the T-score as the standard for defining BMD [3]. The WHO criteria intend to provide a reasonable standard for evaluation of individual BMD values in comparison to existing databases. Comparisons are stated as standard deviation (SD) from normal BMD values obtained from young, healthy persons of the same sex, race, and age. These young normal scores, or T-scores, can then be used to decide whether a patient has a reduced BMD consistent with osteoporosis or osteopenia. The Z-score compares one patient's BMD, in standard deviations, with the mean BMD people of similar age and gender.

Osteoporosis is defined as a BMD of 2.5 SD or more below the young average value, whereas established osteoporosis uses the same threshold, but in the presence of fragility fractures [4]. In case of osteoporosis fracture risk increases continuously with decreasing BMD, but there is no biological break-point to characterize absolutely an individual who will fracture from one who will not.

According to the International Society of Clinical Densitometry (ISCD) measurement of BMD is recommended for women 65 years and older, postmenopausal women under 65 years with risk factors, men 70 years and older, adults with a fragility fracture, adults with a disease or condition associated with low bone mass or bone loss, adults taking medications associated with low bone mass or bone loss, anyone being considered for pharmacological therapy, anyone being treated, to monitor treatment effect, and anyone not receiving therapy in whom evidence of bone loss would lead to treatment [5,6,7,8].

Keywords: Osteoporosis, Bone Mineral Density, Dual Energy X-ray Absorptiometry.

INTRODUCTION

Osteoporosis is the most common systemic skeletal syndrome and it is characterized by reduced bone mass, microarchitectural deterioration of bone tissue, and easy fracture [1]. The underlying mechanism in all cases of osteoporosis is an imbalance between bone resorption and bone formation. Bone is resorbed by osteoclasts cells and subsequently new bone is deposited by osteoblasts cells. It is a “silent” and progressive disease in that it often exists undiagnosed until a fragility fracture occurs.

Osteoporotic fractures can occur in any site. Most commonly affects sites rich in trabecular bone such as hip, spine, forearm and shoulder. The fractures of the hip areas result in considerable morbidity and even mortality, with enormous socio-economic consequences [9]. Approximately 30% of all women over 50 years of age have osteoporosis according to the definition proposed by the WHO [10]. The lifetime risk of sustaining a hip fracture in white women has been estimated to be 15% [11], and the prevalence of vertebral fractures in women over 50 years old approximately 19% [12].

It is well known that a low bone mass is by far the most important determinant of osteoporotic fractures [1]. In recent years, several studies have shown an age-related decrease of BMD that occurs predominantly after the menopause, and association of low BMD values with bone fractures [13,14,15,16]. The fracture risk increases as BMD decreases, but there is no fracture threshold below which fracture risk abruptly increases. Therefore, BMD is best thought of as a continuous risk factor: the lower the BMD, the higher the risk of fracture [17].

Whether a fracture is sustained depends on a variety of factors including the propensity to fall and the response to falling [18,19]. The fracture risk is greater with increasing age and it is accompanied by higher risk of falls. Risk factors of falling also include impaired gait or balance and lower body muscle weakness; poor vision/cataracts; malnutrition; excessive alcohol intake; certain medical conditions such as arthritis, diabetes, postural hypotension, cognitive impairment, peripheral neuropathy; polypharmacy; certain medications such as psychoactive medications, antihypertensives; footwear with slippery soles; high heels, factors in home such as poor lighting, loose rugs, loose cabling, uneven or wet surfaces, bathtubs without handrails or bath mat, clutter at floor level, stepping over pets and environmental factors such as wet or cracked paving or steps, ice.

The probability of sustaining osteoporotic fractures varies markedly in different regions of the world. In Europe the highest risks of the hip fracture are seen in Norway, Sweden, Iceland and Denmark, whereas Germany, Switzerland, Finland, Greece, The Netherlands, Hungary, Italy, the UK and Portugal have been described as "high risk" countries defined as having a hip fracture probability that lies between 50% and 75% of the risk that is observed in Sweden [20]. For the year 2000 in Europe the number of osteoporotic fractures in men was estimated 1,053,172 of which 178,777 were hip fractures and 163,151 were clinical spine fractures. Among women there were estimated 2,739,863 fractures, 711,223 involved the hip and 406,493 the spine. The combined costs in men and women for osteoporotic fractures were €36,248 million, of which €24,353 million were for the hip fracture, €719 million for vertebral fracture and €11,177 million for other osteoporotic fracture. Costs were approximately 3-fold higher in women than in men [21].

RISK FACTORS FOR OSTEOPOROSIS AND RELATED FRACTURES:

The first step in the management is a thorough medical history. The International Osteoporosis Foundation (IOF) has identified several risk factors for osteoporosis and related fractures in white postmenopausal women [7,22,23].

Major risk factors for osteoporotic fracture with relative risk ≥ 2 have been: age > 70 years old, menopause < 45 years, hypogonadism, personal history of fragility fracture, history of hip fracture in parents, use of oral glucorticoid therapy for more than 3 months, malabsorption, high bone turnover, anorexia nervosa, BMI < 18 (overweight protects against osteoporosis, either by increasing load or through the hormone leptin), immobilization, chronic renal failure, for patients on dialysis and transplantation [5]. During physical activity, bone performs remodeling in response to physical stress; people who remain physically active throughout life have a lower risk of osteoporosis.

Moderate risk factors with relative risk 1-2 include: estrogen deficiency at an early age (<45 years), lifelong low calcium intake < 500 mg/d, primary hyperparathyroidism, rheumatoid arthritis, Bechterew disease, anticonvulsivants, hyperthyroidism, diabetes mellitus, smoking and alcohol excess in amounts >2 drinks per day [5]. It is already known that tobacco smoking inhibits the activity of osteoblasts. On the other hand, small amount of alcohol does not increase osteoporosis risk and may even be beneficial, but chronic heavy drinking, especially at a younger age increases risk significantly.

Other medical conditions associated with increased risk of osteoporosis are: chronic obstructive pulmonary disease, gastrectomy, multiple myeloma, dementia and celiac disease. Several medications, in addition to oral glucocorticoids, have been implicated with osteoporosis and include: GnRH agonists, excessive T4 doses, long-term phenytoin therapy and lithium [7].

According to the IOF risk factors that provide indications for the diagnostic use of bone densitometry include: 1) radiographic evidence of osteopenia or vertebral deformity or both, 2) previous fragility fracture, 3) loss of height or thoracic kyphosis and vertebral deformities confirmed by radiography and 4) presence of strong risk factors such as anorexia nervosa, malabsorption syndromes, primary hyperparathyroidism, post-transplantation, chronic renal failure, hyperthyroidism, prolonged immobilization, Cushing's syndrome, oestrogen deficiency, corticosteroid therapy, premature menopause < 45 years, maternal family history of hip fracture, long-term secondary amenorrhea > 1 year, low bone mass index (< 19 kg/m2), primary hypogonadism and any other disorder associated with osteoporosis [24].

For the assessment of osteoporosis, according to the ISCD, estimation of BMD is recommended in the following situations: women 65 years and older; postmenopausal women under 65 years with risk factors; men 70 years and older; adults with a fragility fracture; adults with a disease or condition associated with low bone mass or bone loss; adults taking medications associated with low bone mass or bone loss; anyone being considered for pharmacological therapy; anyone being treated, to monitor treatment effect; and anyone not receiving therapy in whom evidence of bone loss would lead to treatment [5,6,7,8].

Dual Energy X-Ray Absorptiometry Technique (DXA): Clinical Utility and Diagnostic Ability:

Dual Energy X-ray Absorptiometry (DXA) is the most widely applied technique for evaluation of BMD. Two X-ray beams of different energy levels are applied to scan the region of interest. The X-ray is generated by a tube, which is located below the supine patient, travels upward through the body of the patient and is detected above by banks of electronic detectors which are located above the patient. A computerized image is generated, which the radiologist uses to identify regions of interest. The bone reduces the signal of the higher-energy X-ray, whereas soft tissues allow the signal to pass through.

The human bone is composed of mineral, principally calcium hydroxyapatite, embedded in type I collagen and specialized proteins that make up the bone matrix. Calcium absorbs much more radiation than protein or soft tissue. The amount of x-ray energy that is absorbed by calcium, in a section, reflects the bone mineral content (BMC). BMC divided by the area or volume of the bone estimates BMD. DXA estimates the average concentration of bone mineral in the area that is being scanned and allows calculation of BMD in g/cm^2 and BMC in grams. Because DXA is a projectional technique, the measured bone density does not reflect true volumetric density but rather an area density, calculated as the quotient of the BMC and the area [25].

Early in life, more bone tissue is formed faster than it is resorbed, allowing the skeleton to grow. Approximately at the age of 30, BMD is at its lifetime best, or "peak bone mass". After this peak, bone remains in equilibrium until about age 50 in women and 60 in men. After that, bone is absorbed faster than it is formed. The resulting bone loss affects both women and men. In women, this decline is accelerated by menopause. The choice of the appropriate measurement sites may vary depending on the specific circumstances of the patient [26].

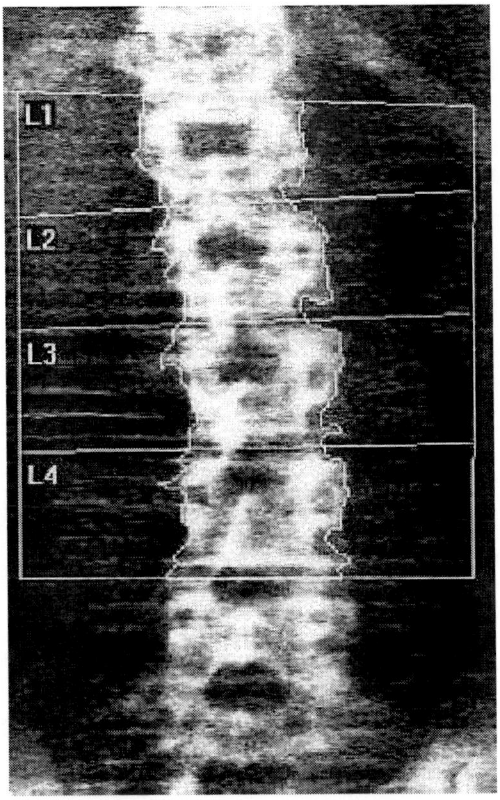

Figure 1. DXA lumbar spine. Posteroanterior projection shows regions of interest from L1 to L4.

DXA scans of the spine can focus on either a posteroanterior projection or a lateral view of the lumbar vertebrae. Vertebral bodies are largely made of trabecular bone that is more sensitive to the effects of hormones and drugs than cortical bone. Therefore, spine BMD tends to change more in response to some medical conditions, such as corticosteroid excess, and to treatments than does BMD of other sites. Depending on the particular equipment, measurements can be obtained either from the L1 to L4 region, or from L2 to L4 (Figure 1). Patient positioning and selection of region of interest (ROI) require precision and careful evaluation by the radiologist for each individual study. The patient is positioned supine on the scanning table. For the examination of the spine, the hips and knees are flexed over a support so as to eliminate the lumbar lordosis and flatten the spine to the table top. The lumbar spine should be straight and centered in the image, with visualization of the last rid pair and the upper sacrum. All evaluable vertebrae should be used for BMD measurement whereas segments with local structural changes or overlying artifacts should be excluded from the BMD analysis. According to the ISCD recommendations we can use three vertebrae if four cannot be used and two if three cannot be used, but the BMD analysis should not be made using a single vertebra. In this case the diagnosis should be based on a different valid skeletal site. Besides anatomically abnormal vertebra may be excluded from analysis if there is more than a 1.0 T-score difference between the vertebra in question and adjacent vertebrae or if vertebral compression fracrure exists [7]. Because of the increased prevalence of degenerative spinal changes and aortic calcification, falsely elevated BMD values can be obtained particularly when posteroanterior spine scans are used in the elderly. Consequently, spine BMD values are increased by degenerative arthritis and therefore tend to increase after age 65 years rather than decrease, as seen in other BMD sites measurements. In summary, the limitations of measuring bone density of the vertebra in the posteroanterior projection include patient age above 65 years, the presence of osteophytes, calcification of paraspinal ligaments, vertebral compression fractures, aortic calcification and vertebral scoliosis [26].

In these patients, lateral spine scans or hip scans may be more reliable and sensitive. Lateral scans of the vertebra eliminate the potential artefacts of osteophytes or aortic calcifications. The limitations of lateral scans include the increased amount of soft tissue in this projection, and the overlap of the ribs and pelvis which decrease the number of vertebrae that can be analysed, thus affecting the precision of the measurements [27] (Figure 2). Lateral spine should not be used for diagnosis, but may have a role in monitoring.

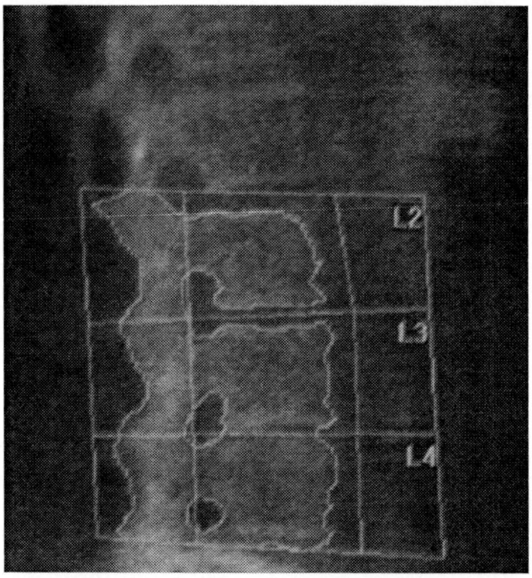

Figure 2. DXA lumbar spine, lateral scan. Such scans can exclude hyperostotic changes and measure integral bone density with cortical/trabecular ratio of 10/90 in the lateral lumbar spine projection.

Scans of the hip include the femoral neck, the trochanteric and intertrochanteric region, Ward's triangle and/or the entire hip. By using a large region of scanning in the total hip, measurement errors can be minimized. For scanning of the femoral neck, the leg is slightly abducted and internally rotated by use of a positioning device. In this position, the femoral shaft should be parallel to the long axis of the image with only a small amount of the lesser trochanter visualized (Figure 3). Because BMD at the hip is the best predictor of hip fracture, hip BMD is particularly useful in women older than 65 years, since risk of hip fracture rises rapidly after age 65. Studies have demonstrated that the use of hip strength analysis (generated by newly developed DXA software) together with densitometric measurements of the bone mass might improve the assessment of the hip better than BMD alone. The use of a dual-femur leg positioned and software allows the simultaneous bilateral measurement of the femoral bone mineral density and thus helped eliminate the error associated with the repositioning needed during single femur scan and decreases precision errors by approximately 25% compared with single femur results (Figure 4) [28]. Recent studies have shown that variation in geometrical measurements of the hip, such as increased hip axis length (HAL) of femoral neck-shaft angle, was associated with increased fracture risk. The HAL was evaluated as the linear distance from the pelvic rim to the lateral edge of the femur below the greater trochanter and along the femoral neck axis [29]. A limitation of hip measurements includes the variability of different areas of the femur in regard to the percentage of cancellous bone and thus the potential risk of fracture [30], the presence of metal prostheses, osteoarthritis, recent hip fracture and fibrodysplasia ossificans progressiva.

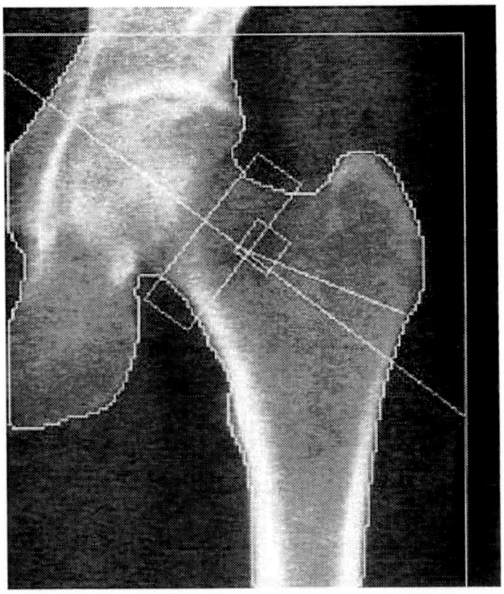

Figure 3. Posteroanterior DXA image of the left hip showing ROIs analyzed: femoral neck, greater trochanter and total hip.

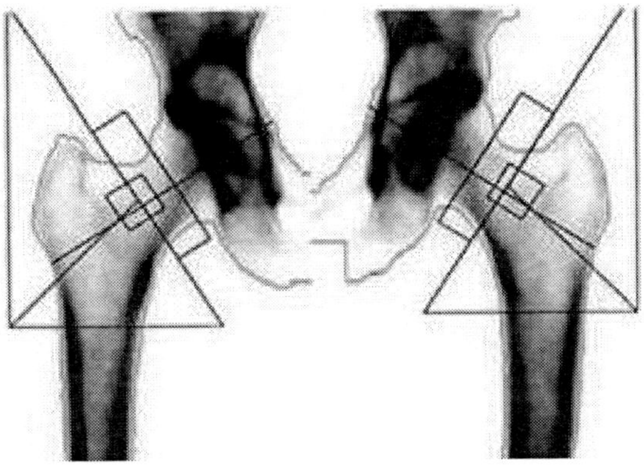

Figure 4. Posteroanterior DXA image of dual-femur. Such scans decrease precision errors.

For whole-body scanning, it is imperative that all parts of the body, including the arms, are included in the scan field for precise results. Whole-body scanning provides total body BMD and BMC but also allows assessments of subregions with appropriately drawn ROIs (Figure 5).

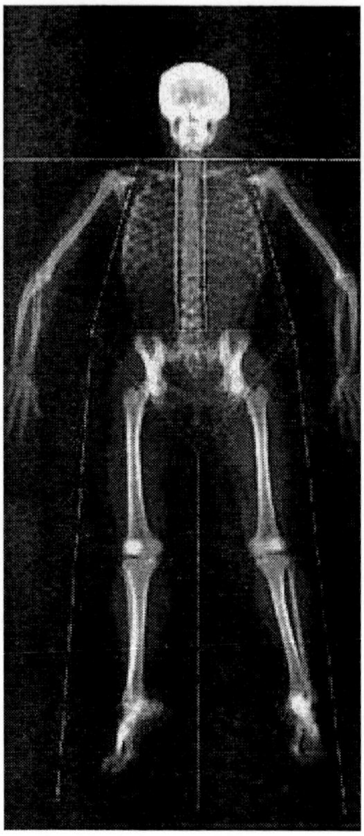

Figure 5. DXA whole-body scan with subregions of interest: head, chest, pelvis and extremities. With appropriate software programs information on whole and regional body composition (lean and fat mass) can be obtained.

For scanning in the forearm, the patient is sitting on a chair next to the scanner table, with the forearm resting on the table top, the hand pronated and, on some scanners, secured on a positioning board and restraining strap. Scan in the forearm include the 33% of the non-dominant radius (sometimes called one-third radius) for diagnosis (Figure 6). DXA of the forearm should be performed if hip and/or spine cannot be measured or interpreted, in hyperparathyroidism and in overweighted patients who exceed the weight limit of DXA tables.

There are other important limitations to DXA. Because BMD is the average on two-dimensional projection of the bone, and variations in the third dimension are ignored, the estimated BMD can be strongly altered by the size of the bone. Therefore if a large and a small bone have the same mineral density, the larger one will appear to have a higher BMD. This potential source of systematic error is especially important when patients with different body size are compared. In addition, DXA does not provide any information regarding the geometric distribution of trabecular and cortical bone, whereas the geometric component of bone competence is completely ignored. Finally, these measurements are strongly influenced by the composition of the soft tissue surrounding the bone, compromising accuracy in frail older women in whom the magnitude of the measurement error can be as high as 20% [31].

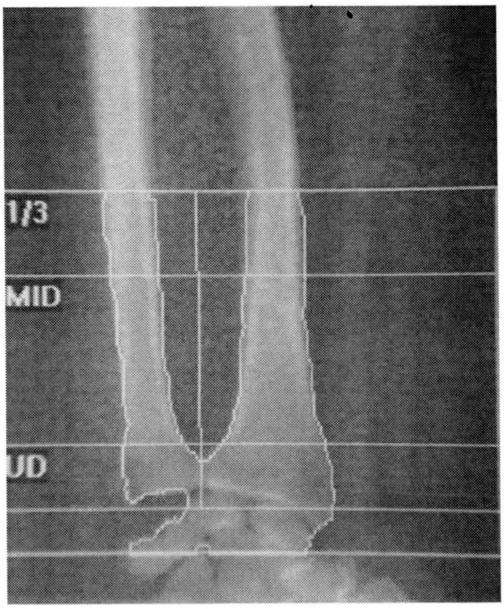

Figure 6. DXA forearm shows region of interest: ultradistal (UD), distal shaft (MID) and shaft (1/3).

The method emits high and low X-ray energy and measures the difference in tissue attenuation of each, allowing separation of soft tissue density from bone density. This separation is particularly important since there is individual variability in the soft tissue content around the hip and spine. The attenuation of X-rays is also distinctly different between normal bone and osteoporotic bone. DXA measurements can neither sufficiently differentiate between cortical and trabecular bone, nor give details with respect to bone architecture [32,33,34].

Each patient's bone density is plotted against a healthy young adult or against age-matched control data. In 1994, the WHO chose the T-score as its standard for defining BMD [3]. The WHO criteria are intended to provide a reasonable standard for evaluation of individual BMD values in comparison to existing databases. Comparisons are stated as standard deviation/SD from normal BMD values obtained from young, healthy persons of the same sex, race, and age. An SD represents the normal variability in a measurement in a young normal population, and these may vary from technique to technique and among various reference populations that are used to define normal values.

The young normal scores, or T-scores, can be used to decide whether a patient has a reduced BMD consistent with osteoporosis or osteopenia. The Z-score compares one patient's BMD, in standard deviations, with the mean BMD for people of similar age and gender. Most densitometry equipment contains software that calculates T-scores and Z-scores automatically. The T-score is defined by the formula: Patient's BMD Young adult BMD/1SD of Young adult Mean BMD and the Z-score by the formula: Patient's BMD-Age matched Mean BMD/1SD of age-matched Mean BMD.

A normal BMD is one that is within 1 SD of the young adult reference range (T-score > –1), osteopenia a BMD more than 1 SD but less than 2.5 SD below the young adult mean (T-score between –1 and –2.5), osteoporosis the BMD value of 2.5 SD or more below the young adult mean (T-score < –2.5) and severe/established osteoporosis the BMD value of 2.5 SD or more below the young adult mean in the presence of one or more fragility fractures [35] (Figure 7). The term "osteopenia" has limited value because it encompasses a broad range of patients, including some with a relatively high risk for their age and others whose risk is lower than average for their age.

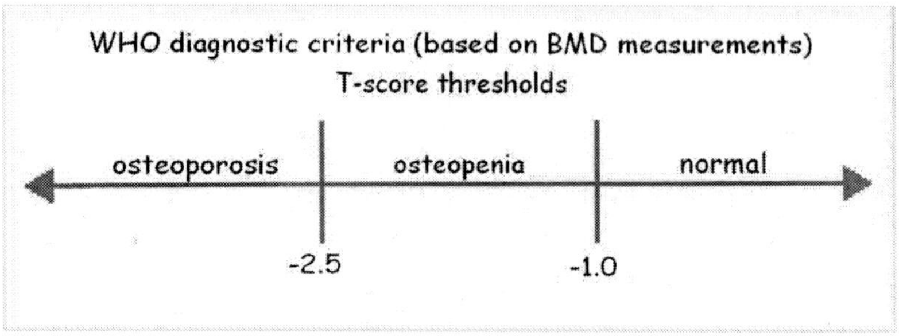

Figure 7. WHO diagnostic criteria, based on BMD measurements.

Because BMD declines with age, T-scores are consistently lower than Z-scores about after the age of 40 years, and the difference increases with age. It is important to mention that men have higher BMD than women, and African Americans and Latinos have higher BMD than Caucasians [36]. Asians tend to have slightly lower BMD than whites mainly because of their smaller size [37,38]. Densitometers report T-score and Z-score that are specific to the patient's sex, and usually manufacturers report values compared with those of patients of the same race. Although men and nonwhite women have a lower overall fracture rate than white women, there are insufficient data on which to base recommendations about BMD. Moreover, there is a controversy about what levels of BMD should be considered osteoporotic and what values should trigger a recommendation for treatment in men and nonwhite women population [17].

DXA examinations normally should be including hip and anteroposterior spine BMD as one measurement in all patients. Because of the stronger relationship of hip BMD to hip fracture and weaker influence of degenerative arthritis after age of 65 years, it is reasonable to give more weight to the results of hip BMD measurements. According to ISCD and IOF recommendations, the decision should be based on the lowest BMD values of the lumbar spine, total hip or femoral neck. If hip or spine BMD has been measured, there is generally no reason to measure a peripheral site.

In regard to BMD reporting in postmenopausal women and in men aged 50 years and older T-scores are preferred and the WHO densitometric classification is applicable.

It should be noted that the WHO classification should not be applied to healthy premenopausal women or healthy men under the age of 50. The diagnosis of osteoporosis in healthy premenopausal women or healthy men under the age of 50 should not be made on the basis of densitometric criteria alone. In these patients, Z-scores, not T-scores are preferred. A

Z-score of -2.0 or lower is defined as "below the expected range for age" and a Z-score above -2.0 is "within the expected range for age" [39] (Figure 8).

In the children are considered the preferred skeletal sites for measurement the spine and whole-body. The value of BMD to predict fractures in children is not yet clearly determined. The T-score should not be included in the pediatric DXA report. Because the T-score is a measure of bone density lose since early adulthood its use in children whose BMD has yet to peak will always yield a low result. Z-score must be interpreted in light of the best available pediatric data bases of age-matched controls and the reference database should be cited in the report. Terminology such as "low bone density for chronologic age" or "below the expected range for age" may be used if the Z-score is below -2.0. It is important to mention that in children the diagnosis of osteoporosis should not be made on DXA results alone, but should take into account other patient factors [39].

Risk factors used in the calculation of 10-year risk of fracture include: the femoral neck T-score, the patients age, history of previous low trauma fracture, low BMI, ever steroid exposure, family history of hip fracture, current cigarette smoking, high alcohol intake > 2 units/day (1 unit: 8 gm alcohol ~1/2 pt. beer ~ glass wine) [40,41].

If DXA investigations are repeated, anteroposterior spine and total hip measurements should be used to follow response to treatment. For bone loss monitoring BMD testing should be performed every two years. All patients receiving pharmacologic intervention should have BMD testing two years after starting therapy and ever two years thereafter [42].

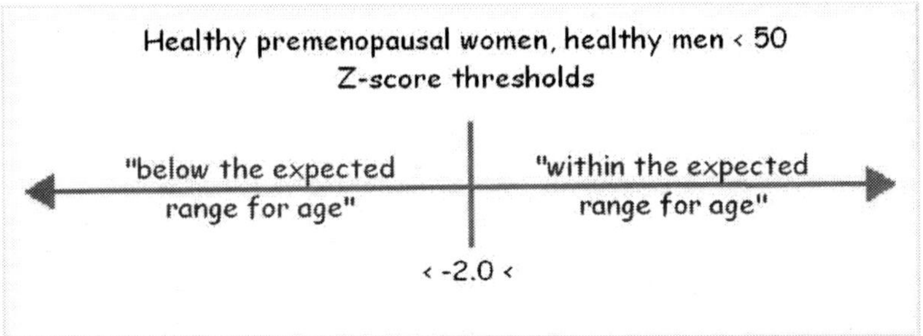

Figure 8. BMD reporting in females prior to menopause and in male younger than age 50.

ERRORS, ARTEFACTS AND RADIATION DOSE:

Error and artefacts in DXA are correlated to the calibration and the quality assurance of the equipment, patient positioning, image analysis, operator variability, anatomical problems of the patient, misunderstanding of data, as well as the age and ethnicity of the patient. During the examination the patient lies almost fully clothed on a padded table while the system scans one or more areas of bone [26]. A complete DXA examination, including patient preparation, image acquisitions, analysis, printouts and report generation, is typically performed in 20-25 minutes.

While DXA uses X-rays, the amount of radiation is very low, less than one-tenth the dose of a standard chest X-ray. Although it is recommended that the radiologist is positioned at least 2 m from the scanning table when the scanner is in use [9]. It is also very important that women should always inform their radiologist if there is any possibility that they are pregnant. DXA is a high precision and accuracy technique, with high resolution and well-documented correlation to fracture risk [26].

As any medical device using radiation, DXA requires testing after installation in order to ensure that the system is functioning properly and the radiation dose is within the specified limits. This is carried out by a medical physicist at the time of installation, who should review these data and compare the results with the specifications of the instrument given by the manufacturer. At times, it may be necessary to repeat some measurements, particularly if a new brand of instrument is installed. It may also be necessary to evaluate the instrument for new applications or to determine measurement errors under certain experimental conditions. Besides these occasional evaluations, there are also daily quality control requirements. Instrument calibration and, if indicated, radiation dose to the patient should be measured after each major maintenance or repair [43].

Conclusion

Since its commercial inception in 1987, DXA has become the "gold standard" technique for the diagnosis of the osteoporosis [44]. It is painless, requires no injections or other invasive procedures, sedation, special diet or any other prior preparation. The method aids in the investigation and differential diagnosis of patients with radiographic osteopenia or medical condition compatible with primary osteoporosis [45]. Thus DXA is the best available index for the estimation of fracture risk as well as an important tool in therapeutic management.

References

[1] Consensus Development Conference: Diagnosis, Prophylaxis, and Treatment of Osteoporosis, *Am J Med.* 1993;94:646-650. WHO Study Group 1994.

[2] Position statement: executive summary. The Writing Group for the International Society for Clinical Densitometry (ISCD) Position Development Conference. *J Clinical Densitom.* 2004;7:7-12.

[3] Assessment of fracture risk and its application to screening for postmenopausal osteoporosis. Report of a WHO Study Group. World Health Organ *Tech Rep Ser.* 1994;843:1-129.

[4] Kanis JA, Gluer CC for the Committee of Scientific Advisors, International Osteoporosis Foundation. An update on the diagnosis and assessment of osteoporosis with densitometry. *Osteoporos Int.* 2000;11:192-202.

[5] Brown JP, Josse RG for the Scientific Advisory Council of the Osteoporosis Society of Canada. Clinical practice guidelines for the diagnosis and management of osteoporosis in Canada. *CMAJ.* 2002;167(Suppl.10):S1-S31.

[6] National Osteoporosis Foundation. Osteoporosis. Review of the evidence for prevention, diagnosis, treatment and cost-effectiveness analysis. *Osteoporos Int.* 1998;8(Suppl 4):S7-S80.

[7] Lewiecki EM, Watts NB, McClung MR, Petak SM, Bachrach LK, Shepherd JA, Downs RW. International Society for Clinical Densitometry: Official positions of the International Society for Clinical Densitometry. *J Clin Endocrinol Metab.* 2004; 89:3651-3655.

[8] Lawrence GR. Screening for Osteoporosis. *N Engl J Med.* 2005;353:164-171.

[9] Adams JE. Single- and Dual-Energy: X-Ray Absorptiometry. In: Genant HK, Guglielmi G, Jergas M. Bone Densitometry and Osteoporosis. *Springer* 1998.

[10]Genant HK, Cooper C, Poor G, Reid I, Ehrlich G, Kanis JA, Nordin BE, Barrett-Connor E, Bonjour JP, Dawson-Hughes B, Delmas PD, Dequeker J, Ragi Eis S, Gennari C, Johnell O, Johnston CC Jr, Lau EM, Liberman UA, Lindsay R, Martin TJ, Masri B, Mautalen CA, Meunier PJ, Kahaltaev N. Interim report and recommendations of the World Health Organization Task-Force for Osteoporosis. *Osteoporos Int.* 1999;10:259-264.

[11]Cummings SR, Kelsey JL, Nevitt MC, O'Dowd KJ. Epidemiology of osteoporosis and osteoporotic fractures. *Epidemiol Rev.* 1985;7:178-208.

[12]Melton LJ, Lane AW, Cooper C, Eastell R, O'Fallon WM, Riggs BL. Prevalence and incidence of vertebral deformities. *Osteoporos Int.* 1993;3:113-119.

[13]Riggs BL, Wahner HW, Seeman E, Offord KP, Dunn WL, Mazess RB, Johnson KA, Melton LJ III. Changes in bone mineral density of the proximal femur and spine with aging. *J Clin Invest.* 1982;70:716-723.

[14]Riggs BL, Wahner HW, Melton LJ III, Richelson LS, Judd HL, Offord KP. Rates of bone loss in the appendicular skeletons of women: Evidence of substantial vertebral bone loss before menopause. *J Clin Invest.* 1986;77:1487-1491.

[15]Gotfrensen A, Nilas L, Podenphant J, Haldberg A, Christiansen C. Regional bone mineral in healthy and osteoporotic women: A cross-sectional study. *Scan J Clin Lab Invest.* 1989;49:739-749.

[16]Ravn P, Hetland ML, Overgaard K, Christiansen C. Premenopausal and postmenopausal changes in bone mineral density of the proximal femur measured by dual-energy X-ray absorptiometry. *J Bone Miner Res.* 1994;9:1975-1980.

[17]Cummings SR, Bates D, Black DM. Clinical Use of Bone Densitometry. *JAMA.* 2002;288:1889-1897.

[18]Prudham G, Evans JG. Factors associated with falls an the elderly: a community study. *Age Ageing.* 1981;10:141-146.

[19]Kelsey JL, Hoffmann S. Risk factors of the hip fractures. *N Engl J Med.* 1987;316:404-406.

[20]Kanis JA, Johnell O, De Laet C et al. International variations in hip fracture probabilities: implications for risk assessment. *J Bone Miner Res.* 2002b;17:1237-1244.

[21]Kanis JA, Johnell O. Requirements for DXA for the management of osteoporosis in Europe. *Osteoporos Int.* 2005;16(3):229-238.

[22]National Osteoporosis Foundation 2003. Physician's guide to prevention and treatment of osteoporosis. National Osteoporosis Foundation, Washington DC.

[23]National Osteoporosis Foundation. Physician's Guide to prevention and treatment of osteoporosis. Excerpta Medica, Belle Meade, NJ;1998.

[24]Kanis JA. Diagnosis of osteoporosis and assessment of fracture risk. *Lancet.* 2002;359:1929-1936.

[25]Genant HK. Measurement of axial and bone mass by DXA. Bone mass measurement in osteoporosis and other bone diseases. National Osteoporosis Foundation; November 1995.

[26]Baltas CS, Balanika AP, Raptou PD, Tournis S, Lyritis GP. Clinical practice guidelines proposed by the Hellenic Foundation of Osteoporosis for the management of osteoporosis based on DXA results. *J Musculoskelet Neuronal Interact.* 2005;5(4):388-92.

[27]Rizzoli R, Slosman D, Bonjour J. The role of dual energy X-ray absorptiometry of lumbar spine and proximal femur in the diagnosis and follow-up of osteoporosis. *Am J Med.* 1995;98:33S-36S.

[28]Shepherd JA, Fan B, Lu Y, Lewiecki EM, Miller P, Genant HK. Comparison of bone mineral density precision for Prodigy and Delphi spine and femur scans. *Osteoporos Int.* 2006;17(9):1303-1308.

[29]Ahlborg HG, Nguyen ND, Nguyen TV, Center JR, Eisman JA. Contribution of hip length indices to hip fracture risk in elderly men and women. *J Bone Miner Res.* 2005;10:1820-1827.

[30]Wahner HW. Use of densitometry in the management of osteoporosis. In: Meunier PJ (ed) Osteoporosis: Diagnosis and Management. 1st ed. Martin Duntz, London;1998.

[31]Russo CR, Lauretani F, Bandinelli S, Bartali B, Di Iorio A, Volpato S, Guralnik JM, Harris T, Ferrucci L. Aging bone in men and women: beyond changes in bone mineral density. *Osteoporos Int.* 2003;14:531-538.

[32]Milos G, Spindler A, Ruegsegger P, Seifert B, Muhlebach S, Uebelhart D, Hauselmann HJ. Cortical and trabecular bone density and structure in anorexia nervosa. *Osteoporos Int.* 2004;Sep 28.

[33]Boyanov MA, Popovanov PR, Roux C. Separate assessment of forearm cortical and trabecular bone density from standard densitometry data. *Ann Med.* 2001;33:497-506.

[34]Hergenroeder AC. Bone mineralization, hypothalamic amenorrhea, and sex steroid therapy in female adolescents and young adults. *J Pediatr.* 1995;126:683-689.

[35]Kanis JA. Assessment of fracture risk and its application to screening for postmenopausal osteoporosis: Synopsis of a WHO report. *Osteoporos Int.* 1994; 4:368-381.

[36]Looker AC, Orwoll ES, Johnston CC, et al. Prevalence of low femoral bone density in older U.S. adults from NHANES III. *J Bone Miner Res.* 1997;12:1761-1768.

[37]Russell-Aulet M, Wang J, Thornton J, Colt EWD, Pierson RN Jr. Bone mineral density and mass by total-body dual-photon absorptiometry in normal white and Asian men. *J Bone Miner Res.* 1991;6:1109-1113.

[38]Russell-Aulet M, Wang J, Thornton JC, Colt EWD, Pierson RN Jr. Bone mineral density and mass in a cross-sectional study of white and Asian women. *J Bone Miner Res.* 1993;8:575-582.

[39]The writing group for the ISCD Position Development Conference. Diagnosis of osteoporosis in men, premenopausal women and children. *J Clin Densitom.* 2004;7:17-26.

[40]Kanis JA, Johnell O, Oden A, De Laet C, Jonsson B, Dawson A. Ten year risk of osteoporotic fracture and the effect of risk factors on screening strategies. *Bone* 2002;30:251-258.

[41]Kanis JA, Borgstrom F, De Laet C, Johansson M, Johnell O, Jonsson B, Oden A, Zethraeus N, Pfleger B, Khaltaev N. Assessment of fracture risk. *Osteoporos Int.* 2005;16(6):581-589.

[42]Barclay L. National Osteoporosis Foundation Issues Guidelines for Osteoporosis Management. *Osteoporos Int.* published online February 22, 2008.

[43]Wahner HW, Fogelman I. The evaluation of osteoporosis: DEXA in clinical practice, Chapter 5, Mayo Foundation and Ignac Fogelman;1994.

[44]Laboratory assessment of osteoporosis and quality assurance guidelines. Hellenic Foundation of Osteoporosis. Athens, 2005.

[45]Jergas M, Genant HK. Spinal and femoral DXA for the assessment of spinal osteoporosis. *Calcif Tiss Int.* 1997;61:351-357.

In: Osteoporosis: Etiology, Diagnosis and Treatment
Editors: Bilar E. Mattingly and Albert C. Pillare
ISBN 978-1-60692-397-9

Chapter 3

NUTRITIONAL TREATMENT IN OSTEOPOROSIS

Cristina Palacios
University of Puerto Rico, San Juan, PR 00935

ABSTRACT

This chapter discusses the steps in the nutritional assessment of osteoporotic patients. It focuses on the nutritional clinical history, but anthropometry and diagnostic tests are also described. Within the former, familiar and personal health history important in bone metabolism are described. In addition, different nutritional questionnaires are discussed in assessing diet in osteoporotic patients. This chapter also emphasizes on the nutritional requirements for bone health and osteoporosis, focuzing on the key bone nutrients such as protein, calcium, phosphorus, magnesium, fluoride and vitamin D. Other nutrients important to bone are also discussed, such as zinc, copper, boron, manganese, potassium, vitamins A, K, C and the B vitamins. Nutritional recommendations on how to reach these requirements through diet are given, as well as the use of nutritional supplements for osteoporotic patients. The substances and the nutrients that interfere with calcium metabolism, as well as in the metabolism of other important bone nutrients are also described, along with nutritional recommendations to avoid these interactions. In conclusion, this review paper gives insights to the nutritional management of osteoporosis, a very important complement to medical and technology therapies.

INTRODUCTION

The nutritional assessment and recommendations are important components in the treatment of osteoporosis. The first step in the assessment is to know the clinical history of the patient, along with the current and past food consumption, exercise habits, anthropometric measurements and diagnostic tests. This assessment should lead to establishing the nutritional goals for an osteoporotic patient. The goals include: aiming to meet the nutritional requirements of nutrients important to bone health through a nutritional plan, reinforced with nutritional supplements; limiting the consumption of certain foods and substances that interfere with bone metabolism, such as foods high in sodium, caffeine, oxalate and alcohol; and promoting exercise, particularly high impact or strength training exercise.

A balanced diet with adequate intakes of calcium, vitamin D, magnesium, phosphorous and other important nutrients for bone health, in combination with outdoors physical activity and healthy lifestyle choices are associated with osteoporosis prevention. If osteoporosis is already present, these recommendation along with the addition of certain supplements may help prevent further bone loss and in some cases even restore bone mass.

1. Nutritional Assessment of Osteoporotic Patients

- Clinical history

The clinical history is the first step to asses the nutritional status of a patient. Personal and familiar health history is very important in determining the genetic background of a patient with osteoporosis, given that 60-80% of peak bone mass is explained by genetics [1] and possibly also rates of bone loss.

- Familiar health history

This part of the assessment should ask about the following aspects in first-degree relatives.

  - Age of menopause
  - Age of appearance of osteoporosis or other bone related diseases (if applicable)
  - Previous fractures, including frequency, age and site each fracture. This is a major risk factor for osteoporosis.

- Personal health history

A comprehensive personal health history should be done, including:

  - Age: women older than – years and men older than 70 years are at increased risk factor for osteoporosis [2].
  - Age of menopause: early menopause is a risk factor for osteoporosis. The cause of early menopause should be further elucidated (natural or by ovariectomy).
  - Weight loss: the amount of weight loss, as well as the timing should be included in this section. A 10% weight loss is associated with low bone mass and osteoporosis [2].
  - Hormonal conditions that could affect bone: patients should be asked if they have hyperthyroidism, hypothyroidism, hyperparathyroidism, cushing's syndrome, etc.
  - Use of medications that could affect bone metabolism: patients should be asked if they use corticoesteroids, thyroxine, heparin, aluminum antiacids, chemotherapy, litum, anticonvulsionist and thiazide diuretics.

- Pregnancy and breastfeeding: this section should include age of last pregnancy and duration of breastfeeding. Although cross-sectional studies have indicated that parity and duration of breastfeeding results in similar or higher BMD and similar or lower fracture risk than their peers who have not given birth [3], women who breastfeed after age 40 may not recuperate from the bone loss due to lactation before entering menopause.
- Smoking habits: it should ask frequency and amount of cigarettes used currently and in the past. A smoking history, as well as current smoking is associated with increased risk of osteoporotic fractures [4,5].
- Alcohol intake: it should ask type, frequency and amount of alcohol intake currently and in the past. A high alcohol intake is associated with increased risk of osteoporotic fractures [6], while moderate drinking (0.5 to 1 drink/d) appears to be protective of hip fractures [7].
- Sun exposure: to estimate vitamin D status, the following questions should be included: timing, amount and frequency of sun exposure, use of sunblock, hats and clothing.
- Recurrent falls
- Home conditions: presence of stairs, railways, night lights, rugs, etc.

- Food consumption

Nutrition is an important determinant in bone health. Several methods could be used to estimate food intake and to calculate nutrient adequacy based on requirements by sex and age. Special emphasis should be made on food intake rich in nutrients important for bone, i.e. calcium, protein, phosphorus, magnesium, fluoride, vitamin D, among others (more on next section).

- Food intake diary

A dairy is given to a patient to complete at home during 3 or more days. If a 3 day diary is given, 2 days should be completed during the weekdays and 1 day during the weekend. Studies have found that a good estimation of calcium intake should include 7-10 days of food intake diary [8]. This diary typically includes time and place of all foods and beverages consumed, brand, amount and type of preparation. Written instructions should be given to the patient and reminder calls should be made to return the completed dairy. The analysis of a food intake dairy requires access to a food nutrient database and it is time consuming. Alternatively, the analysis could be done based on the number of portions by food groups and comparing it to the Food Guide Pyramide [9].

- Food recalls

Food recalls is similar to the food intake dairy, except it only includes the foods and beverages consumed on the previous 24-h. It should always ask if it represents a usual day. Since a single 24-h food recall usually does not represente a patient's typical diet, an additional recall could be included asking the foods consumed on a typical day. The analysis of a food recall also requires access to a food nutrient database but since it only analysis a day of food intake, it is less time consuming. It could also be analyzed based on number of portions by food groups and comparing it to the Food Guide Pyramide [9].

- Food frequency questionnaire (FFQ)

This type of questionnaire is very useful and simple to complete. For osteoporotic patients, a semi-quantitative questionnaire of foods rich in calcium could be used. For this questionnaire, a fixed amount or portion is given and the frequency is established based on this portion for the last month. The frequency could be measured by: > 3 or 1-2 per day, 4-6, 2-3 or 1 per week and 2-3 or 1 per month and nevere. In addition, other foods that affect calcium metabolism could be included, such as caffeine intake, soda consumption, and salty foods. Although nutritional supplements were asked on personal health history, it could be added again to check for compliance and for other supplements not reported before. The food frequency questionnaire is easy to analyze, since it only requires calculating the amount of calcium and other nutrients, such as vitamin D and magnesium, from the portions of foods included using a food database once. Depending on the answer, the frequency is adjusted with the amount of nutrient provided by the portion size. Several studies have validated FFQ for calcium intake in adults [10], in postmenopausal women [11] and in the elderly [12].

- Past consumption

Although recent food consumption provides information on actual nutritional status, past intakes of certain nutrients is very important in bone health, since osteoporosis is considered a child disease. Forty percent of bone mass is acquired in 3-4 years during adolescence [13], therefore, nutrient intakes during this stage of life is crucial in the development of osteoporosis later in life. Past consumption of foods rich in calcium could be estimated by a FFQ of dairy products consumed in childhood (5-12 y), adolescence (13-17 y), young adulthood (18-35 y), middle adulthood (36-65 y) and later adulthood (>65 y) [14].

- Exercise patterns

Exercise or physical activity is an important component of bone health. In fact, physical inactivity is a risk factor for low bone mass [2]. The type of physical activity influences bone mass and it is well established that high impact exercises (i.e. running and jumping) are important for building bone mass [15]. However, other type of exercise also benefits bone. Resistive training has been shown to improve prevent bone mass loss and even build bone mass in young and healthy older men and women ([16,17].

Exercise or physical activity patterns could be estimated from questionnaires or measured using pedometers or accelerometers.

- Physical activity recalls

There are several questionnaires reported in the literature to estimate physical activity. The 24-h physical activity recall records the hours spent on sedentary, light, moderate or heavy physical activity in 24 hours [18]. The International Physical Activity Questionnaire (IPAQ) is another instrument to estimate 7-day patterns of time spent sleeping, performing light, moderate or heavy physical activity [19]. Alternatively, a dairy log of physical activity can be given to the patient to monitor during several days or during 1 week all the activities performed. These questionnaires only provide an estimate of physical activity on a given day or week.

- Pedometer and accelerometer

The pedometer is a small instrument, similar to a beeper that registers the amount of steps given over a specified time interval. It is usually placed around the waist for about 1 week. The total number of steps are recorded and compared to international standards [20]. The accelerometers are similar instruments to pedometers as they also measure physical activity continuously over a specified time interval. However, contrary to pedometers, accelerometers can estimate the physical activity intensity and they are much more expensive. These instruments are more reliable than questionnaires for measuring physical activity [21,22].

- Anthropometry

Anthropometry is very useful in providing information of past nutritional history. The most frequently measurements are:

- Weight

Weight should be measured while wearing light clothing, no shoes, socks, sweater, coat, belt and other accessories. Pockets should be emptied before. The patient should stand upright on a calibrated balance, with both feet parallel and looking straight. The measurement is taken while the patient is holding a deep breath. It should be recorded in kilograms (kg).

- Standing Height

To measure standing height, a wall stadiometer should be used. The patient should stand erect, with heals together and touching the wall, buttocks and upper part of the back in contact with the vertical wall, arms at both side and chin parallel to the floor. The measurement is taken while the patient is holding a deep breath with the help of a set-square positioned over the head and aligned to the wall.

In addition, past height measurements should be asked and recorded, along with the age at which height shortening started (if applicable). A decrease in standing height is a physical sign of osteoporosis and is often the reason for a patient to seek medical attention.

- Body mass index (BMI)

BMI is calculated with the following formula: kg/m^2. A low BMI ($<22\ kg/m^2$) is a major risk factor for low bone mass in men and women [2,23,24].

- Fat and muscle mass

A low fat mass is associated with lower bone mass and low muscle mass is associated with an increased risk of fractures [25]. In addition, as fat mass is lost as a result of a weight loss program, bone mass also decreases [2].

Fat and muscle mass could be measured easily by bioelectrical impedance. Alternatively, if a dual-energy absorptiometry (DEXA) is done for measuring bone mass, a whole body scanning could be added to obtain whole body fat and muscle mass as well.

- Diagnostic tests

    - Bone densitometry

This is the technique most commonly used and recommended by physicians to measure bone mass. It provides the bone mineral density (BMD) by site (spine, femur, hip, arm, heel etc) or whole body depending on the instrument used. Such instruments include DEXA, single-energy x-ray absorptiometry, radiographic absorptiometry, quantitative computed tomography and ultrasound densitometry. Most of these instruments expose the patient to small amount of radiation while scanning the body or specific site during a short period of time. DEXA is the most commonly and preferred method by physicians. It is usually performed on the spinal, hip and arm, which are the areas most frequently fractured.

Bone densitometry is very useful because it classifies bone mass in normal, osteopenia and level of osteoporosis (Table I), therefore helping in predicting fracture risk.

Table I. Diagnostic criteria for osteoporosis based on BMD (World Health Organization [26])

Normal	BMD is within 1 SD of a young normal adult
Osteopenia (low bone mass)	BMD is between 1 and 2.5 SD below that of a young normal adult
Osteoporosis	BMD is 2.5 SD or more below that of a young normal adult
Severe osteoporosis	BMD is 2.5 SD or more below that of a young normal adult, with 1 or more fractures.

BMD: bone mineral density;
SD: standard deviation.

Table II. Biochemical biomarkers of bone turnover

Resorption	Formation
• **Urine:** - Calcium - Hydroxiproline - Deoxypyridinoline - N-telopeptide collagen cross link type I - C-terminal cross-linked telopeptides of type I collagen	• **Serum:** - Bone-specific alkaline phosphatase - Osteocalcin and total carboxylated osteocalcin - Procollagen type I N-terminal peptide
• **Serum:** - C-terminal cross-linked telopeptides of type I collagen - Tartrate-resistant acid phosphatase	

    - Serum and urine biochemical biomarkers

Biochemical biomarkers of bone turnover help identify an increase or decrease in bone resorption or formation by measuring enzymes directly related to osteoblast (bone forming cells) or osteoclast (bone resorpting cells) or by measuring circulating constituyents of bone matrix in urine and blood (Table II).

2. Nutrients Involved in Bone Health

Because bone undergoes continuous remodeling, an adequate supply of nutrients important to bone is needed to support bone formation. There are numerous nutrients involved in bone health, and they interact among each other in a complex way on bone metabolism.

The main nutrients that affect bone directly are protein, calcium, phosphorus, magnesium, fluoride and vitamin D. These nutrients, with the exception of protein, were taken together in consideration for their effects on bone health when establishing the Dietary Refereces Intakes (DRI) in 1997 [27].

Other nutrients, such as several of the trace minerals, may also be important in maintaining bone quality through their role as metallo-enzymes in the synthesis of collagen and other proteins that form the structure of bone. Certain vitamins are also involved as co-factors or modulators in bone metabolism, while the consumption of certain substances negative effects on calcium metabolism.

Bone Nutrients

- Protein

The role of protein on bone has been recognized for many years, as protein is part of the organic matrix of bone for collagen structure and is essential to maintain the production of hormones and growth factors that modulate bone synthesis. However, protein may be both beneficial and detrimental bone, depending on the amount and the source of dietary protein, as well as the total calcium intake, among other factors [28].

Balance studies have shown that a high protein diet increases urinary calcium excretion, but intestinal calcium absorption is also increased [29,30], therefore, calcium balance is not necessarily negative. In fact, protein intake has shown to increase insulin-like growth factor I (IGF-I), which is known to be osteotrophic [31] and together with a high calcium intake it increases bone mass in postmenopausal women [32] and in the elderly [33]. Furthermore, protein supplementation alone [34] or along with calcium [35] has shown to reduce hip fractures in elderly.

The source of protein has also been linked to bone health as well; however, the results have been contradictory. Some studies show an increase in urinary calcium excretion with animal protein diets but others have not found this effect [28]. Furthermore, a high animal protein may induce bone loss and this could be explained by the bone mobilization of skeletal salts to balance the endogenous acid generated from acid-forming foods [36]. This could be easily offset by increasing fruits and vegetable consumption [37].

- Calcium

Calcium has been traditionally linked to bone health, however, is not the only nutrient affecting bone. Although calcium deficiency not always leads to osteoporosis, it is an important factor in the progression of osteoporosis.

Calcium is one of the main bone-forming minerals and 99% of the body's calcium resides in the skeleton. There is enough evidence to sustain that an adequate calcium intake during adolescence leads to peak bone mass in adolescence [38,39] and prevents bone loss during menopause [40,41].

Around menopause calcium intake is important to replace calcium lost by resorption. However, studies have found that during this period of rapid bone resorption, bone mass is less responsive to calcium supplementation [40,41]. Several years after menopause, studies have shown that calcium supplementation is beneficial to bone mass [40-43]. A meta-analysis of 15 randomized clinical trials of calcium suplementation in 1806 postmenopausal women showed that calcium increased bone mass in about 1.6 to 2% [44].

Calcium supplementation has also shown to reduce modestly fracture risk. Several meta-analysis of calcium supplementation in older adults have reported a reduction in vertebral and non-vertebral fracture risk of 23% and 14%, respectiverly [44], 12% in all types of fractures [45] or a reduction in the relative risk of hip fractures [46]. Those with good adherence to the treatment have shown higher fracture reduction [45]. These studies also indicate that a dose higher than 1200 mg/d is more effective for bone health. However, the Women Health Initiative study found no significant reduction in hip fractures with 1000 mg/d of calcium supplementation in more than 32,000 women after 7 years [47].

- Phosphorus

Phosphorus is an important component of the bone mineral, as most of it is calcium phosphate. Together with calcium, they affect the levels of parathyroid hormone (PTH), the most important regulator of bone metabolism. When PTH levels increases bone resoprtion increases, resulting in bone mass loss.

Studies have shown that phosphorus and calcium intake interact depending on the level of their intakes. Low phosphorus intake impairs bone mineralization; however, because phosphorus is very widely distributed in plant and animal foods, dietary deficiency is not a concern.

On the other hand, a diet high in phosphorus and low in calcium increases parathyroid hormone (PTH) levels in young adults in a dose response way [48,49]. In addition, short term high phosphorus intake decreases the markers of bone formation and increases the markers of bone resorption [48,49]. Further studies from this group showed that when subjects consumed a diet high in phosphorus together with high calcium intakes, PTH levels and bone resorption decreased, however, bone formation was unaffected [48,49]. Therefore, a very high phosphorus intake, regardeless of calcium intake, is not benefitial for bone.

Phosphorus content is very high in carbonated drinks, and its consumption has been increasingly worldwide. Studies have related the consumption of these drinks to higher fracture rates and lower bone mass in children and young adults [50,51]. However, Heaney and Rafferty [52,53] showed negligible effects on calcium excretion with consumption of these drinks and concluded that the skeletal effects of carbonated beverage consumption are likely due primarily to milk displacement. More studies are needed in older adults to elucidate the effect of a high phosphorus intake on bone mass and osteoporosis.

- Magnesium

Magnesium is another mineral involved in several processes in bone metabolism. It acts directly increasing bone quality by decreasing the size of the hydroxyapatite crystals to prevent brittle bone, but it also acts indirectly through its role in ATP metabolism, as a cofactor of several proteins and hormones, such as parathyroid hormone and 1,25 vitamin D, and as a buffer for the acid produced by the typical Western diet.

Magnesium deficiency could affect bone growth, osteoblastic and osteoclastic activity, osteopenia, bone fragility, and alter calcium metabolism by means of affecting calciotropic hormones [53].

On the other hand, a high dietary magnesium intake or the use of magnesium supplementation in the diet appears to benefit bone. Epidemiologic studies have found positive associations between high magnesium intakes and bone mass in adults, older adults and the elderly from different countries [37,54,55,56,57]. A few clinical studies in different age groups have also found benefitial effects of magnesium supplementation on BMD [58,59,60] and in the markers of bone turnover [61].

- Fluoride

Fluoride acts on bone by increasing the recruitment of osteoblast cells, possibly by inhibiting the activity of osteoblastic acid phosphatase [62]. In addition, fluoride can replace the hydroxyl group to form fluorapatite instead of hydroxyapatite. By doing this, the crystals become larger and stable, which can possibly lead to an increase in resistance to osteoclastic resorption [62]. [63,64] However, excessive fluoride produces bone that is abnormal, with very large crystals that result in brittle bone.

Since water has been fluoridated for many years, several population studies have been able to determine the effects of fluoridation on bone health. Populations with fluoridated water at 1 ppm have reduced overall fracture risk [63,65], while those with fluoridated water at >4.32 ppm were found to have higher facture risk [63].

Clinical studies using fluoride salt supplementation have also found conflicting results, mainly depending on the dose used [66]. Supplementation with >50 mg/d of fluoride salts have not found decrease on fracture rates, despite increases in bone mass [67,68]. However, others have found that levels of 11-20 mg/d appear to decrease vertebral fracture risk and increase bone mass at different sites [69,70].

- Vitamin D

Vitamin D is an essential precursor of 1,25-dihydroxyvitamin D (1,25-dihydroxycholecalciferol, calcitriol), the steroid hormone involved in maintaining the serum calcium at a physiologically acceptable level. One way of doing this is by directly increasing the efficiency of intestinal calcium transport, and thus, increasing calcium absorption into the blood.

Numerous studies worldwide have reported a high prevalence of vitamin D deficiency in different populations. Specifically, the elderly are at higher risk for vitamin D deficiency because of decreased renal hydroxylation of vitamin D, poor nutrition, scarce exposition to sunlight and a decline in the synthesis of vitamin D in the skin [71]. The prevalence of vitamin D deficiency has been estimated between 20 and 60% in US adults over 50 y [72] and 64% in postmenopausal women with osteoporosis from a study in 18 countries [73].

Health care professionals have not paid attention to vitamin D status and measurement of serum 25 (OH)D level, the only way to determine vitamin D status, is seldom performed in the clinical setting. Vitamin D deficiency has been linked to lower bone mass and higher risk of falls and fractures [74,75]. In addition, randomized clinical trials have shown a positive relationship between the use of vitamin D supplements and gains in bone mass and lower fracture rates [74,76-79].

Trace Minerals

Zinc is a constituent mineral of the bone matrix. It also affects bone metabolism indirectly through its role in modulating osteoblastic activity, collagen synthesis, and alkaline phosphatase activity [80] by activating several metallo-enzymes. An epidemiological study related low zinc intake (about 10 mg/d) with doubled risk of fracture compared to much greater intakes [81]. Clinical studies have related low serum zinc levels and excessive urinary zinc excretion to osteoporosis [82,83,84]. In addition, several randomized clinical trials of copper supplementation showed gains in bone mass in postmenopausal women [85] and increases in the markers of bone formation in men [86], while low levels resulted in undesirable changes in circulating calcitonin and osteocalcin in postmenopausal women [87].

Copper is another trace mineral that affects bone by its role as a co-factor of certain enzymes involved in bone metabolism, i.e. lysyl oxidase, superoxide dismutase, ceruloplasmin. Lysyl oxidase is involved in cross-linking of collagen fibers. A case-control study found that copper serum levels were lower in elderly osteoporotic patients compared to controls [88]. Clinical trials of copper supplementation have reported a reduction of bone loss with 1mg/d of copper in perimenopausal [89] and 3 mg/d of copper in postmenopausal women [85], with no effects on the markers of bone turnover in young adults with either 3 or 6 mgd of copper [90,91].

Boron plays a regulatory role in the metabolism of minerals and bone throught its role in steroid hormones, such as testosterone and beta-oestradiol. The few studies done with boron supplementation showed that boron increases serum estradiol levels and decreases urinary excretion of calcium and magnesium [92] and increases calcium absorption [93] in peri- and postmenopausal women. Boron may be also related to vitamin D function, as shown in animal studies [94].

Manganese is an important cofactor of glycosyltransferases, enzymes required for the synthesis of proteoglycans, which are integral components of bone and cartilage. There is only one study to date reporting a beneficial effect of manganese supplementation on bone in postmenopausal women over a 2 year period [85]. However, this study used a combination of manganese, calcium, copper, and zinc supplementation; therefore, more studies are needed to determine the role of manganese on bone.

Iron is a cofactor in enzymes involved in collagen bone matrix synthesis, i.e. prolyl and lysyl hydroxylases and in vitamin D metabolism, i.e. 25-hydroxycholcalciferol hydroxylase.

Iron-deficient animals have lower bone mass and mechanical strength compared to iron-replete rats and a trend has been found between serum ferritin and radius BMD in girls [95].

Strontium is a trace element closely chemically related to calcium. About 99% of strontium is located in bone and studies in vitro show that strontium stimulates bone formation [96]. In humans, most studies have been done with strontium ranelate, a salt used therapeutically to treat osteoporosis. Such studies have shown a reduction in fracture and increases in BMD in different sites rates in postmenopausal women [97-99]. Most studies using strontium ranelate as a treatment for osteoporosis have been done in Europe.

Other Minerals

Silicon may affect bone by stimulating human osteoblasts and by being involved in the cross-linking and stabilization of collagen and matrix mineralization [100,101]. The only study published to date relating silicon to bone was an epidemiological study on the Framingham Offspring Cohort [101]. This study showed that intakes of 45 mg/d were associated with higher BMD at the hip sites for men and premenopausal women, but not for postmenopausal women.

Potassium affects bone metabolism by several mechanisms. Potasium intake promotes an alkaline environment, thereby decreasing the needs for skeletal salts to balance the acid generated from typical western diets high in meats. This alkine environment may also inhibit osteoclastic bone resorption and possibly stimulate bone formation. Several cross-sectional and population studies have shown a positive association between potassium intake and bone mass in perimenopausal and early post-menopausal women [37,102,103] and in the elderly [55,104]. In addition, clinical studies show that potassium bicarbonate supplementation reduces urinary calcium excretion and improves calcium balance in adults [105-107]. Furthermore, combined treatment of calcium and potassium citrate supplementation resulted in decreased bone resorption markers and increased calcium absorption in postmenopausal women [108,109].

Other Vitamins

Vitamin K is a cofactor of γ-carboxylase, an enzyme necessary for the formation of γ-carboxyglutamyl (GLA) residues in bone proteins. There are 3 vitamin K depedent proteins, osteocalcin, the principal and most abundant noncollagenous protein of bone, matrix GLA protein and protein S. Under-γ-caboxylated osteocalcin is considered a sensitive marker of vitamin K status in bone. Vitamin K deficiency increases undercarboxylated osteocalcin, a less fully functional form. Population studies have also shown an inverse association between low vitamin K intake and higher fracture risk [108,110] and lower BMD [111] and with under-carboxilated osteocalcin levels and fractures [112,113] and bone mass [114]. A meta-analysis of clinical trials of vitamin K supplementation reported significant gains in bone mass and reduction of fractures, primarily with the use of 45 mg/d of menaquinone [115]. However, these studies used therapeutical doses. Recent studies supplementing pre and postmenopausal women with lower doses (80-500 mcg/d) of vitamin K (phylloquinone), plus calcium and vitamin D, showed only modest or no effects on bone compared to controls, although benefits on under-γ-caboxylated osteocalcin levels were detected [116-119]. Thus, the evidence appears to favor therapeutical doses of vitamin K for bone health.

Vitamin C is a cofactor in the hydroxylation of lysine and proline, and therefore is required in the cross-linking of collagen fibrils in bone. Vitamin C stimulates alkaline phosphatase activity, a marker for osteoblast formation. The only studies reported to date are population studies, in which high vitamin C intakes have been relatd to higher bone mass [120,121] and long term use of vitamin C supplements to higher BMD [122] in postmenopausal women.

Vitamin A is thought to be directly involved in bone remodeling as osteoblasts and osteoclasts have nuclear receptors for retinoic acid. Population studies have found that very high intakes of retinol and high serum retinol levels are related to lower BMD and higher fracture risk [123,124], but low intakes are too [125], showing a U-shape relationship [126]. A review of 20 clinical studies also found that high retinol intake from diet or supplements (twice the recommendation) and high retinol levels were negatively associated with BMD and fracture risk, but not with beta-carotene intake [127]. However, a large prospective study in elderly found no relationship [128].

The B vitamins appear to be indirectly involved with bone metabolism. Most studies reported to date relate the intakes of some of the B vitamins to BMD or fractures, together with the intakes of key nutrients for bone. Therefore, it is difficult to determine their role in bone health. For example, thiamin, riboflavin, and niacin are involved in energy metabolism; vitamin B6 is involved in osteoblast NADPH concentrations, essential for the vitamin K cycle, while folic acid is involved in the transfer of one-carbon units. Small cross-sectional studies have found positive associations between riboflavin and niacin intake and higher BMD in pre-menopausal women [129,130], while thiamin and vitamin B6 intake were found significantly lower in hip fracture patients compared with age-matched counterparts [131]. A 4-yr clinical trial in postmenopausal women found folate intake significantly correlated with changes in radius BMC [132], while a population-based prospective study in the elderly found folate serum level, as well as homocysteine levels, significantly related to fracture risk in women [133] .

Vitamin B12 is a cofactor on osteoblast-related proteins, such as bone alkaline phosphatase and osteocalcin. Its role on bone health has been directly determined from studies in men and women form the Framingham Offspring Osteoporosis Study and in frail elderly people. Such studies found that osteoporosis occurred more often among men and women with marginal or deficient vitamin B12 status compared to those with a normal status [134,135].

Other Nutrients

Sodium intake has been considered a risk factor for osteoporosis since population studies [136-138] as well as short-term interevention studies in post-menopausal women [139-141] show increase urinary calcium loss with sodium intake. Studies relating sodium with markers of bone turnover have been inconclusive [137,140,142]. It has been proposed that this calcium loss could be compensated for by increased intestinal calcium absorption. However, a recent kinetic study in postmenopausal women showed that bone calcium balance was negative while consuming diets high in sodium, with no compensation in calcium absorption efficiency [143]. This study and others have also shown that only those salt sentive respond to a sodium challenge by increasing urinary calcium. In addition, a longitudinal study of postmenopausal women showed a negative correlation between urinary sodium excretion and bone loss of the hip and concluded that bone loss could have been prevented by either a daily dietary calcium increase of 891 mg calcium or by halving the daily sodium excretion [144]. Further studies are needed to clarify the role of sodium and fracture risk.

Caffeine intake has been implicated as a risk factor in osteoporosis. An analysis of the Framingham Study found that consumption greater than two cups of coffee per day (four cups of tea) increased the risk of fracture [145]. This has been explained by the acutely calciuric effect of caffeine intake. However, double-blind, placebo-controlled crossover trials failed to detect significant changes in calcium balance [146]. Daily consumption of caffeine equivalent to 2-3 cups of coffee accelerated bone loss from the spine and total body in postmenopausal women who consumed less than 744 mg calcium/day [147]. Therefore, more important than caffeine intake is calcium intake on bone.

3. Nutritional Requirements and Recommendations for Osteoporotic Patients

The Dietary Reference intakes (DRI) are the levels established by the Food and Nutrition Board to prevent deficits and promote health. However, for the nutrients related to bone health, these levels are not always appropriate. This section will discuss the current DRIs in light of the evidence associated with bone benefits and practical recommendations for osteoporotic patients.

Nutritional Requirements and Levels Associated with Bone Health

- Protein: the DRI was established at 0.8 grams of protein per kilogram of body weight [148]. However, protein intakes of about 1.0 to 1.5 g per kilogram of body weight has been associated with normal calcium and bone metabolism, while intakes below 0.8 g per kilogram of body weight increase the level of parathyroid hormone, thus, increasing bone resorption [29].
- Calcium: the DRI is 1000 mg/d for adults and increases to 1200 mg/d for 51 y and older adults [27], due to lower absorption efficiency. Calcium intake in the US is well below these levels. The National Center for Health Statitics reported a mean calcium intake of 744 mg/d and 969 mg/d in adults aged 40-59 y and 660 mg/d and 797 mg/d in >60 y, in females and males, respectively [149]. The main dietary sources of calcium are dairy products. Other foods include low oxalate containing vegetables (i.e. broccoli, turnip greens, chinese cabbage/bok choy, kale, etc.), salmon and sardines canned with bones, calcium fortified products (juice, soy and rice beverages, waffles, etc.). Older adults and those with osteoporosis may need calcium supplementation to reach the DRI. As mentioned before, calcium supplementation of 1200 mg/d or higher reduces fracture risk. In addition, a high calcium intake potentiates the positive effect of estrogen replacement therapy on bone mass at all skeletal sites [150]. Furtheremore, a high calcium intake is crucial if patients are treated with fluoride, because this type of treatment may result in calcium deficiency, which responds to calcium supplementation [151].

- Phosphorus: the DRI is 700 mg/d for adults and 580 mg/d for 51 y and older [27]. Phosphorus is widely distributed in plant and animal foods; therefore, the concern is in excess intake rather than deficiency. It is found in grains, cereals, meats, fish and egg products, milk products, nuts and seeds, and certain beverages.
- Magnesium: the DRI is 320 and 420 mg/d in >30y, in females and males, respectively [27]. A national study in US adults found intakes below this recommendation, at 237 mg/d in women and 326 mg/d in men [152]. Although these intakes will not lead to magnesium deficiency, it could affect bone. The studies discussed previously relating magnesium to bone indicate that an intake close to the recommended levels are related to greater BMD and lower bone resorption in adults. Since magnesium is found primarily in nuts and seeds, supplementation is recommended as part of the nutritional therapy in osteoporosis.
- Fluoride: the DRI is 3 mg/d in women and 4 mg/d in men [27]. The most common sources of fluoride are the water supply and the use of fluoridated water in the processing of foods as well as toothpaste and mouthwashes. Fluoride consumption at levels close to the recommendation results in bone mass gain and lower fracture risk in adults [63].
- Vitamin D: the DRI is 400 mg/d for 51-70 y, and 600 for >70 y [27]. However, these levels may be inadequate in preventing fractures [153], especially if a person has no exposure to sunlight [154,155]. Without exposure to sunlight, a higher level of intake (>1000 IU vitamin D/d) has been proposed [156]. Elders with osteoporosis may also need higher levels, since supplementation with 800 IU/d and calcium was found not enough to prevent subsequent fractures [157]. The natural sources of vitamin D are limited to oily fish, such as salmon and mackerel and cod liver oil. Other sources include fortified foods (milk, some cereals, and some bread) and supplements. However, sun exposure is the main and easiest source of vitamin D precursors. With only two to three times per week of sun exposure on the hands, arms, face, or back is more than adequate to meet vitamin D requirements and to store enough for other days of no sun exposure [72].
- Zinc: the DRI for zinc is 8 mg/d in women and 11 mg/d in men and National surverys found intake to be close to recommendations [158]. However, these levels have been associated with increased fracture risk [81], while 15 mg/d may lead to gains in bone mass [85] and 50 mg/d to increases in the markers of bone formation [86]. Since the elderly may be at high risk of zinc deficiency, zinc supplementation may be beneficial. Zinc is found primarily in shellfish, beef, and other red meats, as well as in nuts and legumes.
- Copper: the DRI is 900 mg/d in adults [158,158]. The studies discussed in the previous section showed that higher levels (1-3 mg/d) may be needed to prevent bone loss, although more studies are needed. Good sources of copper include organ meats, shellfish, nuts, seeds, wheat bran cereals and whole grain products. Adults in the US consumed approximately 1.0 to 1.1 mg in women and 1.2 to 1.6 mg in men [158,158]..

- Boron: the upper limit is 20 mg/d [158,158], however, the level associated with bone mass gain is about 3 mg/d [93]. Boron is obtained from a diet rich in fruits, vegetables, nuts and legumes.
- Manganese: the DRI is 1.8 mg/d in women and 2.3 mg/d in men and estimated average intakes range from 2.1-2.3 mg/day for men and 1.6-1.8 mg/day for women [158]. However, higher levels (5 mg/d) appear to result in bone mass gain [85]. Good sources of manganese include whole grains, nuts, leafy vegetables, and teas.
- Strontium: since strontium is not an essential mineral, no DRI has been established and no level of intake has been related to bone health. Strontium is found in plant foods, dairy products, nuts and seawater.
- Silicon: as with strontium, there is no DRI established for silicon. Intakes about 45 mg/d could be beneficial for bone, which is close to regular intakes in the Western world (20-50 mg/day) [159]. The main sources of silicon are cereals and grains, some fruits vegetables and unfiltered water.
- Potassium: the levels recommended are 4700 mg/d for ages 19 and older. The studies discussed earlier showed that such high levels benefit bone. Since potassium is found mainly in fruits and vegetables, it could be a marker for the consumption of these food groups.
- Vitamin C: the DRI is 75 mg/d in women and 90 mg/d in men [160]. However, in postmenopausal women greater BMD was reported as vitamin C intake increased from 0, 500 and 1000 mg/d from supplements [121]. Vitamin C content is very high in mango, guava, berries, orange, grapefruit, tomato, sweet red pepper, among others.
- Vitamin K: the recommendation is 90 mcg/d in women and 120 mcg/d in men [158]. Although the evidence does not favor vitamin K supplementation in dose attainable in the diet, the epidemiological evidence report that intakes <109 mcg/d are related to lower BMD and higher fracture risks [110,111]. Good sources of vitamin K include green leafy vegetables and some vegetable oils (soybean, cottonseed, canola, and olive).
- Vitamin A: the DRI is 2333 IU in women and 3000 IU in men [158]. Intakes much lower or twice the recommendations may lead to adverse effects on bones, while intakes close to these recommended levels are associated with bone maintenance [125]. Retinol is found in animal foods such as cod liver oil, egg and dairy products while carotenoids are found in yellow, orange and green vegetables.
- B vitamins: good sources for most B vitamins include cereals, legumes and seeds. There is little evidence to determine the appropriateness of these B vitamins' recommended levels for optimal bone health.

Diet Recommendations

- 3 servings of dairy products (1 cup of milk and yogurt, and 2 slices of cheese) are needed daily to meet most calcium, phosphorus and vitamin D requirements. These will also provide zinc, magnesium, vitamin A and strontium.

- 5 fruits and vegetables daily provide an alkaline based diet, because of a high load of potassium. In addition, these provide vitamin C, vitamin A, magnesium, manganese, vitamin K, boron, silicon and strontium.
- 2 servings of beef, fish or poultry, and a serving of nuts provide zinc, magnesium, copper, phosphorus, manganese, iron and strontium.
- 1 serving of legumes and 3-4 servings of whole cereals provides the B vitamins and additional magnesium, zinc, vitamin K, manganese, copper and silicon.

Supplement Recommendations

With the combinations of food groups mentioned above, the DRI for most nutrients important to bone are met. However, the studies show that intakes of some nutrients provide bone health benefits beyond these levels. In the case of osteoporotic patients, calcium, vitamin D and magnesium supplements are recommended. In addition, zinc and vitamin C supplements may add further bone benefits.

Within calcium supplements, most have similar levels of bioavailability [161]. Most important is the level of the dose and the consumption with other foods, to maximize bioavailability. Doses higher than 500 mg/d may decrease absorption efficiency, therefore, calcium supplements of 500 mg/d are recommended with foods.

For vitamin D, doses 400-1000 IU are recommended [72].The lower levels may have higher bioavailability but need to be consumed twice a day. Those with limited or no sun exposure may require higher levels. Vitamin D supplements may be combined with calcium and magnesium. Osteoporotic patients may need to consume this combination twice a day, on separate meals.

Other Recommendations

- Salty foods should be avoided to prevent futher urinary calcium loss.
- Caffeine intake should be limited to 1 or 2 cups daily if dripped and to ½ cup daily if expresso.
- High oxalate foods should be consumed at different meals from dairy products because oxalate is a potent inhibitor of calcium absorption.
- Exercise is important to increase muscle mass and strength, which may help prevent falls and fractures.There are two types of exercise that benefit bone: weight bearing, such as walking, dancing, climbing stairs, and, resistance training, such as weight-lifting. Training should be 30-min long, at least 3 times a week and continuous to induce changes on bone.

CONCLUSION

The nutritional assessement and recommendations are key in the prevention and treatment of osteoporosis and should be included routinely in the clinical practice. These important components help identify nutritional and exercise habits and lifestyle choices that affect bone health for establishing the nutritional goals in the treatment of osteoporosis.

The key bone nutrients, protein, calcium, phosphorus, magnesium, vitamin D and fluoride are part of the bone matrix and have been widely recognized. However, other nutrients have shown to be directly or indirectly involved in bone metabolism (zinc, copper, manganese, boron, silicon, strontium, vitamin A, C and K, and the B vitamins). Although the evidence of the effect of any nutrient on bone in many cases is weak, when combined they could impact significantly bone health. Some of these nutrients have recommended intake levels lower than evidenced in the literature for bone health. In addition, most of these nutrients are not consumed by the population at the levels shown to exert bone mass gains and fracture prevention. More studies are needed to determine the optimal level of these nutrients combined in the diet for bone health.

Although genetics determine in great proportion bone mass, a balance diet, regular exercise and healthy lifestyle choices throught the life cycle are important in bone health.

REFERENCES

[1] Bonjour JP, Chevalley T, Rizzoli R, Ferrari S: Gene-environment interactions in the skeletal response to nutrition and exercise during growth. *Med Sport Sci* 2007, 51:64-80.

[2] Liu H, Paige NM, Goldzweig CL, Wong E, Zhou A, Suttorp MJ, Munjas B, Orwoll E, Shekelle P: Screening for osteoporosis in men: a systematic review for an American College of Physicians guideline. *Ann Intern Med* 2008, 148(9):685-701.

[3] Karlsson MK, Ahlborg HG, Karlsson C: Maternity and bone mineral density. *Acta Orthop* 2005, 76(1):2-13.

[4] Law MR, Hackshaw AK: A meta-analysis of cigarette smoking, bone mineral density and risk of hip fracture: recognition of a major effect. *BMJ* 1997, 315(7112):841-846.

[5] Kanis JA, Johnell O, Oden A, Johansson H, De Laet C, Eisman JA, Fujiwara S, Kroger H, McCloskey EV, Mellstrom D, Melton LJ, Pols H, Reeve J, Silman A, Tenenhouse A: Smoking and fracture risk: a meta-analysis. *Osteoporos Int* 2005, 16(2):155-162.

[6] Kanis JA, Johansson H, Johnell O, Oden A, De Laet C, Eisman JA, Pols H, Tenenhouse A: Alcohol intake as a risk factor for fracture. *Osteoporos Int* 2005, 16(7):737-742.

[7] Berg KM, Kunins HV, Jackson JL, Nahvi S, Chaudhry A, Harris KA,Jr, Malik R, Arnsten JH: Association between alcohol consumption and both osteoporotic fracture and bone density. *Am J Med* 2008, 121(5):406-418.

[8] Basiotis PP, Welsh SO, Cronin FJ, Kelsay JL, Mertz W: Number of days of food intake records required to estimate individual and group nutrient intakes with defined confidence. *J Nutr* 1987, 117(9):1638-1641.

[9] [http://www.nal.usda.gov/fnic/foodcomp/search/]

[10] Sebring NG, Denkinger BI, Menzie CM, Yanoff LB, Parikh SJ, Yanovski JA: Validation of three food frequency questionnaires to assess dietary calcium intake in adults. *J Am Diet Assoc* 2007, 107(5):752-759.

[11] Roddam AW, Spencer E, Banks E, Beral V, Reeves G, Appleby P, Barnes I, Whiteman DC, Key TJ: Reproducibility of a short semi-quantitative food group questionnaire and

its performance in estimating nutrient intake compared with a 7-day diet diary in the Million Women Study. *Public Health Nutr* 2005, 8(2):201-213.

[12] Dumartheray EW, Krieg MA, Cornuz J, Whittamore DR, Lovell DP, Burckhardt P, Lanham-New SA: Validation and reproducibility of a semi-quantitative Food Frequency Questionnaire for use in elderly Swiss women. *J Hum Nutr Diet* 2006, 19(5):321-330.

[13] Teegarden D, Proulx WR, Martin BR, Zhao J, McCabe GP, Lyle RM, Peacock M, Slemenda C, Johnston CC, Weaver CM: Peak bone mass in young women. *J Bone Miner Res* 1995, 10(5):711-715.

[14] Kalkwarf HJ, Khoury JC, Lanphear BP: Milk intake during childhood and adolescence, adult bone density, and osteoporotic fractures in US women. *Am J Clin Nutr* 2003, 77(1):257-265.

[15] Borer KT: Physical activity in the prevention and amelioration of osteoporosis in women : interaction of mechanical, hormonal and dietary factors. *Sports Med* 2005, 35(9):779-830.

[16] Ryan AS, Ivey FM, Hurlbut DE, Martel GF, Lemmer JT, Sorkin JD, Metter EJ, Fleg JL, Hurley BF: Regional bone mineral density after resistive training in young and older men and women. *Scand J Med Sci Sports* 2004, 14(1):16-23.

[17] Ryan AS, Treuth MS, Hunter GR, Elahi D: Resistive training maintains bone mineral density in postmenopausal women. *Calcif Tissue Int* 1998, 62(4):295-299.

[18] Pereira MA, FitzerGerald SJ, Gregg EW, Joswiak ML, Ryan WJ, Suminski RR, Utter AC, Zmuda JM: A collection of Physical Activity Questionnaires for health-related research. *Med Sci Sports Exerc* 1997, 29(6 Suppl):S1-205.

[19] [http://www.ipaq.ki.se/ipaq.htm]

[20] Tudor-Locke C, Bassett DR,Jr, Rutherford WJ, Ainsworth BE, Chan CB, Croteau K, Giles-Corti B, Le Masurier G, Moreau K, Mrozek J, Oppert JM, Raustorp A, Strath SJ, Thompson D, Whitt-Glover MC, Wilde B, Wojcik JR: BMI-referenced cut points for pedometer-determined steps per day in adults. *J Phys Act Health* 2008, 5 Suppl 1:S126-39.

[21] Strycker LA, Duncan SC, Chaumeton NR, Duncan TE, Toobert DJ: Reliability of pedometer data in samples of youth and older women. *Int J Behav Nutr Phys Act* 2007, 4:4.

[22] Togo F, Watanabe E, Park H, Yasunaga A, Park S, Shephard RJ, Aoyagi Y: How many days of pedometer use predict the annual activity of the elderly reliably? *Med Sci Sports Exerc* 2008, 40(6):1058-1064.

[23] Waugh EJ, Lam MA, Hawker GA, McGowan J, Papaioannou A, Cheung AM, Hodsman AB, Leslie WD, Siminoski K, Jamal SA: Risk factors for low bone mass in healthy 40-60 year old women: A systematic review of the literature. *Osteoporos Int* 2008, .

[24] Coin A, Perissinotto E, Enzi G, Zamboni M, Inelmen EM, Frigo AC, Manzato E, Busetto L, Buja A, Sergi G: Predictors of low bone mineral density in the elderly: the role of dietary intake, nutritional status and sarcopenia. *Eur J Clin Nutr* 2008, 62(6):802-809.

[25] Crepaldi G, Romanato G, Tonin P, Maggi S: Osteoporosis and body composition. *J Endocrinol Invest* 2007, 30(6 Suppl):42-47.

[26] World Health Organization (WHO): Assessment of fracture risk and its application for screening for postmenopausal osteoporosis. 1994, 843:.

[27] Standing Committee on the Scientific Evaluation of Dietary Reference Intakes,Food and Nutrition board,Institute of Medicine,: *Dietary reference Intakes for calcium, phosphorus, magnesium, vitamin D, and Flouride:* Washington, DC: National Academy Press; 1997.

[28] Heaney RP, Layman DK: Amount and type of protein influences bone health. *Am J Clin Nutr* 2008, 87(5):1567S-1570S.

[29] Kerstetter JE, O'Brien KO, Insogna KL: Dietary protein, calcium metabolism, and skeletal homeostasis revisited. *Am J Clin Nutr* 2003, 78(3 Suppl):584S-592S.

[30] Kerstetter JE, Allen LH: Protein intake and calcium homeostasis. *Adv Nutr Res* 1994, 9:167-181.

[31] Dawson-Hughes B: Calcium and protein in bone health. *Proc Nutr Soc* 2003, 62(2):505-509.

[32] Munger RG, Cerhan JR, Chiu BC: Prospective study of dietary protein intake and risk of hip fracture in postmenopausal women. *Am J Clin Nutr* 1999, 69(1):147-152.

[33] Hannan MT, Tucker KL, Dawson-Hughes B, Cupples LA, Felson DT, Kiel DP: Effect of dietary protein on bone loss in elderly men and women: the Framingham Osteoporosis Study. *J Bone Miner Res* 2000, 15(12):2504-2512.

[34] Delmi M, Rapin CH, Bengoa JM, Delmas PD, Vasey H, Bonjour JP: Dietary supplementation in elderly patients with fractured neck of the femur. *Lancet* 1990, 335(8696):1013-1016.

[35] Schurch MA, Rizzoli R, Slosman D, Vadas L, Vergnaud P, Bonjour JP: Protein supplements increase serum insulin-like growth factor-I levels and attenuate proximal femur bone loss in patients with recent hip fracture. A randomized, double-blind, placebo-controlled trial. *Ann Intern Med* 1998, 128(10):801-809.

[36] Spence LA, Lipscomb ER, Cadogan J, Martin B, Wastney ME, Peacock M, Weaver CM: The effect of soy protein and soy isoflavones on calcium metabolism in postmenopausal women: a randomized crossover study. *Am J Clin Nutr* 2005, 81(4):916-922.

[37] New SA, Robins SP, Campbell MK, Martin JC, Garton MJ, Bolton-Smith C, Grubb DA, Lee SJ, Reid DM: Dietary influences on bone mass and bone metabolism: further evidence of a positive link between fruit and vegetable consumption and bone health? *Am J Clin Nutr* 2000, 71(1):142-151.

[38] Johnston CC,Jr., Miller JZ, Slemenda CW, Reister TK, Hui S, Christian JC, Peacock M: Calcium supplementation and increases in bone mineral density in children. *N Engl J Med* 1992, 327(2):82-87.

[39] Lloyd T, Andon MB, Rollings N, Martel JK, Landis JR, Demers LM, Eggli DF, Kieselhorst K, Kulin HE: Calcium supplementation and bone mineral density in adolescent girls. *JAMA* 1993, 270(7):841-844.

[40] Reid IR, Ames RW, Evans MC, Gamble GD, Sharpe SJ: Long-term effects of calcium supplementation on bone loss and fractures in postmenopausal women: a randomized controlled trial. *Am J Med* 1995, 98(4):331-335.

[41] Dawson-Hughes B, Dallal GE, Krall EA, Sadowski L, Sahyoun N, Tannenbaum S: A controlled trial of the effect of calcium supplementation on bone density in postmenopausal women. *N Engl J Med* 1990, 323(13):878-883.

[42] Aloia JF, Vaswani A, Yeh JK, Ross PL, Flaster E, Dilmanian FA: Calcium supplementation with and without hormone replacement therapy to prevent postmenopausal bone loss. *Ann Intern Med* 1994, 120(2):97-103.

[43] Prince R, Devine A, Dick I, Criddle A, Kerr D, Kent N, Price R, Randell A: The effects of calcium supplementation (milk powder or tablets) and exercise on bone density in postmenopausal women. *J Bone Miner Res* 1995, 10(7):1068-1075.

[44] Shea B, Wells G, Cranney A, Zytaruk N, Robinson V, Griffith L, Hamel C, Ortiz Z, Peterson J, Adachi J, Tugwell P, Guyatt G, Osteoporosis Methodology Group, Osteoporosis Research Advisory Group: Calcium supplementation on bone loss in postmenopausal women. *Cochrane Database Syst Rev* 2004, (1)(1):CD004526.

[45] Tang BM, Eslick GD, Nowson C, Smith C, Bensoussan A: Use of calcium or calcium in combination with vitamin D supplementation to prevent fractures and bone loss in people aged 50 years and older: a meta-analysis. *Lancet* 2007, 370(9588):657-666.

[46] Boonen S, Lips P, Bouillon R, Bischoff-Ferrari HA, Vanderschueren D, Haentjens P: Need for additional calcium to reduce the risk of hip fracture with vitamin d supplementation: evidence from a comparative metaanalysis of randomized controlled trials. *J Clin Endocrinol Metab* 2007, 92(4):1415-1423.

[47] Jackson RD, LaCroix AZ, Gass M, Wallace RB, Robbins J, Lewis CE, Bassford T, Beresford SA, Black HR, Blanchette P, Bonds DE, Brunner RL, Brzyski RG, Caan B, Cauley JA, Chlebowski RT, Cummings SR, Granek I, Hays J, Heiss G, Hendrix SL, Howard BV, Hsia J, Hubbell FA, Johnson KC, Judd H, Kotchen JM, Kuller LH, Langer RD, Lasser NL, Limacher MC, Ludlam S, Manson JE, Margolis KL, McGowan J, Ockene JK, O'Sullivan MJ, Phillips L, Prentice RL, Sarto GE, Stefanick ML, Van Horn L, Wactawski-Wende J, Whitlock E, Anderson GL, Assaf AR, Barad D, Women's Health Initiative Investigators: Calcium plus vitamin D supplementation and the risk of fractures. *N Engl J Med* 2006, 354(7):669-683.

[48] Calvo MS, Kumar R, Heath H: Persistently elevated parathyroid hormone secretion and action in young women after four weeks of ingesting high phosphorus, low calcium diets. *J Clin Endocrinol Metab* 1990, 70(5):1334-1340.

[49] Kemi VE, Karkkainen MU, Lamberg-Allardt CJ: High phosphorus intakes acutely and negatively affect Ca and bone metabolism in a dose-dependent manner in healthy young females. *Br J Nutr* 2006, 96(3):545-552.

[50] Wyshak G, Frisch RE: Carbonated beverages, dietary calcium, the dietary calcium/phosphorus ratio, and bone fractures in girls and boys. *J Adolesc Health* 1994, 15(3):210-215.

[51] Petridou E, Karpathios T, Dessypris N, Simou E, Trichopoulos D: The role of dairy products and non alcoholic beverages in bone fractures among schoolage children. *Scand J Soc Med* 1997, 25(2):119-125.

[52] Heaney RP, Rafferty K: Carbonated beverages and urinary calcium excretion. *Am J Clin Nutr* 2001, 74(3):343-347.

[53] Fatemi S, Ryzen E, Flores J, Endres DB, Rude RK: Effect of experimental human magnesium depletion on parathyroid hormone secretion and 1,25-dihydroxyvitamin D metabolism. *J Clin Endocrinol Metab* 1991, 73(5):1067-1072.

[54] New SA, Bolton-Smith C, Grubb DA, Reid DM: Nutritional influences on bone mineral density: a cross-sectional study in premenopausal women. *Am J Clin Nutr* 1997, 65(6):1831-1839.

[55] Tucker KL, Hannan MT, Chen H, Cupples LA, Wilson PW, Kiel DP: Potassium, magnesium, and fruit and vegetable intakes are associated with greater bone mineral density in elderly men and women. *Am J Clin Nutr* 1999, 69(4):727-736.

[56] Bass M, Ford MA, Brown B, Mauromoustakos A, Keathley RS: Variables for the prediction of femoral bone mineral status in American women. *South Med J* 2006, 99(2):115-122.

[57] Tranquilli AL, Lucino E, Garzetti GG, Romanini C: Calcium, phosphorus and magnesium intakes correlate with bone mineral content in postmenopausal women. *Gynecol Endocrinol* 1994, 8(1):55-58.

[58] Abraham GE, Grewal H: A total dietary program emphasizing magnesium instead of calcium. Effect on the mineral density of calcaneous bone in postmenopausal women on hormonal therapy. *J Reprod Med* 1990, 35(5):503-507.

[59] Stendig-Lindberg G, Tepper R, Leichter I: Trabecular bone density in a two year controlled trial of peroral magnesium in osteoporosis. *Magnes Res* 1993, 6(2):155-163.

[60] Sojka JE, Weaver CM: Magnesium supplementation and osteoporosis. *Nutr Rev* 1995, 53(3):71-74.

[61] Dimai HP, Porta S, Wirnsberger G, Lindschinger M, Pamperl I, Dobnig H, Wilders-Truschnig M, Lau KH: Daily oral magnesium supplementation suppresses bone turnover in young adult males. *J Clin Endocrinol Metab* 1998, 83(8):2742-2748.

[62] Kleerekoper M: The role of fluoride in the prevention of osteoporosis. *Endocrinol Metab Clin North Am* 1998, 27(2):441-452.

[63] Li Y, Liang C, Slemenda CW, Ji R, Sun S, Cao J, Emsley CL, Ma F, Wu Y, Ying P, Zhang Y, Gao S, Zhang W, Katz BP, Niu S, Cao S, Johnston CC,Jr: Effect of long-term exposure to fluoride in drinking water on risks of bone fractures. *J Bone Miner Res* 2001, 16(5):932-939.

[64] Li JY, Specker BL, Ho ML, Tsang RC: Bone mineral content in black and white children 1 to 6 years of age. Early appearance of race and sex differences. *Am J Dis Child* 1989, 143(11):1346-1349.

[65] Lehmann R, Wapniarz M, Hofmann B, Pieper B, Haubitz I, Allolio B: Drinking water fluoridation: bone mineral density and hip fracture incidence. *Bone* 1998, 22(3):273-278.

[66] Demos LL, Kazda H, Cicuttini FM, Sinclair MI, Fairley CK: Water fluoridation, osteoporosis, fractures--recent developments. *Aust Dent J* 2001, 46(2):80-7; quiz 143.

[67] Meunier PJ, Sebert JL, Reginster JY, Briancon D, Appelboom T, Netter P, Loeb G, Rouillon A, Barry S, Evreux JC, Avouac B, Marchandise X: Fluoride salts are no better

at preventing new vertebral fractures than calcium-vitamin D in postmenopausal osteoporosis: the FAVOStudy. *Osteoporos Int* 1998, 8(1):4-12.

[68] Riggs BL, Hodgson SF, O'Fallon WM, Chao EY, Wahner HW, Muhs JM, Cedel SL, Melton LJ,3rd: Effect of fluoride treatment on the fracture rate in postmenopausal women with osteoporosis. *N Engl J Med* 1990, 322(12):802-809.

[69] Reginster JY, Meurmans L, Zegels B, Rovati LC, Minne HW, Giacovelli G, Taquet AN, Setnikar I, Collette J, Gosset C: The effect of sodium monofluorophosphate plus calcium on vertebral fracture rate in postmenopausal women with moderate osteoporosis. A randomized, controlled trial. *Ann Intern Med* 1998, 129(1):1-8.

[70] Ringe JD, Kipshoven C, Coster A, Umbach R: Therapy of established postmenopausal osteoporosis with monofluorophosphate plus calcium: dose-related effects on bone density and fracture rate. *Osteoporos Int* 1999, 9(2):171-178.

[71] Gennari C: Calcium and vitamin D nutrition and bone disease of the elderly. *Public Health Nutr* 2001, 4(2B):547-559.

[72] Holick MF: Vitamin D: the underappreciated D-lightful hormone that is important for skeletal and cellular health. *Current Opinion in Endocrinology & Diabetes* 2002, 9(1):87-98.

[73] Lips P, Hosking D, Lippuner K, Norquist JM, Wehren L, Maalouf G, Ragi-Eis S, Chandler J: The prevalence of vitamin D inadequacy amongst women with osteoporosis: an international epidemiological investigation. *J Intern Med* 2006, 260(3):245-254.

[74] Cranney A, Horsley T, O'Donnell S, Weiler H, Puil L, Ooi D, Atkinson S, Ward L, Moher D, Hanley D, Fang M, Yazdi F, Garritty C, Sampson M, Barrowman N, Tsertsvadze A, Mamaladze V: Effectiveness and safety of vitamin D in relation to bone health. *Evid Rep Technol Assess (Full Rep)* 2007, (158)(158):1-235.

[75] Bischoff-Ferrari HA, Dawson-Hughes B, Willett WC, Staehelin HB, Bazemore MG, Zee RY, Wong JB: Effect of Vitamin D on falls: a meta-analysis. *JAMA* 2004, 291(16):1999-2006.

[76] Bischoff-Ferrari HA, Dietrich T, Orav EJ, Dawson-Hughes B: Positive association between 25-hydroxy vitamin D levels and bone mineral density: a population-based study of younger and older adults. *Am J Med* 2004, 116(9):634-639.

[77] Chapuy MC, Pamphile R, Paris E, Kempf C, Schlichting M, Arnaud S, Garnero P, Meunier PJ: Combined calcium and vitamin D3 supplementation in elderly women: confirmation of reversal of secondary hyperparathyroidism and hip fracture risk: the Decalyos II study. *Osteoporos Int* 2002, 13(3):257-264.

[78] Dawson-Hughes B, Harris SS, Krall EA, Dallal GE: Effect of calcium and vitamin D supplementation on bone density in men and women 65 years of age or older. *N Engl J Med* 1997, 337(10):670-676.

[79] Ooms ME, Roos JC, Bezemer PD, van der Vijgh WJ, Bouter LM, Lips P: Prevention of bone loss by vitamin D supplementation in elderly women: a randomized double-blind trial. *J Clin Endocrinol Metab* 1995, 80(4):1052-1058.

[80] Colpan L, Gur A, Cevik R, Nas K, Sarac AJ: The effect of calcitonin on biochemical markers and zinc excretion in postmenopausal osteoporosis. *Maturitas* 2005, 51(3):246-253.

[81] Elmstahl S, Gullberg B, Janzon L, Johnell O, Elmstahl B: Increased incidence of fractures in middle-aged and elderly men with low intakes of phosphorus and zinc. *Osteoporos Int* 1998, 8(4):333-340.

[82] Relea P, Revilla M, Ripoll E, Arribas I, Villa LF, Rico H: Zinc, biochemical markers of nutrition, and type I osteoporosis. *Age Ageing* 1995, 24(4):303-307.

[83] Atik OS: Zinc and senile osteoporosis. *J Am Geriatr Soc* 1983, 31(12):790-791.

[84] Mutlu M, Argun M, Kilic E, Saraymen R, Yazar S: Magnesium, zinc and copper status in osteoporotic, osteopenic and normal post-menopausal women. *J Int Med Res* 2007, 35(5):692-695.

[85] Strause L, Saltman P, Smith KT, Bracker M, Andon MB: Spinal bone loss in postmenopausal women supplemented with calcium and trace minerals. *J Nutr* 1994, 124(7):1060-1064.

[86] Peretz A, Papadopoulos T, Willems D, Hotimsky A, Michiels N, Siderova V, Bergmann P, Neve J: Zinc supplementation increases bone alkaline phosphatase in healthy men. *J Trace Elem Med Biol* 2001, 15(2-3):175-178.

[87] Nielsen FH, Milne DB: A moderately high intake compared to a low intake of zinc depresses magnesium balance and alters indices of bone turnover in postmenopausal women. *Eur J Clin Nutr* 2004, 58(5):703-710.

[88] Conlan D, Korula R, Tallentire D: Serum copper levels in elderly patients with femoral-neck fractures. *Age Ageing* 1990, 19(3):212-214.

[89] Eaton-Evans J, Mellwrath EM, Jackson WE, McCartney H, Strain JJ: Copper supplementation and the maintenance of bone mineral density in middle-aged women. *J Trace Elem Exp Med* 1996, 9:87-94.

[90] Baker A, Turley E, Bonham MP, O'Connor JM, Strain JJ, Flynn A, Cashman KD: No effect of copper supplementation on biochemical markers of bone metabolism in healthy adults. *Br J Nutr* 1999, 82(4):283-290.

[91] Cashman KD, Baker A, Ginty F, Flynn A, Strain JJ, Bonham MP, O'Connor JM, Bugel S, Sandstrom B: No effect of copper supplementation on biochemical markers of bone metabolism in healthy young adult females despite apparently improved copper status. *Eur J Clin Nutr* 2001, 55(7):525-531.

[92] Nielsen FH, Hunt CD, Mullen LM, Hunt JR: Effect of dietary boron on mineral, estrogen, and testosterone metabolism in postmenopausal women. *FASEB J* 1987, 1(5):394-397.

[93] Beattie JH, Peace HS: The influence of a low-boron diet and boron supplementation on bone, major mineral and sex steroid metabolism in postmenopausal women. *Br J Nutr* 1993, 69(3):871-884.

[94] Hunt CD, Herbel JL, Idso JP: Dietary boron modifies the effects of vitamin D3 nutrition on indices of energy substrate utilization and mineral metabolism in the chick. *J Bone Miner Res* 1994, 9(2):171-182.

[95] Ilich-Ernst JZ, McKenna AA, Badenhop NE, Clairmont AC, Andon MB, Nahhas RW, Goel P, Matkovic V: Iron status, menarche, and calcium supplementation in adolescent girls. *Am J Clin Nutr* 1998, 68(4):880-887.

[96] Dahl SG, Allain P, Marie PJ, Mauras Y, Boivin G, Ammann P, Tsouderos Y, Delmas PD, Christiansen C: Incorporation and distribution of strontium in bone. *Bone* 2001, 28(4):446-453.

[97] Meunier PJ: Strontium ranelate: new therapeutic agent for postmenopausal osteoporosis. *Med Sci (Paris)* 2004, 20(6-7):631-633.

[98] Seeman E, Devogelaer JP, Lorenc R, Spector T, Brixen K, Balogh A, Stucki G, Reginster JY: Strontium ranelate reduces the risk of vertebral fractures in patients with osteopenia. *J Bone Miner Res* 2008, 23(3):433-438.

[99] O'Donnell S, Cranney A, Wells GA, Adachi JD, Reginster JY: Strontium ranelate for preventing and treating postmenopausal osteoporosis. *Cochrane Database Syst Rev* 2006, (4)(4):CD005326.

[100] Jugdaohsingh R: Silicon and bone health. *J Nutr Health Aging* 2007, 11(2):99-110.

[101] Jugdaohsingh R, Tucker KL, Qiao N, Cupples LA, Kiel DP, Powell JJ: Dietary silicon intake is positively associated with bone mineral density in men and premenopausal women of the Framingham Offspring cohort. *J Bone Miner Res* 2004, 19(2):297-307.

[102] New SA, MacDonald HM, Campbell MK, Martin JC, Garton MJ, Robins SP, Reid DM: Lower estimates of net endogenous non-carbonic acid production are positively associated with indexes of bone health in premenopausal and perimenopausal women. *Am J Clin Nutr* 2004, 79(1):131-138.

[103] Macdonald HM, New SA, Fraser WD, Campbell MK, Reid DM: Low dietary potassium intakes and high dietary estimates of net endogenous acid production are associated with low bone mineral density in premenopausal women and increased markers of bone resorption in postmenopausal women. *Am J Clin Nutr* 2005, 81(4):923-933.

[104] Zhu K, Devine A, Prince RL: The effects of high potassium consumption on bone mineral density in a prospective cohort study of elderly postmenopausal women. *Osteoporos Int* 2008,

[105] Sebastian A, Morris RC,Jr: Improved mineral balance and skeletal metabolism in postmenopausal women treated with potassium bicarbonate. *N Engl J Med* 1994, 331(4):279.

[106] Lemann J,Jr, Pleuss JA, Gray RW, Hoffmann RG: Potassium administration reduces and potassium deprivation increases urinary calcium excretion in healthy adults [corrected. *Kidney Int* 1991, 39(5):973-983.

[107] Lemann J,Jr, Pleuss JA, Gray RW: Potassium causes calcium retention in healthy adults. *J Nutr* 1993, 123(9):1623-1626.

[108] Booth SL, Tucker KL, Chen H, Hannan MT, Gagnon DR, Cupples LA, Wilson PW, Ordovas J, Schaefer EJ, Dawson-Hughes B, Kiel DP: Dietary vitamin K intakes are associated with hip fracture but not with bone mineral density in elderly men and women. *Am J Clin Nutr* 2000, 71(5):1201-1208.

[109] Sakhaee K, Maalouf NM, Abrams SA, Pak CY: Effects of potassium alkali and calcium supplementation on bone turnover in postmenopausal women. *J Clin Endocrinol Metab* 2005, 90(6):3528-3533.

[110] Feskanich D, Weber P, Willett WC, Rockett H, Booth SL, Colditz GA: Vitamin K intake and hip fractures in women: a prospective study. *Am J Clin Nutr* 1999, 69(1):74-79.

[111] Booth SL, Broe KE, Gagnon DR, Tucker KL, Hannan MT, McLean RR, Dawson-Hughes B, Wilson PW, Cupples LA, Kiel DP: Vitamin K intake and bone mineral density in women and men. *Am J Clin Nutr* 2003, 77(2):512-516.

[112] Szulc P, Chapuy MC, Meunier PJ, Delmas PD: Serum undercarboxylated osteocalcin is a marker of the risk of hip fracture: a three year follow-up study. *Bone* 1996, 18(5):487-488.

[113] Luukinen H, Kakonen SM, Pettersson K, Koski K, Laippala P, Lovgren T, Kivela SL, Vaananen HK: Strong prediction of fractures among older adults by the ratio of carboxylated to total serum osteocalcin. *J Bone Miner Res* 2000, 15(12):2473-2478.

[114] Szulc P, Arlot M, Chapuy MC, Duboeuf F, Meunier PJ, Delmas PD: Serum undercarboxylated osteocalcin correlates with hip bone mineral density in elderly women. *J Bone Miner Res* 1994, 9(10):1591-1595.

[115] Cockayne S, Adamson J, Lanham-New S, Shearer MJ, Gilbody S, Torgerson DJ: Vitamin K and the prevention of fractures: systematic review and meta-analysis of randomized controlled trials. *Arch Intern Med* 2006, 166(12):1256-1261.

[116] Booth SL, Dallal G, Shea MK, Gundberg C, Peterson JW, Dawson-Hughes B: Effect of vitamin K supplementation on bone loss in elderly men and women. *J Clin Endocrinol Metab* 2008, 93(4):1217-1223.

[117] Bolton-Smith C, McMurdo ME, Paterson CR, Mole PA, Harvey JM, Fenton ST, Prynne CJ, Mishra GD, Shearer MJ: Two-year randomized controlled trial of vitamin K1 (phylloquinone) and vitamin D3 plus calcium on the bone health of older women. *J Bone Miner Res* 2007, 22(4):509-519.

[118] Kruger MC, Booth CL, Coad J, Schollum LM, Kuhn-Sherlock B, Shearer MJ: Effect of calcium fortified milk supplementation with or without vitamin K on biochemical markers of bone turnover in premenopausal women. *Nutrition* 2006, 22(11-12):1120-1128.

[119] Bugel S, Sorensen AD, Hels O, Kristensen M, Vermeer C, Jakobsen J, Flynn A, Molgaard C, Cashman KD: Effect of phylloquinone supplementation on biochemical markers of vitamin K status and bone turnover in postmenopausal women. *Br J Nutr* 2007, 97(2):373-380.

[120] Hall SL, Greendale GA: The relation of dietary vitamin C intake to bone mineral density: results from the PEPI study. *Calcif Tissue Int* 1998, 63(3):183-189.

[121] Morton DJ, Barrett-Connor EL, Schneider DL: Vitamin C supplement use and bone mineral density in postmenopausal women. *J Bone Miner Res* 2001, 16(1):135-140.

[122] Leveille SG, LaCroix AZ, Koepsell TD, Beresford SA, Van Belle G, Buchner DM: Dietary vitamin C and bone mineral density in postmenopausal women in Washington State, USA. *J Epidemiol Community Health* 1997, 51(5):479-485.

[123] Melhus H, Michaelsson K, Kindmark A, Bergstrom R, Holmberg L, Mallmin H, Wolk A, Ljunghall S: Excessive dietary intake of vitamin A is associated with reduced bone mineral density and increased risk for hip fracture. *Ann Intern Med* 1998, 129(10):770-778.

[124] Michaelsson K, Lithell H, Vessby B, Melhus H: Serum retinol levels and the risk of fracture. *N Engl J Med* 2003, 348(4):287-294.

[125] Promislow JH, Goodman-Gruen D, Slymen DJ, Barrett-Connor E: Retinol intake and bone mineral density in the elderly: the Rancho Bernardo Study. *J Bone Miner Res* 2002, 17(8):1349-1358.

[126] Opotowsky AR, Bilezikian JP, NHANES I follow-up study: Serum vitamin A concentration and the risk of hip fracture among women 50 to 74 years old in the United States: a prospective analysis of the NHANES I follow-up study. *Am J Med* 2004, 117(3):169-174.

[127] Crandall C: Vitamin A intake and osteoporosis: a clinical review. *J Womens Health (Larchmt)* 2004, 13(8):939-953.

[128] Barker ME, McCloskey E, Saha S, Gossiel F, Charlesworth D, Powers HJ, Blumsohn A: Serum retinoids and beta-carotene as predictors of hip and other fractures in elderly women. *J Bone Miner Res* 2005, 20(6):913-920.

[129] Shono N, Kugino K, Yoshida S, Nakayama M, Ueno H, Nishizumi M: Bone mineral density by ultrasonic measurement in pre- and postmenopausal women--relationship with sex hormones and nutritional states. *Nippon Eiseigaku Zasshi* 1997, 51(4):755-762.

[130] Sasaki S, Yanagibori R: Association between current nutrient intakes and bone mineral density at calcaneus in pre- and postmenopausal Japanese women. *J Nutr Sci Vitaminol* (Tokyo) 2001, 47(4):289-294.

[131] Lumbers M, New SA, Gibson S, Murphy MC: Nutritional status in elderly female hip fracture patients: comparison with an age-matched home living group attending day centres. *Br J Nutr* 2001, 85(6):733-740.

[132] Freudenheim JL, Johnson NE, Smith EL: Relationships between usual nutrient intake and bone-mineral content of women 35-65 years of age: longitudinal and cross-sectional analysis. *Am J Clin Nutr* 1986, 44(6):863-876.

[133] Gjesdal CG, Vollset SE, Ueland PM, Refsum H, Meyer HE, Tell GS: Plasma homocysteine, folate, and vitamin B 12 and the risk of hip fracture: the hordaland homocysteine study. *J Bone Miner Res* 2007, 22(5):747-756.

[134] Dhonukshe-Rutten RA, Lips M, de Jong N, Chin A Paw MJ, Hiddink GJ, van Dusseldorp M, De Groot LC, van Staveren WA: Vitamin B-12 status is associated with bone mineral content and bone mineral density in frail elderly women but not in men. *J Nutr* 2003, 133(3):801-807.

[135] Tucker KL, Hannan MT, Qiao N, Jacques PF, Selhub J, Cupples LA, Kiel DP: Low plasma vitamin B12 is associated with lower BMD: the Framingham Osteoporosis Study. *J Bone Miner Res* 2005, 20(1):152-158.

[136] Dawson-Hughes B, Fowler SE, Dalsky G, Gallagher C: Sodium excretion influences calcium homeostasis in elderly men and women. *J Nutr* 1996, 126(9):2107-2112.

[137] Jones G, Beard T, Parameswaran V, Greenaway T, von Witt R: A population-based study of the relationship between salt intake, bone resorption and bone mass. *Eur J Clin Nutr* 1997, 51(8):561-565.

[138] Goulding A: Fasting urinary sodium/creatinine in relation to calcium/creatinine and hydroxyproline/creatinine in a general population of women. *N Z Med J* 1981, 93(683):294-297.

[139] Zarkadas M, Gougeon-Reyburn R, Marliss EB, Block E, Alton-Mackey M: Sodium chloride supplementation and urinary calcium excretion in postmenopausal women. *Am J Clin Nutr* 1989, 50(5):1088-1094.

[140] Evans CE, Chughtai AY, Blumsohn A, Giles M, Eastell R: The effect of dietary sodium on calcium metabolism in premenopausal and postmenopausal women. *Eur J Clin Nutr* 1997, 51(6):394-399.

[141] Lietz G, Avenell A, Robins SP: Short-term effects of dietary sodium intake on bone metabolism in postmenopausal women measured using urinary deoxypyridinoline excretion. *Br J Nutr* 1997, 78(1):73-82.

[142] Ginty F, Flynn A, Cashman KD: The effect of dietary sodium intake on biochemical markers of bone metabolism in young women. *Br J Nutr* 1998, 79(4):343-350.

[143] Teucher B, Dainty JR, Spinks CA, Majsak-Newman G, Berry DJ, Hoogewerff JA, Foxall RJ, Jakobsen J, Cashman KD, Flynn A, Fairweather-Tait SJ: Sodium and Bone Health: The Impact of Moderately High and Low Salt Intakes on Calcium Metabolism in Postmenopausal Women. *J Bone Miner Res* 2008, .

[144] Devine A, Criddle RA, Dick IM, Kerr DA, Prince RL: A longitudinal study of the effect of sodium and calcium intakes on regional bone density in postmenopausal women. *Am J Clin Nutr* 1995, 62(4):740-745.

[145] Kiel DP, Felson DT, Hannan MT, Anderson JJ, Wilson PW: Caffeine and the risk of hip fracture: the Framingham Study. *Am J Epidemiol* 1990, 132(4):675-684.

[146] Barger-Lux MJ, Heaney RP, Stegman MR: Effects of moderate caffeine intake on the calcium economy of premenopausal women. *Am J Clin Nutr* 1990, 52(4):722-725.

[147] Harris SS, Dawson-Hughes B: Caffeine and bone loss in healthy postmenopausal women. Am J Clin Nutr 1994, 60(4):573-578.

[148] Standing Committee on the Scientific Evaluation of Dietary Reference Intakes,Food and Nutrition board,Institute of Medicine,: *Dietary Reference Intakes for Energy, Carbohydrate, Fiber, Fat, Fatty Acids, Cholesterol, Protein, and Amino Acids* Washington, DC: National Academy Press; 2005.

[149] Wright JD, Wang CY, Kennedy-Stephenson J, Ervin RB: Dietary intake of ten key nutrients for public health, United States: 1999-2000. *Adv Data* 2003, (334)(334):1-4.

[150] Nieves JW, Komar L, Cosman F, Lindsay R: Calcium potentiates the effect of estrogen and calcitonin on bone mass: review and analysis. *Am J Clin Nutr* 1998, 67(1):18-24.

[151] Dure-Smith BA, Farley SM, Linkhart SG, Farley JR, Baylink DJ: Calcium deficiency in fluoride-treated osteoporotic patients despite calcium supplementation. *J Clin Endocrinol Metab* 1996, 81(1):269-275.

[152] Ford ES, Mokdad AH: Dietary magnesium intake in a national sample of US adults. *J Nutr* 2003, 133(9):2879-2882.

[153] Bischoff-Ferrari HA, Willett WC, Wong JB, Giovannucci E, Dietrich T, Dawson-Hughes B: Fracture prevention with vitamin D supplementation: a meta-analysis of randomized controlled trials. *JAMA* 2005, 293(18):2257-2264.

[154] Heaney RP, Davies KM, Chen TC, Holick MF, Barger-Lux MJ: Human serum 25-hydroxycholecalciferol response to extended oral dosing with cholecalciferol. *Am J Clin Nutr* 2003, 77(1):204-210.

[155] Heaney RP, Dowell MS, Hale CA, Bendich A: Calcium absorption varies within the reference range for serum 25-hydroxyvitamin D. *J Am Coll Nutr* 2003, 22(2):142-146.

[156] Holick MF: Sunlight and vitamin D for bone health and prevention of autoimmune diseases, cancers, and cardiovascular disease. *Am J Clin Nutr* 2004, 80(6 Suppl):1678S-88S.

[157] Grant AM, Avenell A, Campbell MK, McDonald AM, MacLennan GS, McPherson GC, Anderson FH, Cooper C, Francis RM, Donaldson C, Gillespie WJ, Robinson CM, Torgerson DJ, Wallace WA, RECORD Trial Group: Oral vitamin D3 and calcium for secondary prevention of low-trauma fractures in elderly people (Randomised Evaluation of Calcium Or vitamin D, RECORD): a randomised placebo-controlled trial. *Lancet* 2005, 365(9471):1621-1628.

[158] Standing Committee on the Scientific Evaluation of Dietary Reference Intakes,Food and Nutrition board,Institute of Medicine,: *Dietary Reference Intakes for Vitamin A, Vitamin K, Arsenic, Boron, Chromium, Copper, Iodine, Iron, Manganese, Molybdenum, Nickel, Silicon, Vanadium, and Zinc:* Washington, DC: National Academy Press; 2000.

[159] Jugdaohsingh R, Anderson SH, Tucker KL, Elliott H, Kiel DP, Thompson RP, Powell JJ: Dietary silicon intake and absorption. *Am J Clin Nutr* 2002, 75(5):887-893.

[160] Standing Committee on the Scientific Evaluation of Dietary Reference Intakes,Food and Nutrition board,Institute of Medicine,: *Dietary Reference Intakes for Vitamin C, Vitamin E, Selenium, and Carotenoids:* Washington, DC: National Academy Press; 2000.

[161] Heaney RP: In *Calcium in Human Health.* Edited by Weaver CM, Heaney RP. Totowa, NJ.: Humana Press; 2005:

In: Osteoporosis: Etiology, Diagnosis and Treatment
Editors: Bilar E. Mattingly and Albert C. Pillare
ISBN 978-1-60692-397-9

Chapter 4

A NARRATIVE REVIEW OF GLUCOCORTICOID-INDUCED BONE LOSS

Ionnis Ilias[1], Konstantinos Michalakis[1] and Salvatore Alesci[2]
[1]Elena Venizelou Hospital, Athens, Greece;
[2]Wyeth Research, Discovery Transplantational Medicine, Collegeville PA-19426, USA.

ABSTRACT

In this chapter we discuss the epidemiology, pathogenesis and management of glucocorticoid-induced osteoporosis. One third to almost half of patients with endogenous or exogenous hypercortisolemia (particularly patients affected by rheumatoid arthritis and treated with synthetic glucocorticoids) presents bone loss. Trabecular bones (such as the ribs and vertebral bodies) are more affected but corical bones (such as the upper femur) are not spared. Bone turnover markers and assessments of bone mineral density (BMD) assist in the evaluation of bone loss. Glucocorticoids stimulate bone resorption and suppress bone formation. Even during the first few months after glucocorticoid administration bone loss is rapid. Nevertheless, only few patients on steroids receive prophylaxis or treatment for glucocorticoid-induced bone loss,which is required even when BMD measurements point to osteopenia (a milder form of bone loss) rather than osteoporosis. Lifestyle changes, calcium and vitamin D, bisphosphonates, are currently standard therapy for most cases of glucocorticoid-induced osteoporosis. Recent studies indicate that parathyroid hormone (PTH) might also offer a valid therapeutic option.

INTRODUCTION AND EPIDEMIOLOGY

In adults aged 20 to 45 years, glucocorticoid (GC) administration is the most common cause of osteoporosis (OP) [1,2]. Bone loss may occur with or without other manifestations and its severity is dependent on both the dose and duration of GC treatment [3]. In a retrospective study done in the United Kingdom the prevalence of chronic use of oral GCs in the general population was 0.5%, although the prevalence was higher in women over 55 years (1.7%) and reached 2.5% in subjects older than 70 years [4,5]. Interestingly, only 4%-14% of patients on oral steroids were given treatment for osteoporosis, thus pointing to a likely underestimation of GCOP [4]. Bone loss is observed in up to 30-50% of patients with GC excess (either endogenous -caused by Cushing's syndrome - or iatrogenic – caused by exogenous GC therapy) [6-8]. One way to assess future bone loss is by measuring daily GC dosage, although cumulative GC dose (g/year) is more predictive for this purpose [9,10]. A total dose greater than 30 g of prednisone per year is associated with a very high incidence of OP (78%) and fractures (53%)

Bone loss begins a few weeks after GC treatment and is rapid in the first few months, continuing at a slower rate after a year of treatment(GC dose attenuation, or development of some degree of tolerance to GCs may be implicated) [11,12].

Fractures occur in 30% to 50% of patients taking GCs [13-15]; fractures may occur at lower bone mineral density (BMD) values compared to postmenopausal women with OP [15-17]. Patients with rheumatoid arthritis on GCs manifest higher fracture rates compared to age-matched controls [18]. However, fracture thresholds in patients with asthma or autoimmune diseases treated with GCs are higher than in postmenopausal women [19,20]. Yet, in another study patients treated with GCs had the same incidence of fractures when compared to BMD-matched controls [21]. Thus, there is no consensus on whether GC treatment may favor fractures. In retrospective cohort studies of oral corticosteroid users and matched controls the relative risk of fractures on oral GCs ranged from 1.61 to 2.63 [22]. Fracture risk was higher in patients taking higher doses of GCs and returned to baseline values after terminating treatment [10,22].

Cofactors Contributing to GCOP

Various factors can add to the effects of GC on bone loss: irreversible causes, such as race, sex, advancing age, menopausal status, family history of OP and fractures and secondary causes of OP, such as hyperthyroidism, hyperparathyroidism, rheumatoid arthritis and renal failure [23]. Modifiable risk factors for GCOP include low calcium and high sodium intake [24], decreased daily physical activity/immobilization, high caffeine intake (when calcium intake is low) [25], and tobacco and alcohol use [23,26,27]. The effect of GC on BMD may be influenced or worsened by other co-administered medications (i.e., as methotrexate, cyclosporine, heparin, medroxyprogesterone acetate, GnRH analogs, levothyroxine, anticonvulsants) or radiotherapy. In adult women with classical congenital adrenal hyperplasia (CAH) that are treated chronically with high GCs doses, BMD may be low, possibly due to the iatrogenic suppression of adrenal androgens [28]. Postmenopausal women on GCs have more fractures than premenopausal women (because of already lower bone mass when starting GC therapy) [15,29]. Bone loss is more rapid in young men treated with GCs than in older men, premenopausal or postmenopausal women.Patients with sarcoidosis and those on steroids to prevent post-transplantation heart or kidney rejection, are also more prone to show rapid bone loss [30-32].

Although ccumulative GC dose is thought to be the determinant of bone loss, some patients on a low GC dose show increased bone loss compared to others on a higher GC dose [33]. This, may in part be due to genetic differences. Indeed, a polymorphism in the glucocorticoid receptor (GR) gene leads to increased *in vivo* sensitivity to GCs (these individuals are heterozygous for a polymorphism at nucleotide 1,220, resulting in an Asparagine-to-Serine change at codon 360) [34,35].

BIOLOGICAL AND MOLECULAR SKELETAL MECHANISMS OF GCOP

The effects GCs are more prominent on trabecular bones and the cortical rim of vertebral bodies, whereas the cortical component of long bones (radius, humerus) is less affected. [36-39]. Consistently, in patients on GC therapy, lumbar BMD shows significantly lower values than at the distal radius, and bone loss is also noted in the proximal femur (particularly at the trabecular bone-rich Ward's triangle) [40,41]. After prolonged GC administration, cortical bone becomes increasingly affected and long bones become more fragile as well.

Decreased trabecular volume, increased bone resorption and a decline in bone formation are noted in bone biopsies of patients on GCs for more than one year: bone tissue loss is more prominent in the metaphyses than in the diaphyses [13,42,43]. GCOP differs from post-menopausal OP in its microanatomical appearance: in the former the number of trabeculae and their surface area are relatively preserved, and individual plates are very thin (trabecular attenuation), whereas in the latter trabecular width is relatively preserved but in the lamellae a loss of trabecular surface and continuity is observed [44].

Formation of the GC-GR complex leads to activation or repression of target gene expression. Activation requires binding of a dimerized receptors to GC-responsive elements (GREs) in the promoters of target genes; repression results from interaction between GR monomers and transcription factors [45]. The translation of GR mRNAs produces two GR isoforms, GRα (which is transcriptionally active) and GRβ, which heterodimerizes with GRα and inhibits its transcriptional activity [46]. Normal human osteoblasts show GRα expression, while osteoclasts do not express GRα (since thay predominatly express GRβ). Both osteoblasts and osteoclasts also express mineralocorticoid receptors (MRs) that bind to cortisol and form heterodimers with both GRα and GRβ [47]. At physiologic concentrations cortisol modulates negatively the secretion of interleukin-11 (IL-11), which in turn decreases GR expression [48]. Another cytokine, IL-6, upregulates the number of GRs in human osteoblasts [49,50]. Thus, cytokines seem to modulate bone sensitivity to GCs through autocrine/paracrine loops [51].

Apoptosis of osteoblasts and mature osteocyte is increased by GCs via activation of caspase 3 [52-54]. This apoptotic process may involve decreased expression of the Bcl-2 gene and increased expression of the Bax gene [55]. GCs may induce repression of bone morphogenic protein-2 (BMP-2); they may also induce expression of core binding factor a1 (Cbfa1) and reduce osteoblast differentiation [55]. GCs also modify the expression of osteoblast-specific genes, such as osteocalcin. During bone development, osteocalcin expression is tightly regulated by GCs, and multiple GREs have been identified on the human and rat osteocalcin promoter region [56,57]. Many facets of bone metabolism (osteoblast differentiation and function, bone development and peak bone mass) are mediated by the Wnt signaling pathway [58]. This pathway may be related to the response to mechanical loading [58]; GC-induced inhibition of skeletal growth may be mediated by their effects on Wnt signaling [59].

Bone matrix formation [60,61] is inhibited by GCs since they increase the synthesis of collagenase 3 (or MMP-13; a metalloproteinase that cleaves collagen fibrils) and suppress the synthesis of β-1 integrin and type I collagen (major components of the matrix).

The effects of GCs on osteoclasts are not well studied since osteoclast isolation from bone is technically difficult. Transgenic mouse technology has allowed the generation of two osteoclastic cell lines [62]. Contrary to older studies, more recent research indicates that GCs may stimulate bone resorption [63-65]. Although GCs stimulate osteoclast differentiation by altering the expression of N-acetylglucosamine and N-acetylgalactosamine [66] they cannot affect directly the bone-resorbing activity of mature osteoclasts (since these cells do not appear to have functional GRs) [67]. In subjects with lower BMD, higher expression of the GR gene may increase their monocytes'/macrophages' sensitivity to differentiate into osteoclasts [68].

GCs inhibit the production of IL-1 and IL-6 (that inhibit bone formation and induce bone resorption) and TGF-β (which inhibits IL-1-induced bone resorption and stimulates osteoblast activity) [69-73]. GCs increase the expression of receptor activator of the nuclear factor-κB ligand (RANKL) and colony-stimulating factor-1 (CSF-1) but they also lower osteoprotegerin (OPG) expression in human preosteoblasts or osteoblasts [51,74,75]. The net result is an increase in RANKL/OPG ratio, leading to osteoclast differentiation and bone resorption [76].

Insulin-like growth factors (IGFs)–I and –II increase osteoblast replication, type I collagen synthesis and matrix apposition rates, and decrease collagenase-3 (metalloproteinase-13) expression by osteoblasts [77,78]. GCs decrease synthesis of IGF-I and IGF-II receptor expression in osteoblasts [79-81].

Hepatocyte growth factor (HGF) is produced by both osteoblasts and osteoclasts, stimulating osteoblastic function and suppressing bone resorption [82,83]. GCs inhibits HGF release *in vitro* [84,85].

Prostaglandins (PGs; and PGE_2 in particular) stimulate bone collagen and non-collagen protein synthesis [86-88]. PGs inhibit directly the activity of isolated osteoclasts and increase bone resorption (apparently via promotion of osteoclastogenesis). GCs interfere with the production of PGE_2, by decreasing the expression of cyclooxygenases (that convert arachidonic acid into PGs and more particularly inducible prostaglandin synthase-2; PGHS-2) [89,90].

Extraskeletal Mechanisms of GCOP

GCs impair intestinal calcium absorption [91-98]. Acting directly on bowel mucosa, high doses of GCs (>10 mg prednisolone/day) not only decrease calcium absorption but cause secondary hyperparathyroidism and elevation of plasma $1,25(OH)_2$ vitamin D [99]. Patients on GCs have increased renal calcium loss [100]. Thus, hypercalciouria in patients with Cushing's syndrome may be due either to increased bone resorption or decreased renal tubular reabsorption. On long-term GC therapy, hypercalciuria is most likely due to increased skeletal mobilization of calcium and decreased renal tubular reabsorption. GC-induced decreases in bone formation lower calcium uptake by newly formed bone and elevate the filtered load of calcium. .

GCs also lower tubular reabsorption of phosphate (inducing secondary hyperparathyroidism) and decrease phosphate uptake in the proximal tubule (resulting in increased acid secretion and phosphaturia) [101-103].

Apart from GC-induced secondary hyperparathyroidism, a direct stimulatory effect of GCs on PTH secretion may exist; in fact, chronic GC administration reduces the tonic secretion of PTH and increases its pulses while responses to PTH may be increased by GCs [101,104-106].

GCs inhibit gonadotropin secretion but also may act directly on the gonads (there is a GC-responsive upstream promoter region in the cholesterol side-chain cleavage gene) [107]. High-dose GC therapy in men or women may lower sex steroid production [108-110], while in postmenopausal women the effect of GC superimposes on that of estrogen deficiency vis-à-vis bone loss [111,112].

Growth hormone (GH) increases bone formation (via direct interaction with GH receptors on osteoblasts and through induction of endocrine and autocrine/paracrine IGF-I) [113]. In patients with GCOP a lower GH response to growth hormone–releasing hormone (GHRH) and a positive correlation between GH increment and osteocalcin are observed. Through an upregulatory effect on GH receptor, bone sensitivity to GH may be reduced by GCs [114].

GC-induced myopathy is attributed to increased protein catabolism and inhibition of glycogen synthesis. The association between steroid myopathy and OP is strong [115]. Muscle biopsies of GC-treated patients show selective atrophy of type IIa muscle fibers, along with a relative increase in the number of type IIb fibers and a decrease in the number of type I fibers [116-118].

Diagnosis of GCOP

All patients on long-term GC treatment should be suspected as suffering from GCOP. Bone loss depends on the dose, route and duration of GC administration [119-121]. Postmenopausal women, transplant recipients and patients with sarcoidosis have a high risk for GCOP [119-123].

When first examining the patient, special care should be given to cushingoid clinical features, including skin atrophy with increased fragility and ecchymoses, truncal obesity, fluid retention, hyperglycemia, and symptoms of vertebral compression and myopathy. Brief exposure to GCs may trigger myopathy that is not always dose-dependent, and may be difficult to differentiate from inflammatory myopathy. Myalgias or abrupt proximal muscle weakness can be characteristics of myopathy [115]. In the laboratory work-up of GC myopathy, creatinuria is noted whereas creatine kinase, aspartate aminotransferase and aldolase may be normal [115,116].

Another issue for potential evaluation is gonadal function. Both men and women on long-term GCs often may be hypogonadic, presenting with decreased libido and sexual activity and/or infertility. In premenopausal women menstrual cycle regularity should be assessed.

Apart from clinical evaluation, laboratory evaluation for GCOP should include total blood cell count, markers of renal and liver function, serum electrophoresis, serum and 24-hour urine calcium, serum levels of 25-hydroxyvitamin D, alkaline phosphatase, parathyormone, estradiol (in women), total and free testosterone (in men) and thyroid-stimulating hormone [119-121,124].

A dose-dependent decrease in serum osteocalcin is found in patients receiving GCs; this is a good indicator of the degree of inhibition of osteoblastic activity [125,126]. Other markers of bone formation (including procollagen type I carboxy-propeptide and total and bone specific alkaline phosphatase) are also lower under GC therapy [127,128]. Baseline levels of osteocalcin do not always correlate with subsequent bone loss under GC therapy [129-131]. In some studies, markers of bone resorption (like urinary collagen N-telopeptides [NTX]) are high [102,132-134]. Thus, the measurement of serum markers of bone formation and resorption is not so helpful, and may not be advised for all patients in clinical routine [123].

Dual-energy X-ray absorptiometry (DEXA) and less often quantitative computed tomography (QCT) are used for the imaging evaluation of GCOP; vertebral compression fractures are detected by classic X-ray studies. Although both DEXA and QCT can measure cortical and trabecular bone density, the latter is used to evaluate solely trabecular bone density [135,136]. DEXA also helps estimate the fracture risk, and judges the efficacy of treatment (with minimal irradiation dose) [124,137,138]. BMD measurment techniques that focus on the vertebral body and exclude the cortical bone of posterior processes, such as lateral DEXA scanning, are more sensitive in detecting GCOP [39,139]. However, the selection of a BMD assessment method is influenced by the presence of vertebral deformities, osteophytes, or of calcifications in the aorta. In case of marked osteophytosis or scoliosis of the spine, proximal femoral densitometry (in the femoral neck) should be preferred [40].

Whether subjects with GCOP suffer fractures at a higher threshold of BMD compared to those affected by age-related or postmenopausal OP, is a field of debate [19,21]. The American College of Rheumatology (ACR) has defined the T-score cut off to – 1.0 SD [121], whereas a T-score threshold value of – 1.5 SD is usually the cutoff for GCOP in Europe [4]. The ACR recommends BMD baseline measurements at the lumbar spine and/or hip before starting any GC treatment longer than 6 months [121]. Follow-up measurements should be done at 6-month intervals from the baseline assessment or at 12 month intervals if the patient is receiving therapy to prevent bone loss [140]. For patients on chronic treatment with GC doses higher than 7.5 mg/day of prednisolone or equivalent, Medicare approves regular BMD evaluation [141].

The data available for evaluation of bone loss in GC-treated patients with quantitative ultrasound (QU) evaluations at the heel and hand phalanges are very limited [142,143].

MANAGEMENT OF GCOP

Prevention of GCOP

Guidelines for the prevention and treatment of GCOP from the ACR [121] are made available by the UK Consensus group in Management of GCOP [140], the Belgian Bone Club [144] and the Spanish Society of Internal Medicine [145]. Although 0,5% of the general population and 2% of medical outpatients received prolonged steroid therapy at some time, only a minority are considered for medical meausures to prevent GCOP [146]. Prevention of GCOP should start as soon as GCs are administered. Apart from specialized guidelines regarding the tolerability of GCs, general measures include: sufficient nutrition with adequate dietary calcium and vitamin D intake [147], encouragement of appropriate physical activity (30 minute - 3 times per week), restriction of tobacco use (tobacco has anti-osteoblastic activity), alcohol cessation (although social use of 1 glass of wine/day may be of some benefit), management of factors predisposing to falls (eye disease, neurologic diseases, cardiac arrhythmias, seizures or strokes).

As noted above, bone loss is more rapid in the first months of GC therapy. The minimal effective GC dose should be used, with the option of alternate-day therapy to preserve the normal response of the hypothalamo-pituitary-adrenal axis and avoid down regulation of GC receptors. GCs with shorter half-life topical or inhaled preparations (whenever possible) should be preferred. The choice of the lowest GC dose is based on common sense and depends on the individual practitioner's decision [148]. Grossly, there is no real evidence-based indication of a precise dose of GC in the numerous conditions necessitating this therapy, even though many recommendations exist.

The issue a "safe dose" when treating with oral GCs is controversial [17]. Prednisone given at low doses (5-9 mg/d) may affect BMD whereas lower doses (1-4 mg/d) have very little or no effect [149]. Nevertheless, a single oral dose of 2.5 mg of prednisone has an almost immediate negative effect on osteocalcin secretion [150]. Alternate-day GC administration may prevent growth retardation in children less than a daily regimen but not bone loss [33,147,151]. Because rates of bone loss are greater in the first few months of glucocorticoid administration, treatment for periods as short as 3 months, may result in increased fracture risk and thus the need for prevention of bone loss and fractures should be carefully assessed in this situation [147].

Several trials have attempted to define the relationship between inhaled glucocorticoids (mainly in asthma and COPD patients) and the development of osteoporosis. Either because of study design defaults or because of the small number of participants, those studies have proven to be inadequate [152]. Nevertheless, increasing evidence seems to point towards a relationship between use of inhaled glucocorticoids and reduced BMD [153]. Inhaled GCs should be used in the lowest possible dose and for a short duration of therapy [152]. The newest inhaled GCs (such as budesonide), seem to have less adverse effects on the bone, as indicated by bone markers [154,155]. Dosing of inhaled GCs is important: beclomethasone dipropionate or budesonide given at low doses for more then one year did not affect spine BMD in asthmatic subjects [155]. However, patients treated with high doses of inhaled budesonide or beclomethasone (1.5 mg/day, for at least 12 months) and without prior oral GC treatment for more than 1 month, had a significant decrease in bone mineral density (BMD) and bone formation markers, with no changes in bone resorption markers [156]. In a recent study, inhaled GCs in adults with chronic pulmonary disease were not associated with increased fracture risk (and no dose-response relationship was naoted) [157]. Moreover, in children treated with beclomethasone for bronchial asthma, analysis after adjustment for the severity of the underlying disease did not show any association between inhaled GCs and fracture risk [158]. Consequently, in children, other factors, such as excess body weight, low muscle mass and limited exercise capacity may predispose to low BMD [159].

Treatment of GCOP

The aim should be to minimize bone loss, increase BMD and, at least partially, reverse the effects of GC excess. Treatment should be given for as long as GC therapy is administered.

Patients given GCs should receive supplementation with 1,500 mg/d of calcium and 800 IU/d of vitamin D (0.5-1 μg/day of α-calcidiol or 0.5 of μg/day calcitriol, 35-40 μg/d of calcidiol, 0,1 mg every other day of dihydrotachysterol) [121,160]. Active metabolites of vitamin D (α-calcidiol and calcitriol) are more effective than vitamin D in maintaining bone density during medium-to-high dose GC treatment [161-163]. Alfacalcidol (1.0 μg; plus 500 mg calcium/day) produced a larger increase in lumbar BMD than plain cholecalciferol (1000IU; plus 500 mg calcium/day), but no difference was observed on hip BMD or on fracture rate [164]. Treatment with active (more polar) forms of vitamin D may lead to hypercalciuria and hypercalcemia; consequently, periodic assessment of serum calcium and creatinine levels at the beginning of the therapy, after 2-4 weeks, and thereafter every 2-3 months is advised [165,166]. If adverse effects develop, the dose of activated vitamin D should be reduced [146]. Calcium and vitamin D alone, can reduce early bone loss, but to prevent a fracture, they should be used along with a bisphosphonate [167]. Thiazide diuretics lower urinary calcium excretion. Chronic treatment with thiazides decreased the incidence of hip fracture in elderly patients, and increased BMD in the general population [168-170]. Despite these findings, there are currently no studies to evaluate the long-term effect of thiazide diuretics on BMD in patients treated with GCs.

Bisphosphonates (such as alendronate, etidronate, pamidronate, ibandronate, clodronate or risedronate) are synthetic, stable pyrophosphate analogues that are potent inhibitors of bone resorption [152]. They decrease the resorptive activity of osteoclasts, increase osteoclast apoptosis and decrease osteoblast and osteocyte apoptosis [171]. They are effective preventing and treating GCOP [172]. Treatment with alendronate for 18/24 months increased total body BMD, and significantly decreased risk of vertebral fractures in patients taking GC [173,174]. In a one-year study with risedronate in patients taking prednisone (7.5 mg/day for at least 6 months) an increase in lumbar spine and femoral neck BMD and a 70% decrease in the relative risk of vertebral fractures was seen [175]. Cyclic etidronate (400 mg/day for 14 days every three months for one year) prevented bone loss in patients taking GCs for rheumatoid arthritis and polymyalgia rheumatica, and reversed OP in patients on chronic treatment with prednisone [176,177]. Both oral (150 mg/day) and intermittent i.v. (30 mg every three months for one year) pamidronate disodium increased BMD at the spine and the hip in patients starting long-term GC therapy [178,179]. Clodronate increased BMD in asthmatic patients treated with GCs [180]. Zoledronic acid (a long-acting potent bisphosphonate) given intravenously (4-10 mg once or twice a year) has excellent anti-OP results [181-186]. Drug toxicities were uncommon except a slight increase in non-serious upper GI adverse events. The oral use of these drugs is contraindicated in patients with esophageal motility problems and strictures. Alendronate (5 and 10 mg/day or 70 mg/week) and risedronate (5 mg/day or 35 mg/week) are recommended in the United States to treat men and postmenopausal women starting long-term GC treatment (≥ 5 mg/day) [121]. Ibandronate sodium is given once every month (at 150 mg); it increases BMD and lowers fracture risk similarly to alendronate given once weekly [187]. Published reports on the actions of ibandronate specifically in GCOP are not available.

Bisphosphonates should be used in conjunction with calcium and vitamin D supplementation in the following groups of patients [146]: patients in whom glucocorticoid therapy is newly initiated to prevent bone loss, patients receiving long term glucocorticoid therapy with documented osteoporosis on BMD or presence of osteoporotic fractures and patients on long term glucocortocoid therapy who have had fractures while on HRT or in whom HRT is not tolerated.

Although calcitonin (nasal or subcutaneous), reduces bone loss in patients treated with GCs for asthma or sarcoidosis and decreases OP-related pain [188,189] there is no evidence that it diminishes the risk of osteoporotic fractures. Calcitonin increases lumbar but not femoral neck BMD in patients receiving long term GC therapy [190]. Treatment with nasal calcitonin (200 IU/day) may be considered whenever bisphosphonates are contraindicated or not well tolerated, or in patients with fracture-associated pain (because of its analgesic effect) [148,191]. Other advantages of calcitonin include the non-oral administration (which may be important to patients that receive a lot of per os medications) [148]. Calcitonin is not recommended for prevention of bone loss in patients being initiated on GC treatment [146,152].

Although anabolic medications (sodium fluoride, strontium ranelate, anabolic steroids or recombinant PTH) enhances bone formation [148] most of the information on their use to prevent or treat GCOP comes from small studies. In GC-treated patients (on an average prednisone dose of 1522 mg/day) sodium fluoride (20-50mg/d), given along with calcium, vitamin D, or cyclic etidronate, improved lumbar spine BMD and trabecular bone volume but did not reduce the incidence of fractures; furthermore it induced bone loss at the femoral neck [192,193]. Thus, its use is currently not recommended for GCOP [121]. There are no published studies regarding strontium ranelate and GC-induced osteoporosis [148]. Anabolic steroids have been used for GCOP: cyclic nandrolone decanoate (50 mg i.m. every three weeks for six months) increased the forearm bone density in GC treated women but 10% of them developed virilizing side effects [194]. Similarly, cyclic medroxyprogesterone acetate (200 mg i.m. every 6 weeks for one year) increased lumbar spine BMD in GC-treated men [195]. At present, there are no recommendations on the use of anabolic steroids for GCOP. Recombinant PTH administration (400 IU of PTH 1-34; teriparatide) given to postmenopausal women with GCOP (also on estrogen replacement therapy) increased lumbar spine BMD (as assessed with DEXA and QCT); this increase in BMD was maintained after discontinuation of teriparatide [196,197]. In a recent study of 428 women and men with osteoporosis who had received glucocorticoids for at least 3 months, 50% of them received teriparatide and the other 50% received alendronate: BMD increased more in patients receiving teriparatide than in those receiving alendronate [198]. Teriparatide should be a first-choice therapy (at 20 microg/day sc) for patients with GCOP and fractures [199,200]. The combination of teriparatide and bisphosphonates may lower the effectiveness of the former [201], however bisphosphonates given after stopping teriparatide may help to maintain bone formed by teriparatide [202].

Because hypogonadism frequently occurs on high-dose GC therapy, hormone replacement therapy (HRT) could be considered in postmenopausal women and in men, provided no contraindication to its use exists [121,148,172]. In a retrospective study of postmenopausal women taking GCs BMD was higher in those who were also on estrogens, compared to those who were not on estrogen [203]. In a randomized controlled clinical trial of postmenopausal women on GCs for rheumathoid arthritis, a significant increase in lumbar spine BMD was observed in those given hormone therapy (HT) compared to those given a placebo [204]. Although there is a potential benefit of HT in hypoestrogenic women treated with GCs, a large randomized clinical trial in postmenopausal women treated with a combination of estrogen and progestin planned to last 8.5 years was interrupted after 5 years; the overall treatment risks exceeded the benefits [205]. Despite this, the ACR recommends oral contraceptives (unless contraindicated) in premenopausal women on GCs who develop oligo-amenorrhea [121]. No study exists so far on raloxifene in post-menopausal women on GCs. In women who are suffering from breast cancer and treated with GCs, tamoxifen could be protective for BMD [206]. Adult men with GC excess who develop hypogonadism could also benefit from testosterone replacement: in GC-treated asthmatic men with testosterone deficiency, i.m. testosterone injections increased lumbar spine BMD, but not hip BMD [207]. Data are lacking on the potential benefit of testosterone therapy in GC-treated eugonadal men. Nevertheless, since most studies have shown an increase in prostate size and prostate-specific antigen levels in older men on testosterone supplementation/therapy [208-211], testosterone administration should be monitored with yearly rectal examinations and prostate-specific antigen measurements.

In the future newer selective estrogen receptor modulators (SERMs) and selective GR modulators (SGRMs) may be used for treating GCOP. The latter are selective ligands of the GR that maintain the transrepressive properties of GCs (usually associated with their beneficial anti-inflammatory effect) while lacking their transactivating properties (usually associated with metabolic negative effects, including perhaps those on the bone). The anti-osteoporosis drug armamentarium includes drugs that either inhibit osteoclast resorption or stimulate osteoblast bone forming activity: recombinant osteoprotegrin, antibodies against RANKL, inhibitors of osteoclast enzymes, integrin antagonists, agonists to LRP5, and modulators of the Wnt and BMP pathways [199].

REFERENCES

[1] Khosla, S., et al., Epidemiology and clinical features of osteoporosis in young individuals. *Bone*, 1994; 15: 551-5.

[2] Alesci, S., et al., Glucocorticoid-induced osteoporosis: from basic mechanisms to clinical aspects. *Neuroimmunomodulation*, 2005; 12: 1-19.

[3] Canalis, E., Clinical review 83: Mechanisms of glucocorticoid action in bone: implications to glucocorticoid-induced osteoporosis. *J Clin Endocrinol Metab*, 1996; 81: 3441-7.

[4] Orcel, P., Prise en charge de l'osteoporose cortisonique. *Presse Med*, 2006; 35: 1571-7.

[5] Walsh, L.J., et al., Use of oral corticosteroids in the community and the prevention of secondary osteoporosis: a cross sectional study. *Brit Med J*, 1996; 313: 344-6.

[6] Lukert, B.P. and L.G. Raisz, Glucocorticoid-induced osteoporosis: pathogenesis and management. *Ann Intern Med*, 1990; 112: 352-64.

[7] Henderson, N.K. and P.N. Sambrook, Relationship between osteoporosis and arthritis and effect of corticosteroids and other drugs on bone. *Curr Opin Rheumatol*, 1996; 8: 365-9.

[8] Osella, G., et al., Serum markers of bone and collagen turnover in patients with Cushing's syndrome and in subjects with adrenal incidentalomas. *J Clin Endocrinol Metab*, 1997; 82: 3303-7.

[9] Pearce, G., et al., Corticosteroid-Induced Bone Loss in Men. *J Clin Endocrinol Metab*, 1998; 83: 801-806.

[10] van Staa, T.P., et al., Oral corticosteroids and fracture risk: relationship to daily and cumulative doses. *Rheumatology*, 2000; 39: 1383-1389.

[11] Lo Cascio, V., et al., Bone loss after glucocorticoid therapy. *Calcif Tissue Int*, 1984; 36: 435-8.

[12] van Staa, T.P., The pathogenesis, epidemiology and management of glucocorticoid-induced osteoporosis. *Calcif Tissue Int*, 2006; 79: 129-37.

[13] Adinoff, A.D. and J.R. Hollister, Steroid-induced fractures and bone loss in patients with asthma. *N Engl J Med*, 1983; 309: 265-8.

[14] Michel, B.A., D.A. Bloch, and J.F. Fries, Predictors of fractures in early rheumatoid arthritis. *J Rheumatol*, 1991; 18: 804-8.

[15] Varonos, S., B.M. Ansell, and J. Reeve, Vertebral collapse in juvenile chronic arthritis: its relationship with glucocorticoid therapy. *Calcif Tissue Int*, 1987; 41: 75-8.

[16] Sambrook, P.N., Glucocorticoid osteoporosis. *Curr Pharm Design*, 2002; 8: 1877-1883.

[17] Saag, K.G., Glucocorticoid-induced osteoporosis. *Endocrinol Metab Clin North Am*, 2003; 32: 135-157.

[18] Peel, N.F., et al., Risk of vertebral fracture and relationship to bone mineral density in steroid treated rheumatoid arthritis. *Ann Rheum Dis*, 1995; 54: 801-806.

[19] Luengo, M., et al., Vertebral fractures in steroid dependent asthma and involutional osteoporosis: a comparative study. *Thorax*, 1991; 46: 803-6.

[20] Kaji, H., et al., The threshold of bone mineral density for vertebral fracture in female patients with glucocorticoid-induced osteoporosis. *Endocr J*, 2006; 53: 27-34.

[21] Selby, P.L., et al., Corticosteroids do not alter the threshold for vertebral fracture. *J Bone Miner Res*, 2000; 15: 952-6.

[22] Kanis, J.A., H. Johannsson, and A. Oden, A meta-analysis of prior corticosteroid use and fracture risk. *J Bone Miner Res*, 2004; 19: 893-899.

[23] Dykman, T.R., et al., Evaluation of factors associated with glucocorticoid-induced osteopenia in patients with rheumatic diseases. *Arthritis Rheum*, 1985; 28: 361-8.

[24] Prentice, A., Diet, nutrition and the prevention of osteoporosis. *Public Health Nutr*, 2004; 7: 227-243.

[25] Heaney, R.P., Effects of caffeine on bone and the calcium economy. *Food and Chemical Toxicology*, 2002; 40: 1263-1270.

[26] Heaney, R.P., Long-latency deficiency disease: insights from calcium and vitamin D. *Am J Clin Nutr*, 2003; 78: 912-919.

[27] Packard, P.T. and R.P. Heaney, Medical Nutrition Therapy for Patients with Osteoporosis. *J Am Diet Assoc*, 1997; 97: 414-417.

[28] King, J.A., et al., Long-term corticosteroid replacement and bone mineral density in adult women with classical congenital adrenal hyperplasia. *J Clin Endocrinol Metab*, 2006; 91: 865-9.

[29] Thompson, J.M., et al., Not all postmenopausal women on chronic steroid and estrogen treatment are osteoporotic: predictors of bone mineral density. *Calcif Tissue Int*, 1997; 61: 377-81.

[30] Rich, G.M., et al., Cyclosporine A and prednisone-associated osteoporosis in heart transplant recipients. *J Heart Lung Transplant*, 1992; 11: 950-8.

[31] Rizzato, G., et al., Prednisone-induced bone loss in sarcoidosis: a risk especially frequent in postmenopausal women. *Sarcoidosis*, 1988; 5: 93-8.

[32] Shane, E., et al., Osteoporosis after cardiac transplantation. *Am J Med*, 1993; 94: 257-64.

[33] Ruegsegger, P., T.C. Medici, and M. Anliker, Corticosteroid-induced bone loss. A longitudinal study of alternate day therapy in patients with bronchial asthma using quantitative computed tomography. *Eur J Clin Pharmacol*, 1983; 25: 615-20.

[34] Huizenga, N.A., et al., A polymorphism in the glucocorticoid receptor gene may be associated with and increased sensitivity to glucocorticoids in vivo. *J Clin Endocrinol Metab*, 1998; 83: 144-51.

[35] van Rossum, E.F. and S.W. Lamberts, Polymorphisms in the glucocorticoid receptor gene and their associations with metabolic parameters and body composition. *Recent Prog Horm Res*, 2004; 59: 333-357.

[36] Ehrlich, P.J. and L.E. Lanyon, Mechanical strain and bone cell function: a review. *Osteoporos Int*, 2002; 13: 688-700.

[37] Laan, R.F., et al., Differential effects of glucocorticoids on cortical appendicular and cortical vertebral bone mineral content. *Calcif Tissue Int*, 1993; 52: 5-9.

[38] Reid, I.R. and S.W. Heap, Determinants of vertebral mineral density in patients receiving long-term glucocorticoid therapy. *Arch Intern Med*, 1990; 150: 2545-8.

[39] Reid, I.R., M.C. Evans, and J. Stapleton, Lateral spine densitometry is a more sensitive indicator of glucocorticoid-induced bone loss. *J Bone Miner Res*, 1992; 7: 1221-5.

[40] Reid, I.R., et al., Bone mineral density of the proximal femur and lumbar spine in glucocorticoid-treated asthmatic patients. *Osteoporos Int*, 1992; 2: 103-5.

[41] Sambrook, P., et al., Corticosteroid effects on proximal femur bone loss. *J Bone Miner Res*, 1990; 5: 1211-6.

[42] Dempster, D.W., Bone histomorphometry in glucocorticoid-induced osteoporosis. *J Bone Miner Res*, 1989; 4: 137-41.

[43] Hahn, T.J., V.C. Boisseau, and L.V. Avioli, Effect of chronic corticosteroid administration on diaphyseal and metaphyseal bone mass. *J Clin Endocrinol Metab*, 1974; 39: 274-82.

[44] Aaron, J.E., et al., Contrasting microanatomy of idiopathic and corticosteroid-induced osteoporosis. *Clin Orthop*, 1989 294-305.

[45] Bamberger, C.M., H.M. Schulte, and G.P. Chrousos, Molecular determinants of glucocorticoid receptor function and tissue sensitivity to glucocorticoids. *Endocr Rev*, 1996; 17: 245-61.

[46] Vottero, A. and G.P. Chrousos, Glucocorticoid Receptor beta: View I. *Trends Endocrinol Metab*, 1999; 10: 333-338.

[47] Beavan, S., et al., Colocalization of glucocorticoid and mineralocorticoid receptors in human bone. *J Bone Miner Res*, 2001; 16: 1496-504.

[48] Dovio, A., et al., Autocrine down-regulation of glucocorticoid receptors by interleukin-11 in human osteoblast-like cell lines. *J Endocrinol*, 2003; 177: 109-17.

[49] Masera, R.G., et al., Interleukin-6 upregulates glucocorticoid receptor numbers in human osteoblast-like cells. *Z Rheumatol*, 2000; 59 Suppl 2: II/103-7.

[50] Dovio, A., et al., Autocrine up-regulation of glucocorticoid receptors by interleukin-6 in human osteoblast-like cells. *Calcif Tissue Int*, 2001; 69: 293-8.

[51] Angeli, A., et al., Interactions between glucocorticoids and cytokines in the bone microenvironment. *Ann N Y Acad Sci*, 2002; 966: 97-107.

[52] Weinstein, R.S., et al., Inhibition of Osteoblastogenesis and Promotion of Apoptosis of Osteoblasts and Osteocytes by Glucocorticoids. Potential Mechanisms of Their Deleterious Effects on Bone. *J Clin Invest*, 1998; 102: 274-282.

[53] O'Brien, C.A., et al., Glucocorticoids act directly on osteoblasts and osteocytes to induce their apoptosis and reduce bone formation and strength. *Endocrinology*, 2004; 145: 1835-1841.

[54] Mazziotti, G., et al., Glucocorticoid-induced osteoporosis: an update. *Trends Endocrinol Metab*, 2006; 17: 144-9.

[55] Manolagas, S.C., Birth and death of bone cells: basic regulatory mechanisms and implications for the pathogenesis and treatment of osteoporosis. *Endocr Rev*, 2000; 21: 115-37.

[56] Stromstedt, P.E., et al., The glucocorticoid receptor binds to a sequence overlapping the TATA box of the human osteocalcin promoter: a potential mechanism for negative regulation. *Mol Cell Biol*, 1991; 11: 3379-83.

[57] Heinrichs, A.A., et al., Identification of multiple glucocorticoid receptor binding sites in the rat osteocalcin gene promoter. *Biochemistry*, 1993; 32: 11436-44.

[58] Raisz, L.G., Pathogenesis of osteoporosis: concepts, conflicts, and prospects. *J Clin Invest*, 2005; 115: 3318-25.

[59] Ohnaka, K., et al., Glucocorticoid suppresses the canonical Wnt signal in cultured human osteoblasts. *Biochem Biophys Res Commun*, 2005; 329: 177-81.

[60] Delany, A.M., B.Y. Gabbitas, and E. Canalis, Cortisol downregulates osteoblast alpha 1 (I) procollagen mRNA by transcriptional and posttranscriptional mechanisms. *J Cell Biochem*, 1995; 57: 488-94.

[61] Delany, A.M., et al., Cortisol increases interstitial collagenase expression in osteoblasts by post-transcriptional mechanisms. *J Biol Chem*, 1995; 270: 26607-12.

[62] Roodman, G.D., Cell biology of the osteoclast. *Exp Hematol*, 1999; 27: 1229-41.

[63] Gronowicz, G., M.B. McCarthy, and L.G. Raisz, Glucocorticoids stimulate resorption in fetal rat parietal bones in vitro. *J Bone Miner Res*, 1990; 5: 1223-30.

[64] Lowe, C., D.H. Gray, and I.R. Reid, Serum blocks the osteolytic effect of cortisol in neonatal mouse calvaria. *Calcif Tissue Int*, 1992; 50: 189-92.

[65] Conaway, H.H., D. Grigorie, and U.H. Lerner, Differential effects of glucocorticoids on bone resorption in neonatal mouse calvariae stimulated by peptide and steroid-like hormones. *J Endocrinol*, 1997; 155: 513-21.

[66] Bar-Shavit, Z., et al., Glucocorticoids modulate macrophage surface oligosaccharides and their bone binding activity. *J Clin Invest*, 1984; 73: 1277-83.

[67] Teitelbaum, S.L., et al., Glucocorticoids and bone resorption. *Adv Exp Med Biol*, 1984; 171: 121-9.

[68] Liu, Y.Z., et al., A novel pathophysiological mechanism for osteoporosis suggested by an in vivo gene expression study of circulating monocytes. *J Biol Chem*, 2005; 280: 29011-6.

[69] Heymann, D., et al., Cytokines, growth factors and osteoclasts. *Cytokine*, 1998; 10: 155-68.

[70] Rifas, L., Bone and cytokines: beyond IL-1, IL-6 and TNF-alpha. *Calcif Tissue Int*, 1999; 64: 1-7.

[71] Horowitz, M.C., et al., Control of osteoclastogenesis and bone resorption by members of the TNF family of receptors and ligands. *Cytokine Growth Factor Rev*, 2001; 12: 9-18.

[72] Hofbauer, L.C. and A.E. Heufelder, Clinical review 114: hot topic. The role of receptor activator of nuclear factor-kappaB ligand and osteoprotegerin in the pathogenesis and treatment of metabolic bone diseases. *J Clin Endocrinol Metab*, 2000; 85: 2355-63.

[73] Pfeilschifter, J., S.M. Seyedin, and G.R. Mundy, Transforming growth factor beta inhibits bone resorption in fetal rat long bone cultures. *J Clin Invest*, 1988; 82: 680-5.

[74] Vidal, N.O., et al., Osteoprotegerin mRNA is expressed in primary human osteoblast-like cells: down-regulation by glucocorticoids. *J Endocrinol*, 1998; 159: 191-195.

[75] Bornefalk, E., et al., Serum levels of osteoprotegerin: effects of glucocorticoids and growth hormone. *Bone*, 1998; 23: S486.

[76] Hofbauer, L.C., et al., Stimulation of osteoprotegerin ligand and inhibition of osteoprotegerin production by glucocorticoids in human osteoblastic lineage cells: potential paracrine mechanisms of glucocorticoid-induced osteoporosis. *Endocrinology*, 1999; 140: 4382-9.

[77] Hock, J.M., M. Centrella, and E. Canalis, Insulin-like growth factor I has independent effects on bone matrix formation and cell replication. *Endocrinology*, 1988; 122: 254-60.

[78] Canalis, E., et al., Insulin-like growth factors inhibit interstitial collagenase synthesis in bone cell cultures. *Endocrinology*, 1995; 136: 1348-54.

[79] Delany, A.M., D. Durant, and E. Canalis, Glucocorticoid suppression of IGF I transcription in osteoblasts. *Mol Endocrinol*, 2001; 15: 1781-9.

[80] Bennett, A., et al., Characterization of insulin-like growth factor I receptors on cultured rat bone cells: regulation of receptor concentration by glucocorticoids. *Endocrinology*, 1984; 115: 1577-83.

[81] Rydziel, S. and E. Canalis, Cortisol represses insulin-like growth factor II receptor transcription in skeletal cell cultures. *Endocrinology*, 1995; 136: 4254-60.

[82] Fuller, K., J. Owens, and T.J. Chambers, The effect of hepatocyte growth factor on the behaviour of osteoclasts. *Biochem Biophys Res Commun*, 1995; 212: 334-40.

[83] Sato, T., et al., Hepatocyte growth factor is involved in formation of osteoclast-like cells mediated by clonal stromal cells (MC3T3-G2/PA6). *J Cell Physiol*, 1995; 164: 197-204.

[84] Grano, M., et al., Hepatocyte growth factor is a coupling factor for osteoclasts and osteoblasts in vitro. *Proc Natl Acad Sci U S A*, 1996; 93: 7644-8.

[85] Ferracini, R., et al., The Met/HGF receptor is over-expressed in human osteosarcomas and is activated by either a paracrine or an autocrine circuit. *Oncogene*, 1995; 10: 739-49.

[86] Raisz, L.G., Prostaglandins and bone: physiology and pathophysiology. *Osteoarthr Cartilage*, 1999; 7: 419-21.

[87] Chyun, Y.S. and L.G. Raisz, Stimulation of bone formation by prostaglandin E2. *Prostaglandins*, 1984; 27: 97-103.

[88] Canalis, E., The hormonal and local regulation of bone formation. *Endocr Rev*, 1983; 4: 62-77.

[89] Fuller, K. and T.J. Chambers, Effect of arachidonic acid metabolites on bone resorption by isolated rat osteoclasts. *J Bone Miner Res*, 1989; 4: 209-15.

[90] Klein, D.C. and L.G. Raisz, Prostaglandins: stimulation of bone resorption in tissue culture. *Endocrinology*, 1970; 86: 1436-40.

[91] Wajchenberg, B.L., et al., Effect of dexamethasone on calcium metabolism and 47Ca kinetics in normal subjects. *Acta Endocrinol (Copenh)*, 1969; 61: 173-92.

[92] Morris, H.A., et al., Malabsorption of calcium in corticosteroid-induced osteoporosis. *Calcif Tissue Int*, 1990; 46: 305-8.

[93] Binder, H.J., Effect of dexamethasone on electrolyte transport in the large intestine of the rat. *Gastroenterology*, 1978; 75: 212-7.

[94] Sjoberg, H.E., Retention of orally administered 47-calcium in man under normal and diseased conditions studied with a whole-body counter technique. *Acta Med Scand Suppl*, 1970; 509: 1-28.

[95] Lee, D.B., Unanticipated stimulatory action of glucocorticoids on epithelial calcium absorption. Effect of dexamethasone on rat distal colon. *J Clin Invest*, 1983; 71: 322-8.

[96] Hahn, T.J., et al., Comparison of subacute effects of oxazacort and prednisone on mineral metabolism in man. *Calcif Tissue Int*, 1980; 31: 109-15.

[97] Lekkerkerker, J.F., F. Van Woudenberg, and H. Doorenbos, Influence of low dose of steroid therapy on calcium absorption. *Acta Endocrinol (Copenh)*, 1972; 69: 488-96.

[98] Aloia, J.F., H.M. Semla, and J.K. Yeh, Discordant effects of glucocorticoids on active and passive transport of calcium in the rat duodenum. *Calcif Tissue Int*, 1984; 36: 327-31.

[99] Francis, R.M., A.M. Sutcliffe, and A.C. Scane, Pathogenesis of osteoporosis, In: *Osteoporosis*, J.C. Stevenson and R. Lindsay, Editors. 1998 Chapman & Hall Medical - Lippincott Williams and Wilkins; Philadelphia, Pa: 29-52.

[100] Suzuki, Y., et al., Importance of increased urinary calcium excretion in the development of secondary hyperparathyroidism of patients under glucocorticoid therapy. *Metabolism*, 1983; 32: 151-6.

[101] Au, W.Y., Cortisol stimulation of parathyroid hormone secretion by rat parathyroid glands in organ culture. *Science*, 1976; 193: 1015-7.

[102] Cosman, F., et al., High-dose glucocorticoids in multiple sclerosis patients exert direct effects on the kidney and skeleton. *J Bone Miner Res*, 1994; 9: 1097-105.

[103] Freiberg, J.M., J. Kinsella, and B. Sacktor, Glucocorticoids increase the Na+-H+ exchange and decrease the Na+ gradient-dependent phosphate-uptake systems in renal brush border membrane vesicles. *Proc Natl Acad Sci U S A*, 1982; 79: 4932-6.

[104] Heersche, J.N., et al., Regulation of hormone responsiveness of bone in vitro by corticosteroids, PTH, PGE2, and calcitonin., In: *Hormonal control of calcium metabolism*, R.V. Talmage, D.V. Cohn, and J.L. Mathews, Editors. 1981 Excerpta Medica; Amsterdam: 157-162.

[105] Fucik, R.F., et al., Effect of glucocorticoids on function of the parathyroid glands in man. *J Clin Endocrinol Metab*, 1975; 40: 152-5.

[106] Bonadonna, S., et al., Chronic glucocorticoid treatment alters spontaneous pulsatile parathyroid hormone secretory dynamics in human subjects. *Eur J Endocrinol*, 2005; 152: 199-205.

[107] Urban, R.J. and J.D. Veldhuis, Endocrine control of steroidogenesis in granulosa cells. *Oxf Rev Reprod Biol*, 1992; 14: 225-62.

[108] Crilly, R., et al., Hormonal status in normal, osteoporotic and corticosteroid-treated postmenopausal women. *J R Soc Med*, 1978; 71: 733-6.

[109] Montecucco, C., et al., Sex hormones and bone metabolism in postmenopausal rheumatoid arthritis treated with two different glucocorticoids. *J Rheumatol*, 1992; 19: 1895-900.

[110] MacAdams, M.R., R.H. White, and B.E. Chipps, Reduction of serum testosterone levels during chronic glucocorticoid therapy. *Ann Intern Med*, 1986; 104: 648-51.

[111] Buyon, J.P., et al., Recommendations for exogenous estrogen to prevent glucocorticoid-induced osteoporosis in premenopausal women with oligo- or amenorrhea: comment on the American College of Rheumatology recommendations for the prevention and treatment of glucocorticoid-induced osteoporosis. *Arthritis Rheum*, 1997; 40: 1548-9.

[112] Goulding, A. and E. Gold, Effects of chronic prednisolone treatment on bone resorption and bone composition in intact and ovariectomized rats and in ovariectomized rats receiving beta-estradiol. *Endocrinology*, 1988; 122: 482-7.

[113] Ohlsson, C., et al., Growth hormone and bone. *Endocr Rev*, 1998; 19: 55-79.

[114] King, A.P., et al., Distinct cytoplasmic domains of the growth hormone receptor are required for glucocorticoid- and phorbol ester-induced decreases in growth hormone (GH) binding. These domains are different from that reported for GH-induced receptor internalization. *J Biol Chem*, 1996; 271: 18088-94.

[115] Askari, A., P.J. Vignos, Jr., and R.W. Moskowitz, Steroid myopathy in connective tissue disease. *Am J Med*, 1976; 61: 485-92.

[116] Afifi, A.K., R.A. Bergman, and J.C. Harvey, Steroid myopathy. Clinical, histologic and cytologic observations. *Johns Hopkins Med J*, 1968; 123: 158-73.

[117] Pleasure, D.E., G.O. Walsh, and W.K. Engel, Atrophy of skeletal muscle in patients with Cushing's syndrome. *Arch Neurol*, 1970; 22: 118-25.

[118] Rebuffe-Scrive, M., et al., Muscle and adipose tissue morphology and metabolism in Cushing's syndrome. *J Clin Endocrinol Metab*, 1988; 67: 1122-8.

[119] Anonymous, Consensus development conference: diagnosis, prophylaxis, and treatment of osteoporosis. *Am J Med*, 1993; 94: 646-50.

[120] Anonymous, Osteoporosis prevention, diagnosis, and therapy. *JAMA*, 2001; 285: 785-795.

[121] Anonymous, Recommendations for the prevention and treatment of glucocorticoid-induced osteoporosis: 2001 update. American College of Rheumatology Ad Hoc Committee on Glucocoritcoid-Induced Osteoporosis. *Arthritis Rheum*, 2001; 44: 1496-503.

[122] Gonnelli, S., et al., Prevention of corticosteroid-induced osteoporosis with alendronate in sarcoid patients. *Calcif Tissue Int*, 1997; 61: 382-385.

[123] Adler, R.A. and M.C. Hochberg, Suggested Guidelines for Evaluation and Treatment of Glucocorticoid-Induced Osteoporosis for the Department of Veterans Affairs. *Arch Intern Med*, 2003; 163: 2619-2624.

[124] Eastell, R., et al., A UK Consensus Group on management of glucocorticoid-induced osteoporosis: an update. *J Intern Med*, 1998; 244: 271-92.

[125] Lukert, B.P., J.C. Higgins, and M.M. Stoskopf, Serum osteocalcin is increased in patients with hyperthyroidism and decreased in patients receiving glucocorticoids. *J Clin Endocrinol Metab*, 1986; 62: 1056-8.

[126] Ekenstam, E., G. Stalenheim, and R. Hallgren, The acute effect of high dose corticosteroid treatment on serum osteocalcin. *Metabolism*, 1988; 37: 141-4.

[127] Prummel, M.F., et al., The course of biochemical parameters of bone turnover during treatment with corticosteroids. *J Clin Endocrinol Metab*, 1991; 72: 382-6.

[128] Nielsen, H.K., et al., The effects of high-dose glucocorticoid administration on serum bone gamma carboxyglutamic acid-containing protein, serum alkaline phosphatase and vitamin D metabolites in normal subjects. *Bone Miner*, 1988; 4: 105-13.

[129] Reid, I.R., et al., Low serum osteocalcin levels in glucocorticoid-treated asthmatics. *J Clin Endocrinol Metab*, 1986; 62: 379-83.

[130] Hall, G.M., T.D. Spector, and P.D. Delmas, Markers of bone metabolism in postmenopausal women with rheumatoid arthritis. Effects of corticosteroids and hormone replacement therapy. *Arthritis Rheum*, 1995; 38: 902-6.

[131] Reeve, J., et al., Biochemical prediction of changes in spinal bone mass in juvenile chronic (or rheumatoid) arthritis treated with glucocorticoids. *J Rheumatol*, 1993; 20: 1189-95.

[132] Ton, F.N., et al., Effects of low-dose prednisone on bone metabolism. *J Bone Miner Res*, 2005; 20: 464-470.

[133] Lems, W.F., et al., Changes in (markers of) bone metabolism during high dose corticosteroid pulse treatment in patients with rheumatoid arthritis. *Ann Rheum Dis*, 1996; 55: 288-93.

[134] Gennari, C., et al., Effects of prednisone and deflazacort on mineral metabolism and parathyroid hormone activity in humans. *Calcif Tissue Int*, 1984; 36: 245-52.

[135] Baran, D.T., et al., Diagnosis and management of osteoporosis: guidelines for the utilization of bone densitometry. *Calcif Tissue Int*, 1997; 61: 433-440.

[136] Guglielmi, G. and T.F. Lang, Quantitative computed tomography. *Semin Musculoskelet Radiol*, 2002; 6: 219-227.

[137] Hui, S.L., C.W. Slemenda, and C.C. Johnston, Jr., Baseline measurement of bone mass predicts fracture in white women. *Ann Intern Med*, 1989; 111: 355-61.

[138] Blake, G.M. and I. Fogelman, Applications of bone densitometry for osteoporosis. *Endocrinol Metab Clin North Am*, 1998; 27: 267-88.

[139] Finkelstein, J.S., et al., A comparison of lateral versus anterior-posterior spine dual energy x-ray absorptiometry for the diagnosis of osteopenia. *J Clin Endocrinol Metab*, 1994; 78: 724-30.

[140] Kanis, J.A., D. Torgerson, and C. Cooper, Comparison of the European and USA practice guidelines for Osteoporosis. *Trends Endocrinol Metab*, 2000; 11: 28-32.

[141] Adler, G.S. and A. Shatto, Screening for osteoporosis and colon cancer under Medicare. *Health Care Financ Rev*, 2002; 23: 189-200.

[142] Blanckaert, F., et al., Contribution of calcaneal ultrasonic assessment to the evaluation of postmenopausal and glucocorticoid-induced osteoporosis. *Rev Rhum Engl Ed*, 1997; 64: 305-13.

[143] Daens, S., et al., Efficiency of quantitative ultrasound measurements as compared with dual-energy X-ray absorptiometry in the assessment of corticosteroid-induced bone impairment. *Osteoporos Int*, 1999; 10: 278-83.

[144] Devogelaer, J.P., et al., Evidence-based guidelines for the prevention and treatment of glucocorticoid-induced osteoporosis: a consensus document of the Belgian Bone Club. *Osteoporos Int*, 2006; 17: 8-19.

[145] Sosa Henríquez, M., et al., Guia de prevencion y tratamiento de la osteoporosis inducida por glucocorticoides de la Sociedad Espanola de Medicina Interna. *Rev Clin Esp*, 2008; 208 33-45.

[146] Oak, J., Preventing steroid-induced osteoporosis. *Indian J Dermatol Venereol Leprol* 2008; 74: 5-7.

[147] Compston, J., Management of Glucocorticoid-Induced Osteoporosis – for Neurologists. *Practical Neurology*, 2004; 4: 286-289.

[148] Devogelaer, J.P., Glucocorticoid-Induced Osteoporosis: Mechanisms and Therapeutic Approach. *Rheum Dis Clin N Am* 2006; 32: 733-757.

[149] Martinati, L.C., et al., Longitudinal evaluation of bone mass in asthmatic children treated with inhaled beclomethasone dipropionate or cromolyn sodium. *Allergy*, 1998; 53: 705-8.

[150] Nielsen, H.K., P. Charles, and L. Mosekilde, The effect of single oral doses of prednisone on the circadian rhythm of serum osteocalcin in normal subjects. *J Clin Endocrinol Metab*, 1988; 67: 1025-1030.

[151] Gluck, O.S., et al., Bone loss in adults receiving alternate day glucocorticoid therapy. A comparison with daily therapy. *Arthritis Rheum*, 1981; 24: 892-8.

[152] Gluck, O. and G. Colice, Recognizing and Treating Glucocorticoid-Induced Osteoporosis in Patients With Pulmonary Diseases. *Chest*, 2004; 125: 1859-1876

[153] Wong, C.A., et al., Inhaled corticosteroid use and bone-mineral density in patients with asthma. *Lancet*, 2000; 355 1399-1403.

[154] Bootsma, G.P., et al., Fluticasone propionate does not influence bone metabolism in contrast to beclomethasone dipropionate. *Am J Respir Crit Care Med*, 1996; 153: 924-30.

[155] Luengo, M., et al., Bone mineral density in asthmatic patients treated with inhaled corticosteroids: a case-control study. *Eur Respir J*, 1997; 10: 2110-3.

[156] Ebeling, P.R., et al., Bone mineral density and bone turnover in asthmatics treated with long-term inhaled or oral glucocorticoids. *J Bone Miner Res*, 1998; 13: 1283-9.

[157] Aris, R., J.F. Donohue, and D. Ontjes, Inhaled corticosteroids and fracture risk: having our cake and eating it too. *Chest*, 2005; 127: 5-7.

[158] van Staa, T.P., et al., Are inhaled corticosteroids associated with an increased risk of fracture in children? *Osteoporos Int*, 2004; 15: 785-791.

[159] Pennisi, P., A. Trombetti, and R. Rizzoli, Glucocorticoid-induced osteoporosis and its treatment. *Clin Orthop Relat Res*, 2006; 443: 39-47.

[160] Buckley, L.M., et al., Calcium and vitamin D3 supplementation prevents bone loss in the spine secondary to low-dose corticosteroids in patients with rheumatoid arthritis. A randomized, double-blind, placebo-controlled trial. *Ann Intern Med*, 1996; 125: 961-8.

[161] Reginster, J.Y., et al., Prophylactic use of alfacalcidol in corticosteroid-induced osteoporosis. *Osteoporos Int*, 1999; 9: 75-81.

[162] Amin, S., et al., The role of vitamin D in corticosteroid-induced osteoporosis: a meta-analytic approach. *Arthritis Rheum*, 1999; 42: 1740-51.

[163] Homik, J., et al., Calcium and vitamin D for corticosteroid-induced osteoporosis. *Cochrane Database Syst Rev*, 2000 CD000952.

[164] 164. Ringe, J.D., et al., Treatment of glucocorticoid-induced osteoporosis with alfacalcidol/calcium versus vitamin D/calcium. *Calcif Tissue Int*, 1999 65 337-340.

[165] Dechant, K.L. and K.L. Goa, Calcitriol. A review of its use in the treatment of postmenopausal osteoporosis and its potential in corticosteroid-induced osteoporosis. *Drugs Aging*, 1994; 5: 300-317.

[166] Adverse Drug Reactions Advisory Committee, A., Calcitriol and hypercalcaemia. *Aust Adv Drug React Bull*, 1997; 16: 2.

[167] Homik, J., et al., Bisphosphonates for steroid induced osteoporosis. *Cochrane Database of Systematic Reviews* 1999 CD001347.

[168] LaCroix, A.Z., et al., Thiazide diuretic agents and the incidence of hip fracture. *N Engl J Med*, 1990; 322: 286-90.

[169] Felson, D.T., et al., Thiazide diuretics and the risk of hip fracture. Results from the Framingham Study. *JAMA*, 1991; 265: 370-3.

[170] Cauley, J.A., et al., Effects of thiazide diuretic therapy on bone mass, fractures, and falls. The Study of Osteoporotic Fractures Research Group. *Ann Intern Med*, 1993; 118: 666-73.

[171] Rodan, G.A. and H.A. Fleisch, Bisphosphonates: mechanisms of action. *J Clin Invest*, 1996; 97: 2692-6.

[172] Sambrook, P.N., How to prevent steroid induced osteoporosis. *Ann Rheum Dis*, 2005; 64: 176-8.

[173] Adachi, J.D., et al., Two-year effects of alendronate on bone mineral density and vertebral fracture in patients receiving glucocorticoids: a randomized, double-blind, placebo-controlled extension trial. *Arthritis Rheum*, 2001; 44: 202-11.

[174] de Nijs, R.N., et al., Alendronate or alfacalcidol in glucocorticoid-induced osteoporosis. *N Engl J Med*, 2006; 355: 675-84.

[175] Reid, D.M., et al., Efficacy and safety of daily risedronate in the treatment of corticosteroid-induced osteoporosis in men and women: a randomized trial. European Corticosteroid-Induced Osteoporosis Treatment Study. *J Bone Miner Res*, 2000; 15: 1006-13.

[176] Adachi, J.D., et al., Intermittent etidronate therapy to prevent corticosteroid-induced osteoporosis. *N Engl J Med*, 1997; 337: 382-7.

[177] Struys, A., A.A. Snelder, and H. Mulder, Cyclical etidronate reverses bone loss of the spine and proximal femur in patients with established corticosteroid-induced osteoporosis. *Am J Med*, 1995; 99: 235-42.

[178] Reid, I.R., et al., Two-year follow-up of biphosphonate (APD) treatment in steroid osteoporosis. *Lancet*, 1988; 2: 1144.

[179] Boutsen, Y., et al., Primary prevention of glucocorticoid-induced osteoporosis with intravenous pamidronate and calcium: a prospective controlled 1-year study comparing a single infusion, an infusion given once every 3 months, and calcium alone. *J Bone Miner Res*, 2001; 16: 104-12.

[180] Herrala, J., et al., Clodronate is effective in preventing corticosteroid-induced bone loss among asthmatic patients. *Bone*, 1998; 22: 577-82.

[181] Reid, I.R., et al., Intravenous Zoledronic Acid in Postmenopausal Women with Low Bone Mineral Density. *N Engl J Med*, 2002; 346: 653-661.

[182] Reid, I.R., Bisphosphonates: new indications and methods of administration. *Curr Opin Rheumatol*, 2003; 15: 458-63.

[183] Theriault, R.L., Zoledronic acid (Zometa) use in bone disease. *Expert Rev Anticancer Ther*, 2003; 3: 157-66.

[184] Biskobing, D.M., Novel therapies for osteoporosis. *Expert Opin Investig Drugs*, 2003; 12: 611-21.

[185] Biskobing, D.M., A.M. Novy, and R. Downs, Jr., Novel therapeutic options for osteoporosis. *Curr Opin Rheumatol*, 2002; 14: 447-52.

[186] Doggrell, S.A., Zoledronate once-yearly increases bone mineral density--implications for osteoporosis. *Expert Opin Pharmacother*, 2002; 3: 1007-9.

[187] Miller, P.D., M.R. McClung, and L. Macovei, Monthly oral ibandronate therapy in postmenopausal osteoporosis: 1-year results from the MOBILE study. *J Bone Miner Res*, 2005; 20: 1315-1322.

[188] Luengo, M., et al., Prevention of further bone mass loss by nasal calcitonin in patients on long term glucocorticoid therapy for asthma: a two year follow up study. *Thorax*, 1994; 49: 1099-102.

[189] Montemurro, L., et al., Prevention of corticosteroid-induced osteoporosis with salmon calcitonin in sarcoid patients. *Calcif Tissue Int*, 1991; 49: 71-6.

[190] Ringe, J.D. and D. Welzel, Salmon calcitonin in the therapy of corticoid-induced osteoporosis. *Eur J Clin Pharmacol* 1987; 33: 35-39.

[191] Lyritis, G.P., et al., Analgesic effect of salmon calcitonin in osteoporotic vertebral fractures: a double-blind placebo-controlled clinical study. *Calcif Tissue Int*, 1991; 49: 369-72.

[192] Lems, W.F., et al., Effect of sodium fluoride on the prevention of corticosteroid-induced osteoporosis. *Osteoporos Int*, 1997; 7: 575-82.

[193] Lems, W.F., et al., Is addition of sodium fluoride to cyclical etidronate beneficial in the treatment of corticosteroid induced osteoporosis? *Ann Rheum Dis*, 1997; 56: 357-63.

[194] Adami, S., et al., The prevention of corticosteroid-induced osteoporosis with nandrolone decanoate. *Bone Miner*, 1991; 15: 73-81.

[195] Grecu, E.O., A. Weinshelbaum, and R. Simmons, Effective therapy of glucocorticoid-induced osteoporosis with medroxyprogesterone acetate. *Calcif Tissue Int*, 1990; 46: 294-9.

[196] Lane, N.E., et al., Bone mass continues to increase at the hip after parathyroid hormone treatment is discontinued in glucocorticoid-induced osteoporosis: results of a randomized controlled clinical trial. *J Bone Miner Res*, 2000; 15: 944-51.

[197] Lane, N.E., et al., Parathyroid hormone treatment can reverse corticosteroid-induced osteoporosis. Results of a randomized controlled clinical trial. *J Clin Invest*, 1998; 102: 1627-33.

[198] Saag, K.G., et al., Teriparatide or alendronate in glucocorticoid-induced osteoporosis. *N Engl J Med*, 2007; 357: 2028-2039.

[199] Summey, B.T. and G. Yosipovitch, Glucocorticoid-induced bone loss in dermatologic patients: an update. *Arch Dermatol*, 2006; 142: 82-90.

[200] Hodsman, A.B., D.C. Bauer, and D. Dempster, Parathyroid hormone and teriparatide for the treatment of osteoporosis: a review of the evidence and suggested guidelines for its use. *Endocr Rev*, 2005; 26: 688-703.

[201] Black, D.M., S.L. Greenspan, and K.E. Ensrud, The effects of parathyroid hormone and alendronate alone or in combination in postmenopausal osteoporosis. *N Engl J Med*, 2003; 349: 1207-1215.

[202] Rittmaster, R.S., M. Bolognese, and M.P. Ettinger, Enhancement of bone mass in osteoporotic women with parathyroid hormone followed by alendronate. *J Clin Endocrinol Metab*, 2000; 85: 2129-2134.

[203] Lukert, B.P., B.E. Johnson, and R.G. Robinson, Estrogen and progesterone replacement therapy reduces glucocorticoid-induced bone loss. *J Bone Miner Res*, 1992; 7: 1063-9.

[204] Hall, G.M., et al., Effect of hormone replacement therapy on bone mass in rheumatoid arthritis patients treated with and without steroids. *Arthritis Rheum*, 1994; 37: 1499-505.

[205] Rossouw, J.E., et al., Risks and benefits of estrogen plus progestin in healthy postmenopausal women: principal results From the Women's Health Initiative randomized controlled trial. *JAMA*, 2002; 288: 321-33.

[206] Fentiman, I.S., et al., Tamoxifen protects against steroid-induced bone loss. *Eur J Cancer*, 1992; 28 684-685.

[207] Reid, I.R., et al., Testosterone therapy in glucocorticoid-treated men. *Arch Intern Med*, 1996; 156: 1173-7.

[208] Gruenewald, D.A. and A.M. Matsumoto, Testosterone Supplementation Therapy for Older Men: Potential Benefits and Risks. *J Am Geriatr Soc*, 2003; 51: 101-115.

[209] Oettel, M., The endocrine pharmacology of testosterone therapy in men. *Naturwissenschaften*, 2004; 91: 66-76.

[210] Hafez, B. and E.S. Hafez, Andropause: endocrinology, erectile dysfunction, and prostate pathophysiology. *Arch Androl*, 2004; 50: 45-68.

[211] Rhoden, E.L. and A. Morgentaler, Risks of testosterone-replacement therapy and recommendations for monitoring. *N Engl J Med*, 2004; 350: 482-92.

In: Osteoporosis: Etiology, Diagnosis and Treatment
Editors: Bilar E. Mattingly and Albert C. Pillare
ISBN 978-1-60692-397-9

Chapter 5

SECONDARY BONE LOSS AFTER STROKE: CHARACTERISTICS AND MANAGEMENT

Marco Y. C. Pang
Department of Rehahbilitation Sciences,
Hong Kong Polytechnic University,
Hong Kong, China.

ABSTRACT

Individuals with stroke sustain a much higher risk of fragility fractures than the reference population. Secondary bone loss is a common phenomenon following a stroke and is a major contributing factor to the exaggerated rate of bone fractures. The pattern of bone loss in stroke survivors follows a distinct pattern, with the paretic (weaker) side sustaining a much higher degree of bone loss than the non-paretic side. In addition to progressive decline in bone mass, stroke-induced alterations in bone geometry may also compromise bone strength. Various demographic and physiological factors have been associated with bone status in individuals with stroke. There is also some evidence that certain pharmacological and non-pharmacological interventions may improve bone health and decrease the incidence of fractures in stroke patients. This chapter will review the research findings on the specific bone changes after stroke, the determinants of bone status post-stroke, as well as the current evidence on the use of different pharmacological and non-pharmacological treatments to improve bone health in stroke patients.

INTRODUCTION

Stroke is one of the most common chronic conditions among older adults [1]. Stroke patients may sustain a variety of physical deficits such as muscle weakness, poor balance, hemineglect, and spasticity. Unfortunately, many stroke patients continue to live with different degrees of residual impairment and disability [2-3]. Traditional rehabilitation of stroke patients has primarily focused on the recovery of motor function and performance of daily activities. Bone health, on the other hand, is often an overlooked area in the management of stroke patients [4]. Ample literature suggests that pronounced, unfavorable bone alterations occur following the onset of stroke. There is also increasing evidence that specific pharmacological and non-pharmacological interventions may aid in counteracting the detrimental effects of stroke on bone health. This chapter will provide a comprehensive review of the specific bone changes following a stroke, and the management of secondary bone loss in stroke patients.

Fragility Fractures in Stroke Patients

It is well known that stroke is a major risk factor for fragility fractures (i.e., fractures that occur as a result of a fall from standing height or less) [5-7]. Among patients who undergo surgery for hip fractures, the prevalence of stroke has been reported to range from 8.1% to 38.5% [5, 8-11]. After hospitalization for stroke, there is an acute as well as a long-term increase in fracture risk. Within the first year of hospitalization for stroke, the risk of fracture is increased by more than 7 fold, when compared with the reference population [12]. The excess risk for hip fracture remains 23% higher 8 years after the onset of stroke [12]. Other studies have shown that the fracture rate is approximately 3–4%, 15%, and 24% after 1 year, 5 years, and 10 years post-stroke, respectively [13-14], yielding an incidence rate of 37 fractures per 1000 person-years [13]. Overall, these epidemiological findings point to the pronounced effect of stroke on elevating the risk of fragility fractures.

The majority of fractures in stroke patients occur on the paretic (weaker) side (58–82%) [8,10-11,15], which is probably related to the fact that most stroke patients tend to land sideways toward the paretic side in accidental falls [16]. The median onset of the first fracture is in the chronic stage of stroke recovery, around 2–3 years post-stroke [5, 13]. Among the various skeletal sites, hip fracture is the most common, accounting for 30–58% of all fractures [12-13,15]. The wrist is the second most common site for fragility fractures (14–24%) in stroke patients [13,15].

Fragility fractures post-stroke could lead to devastating consequences for the patients themselves, their families and for society [17]. It is known that the risk of mortality is significantly increased after a hip fracture [18], and that the risk is greatest within the first six months after fracture and persists for the following six years [18]. However, for individuals with a previous stroke, a hip fracture would further reduce the survival. Ramnemark et al. [5] found that among patients with hip fractures and a stroke history, the one-year mortality rate is 29.3%, which is significantly higher than those without stroke history (16.8%) [5]. These patients also have reduced ability to regain independent mobility status when compared with hip-fractured patients without a history of stroke [5]. Among the hip-fractured patients who were previously independently mobile, 69% of patients with no stroke history could mobilize independently whereas only 38% of the patients with a stroke history could regain independent mobility status at discharge [5]. Hip fracture in the stroke population is also associated with a prolonged period of hospital stay [19]. Di Monaco et al. [19] showed that hip-fracture patients who also have a neurological condition (including stroke) have a significantly longer period of hospital stay (by a mean of 3.8 days) than their counterparts without any neurological impairment. In terms of the impact of fractures at the societal level, the cost associated with treatment of fractures post-stroke may impose a tremendous financial burden on the health care system [20].

BONE CHANGES FOLLOWING STROKE

Apart from increased incidence of falls [21-27], another major factor associated with the exaggerated rate of fragility fractures in stroke patients is secondary bone loss [4]. While a lot of attention has been directed to the prevention of falls in stroke patients, the area of bone health is often overlooked [4]. Research studies in post-stroke bone health had not started to emerge in greater numbers until the late 1980s, and now we have ample evidence demonstrating that a hemispheric stroke would induce a distinct pattern of changes in bone mass and geometry in various skeletal sites.

Upper Extremities

Secondary bone loss in the paretic upper extremity is substantial after stroke, although differences in the extent of bone loss among the various skeletal sites exist. Most of the previous studies on bone health in stroke patients have used dual-energy X-ray absorptiometry (DXA) to measure areal bone mineral density (aBMD in g/cm^2). Ramnemark [28] followed a group of 24 stroke patients for one year, and found that the aBMD is reduced by 3.6%, 5.8% and 8.6% in the total arm, humerus, and ultradistal radius, respectively. In another prospective study, Jorgensen and Jacobsen [29] showed that the aBMD of the proximal humerus sustains an average of 17% reduction within the first year post-stroke. These findings have highlighted the pronounced bone loss in the paretic upper extremity after stroke.

In contrast, the aBMD in the non-paretic upper extremity often shows no significant change or may even increase after stroke. For example, Ramnemark [28] has demonstrated that the aBMD values in the non-paretic total arm, humerus, and ultradistal radius all increase significantly at one year follow-up, with a magnitude of gain at 3.6%, 5.8% and 5.5%, respectively. The differential pattern of change on the paretic and non-paretic sides thus explains the results of numerous cross-sectional studies, which show that the aBMD on the paretic side is consistently lower than the non-paretic side within individual patients, regardless of the stage of stroke recovery, or site of measurement in the upper extremities [30-35].

Such a unique pattern of bone density changes may be related to the altered habitual use of the upper extremities. Some stroke patients, particularly those who have severe upper extremity sensorimotor impairment, may choose to use only the more effective non-paretic side to perform daily functional activities, despite the presence of some motor recovery in the paretic upper extremity. This phenomenon, called learned non-use, may promote further disuse of the paretic upper extremity [36-37]. The chronic disuse of the paretic upper extremity, when coupled with increased use of the non-paretic upper extremity, may explain the exaggerated bone loss on the paretic side, and the accompanying increase of aBMD on the non-paretic side [28].

Other studies have examined the upper extremity bone status in chronic stroke patients using peripheral quantitative computed tomography (pQCT), which provides a volumetric bone mineral density (vBMD in mg/cm^3) measure, as well as information on bone geometry [38; 39]. Bone geometry is important as it is a major determinant of bone strength [40] and is useful in the prediction of fracture risk [41]. In a study involving 15 chronic stroke patients, the total bone vBMD has been found to be 15% lower on the paretic side than the non-paretic side at the 4% site of the radius (primarily trabecular bone and a common site of fragility fracture) [38]. At the 30% site of the radius (primarily cortical bone) [39], cortical bone mass, cortical area and cortical thickness on the paretic side are all significantly lower than the non-paretic side [39] (Figure 1). Interestingly, the total bone area shows no significant side-to-side difference. This phenomenon is observed in both male and female chronic stroke patients. Taken together, the findings suggest that endosteal resorption may have occurred after stroke (Figure 2). Such unfavorable bone geometry has resulted in a significantly lower bone strength index on the paretic side [39]. A prospective study is required to investigate the longitudinal changes of bone geometry following stroke and confirm whether endosteal resorption does take place in stroke patients as time progresses.

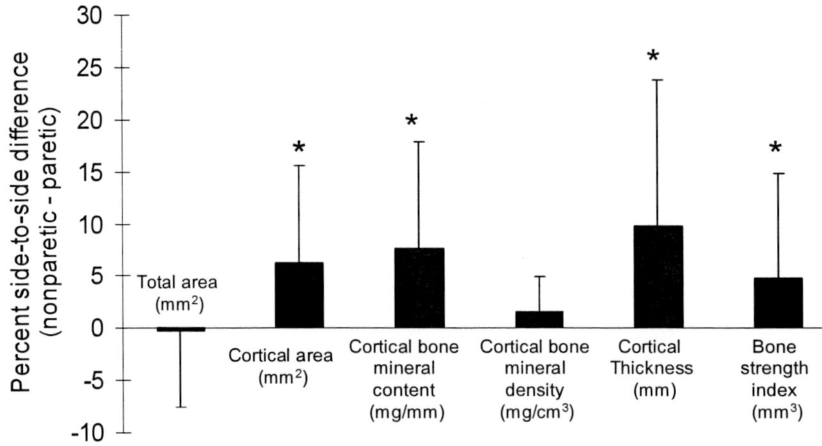

Figure 1. Side-to-side differences of bone parameters at the 30% midshaft radius site as measured by peripheral quantitative computed tomography. Data were collected from 47 chronic stroke patients (19 women). A positive percent difference indicates a higher value on the non-paretic side. The error bar represents one standard deviation. The asterisk (*) sign indicates statistical significance ($p<0.05$). There were significant differences in cortical bone mineral content, cortical bone mineral density, cortical thickness, and bone strength index between the two sides. Total bone area, however, showed no significant side-to-side difference. This phenomenon was found in both men and women [39].

Analysis of biochemical markers for bone turnover has also been used in several studies in the evaluation of upper limb bone loss in stroke patients [42-47]. The level of bone Gla protein (gamma-carboxyglutamate) (a bone formation marker) among stroke patients is either normal or lower than controls [43- 47]. In contrast, a higher level of pyridinoline cross-linked carboxy-terminal telopeptide of type I collagen (ICTP; a bone resorption marker) is consistently found in stroke patients, compared with control subjects. The increased ICTP level is also significantly associated with increased serum ionized calcium concentration in stroke patients [45-46]. These findings indicate that accelerated bone resorption may be the predominant biological process underlying the paretic upper extremity bone loss following a stroke.

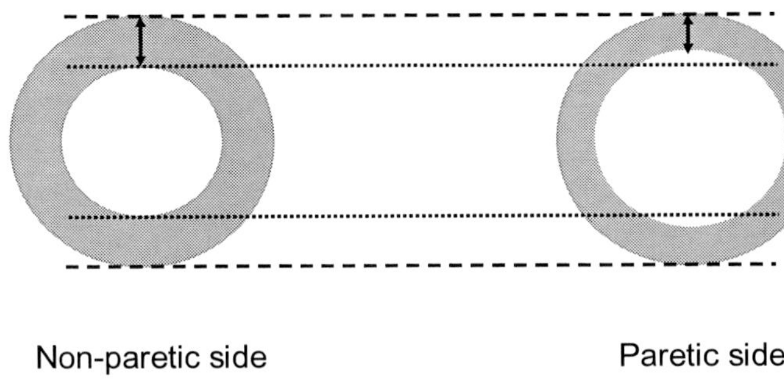

Figure 2. Schematic illustration of the side-to-side difference in bone geometry at the 30% midshaft radius site. A cross-section view of the 30% midshaft radius rate on each side is illustrated. The shaded area represents the cortical bone shell. The differences in geometry between the two sides suggest that endosteal resorption may have occurred in the radius on the paretic side [39].

Lower Extremities

The paretic lower extremity also sustains significant bone loss. The 1-year aBMD decline in total femur and proximal femur has been estimated to be 7.2% and 12.0%, respectively [28]. Such decline in aBMD is clinically relevant, as it has been shown that for every two standard deviations decrease in femoral neck aBMD, the risk of a hip fracture in individuals with a history of stroke is increased by 7-fold [48]. Interestingly, secondary bone loss is also apparent in the non-paretic lower extremity, but to a lesser extent [28,49-51]. The differential rate of bone loss in the two lower extremities would result in a significant side-to-side aBMD difference within individual stroke patients, as reflected by the results obtained from a good number of cross-sectional studies [31,33,52-53,69].

Generally, the side-to-side difference in aBMD in the lower extremities is less pronounced than that in the upper extremities [28,31,33,54]. Hamdy et al. [31] showed that in the upper extremities, the percent side-to-side difference in aBMD was 3.5% and 12.4% for patients with recent strokes (onset <1 year) and remote strokes (onset >1 year), respectively. On the other hand, the percent difference in aBMD between the paretic and non-paretic lower extremities is much less prominent, at 2.6% and 4.3% for patients with recent and remote strokes, respectively [31]. This observation could be explained by two reasons. First, the non-paretic lower extremity tends to sustain bone loss whereas the non-paretic upper extremity tends to gain bone mass [28]. Second, the extent of bone loss in the paretic lower extremity itself is less extensive than the paretic upper extremity. The difference may be related to the extent of limb use, and thus the amount of mechanical loading applied to the limb. As mentioned previously, stroke patients could often successfully perform a variety of daily tasks by only using the non-paretic upper extremity. In contrast, a majority of stroke patients could regain some standing and walking function [3]. The ground reaction forces generated during transfers and ambulation thus provide some mechanical strain to the paretic leg, despite the presence of asymmetry in weight distribution [50,52].

In addition to loss in bone mass, the paretic lower extremity also sustains altered bone geometry. However, unlike the paretic upper extremity, the stroke-induced bone geometric changes in the paretic lower extremity may be gender specific [55]. In a cross-sectional study, Pang et al. [55] have used pQCT to measure the geometric properties at the 30% tibial site (primarily cortical bone) in a group of 55 chronic stroke patients. Both men and women demonstrate a significantly lower cortical bone mineral content on the paretic side than the non-paretic side, indicating the detrimental effect of stroke on cortical bone mass. What is most interesting, however, is that the marrow cavity area on the paretic side is significantly greater than the non-paretic side while the total bone area shows no significant side-to-side difference in men (Figure 3). In contrast, the total bone area on the paretic side is significantly smaller than the non-paretic side while the marrow cavity area has no side-to-side difference in women (Figure 4). Thus, endosteal resorption may be more predominant in men (Figure 5A) whereas periosteal resorption may be the primary process underlying bone loss in women post-stroke (Figure 5B). The gender-specific differences in bone geometry has resulted in a significantly lower tibial bone strength index in women than men, as periosteal resorption would reduce the cross-sectional moment of inertia to a greater extent than endosteal resorption. The exact causes of the observed gender-specific differences in tibial geometry remain elusive. Factors such as genetics, lifestyle, nutritional status, and endogenous sex hormones may well contribute to such phenomenon [55]. It would be important to study the prospective changes in lower extremity bone geometry after stroke and determine how such changes relate to the recovery of functional ability.

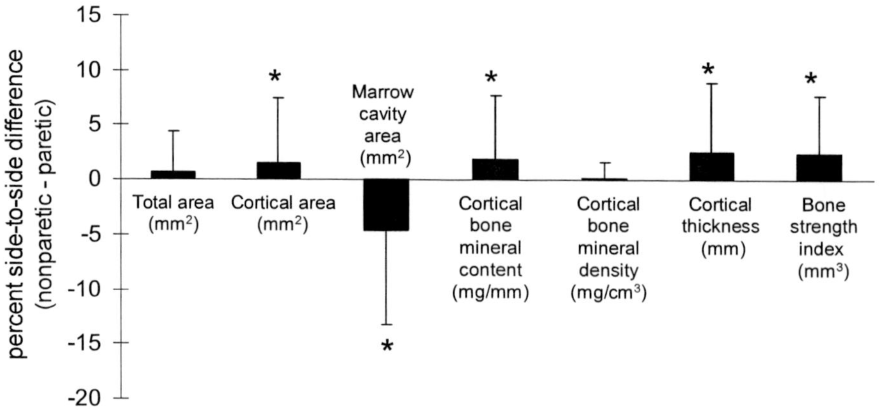

Figure 3. Side-to-side differences of bone parameters at the 30% tibial site in men as measured by peripheral quantitative computed tomography. The same convention is used as in Figure 2. Data were collected from 30 male chronic stroke patients. Significant differences were identified in cortical bone area, cortical bone mineral content, marrow cavity area, cortical thickness, and bone strength index between the two sides. There was no significant side-to-side difference in total bone area [55].

In summary, while numerous studies have described the differences in bone density and geometry between the paretic and non-paretic sides in stroke patients, relatively few studies have described the longitudinal bone changes, with the available studies only documenting the changes within the first year post-stroke. Future studies should address the longitudinal bone changes after the first year post-stroke.

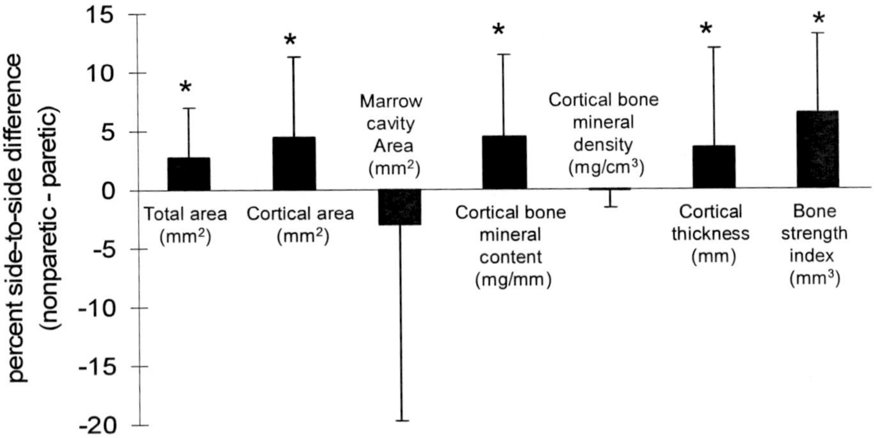

Figure 4. Side-to-side differences of bone parameters at the 30% tibial site in women as measured by peripheral quantitative computed tomography. Data were collected from 25 female chronic stroke patients. Significant differences were identified in total bone area, cortical bone area, cortical bone mineral content, cortical thickness, and bone strength index between the two sides. There was no significant side-to-side difference in marrow cavity area [55].

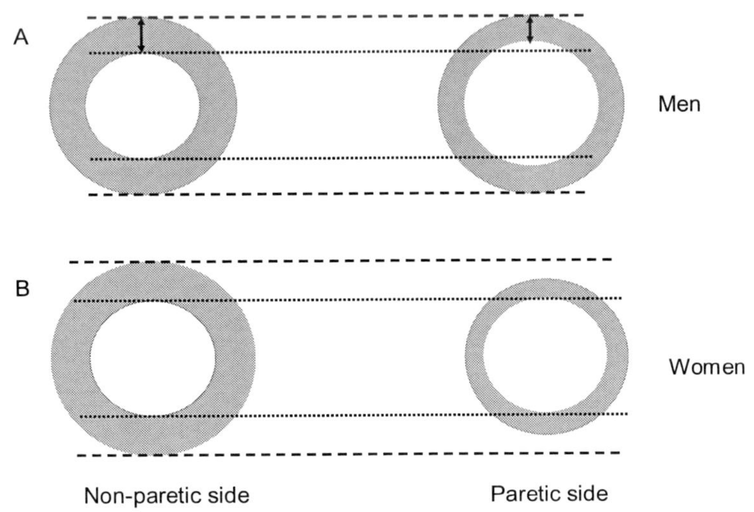

Figure 5. Schematic illustration of the side-to-side difference in bone geometry at the 30% tibial site. A. In men, the differences in geometry between the two sides suggest that endosteal resorption may have occurred in the tibia on the paretic side. B. In women, the side-to-side differences in bone geometry indicate that periosteal resoprtion may have occurred on the paretic side [55].

Factors Underlying Hemiosteoporosis

Although the mechanisms underlying bone loss following a stroke event are not yet fully understood, researchers have identified several factors that may exert important influence on bone health in stroke patients.

Motor Ability and Functional use of Affected Limb

Motor function and ability to use the affected limb in daily activities seems to be a key factor, with a number of cross-sectional studies showing a significant association of motor ability with bone density [39,43-44,46,49-50,54,56-58], bone geometry [39], and level of bone resorption markers [42-43]. Motor function at the early stage of stroke recovery is particularly important in determining bone status at the later stage [29]. In a 1-year prospective study, Jorgensen and Jacobsen [29] showed that those with severe initial upper limb motor deficits have more substantial bone loss (27% decline) in the proximal humerus after 1 year, compared with those who have only mild (4%) or moderate (11%) motor deficits at the beginning.

There may be an interaction between hand dominance and side of paresis in determining the extent of upper extremity bone loss post-stroke. An early study by Naftchi et al. [34] found that bone loss is more substantial for those stroke patients whose paretic side happens to be the non-dominant side, compared with those whose dominant side is affected by stroke. It may be partly explained by the fact that individuals with the non-dominant hand affected by stroke tend to have more severe impairment (i.e. lower muscle strength, more pain and stiffness) than those with the dominant hand affected [59]. It is postulated that if the dominant upper extremity is affected by stroke, individuals may be more motivated to use their dominant hand during the recovery process, because they wish to relearn the "normal ways" of performing daily tasks, just as how they would perform them before stroke. In contrast, if the non-dominant upper extremity is affected by stroke, individuals may have less motivation to use the non-dominant hand because they are not accustomed to using it for daily functional activities [59]. The less frequent utilization of the non-dominant upper extremity may promote a vicious cycle of muscle weakness, stiffness, other secondary complications that may produce pain (i.e. contractures, subluxation, etc.), thereby promoting further bone loss [59].

The importance of early motor recovery on secondary bone loss is also apparent in the lower extremity [49-51]. For example, those stroke patients who are unable to walk at baseline and remain wheelchair-bound at 7 months post-stroke sustain an average of 13% decline in femoral neck aBMD in one year [49]. In contrast, those who are unable to walk at baseline but manage to regain walking function at 2 months post-stroke only lose 8% of the femoral neck aBMD within the same period [49]. Those who are ambulatory throughout the stroke recovery process have the least amount of bone loss at the femoral neck (3%). These findings clearly demonstrate the adverse effects of poor early motor and functional recovery on subsequent bone loss.

Muscle Strength

Another major factor related to bone loss post-stroke is reduced muscle strength. Muscle strength refers to the individual's ability to generate force during a voluntary muscle contraction [60], and the magnitude of force produced is the most common measure of muscle strength [61]. Muscle weakness, reflected by a reduction of the maximum voluntary force when compared to the norm [60], is prevalent among stroke survivors [61] and could be due to several factors. Following a stroke, many changes take place in the neuromuscular system, including reduced descending motor signals to the paretic side [62], decreased number of functioning motor units [63-64], and altered motor unit recruitment and discharge rate in affected muscles [65-67]. Muscle atrophy on the paretic side is also common following stroke [30,68-69]. These factors may reduce the ability of the affected muscles to generate force [30,61,69].

In stroke patients, strong positive associations of muscle strength with bone mass and bone strength index have been found in the paretic upper extremity [30,39,70] and the paretic lower extremity [49,55,69]. The findings in the stroke population are thus consistent with those in other populations, in which a strong muscle-bone relationship has also been identified [71-74]. Muscle forces provide a good source of mechanical strains to the bone tissue. The loss of muscle strength after stroke could substantially decrease the amount of mechanical loading applied to the bone, leading to bone loss.

Spasticity

Spasticity is another impairment observed in many stroke patients. The relationship between spasticity and bone loss is not as clear. At the 30% site of the radius, a pQCT study has shown that a greater side-to-side difference in bone strength index (indicating more severe bone loss on the paretic side) is associated with more severe spasticity [39]. However, in another study using DXA, no significant relationship can be identified between total arm aBMD and spasticity [30]. In the lower extremity, there is also no evidence to show a significant association of bone loss with spasticity [51,69]. The discrepancies in findings may have several explanations. First, spasticity may have differential effect on various skeletal sites at the upper and lower extremities. Second, most of the previous studies used the Modified Ashworth Scale to measure spasticity, which provides only a gross measure of spasticity in the limb, and may not be sensitive enough to detect small differences in spasticity [75]. Third, the relationship between spasticity and bone may be very complex. On one hand, spasticity may impair limb function, and promote disuse [39,59]. Spasticity may also adversely affect walking function [76], thereby promoting bone loss. On the other hand, the tonic muscle activity associated with spasticity may provide a source of mechanical loading, and may thus exert some protective effect on bone. This phenomenon has been demonstrated in spinal cord injured patients. It has been demonstrated that those who suffer flaccid paralysis have considerably more bone loss that those with spastic paralysis [77]. Clearly, further study is required to examine the effects of spasticity on post-stroke bone loss.

Weight Distribution

Many stroke patients demonstrate postural asymmetry while performing a variety of functional activities such as standing or walking, with more weight being borne by the non-paretic side [50,78-79]. Such habitual asymmetrical weightbearing pattern may exert deleterious influence on bone health in the paretic lower extremity. In an elegant study, Jorgensen et al. [50] measured patients' body weight distribution in quiet standing and showed that the 1-year aBMD change of the paretic femoral neck is correlated with the percent weightbearing on the same side (measured at 7 months post-stroke), indicating the importance of weightbearing on bone health. This finding concurs with another study by Worthen et al. [52]. In their study, in addition to ground reaction force magnitude, the number of steps taken during walking tasks outside the laboratory setting was measured by a specific device. Using these parameters, a Bone Density Index (BDI) was computed to indicate the amount of loading each leg is exposed to on a typical day. Interestingly, they found that total femur aBMD on the paretic side is significantly correlated with BDI in chronic stroke patients, again pointing to the importance of loading activities on bone health.

Cardiovascular Fitness

Peak oxygen consumption (VO_2), which is a gold standard for measuring cardiovascular fitness, has been related to BMD in older adults [80], suggesting that cardiovascular mechanisms may also play a role in mediating bone metabolism. Indeed, increasing evidence suggests a link between cardiovascular disease and osteoporosis [81-85]. For example, a strong relationship between aortic calcification and reduced bone mass has been identified in post-menopausal women [83-84]. For each standard deviation decrease in bone mass, there is a 2-fold increase in mortality due to cardiovascular causes in women [86]. BMD has also been found to have an inverse association with low-density lipoprotein-cholesterol but a positive relationship with high-density lipoprotein-cholesterol [87]. The association between osteoporosis and cardiovascular disease is complex and may involve various biological processes [81]. Nevertheless, since bone (particularly the trabecular bone) is a highly vascularized structure and is in close contact with the endothelium, it is not entirely surprising that impaired blood flow could have detrimental effect on bone health [81].

It is possible that the cardiovascular mechanisms may be involved in mediating the unfavorable bone changes after stroke, since stroke patients often have impaired cardiovascular function. In fact, most stroke patients have a positive history of cardiovascular disease [88] or suboptimally controlled cardiovascular risk factors [89]. Stroke patients also tend to have low peak VO_2 values, reflecting poor cardiovascular fitness [90-92]. Moreover, arterial inflow and endothelium-dependent dilation of vasculature in the paretic extremities are often impaired in these patients [93]. Previous studies have indeed identified a positive association of peak VO_2 with hip aBMD [69] and tibial bone strength index [55].

Vitamin D Deficiency

Evidence suggests that vitamin D deficiency may also have an important influence on bone loss in stroke patients. The most potent circulating form of vitamin D is 1,25-dihydroxyvitamin D [1,25-$(OH)_2D$]. 1,25-$(OH)_2D$ is derived from 25-hydroxyvitamin D [25-(OH)D], which is a major circulating form of vitamin D and can be derived from dietary intake or sunlight exposure [94]. Vitamin D deficiency in stroke patients is reflected by the abnormally low serum 25-(OH)D and 1,25-$(OH)_2D$ levels when compared with control subjects [43-46,95-96]. More importantly, vitamin D level is correlated with BMD in the paretic upper extremity [44-46,95] and is an independent determinant of osteopenia in chronic stroke patients [43]. An increased fracture rate is also observed among those stroke patients who have extremely low 25-(OH)D level (<5ng/mL) (96).

Several factors may explain the abnormally low vitamin D level in stroke patients. First, a large proportion of stroke patients have inadequate dietary intake of vitamin D [47,95]. Sato et al. [95] found that the weekly vitamin D intake in stroke patients is significantly lower than control subjects (95), with more than 62% of outpatients and 82% of inpatients consuming less than 100IU of vitamin D per day. Second, stroke patients typically have limited sunlight exposure [47,95]. In one study, almost 90% of stroke patients reported <15 minutes of sunlight exposure during a typical week [47]. Presumably, the limited mobility has prevented these patients from going outdoors, leading to sunlight deprivation [45]. Finally, immobilization-induced bone loss post-stroke leads to an increased serum calcium levels. The elevated ionized calcium in the circulation may inhibit parathyroid hormone secretion, which in turn inhibits the formation of 1,25-$(OH)_2D$ [43- 46].

Vitamin K Deficiency

Vitamin K is important for γ-carboxylation of several bone matrix proteins, which is an essential step for their binding to hydroxyapatite [97- 99]. Vitamin K deficiency has also been associated with hip fracture [100-101] in otherwise healthy adults. Chronic stroke patients have been shown to have significantly lower serum vitamin K_1 level than controls [47]. Vitamin K_1 level is also independently associated with BMD of the second metacarpal on the paretic side [47]. The low vitamin K level, together with vitamin D deficiency, points to the potential influence of poor nutrition on secondary bone loss in stroke patients.

In summary, multiple factors seem to influence bone health post-stroke (Figure 6). Recovery of bodily function, physical activity, and nutrition may all play a role. Effective management of bone loss in stroke patients may thus require a multi-disciplinary approach.

Management of Bone Loss in Stroke Patients

In view of the pronounced bone loss and increased risk of fragility fractures following stroke, it is imperative that proper intervention be devised to enhance bone health in this population. Recent advances have been made in the use of pharmacological and non-pharmacological means to improve bone health and reduce fracture risk in stroke patients.

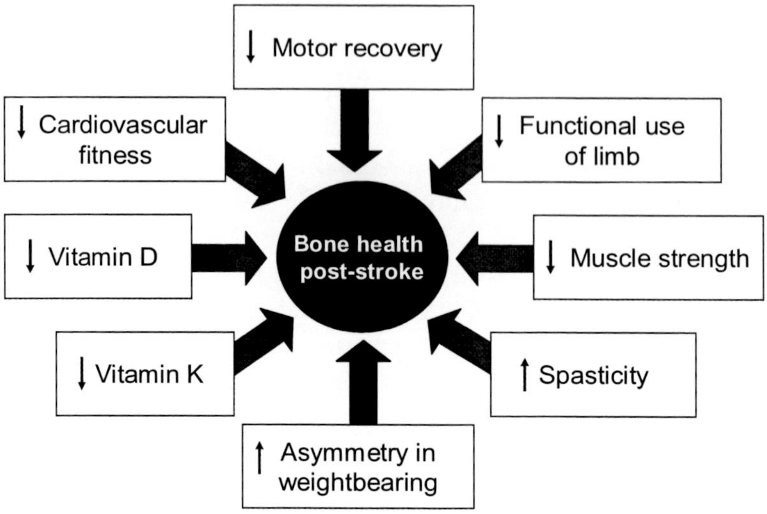

Figure 6. Factors associated with bone health in stroke patients. Multiple factors influence bone health post-stroke.

Bisphosphonates

There is some evidence that bisphosphonates could attenuate bone loss in stroke patients. In a randomized controlled trial (RCT) involving 98 acute stroke patients (mean stroke onset: 7 days), each subject received either etidronate (400mg) or placebo daily for 2 weeks, and followed by a 12-week period in which no medications were given [102]. Each subject underwent a total of four treatment cycles (i.e. 56 weeks). At the end of the treatment period, the BMD of the second metacarpal on the paretic side sustained significantly less decline in the etidronate group (2.3% versus 4.8% in the placebo group). The etidronate group also had significant more reduction in ICTP (a bone resorption marker), and more increase in bone Gla protein (a bone formation marker) than controls. Another study showed that a 2-week administration of etidronate was also effective in suppressing the bone loss in the femoral neck for female subacute stroke patients (mean post-stroke duration: 2.7 months) with low functional ability, but not for those with relatively high functional ability [58]. However, the data need to be interpreted with caution, as the etidronate group also had a significantly lower femoral neck BMD at baseline [58].

Other studies have investigated the effects of risedronate on bone health and fracture risk in subacute stroke patients (mean stroke onset: 90 days)[103-104]. In an 18-month RCT involving 280 male stroke patients who received a daily dose of 2.5mg risedronate sodium and 140 control subjects who received placebo, the risedronate group had a significant 2.5% increase in BMD of the second metacarpal on the paretic side, compared with a 3.5% decline in the placebo group [103]. In addition, the risedronate group also had significantly lower fracture rate than the placebo group (relative risk= 0.19) [103]. Urinary deoxypyridinoline (a bone resorption marker) was also significantly decreased in the risedronate group by 58.7%, compared with only 37.2% decrease in the control group [103]. Similar results have been reported in another RCT involving elderly female stroke patients [104].

While orally-administered bisphosphonates may be effective in suppressing the stroke-induced bone loss, they are contraindicated for patients who have dysphagia or those who are unable to remain upright [105]. Administration of intravenous bisphosphonates such as zoledronate could be an alternative approach for these patients. In a one-year RCT, acute stroke patients were given a single infusion of intravenous zoledronate (4mg) or placebo within 35 days of stroke [106]. After one year, the mean total hip BMD was well maintained in the zoledronate group but significantly decreased by 5.5% in the placebo group. On the non-paretic side, the hip BMD increased by 1.0% in the treatment group versus a 2.7% decrease in the control group. The study thus showed that a single infusion of zoledronate is effective is reducing bone loss in acute stroke patients [106]. However, the study is limited by relatively small sample size (27 subjects). Certain baseline characteristics are also significantly different between the zoledronate group and the control group (e.g. gender proportions, age) [106].

Overall, the available evidence suggests that bisphosphonates could suppress bone loss or even increase BMD in the acute or subacute phase of stroke recovery. The treatment is generally well tolerated, although adverse effects such as abdominal pain [103-104], esophagitis [103; 104], stomach discomfort [58], and peptic ulcer [102] have been reported with oral bisphosphonates. Cases of hypocalcemia, malaise and pyrexia have also been reported with intravenous zoledronate treatment [106]. The risk of hypocalcemia is particularly relevant for those with renal impairment or vitamin D deficiency [106]. Regular assessment of renal function and hydration is recommended by Poole et al. [106] for patients receiving intravenous bisphosphonates.

It is noteworthy that most of the previous studies on bisphosphonates in stroke patients were conducted in Japan. As the epidemiology of factures may vary considerably among different countries, it would be important to evaluate the efficacy of bisphosphonates in other stroke populations. Moreover, most of the trials studied acute or subacute stroke patients, more research is required to establish the efficacy of bisphosphonates in chronic stroke patients.

Vitamin D and Calcium Supplementation

Due to its important role in regulating serum calcium level, it is likely that Vitamin D supplementation may improve bone health in stroke patients [107-109]. In addition, as skeletal muscles express specific receptors for 1,25-$(OH)_2D$, it is suggested that vitamin D may have an additional benefit of enhancing muscle function, thereby reducing falls, and fracture risk [109]. In a two-year RCT involving 96 elderly women with chronic stroke (duration of hospitalization: 2.8 years), the treatment group (48 patients) received 1000IU of ergocalciferol daily while the control group received placebo. At follow-up, the treatment group had significant increase in size and proportion of type II muscle fibers and muscle strength. Such effect on muscle tissue may partly explain the reduced incidence of falls in the treatment group, and hence the lower fracture rate [109]. Another study assessed the efficacy of 1 alpha hydroxyvitamin D_3 and supplemental calcium in chronic stroke patients (mean stroke onset: 4.8 years). After the 6-month treatment period, BMD of the second metacarpal on the paretic side was decreased by as much as 8.9% in the placebo group, compared with only 2.4% decline in the treatment group. The treatment group also had significantly lower hip fracture rate than the placebo group [108]. In summary, vitamin D with or without calcium supplementation may be effective in enhancing BMD and reducing fracture risk in chronic stroke patients.

Sunlight Exposure

It is known that 25-(OH)D, the major circulating form of vitamin D, can be derived from sunlight exposure. As stroke patients typically have very low vitamin D level [43-46,95-96], sunlight exposure could be a viable way to increase vitamin production, thereby enhancing bone health. In a 12-month RCT, a group of 129 chronic stroke patients (mean duration of hospitalization around 4 years) received regular sunlight exposure (15 minutes per day on clear weather days), and another 129 patients did not [110]. At the end of the follow-up period, the BMD of the second metacarpal bone increased by 3.1% in the sunlight-exposed group but decreased by 3.3% in the sunlight-deprived group [110]. In addition, the serum 25-(OH)D level also showed a similar trend, with a significant increase in the sunlight-exposed group, but a significant decrease in the sunlight-deprived group. The sunlight-exposed group also reported a lower fracture risk than the sunlight-deprived group [110].

Vitamin K

Only one study has examined the effects of vitamin K on bone health and fracture risk in chronic stroke patients (mean stroke onset: 13-14 months) [111]. A 12-month RCT has demonstrated that menatetrenone (vitamin K_2) may inhibit bone resorption in the paretic limb. In the study, each of the 54 patients in the treatment group received daily dose of 45mg/day of menatetrenone. At follow-up, the treatment group reported a 4.3% increase in BMD of the second metacarpal on the paretic side, versus a 4.7% decrease in the control group. The vitamin K treatment also resulted in a significant increase in bone Gla protein, with accompanying decrease in ICTP and serum ionized calcium level. However, no beneficial effect on fracture risk was reported [111].

Folate and Mecobalamin

An association between risk of hip fracture and plasma homocysteine level has been previously reported [112-113]. It has been shown that reduction in homocysteine level can be induced by a combination therapy using folate and vitamin B_{12} [114-115]. A RCT involving 628 patients with chronic stroke (stroke onset > 1 year) has been conducted to assess the efficacy of this combination therapy in reducing hip fracture risk [114]. Patients in the treatment group received 5 mg of folate and 1500 μg of mecobalamin (vitamin B_{12}) daily.

The study found that the treatment group had significantly more reduction in homocysteine level than controls. These patients also had a significantly lower incidence of hip fracture (odds ratio=0.2) [116]. However, the treatment did not cause any significant BMD change. The underlying mechanisms of this combination therapy remain unclear.

Exercise

It has long been known that physical inactivity is a risk factor of osteoporosis [117-119] and that mechanical strains can induce bone formation [120]. The ground reaction forces and muscle forces generated during exercise may provide an excellent source of mechanical loading necessary for enhancing bone mass and geometry [121-128]. As mentioned previously, compromised bone health in the stroke population is related to certain modifiable factors such as muscle weakness [30,39,69-70], poor cardiovascular fitness [55,69] and reduced walking ability [39,49,51]. Presumably, a comprehensive exercise program designed to address these various modifiable factors may be a viable way to promote bone health post-stroke. A good number of studies have clearly demonstrated that regular exercise can modify these different factors in stroke patients [129-133]. However, none of these studies have reported on the effects of exercise on bone parameters.

To date, research on exercise and bone health in the stroke population is scarce. Only one RCT has been conducted to examine the effects of regular exercise on bone health in chronic stroke patients [134]. Following a 19-week intensive program (3 one-hour sessions per week) consisting of impact aerobic exercises (i.e. brisk walking, repeated sit-to-stand, stepping onto risers) and other skeletal loading activities, the femoral neck BMD is not significantly changed in the exercise group (0.7% decrease) whereas that in the control group sustains a significant 2.5% decline [134]. The finding thus indicates that the exercise program could maintain BMD in chronic stroke patients.

The same exercise program could also enhance bone geometry at the tibia on the paretic side, as measured by pQCT [135]. The trabecular bone mass is significantly increased at the distal 4% tibial site following the exercise program (Figure 7). At the 50% tibial site, the cortical thickness is well maintained in the exercise group, but not in the control group (Figure 7) [135].

In summary, exercise seems to have beneficial effects on maintaining BMD and enhancing bone geometry in chronic stroke patients. However, whether these changes would translate into a decrease in fracture risk is uncertain. Further study is required to investigate the optimal protocol and dosage of exercise for enhancing BMD and bone geometry in stroke patients. Future studies should also address the effects of exercise on bone health in individuals with acute stroke.

CONCLUSION

Bone health is an extremely relevant issue for stroke survivors, as these individuals often sustain marked secondary bone loss and an exaggerated risk of fragility fractures. More research is needed to determine the rate of bone loss after the first year of stroke, as well as the longitudinal changes in bone geometric properties. Future research should also address the underlying physiological mechanisms underlying bone loss post-stroke. Although the findings from research on bisphosphonates, vitamins, calcium supplementation, and physical exercise seem promising, more investigations are needed to establish the efficacy of various treatment methods and determine the optimal protocol for stroke patients with different disability levels.

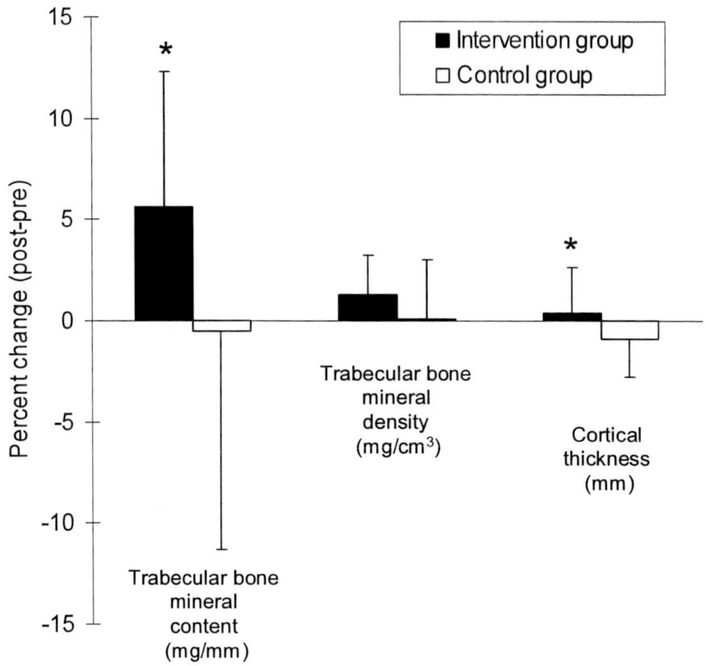

Figure 7. Bone changes in the hemiparetic tibia after a 19-week exercise program as measured by peripheral quantitative computed tomography. A positive value represents a higher value after the exercise program compared with before the exercise program. At the 4% tibial site, there was a significant increase in trabecular bone mineral content for the intervention group. There was also a significant between-group difference in the percent change score of cortical thickness at the 50% tibial site [135].

REFERENCES

[1] Feigin, VL; Lawes, CMM; Bennett, DA; Anderson, CS (2003). Stroke epidemiology: a review of population-based studies of incidence, prevalence, and case-fatality in the late 20th century. *Lancet Neurol*, *l2*, 43-53.

[2] Gresham, GE; Fitzpatrick, TE; Wolf, PA; McNamara, PM; Kannel, WB; Dawber, TR (1975). Residual disability in survivors of stroke--the Framingham study. *N Engl J Med*, *293*, 954-956.

[3] Jørgensen, HS; Nakayama, H; Raaschou, HO; Olsen, TS (1999). Stroke. Neurologic and functional recovery the Copenhagen stroke study. *Phys Med Rehabil Clin N Am, 10*, 887-906.

[4] Poole, KES; Reeve, J; Warburton, EA (2002). Falls, fractures, and osteoporosis after stroke: Time to think about protection? *Stroke, 33*, 1432-1436.

[5] Ramnemark, A; Nilsson, M; Borssén, B; Gustafson, Y (2000). Stroke, a major and increasing risk factor for femoral neck fracture. *Stroke, 31*, 1572-1577.

[6] Wei, TS; Hu, CH; Wang, SH; Hwang, KL (2000). Fall characterisitcs, functional mobility and bone mineral density as risk factors of hip fracture in the community-dwelling anbulatory elderly. *Osteoporos Int. 12*:1050-1055.

[7] Melton, III LJ; Brown, Jr RD; Achenbach, SJ; O'Fallon, WM; WHisnant, JP (2001). Long-term fracture risk following ischemic stroke: a population based study. *Osteoporos Int, 12*, 980-986.

[8] Chiu, KY; Pun, WK; Luk, KDK; Chow, SP (1992). A prospective study on hip fractures in patients with previous cerebrovascular accidents. *Injury, 23*, 297-299.

[9] Peszczynski, M (1957). The fractured hip in hemiplegic patients. *Geriatrics, 12*, 687-690.

[10] Poplingher, AR; Pillar, T (1985). Hip fracture in stroke patients. Epidemiology and rehabilitation. *Acta Orthop Scand, 56*, 226-227.

[11] White, HC. Post-stroke hip fractures. *Arch Orthop Trauma Surg, 107*, 345-347.

[12] Kanis, J; Oden, A; Johnell, O (2001). Acute and long-term increase in fracture risk after hospitalization for stroke. *Stroke, 32*, 702-706.

[13] Ramnemark, A; Nyberg, L; Borssén, B; Olsson, T; Gustafson, Y (1998). Fractures after stroke. *Osteoporos Int, 8*, 92-95.

[14] Whitson HE, Pieper CF, Sanders L, Horner RD, Duncan PW, Lyles KW (2006). Adding injury to insult: Fracture risk after stroke in veterans. *J Am Geriatr Soc, 54*, 1082-1088.

[15] Dennis, MS; Lo, KM; McDowall, M; West, T (2002). Fractures after stroke Frequency, types, and Associations. *Stroke, 33*, 728-734.

[16] Hyndman, D; Ashburn, A; Stack, E (2002). Fall events among people with stroke living in the community: Circumstances of falls and characteristics of fallers. *Arch Phys Med Rehabil, 83*, 165-170.

[17] Cooper C (1997). The crippling consequences of fractures and their impact on quality of life. *Am J Med, 103*, 12S-17S.

[18] Farahmand, BY; Michaelsson, K; Ahlbom, A; Ljunghall, S; Baron, JA (2005). Swedish Hip Fracture Study Group. Survival after hip fracture. *Osteoporos Int, 16*, 1583-1590.

[19] Di Monaco, M; Vallero, F; Di Monaco, R; Mautino, F; Cavanna, A (2003). Functional recovery and length of stay after hip fracture in patients with neurologic impairment. *Am J Phys Med Rehabil, 82*, 143-148.

[20] Braithwaite, RS; Col, NF; Wong, JB (2003). Estimating hip fracture morbidity, mortality and costs. *J Am Geriatr Soc, 51*, 364-370.

[21] Forster, A; Young, J (1995). Incidence and consequences of falls due to stroke: A systematic inquiry. *BMJ. 311*, 83-86.

[22] Sze, KH; Wong, E; Leung, HY; Woo, J (2001). Falls among Chinese stroke patients during rehabilitation. *Arch Phys Med Rehabil*, *82*, 1219-1225.

[23] Nyberg, L; Gustafson; Y (1995). Patient falls in stroke rehabilitation: a challenge to rehabilitation strategies. *Stroke*, *26*, 838-842.

[24] Jorgensen, L; Engstad, T; Jacobsen, BK (2002). Higher incidence of falls in long-term stroke survivors than in population controls: Depressive symptoms predict falls after stroke. *Stroke*, *33*, 542-547.

[25] Tutuarima, JA; van der Meulen, JHP; de Haan, RJ; van Straten, A; Limburg, M (1997). Risk factors for falls of hospitalized stroke patients. *Stroke*, *28*, 297-301.

[26] Lamb, SE; Ferrucci, L; Volapto, S; Fried, LP; Guralnik, JM (2003). Women's Health and Aging Study. Risk factors for falling in home-dwelling older women with stroke: The women's health and aging study. *Stroke*, *34*, 494-501.

[27] Teasell, R; McRae, M; Foley, N; Bhardwaj, A (2002). The incidence and consequences of falls in stroke patients during inpatient rehabilitation: factors associated with high risk. *Arch Phys Med Rehabil*, *83*, 329-333.

[28] Ramnemark, A; Nyberg, L; Lorentzon, R; Englund, U; Gustafson, Y (1999). Progressive Hemiosteoporosis on the paretic side and increased bone mineral density in the nonparetic arm the first year after severe stroke. *Osteoporos Int*, *9*, 269-275.

[29] Jørgensen, L; Jacobsen, BK (2001). Functional status of the paretic arm affects the loss of bone mineral in the proximal humerus after stroke: A 1-year prospective study. *Calcif Tissue Int*, *68*, 11-15.

[30] Pang, MYC; Eng, JJ (2005). Muscle strength is a determinant of bone mineral content in the hemiparetic upper extremity: Implications for stroke rehabilitation. *Bone*, *37*, 103-111.

[31] Hamdy, RC; Krishnaswamy, G; Cancellaro, V; Whalen, K; Harvill, L (1993). Changes in bone mineral content and density after stroke. *Am J Phys Med Rehabil*, *72*, 188-191.

[32] Prince, RL; Price, RI; Ho, S (1988). Forearm bone loss in hemiplegia: A model for the study of immobilization osteoporosis. *J Bone Miner Res*, *3*, 305-310.

[33] Iversen, E; Hassager, C; Christiansen, C (1989). The effect of hemiplegia on bone mass and soft tissue body composition. *Acta Neurol Scand*, *79*, 155-159.

[34] Naftchi, NE; Viau, AT; Marshall, CH; Davis, WS; Lowman, EW (1975). Bone mineralization in the distal forearm of hemiplegic patients. *Arch phys Med Rehabil*, *56*, 487-491.

[35] Ramnemark, A; Nyberg, L; Lorentzon, R; Olsson, T; Gustafson, Y (1999). Hemiosteoporosis after severe stroke, independent of changes in body composition and weight. *Stroke*, *30*, 755-760.

[36] Taub, E; Miller, NE; Novack, TA; Cook, EW 3rd; Fleming, WC ; Nepomuceno, CS; Connell, JS ; Crago, JE (1993). Technique to improve chronic motor deficit after stroke. *Arch Phys Med Rehabil*, *74*, 347-354.

[37] Wolf, SL; Lecraw, DE; Barton, LA; Jann, BB (1989). Forced use of hemiplegic upper extremities to reverse the effect of learned nonuse among chronic stroke and head-injured patients. *Exp Neurol*, *104*, 125-132.

[38] Ashe, MC; Fehling, P; Eng, JJ; Khan, KM; McKay, HA (2006). Bone geometric response to chronic disuse following stroke: A pQCT study. *J Musculoskelet Neuronal Interact*, *6*, 226-233.

[39] Pang, MYC; Ashe, MA; Eng, JJ (2007). Muscle weakness, spasticity and disuse contribute to demineralization and geometric changes in the radius following chronic stroke. *Osteoporos Int*, *18*:1243-1252.

[40] Turner, CH; Burr, DB (1993). Basic biomechanical measurements of bone: a tutorial. *Bone*, *14*, 595-608.

[41] Peacock, M; Turner, CH; Liu, G; Manatunga, AK; Timmerman, L; Johnston, CC (1995). Better discrimination of hip fracture using bone density, geometry, and architecture. *Osteoporos Int*, *5*, 167-173.

[42] Iwamoto, J; Takeda, T; Ichimura, S (2001). Relationships between physical activity and metacarpal bone mass and bone resorption in hemiplegic patients. *J Orthop Sci*, *6*, 227-233.

[43] Sato, Y; Kuno, H; Kaji, M; Oshima, Y; Asoh, T; Oizumi, K (1998). Increased bone resorption during the first year alter stroke. *Stroke*, *29*, 1373-1377.

[44] Sato, Y; Fujimatsu, Y; Kikuyama, M; Kaji, M; Oizumic, K (1998). Influence of immobilization on bone mass and bone metabolism in hemiplegic elderly patients with a long-standing stroke. *J Neurol Sci*, *156*, 205-210.

[45] Sato, Y; Kuno, H; Asoh, T; Honda, Y; Oizumi, K (1999). Effect of immobilization on vitamin D status and bone mass in chronically hospitalized disabled stroke patients. *Age Ageing*, *28*, 265-269.

[46] Sato, Y; Oizumi, K; Kuno, H; Kaji, M (1999). Effect of immobilization upon renal synthesis of 1,25-dihydroxyvitamin D in disabled elderly stroke patients. *Bone*, *24*, 271-275.

[47] Sato, Y; Tsuru, T; Oizumi, K; Kaji, M (1999). Vitamin K deficiency and osteopenia in disuse-affected limbs of vitamin D-deficient elderly stroke patients. *Am J Phys Med Rehabil*, *78*, 317-322.

[48] Browner, WS; Pressman, AR; Nevitt, MC; Cauley, JA; Cummings, SR (1993). Association between low bone density and stroke in elderly women: The study of osteoporotic fractures. *Stroke*, *24*, 940-946.

[49] Jorgensen, L; Jacobsen, BK; Wilsgaard, T; Magnus, JH (2000). Walking after stroke: Does it matter? Changes in bone mineral density within the first 12 months after stroke. A longitudinal study. *Osteoporos Int*, *11*, 381-387.

[50] Jørgensen, L; Crabtree, NJ; Reeve, J; Jacobsen, BK (2000). Ambulatory level and asymmetrical weight bearing after stroke affects bone loss in the upper and lower part of the femoral neck differently: Bone adaptation after decreased mechanical loading. *Bone*, *27*, 701-707.

[51] Jørgensen, L; Jacobsen, BK (2001). Changes in muscle mass, fat mass, and bone mineral content in the legs after stroke: A 1 year prospective study. *Bone*, *28*, 655-659.

[52] Worthen, LC; Kim, CM; Kautz, SA; Lew, HL; Kiratli, BJ; Beaupre, GS (2005). Key characteristics of walking correlate with bone density in individuals with chronic stroke. *J Rehabil Res Dev*, *42*, 761-768.

[53] Takamoto, S; Masuyama, T; Nakajima, M; Seikiya, K; Kosaka, H; Morimoto, S; Ogihara, T; Onishi, T (1995). Alterations of bone mineral density of the femurs in hemiplegia. *Calcif Tissue Int*, *56*, 259-262.

[54] Yavuzer, G; Ataman, S; Süldür, N; Atay, M (2002). Bone mineral density in patients with stroke. *Int J Rehabil Res*, *25*, 235-239.

[55] Pang, MYC; Ashe, MA; Eng, JJ (2008). Tibial bone geometry in chronic stroke patients: influence of sex, cardiovascular health, and muscle mass. *J Bone Miner Res*, 23, 1023-1030.

[56] Liu, M; Tsuji, T; Higuchi, Y; Domen, K; Tsujiuchi, K; Chino, N (1999). Osteoporosis in hemiplegic stroke patients as studied with dual-energy X-ray absorptiometry. *Arch Phys Med Rehabil*, *80*, 1219-1226.

[57] Iwamoto, J; Tsukimura, T; Takeda, T (1999). Bone mineral density of metatarsus in hemiplegic subjects. *Am J Phys Med Rehabil*, *78*, 202-207.

[58] Ikai, T; Uematsu, M; Eun, SS; Kimura, C; Hasegawa, C; Miyano, S (2001). Prevention of secondary osteoporosis postmenopause in hemiplegia. *Am J Phys Med Rehabil*, *80*, 169-174.

[59] Harris, JE; Eng, JJ (2006). Individuals with the dominant hand affected following stroke demonstrate less impairment than those with the nondominant hand affected. *Neurorehabil Neural Repair*, *20*, 380-389.

[60] Bohannon, RW (1995). Measurement, nature, and implications of skeletal muscle strength in persons with neurological disorders. *Clin Biomech*, *10*, 283-292.

[61] McCrea, PH; Eng, JJ; Hodgson, AJ (2003). Time and magnitude of torque generation is impaired in both arms following stroke. *Muscle Nerve*, *28*, 46-53.

[62] Mima, T; Toma, K; Koshy, B; Hallet, M (2001). Coherence between cortical and muscular activities after subcortical stroke. *Stroke*, *32*, 2597-2601.

[63] Hara, Y; Akaboshi, K; Masakado, Y; Chino, N (2000). Physiologic decrease of single thenar motor units in the F-response in stroke patients. *Arch Phys Med Rehabil*, *81*, 418-423.

[64] McComas, AJ; Sica, REP; Upton, ARM; Aguilera, N (1973). Functional changes in motoneurons of hemiparetic patients. *J Neurol Neurosurg Psychiatry*, *36*, 183-193.

[65] Frontera, WR; Grimby, L; Larsson, L (1997). Firing rate of the lower motorneuron and contractile properties of its muscle fibres after upper motorneuron lesion in man. *Muscle Nerve*. *20*, 938-947.

[66] Rosenfalck, A; Andreassen, S (1980). Impaired regulation of force and firing pattern of single motor units in patients with spasticity. *J Neurol Neurosurg Psychiatry*, *43*, 907-916.

[67] Gemperline, JJ; Allen, S; Walk, D; Rymer, WZ (1995). Characteristics of motor unit discharge in subjects with hemiparesis. *Muscle Nerve*, *18*, 1101-1114.

[68] Ryan, AS; Dobrovolny, L; Smith, GV; Silver, KH; Macko, RF (2002). Hemiparetic muscle atrophy and increased intramuscular fat in stroke patients. *Arch Phys Med Rehabil, 83*, 1703-1707.

[69] Pang, MYC; Eng, JJ; McKay, HA; Dawson, AS (2005). Physical fitness is related to hip bone mineral density and leg lean mass in ambulatory individuals with chronic stroke. *Osteoporos Int*, *16*, 1769-1779.

[70] Hamdy, RC; Moore, SW; Cancellaro, VA; Harvill, LM (1995). Long-term effects of strokes on bone mass. *Am J Phys Med Rehabil*, *74*, 351-356.
[71] Ozdurak, RH; Duz, S; Arsal, G; Akinci, Y; Kablan, N; Isikli, S; Korkusuz, F (2003). Quantitative forearm muscle strength influences radial bone mineral density in osteoporotic and healthy males. *Tech Health Care*, *11*, 253-261.
[72] Hughes, VA; Frontera, WR; Dallal, GE; Lutz, KJ; Fisher, EC; Evans, WJ (1995). Muscle strength and body composition: associations with bone density in older subjects. *Med Sci Sports Exerc*, *27*, 967-974.
[73] Di Monaco, M; Di Monaco, R; Manca, M; Cavanna, A (2000). Handgrip strength is an independent predictor of distal radius bone mineral density in postmenopausal women. *Clin Rheumatol*, *19*, 473-476.
[74] Osei-Hyiaman, D; Ueji, M; Toyakawa, S; Takahashi, H; Kano, K (1999). Influence of hand grip strength on metacarpal bone mineral density in postmenopausal Japanese women: a cross-sectional study. *Calcif Tissue Int*, *64*, 263-266.
[75] Bohannon, BW; Smith, MB (1987). Interrater reliability of a Modified Ashworth Scale of muscle spasticity. Phys Ther, *67*, 206-207.
[76] Hsu, AL; Tang, PF; Jan, MH (2003). Analysis of impairments influencing gait velocity and asymmetry of hemiplegic patients after mild to moderate stroke. *Arch Phys Med Rehabil*, *84*, 1185-1193.
[77] Wilmet, E; Ismail, AA; Heilporn, A; Welraeds, D; Bergmann, P (1995). Longitudinal study of the bone mineral content and of soft tissue composition after spinal cord section. *Paraplegia*, *33*, 674-677.
[78] Cheng, PT; Liaw, MY; Wong, MK; Tang, FT; Lee, MY; Lin, PS (1998). The sit-to-stand movement in stroke patients and its correlation with falling. *Arch Phys Med Rehabil*, *79*, 1043-1046.
[79] Eng, JJ; Chu, KS (2002). Reliability and comparison of weight-bearing ability during standing tasks for individuals with chronic stroke. *Arch Phys Med Rehabil*, *83*, 1138-1144.
[80] Vico, L; Pouget, JF; Calmels, P; Chatard, JC; Rehailia, M; Minaire, P; Geyssant, A; Alexandre, C (1995). The relations between physical ability and bone mass in women aged over 65 years. *J Bone Miner Res*, *10*, 374-383.
[81] Whitney, C; Warburton, ER; Frohlich, J; Chan, SY; McKay, H; Khan, K (2004). Are cardiovascular disease and osteoporosis directly linked? *Sports Med*, *34*, 779-807.
[82] Kado, DM; Browner, WS; Blackwell, T; Gore, R; Cummings, SR (2000). Rate of bone loss is associated with mortality in older women: a prospective study. *J Bon Miner Res*, *15*, 1974-1980.
[83] Hak, AE; Pols, HA; van Hemert, AM; Hofman, A; Witteman, JC (2000). Progression of aortic calcification is associated with metacarpal bone loss during menopause: a population-based longitudinal study. *Aterioscler Thromb Vasc Biol*, *20*, 1926-1931.
[84] Kiel, DP; Kauppila, LC; Kauppila, LI; Cupples, LA; Hannan, MT; O'Donnell, CJ; Wilson, PW (2001). Bone loss and the progression of abdominal aortic calcification over a 25 year period: the Framingham Heart Study. *Calcif Tissue Int*, *68*, 271-276.

[85] Rodriguez-Garcia, M; Naves-Diaz, M; Andia, JBC (2005). Bone metabolism, vascular calcifications and mortality: Associations beyond mere coincidence. *J Nephrol, 18*, 458-463.

[86] von der Recke, P; Hansen, M; Hassager, C (1999). The association between low bone mass at the menopause and cardiovascular mortality. *Am J Med, 106*, 273-278.

[87] Yamaguchi, T; Sugimoto, T; Yano, S; Yamauchi, M; Sowa, H; Chen, Q; Chihara, K (2002). Plasma lipids and osteoporosis in postmenopausal women. *Endocr J, 49*, 211-217.

[88] Roth, EJ (1993). Heart disease in patients with stroke: incidence, impact, and implications for rehabilitation. Part I: classification and prevalence. *Arch Phys Med Rehabil, 74*, 752-760.

[89] Kopunek, SP; Michael, KM; Shaughnessy, M; Resnick, B; Nahm, ES; Whitall, J; Goldberg, A; Macko, RF (2007). Cardiovascular risk in survivors of stroke. *Am J Prev Med, 32*, 408-412.

[90] Pang, MYC; Eng, JJ; Dawson, AS (2005). Relationship between ambulatory capacity and cardiorespiratory fitness in chronic stroke: influence of stroke-specific impairments. *Chest, 127*, 495-501.

[91] MacKay-Lyons, MJ; Makrides, L (2002). Exercise capacity early after stroke. Arch *Phys Med Rehabil, 83*, 1697-1702.

[92] MacKay-Lyons, MJ; Makrides, L (2004). Longitudinal changes in exercise capacity after stroke. *Arch Phys Med Rehabil, 85*, 1608-1612.

[93] Wang, JS; Yang, CF; Liaw, MY; Wong, MK (2002). Suppressed cutaneous endothelial vascular control and hemodynamic changes in paretic extremities with edema in the extremities of patients with hemiplegia. *Arch Phys Med Rehabil, 83*, 1017-1023.

[94] Holick, MF. Vitamin D: Photobiology, metabolism, mechanism of action, and clinical applications. In: Favus MJ, editor. *Primer on the metabolic bone diseases and disorders of mineral metabolism. (5th ed)*. Philadelphia: Lippincott Williams & Wilkins; 2003; 129-136.

[95] Sato, Y; Maruoka, H; Oizumi, K; Kikuyama, M (1996). Vitamin D deficiency and osteopenia in the hemiplegic limbs of stroke patients. *Stroke, 27*, 2183-2187.

[96] Sato, Y; Asoh, T; Kondo, I; Satoh, K (2001). Vitamin D deficiency and risk of hip fractures among disabled elderly stroke patients. *Stroke, 32*, 1673-1677.

[97] Heaney, RP. Nutrition and osteoporosis. In: Favus MJ, editor. *Primer on the metabolic bone diseases and disorders of mineral metabolism. (5th ed)*. Philadelphia: Lippincott Williams & Wilkins; 2003; 352-355.

[98] Vermeer, C; Jie, KSG; Knapen, MHJ (1995). Role of vitamin K in bone metabolism. *Annu Rev Nutr, 15*, 1-22.

[99] Shearer, MJ. Vitamin K. *Lancet, 345*, 229-234.

[100] Feskanich, D; Weber, P; Willett, WC; Rockett, H; Booth, SL; Colditz, GA (1999). Vitamin K intakes and hip fractures in women: a prospective study. *Am J Clin Nutr, 64*, 74-79.

[101] Booth, SL; Tucker, KL; Chen, H; Hannan, MT; Gagnon, DR; Cupples, LA; Wilson, PW; Ordovas, J; Schaefer, EJ; Dawson-Hughes, B; Kiel, DP (2000). Dietary vitamin K

intakes are associated with hip fracture but not with bone mineral density in elderly men and women. *Am J Clin Nutr*, *71*, 1201-1208.

[102] Sato, Y; Asoh, T; Kaji, M; Oizumi, K (2000). Beneficial effect of intermittent cyclical etidronate therapy in hemiplegic patients following an acute stroke. *J Bone Miner Res*, *15*, 2487-2494.

[103] Sato, Y; Iwamoto, J; Kanoko, T; Satoh, K (2005). Risedronate sodium therapy for prevention of hip fracture in men 65 years or older after stroke. *Arch Intern Med*, *165*, 1743-1748.

[104] Sato, Y; Iwamoto, J; Kanoko, T; Satoh, K (2005). Risedronate therapy for prevention of hip fracture after stroke in elderly women. *Neurology*, *64*, 811-816.

[105] Myint, PK; Poole, KES; Warburton, EA (2007). Hip fractures after stroke and their prevention. *Q J Med*, *100*, 539-545.

[106] Poole, KES; Loveridge, N; Rose, CM; Warburton, EA; Reeve, J (2007). A single infusion of zoledronate prevents bone loss after stroke. *Stroke*, *38*, 1519-1525.

[107] Sato, Y; Kuno, H; Kaji, M; Saruwatari, N; Oizumi, K (1999). Effect of ipriflavone on bone in elderly hemiplegic stroke patients with hypovitaminosis D. Am *J Phys Med Rehabil*, *78*, 457-463.

[108] Sato, Y; Maruoka, H; Oizumi, K (1997). Amelioration of hemiplegia-associated osteopenia more than 4 years after stroke by 1 alpha-hydroxyvitamin D3 and calcium supplementation. *Stroke*, *28*, 736-739.

[109] Sato, Y; Iwamoto, J; Kanoko, T; Satoh, K (2005). Low-dose vitamin D prevents muscular atrophy and reduces falls and hip fractures in women after stroke: A randomized controlled trial. *Cerebrovasc Dis*, *20*,187-192.

[110] Sato, Y; Metoki, N; Iwamoto, J; Satoh, K. Amelioration of osteoporosis and hypovitaminosis D by sunlight exposure in stroke patients. *Neurology*, *61*, 338-342.

[111] Sato, Y; Honda, Y; Kuno, H; Oizumi, K (1998). Menatetrenone ameliorates osteopenia in disuse-affected limbs of vitamin D- and K-deficient stroke patients. *Bone*, *23*:291-296.

[112] van Meurs, JB; Dhonukshe-Rutten, RA; Pluijm, SM; van der Klift, M; de Jonge, R; Lindemans, J; de Groot, LC; Hofman, A; Witteman, JC; van Leeuwen, JP; Breteler, MM; Lips, P; Pols, HA; Uitterlinden, AG (2004). Homocysteine levels and the risk of osteoporotic fracture. *N Engl J Med*, *350*, 2033-2041.

[113] McLean, RR; Jacques, PF; Selhub, J; Tucker, KL; Samelson, EJ; Broe, KE; Hannan, MT; Cupples, LA; Kiel, DP (2004). Homocysteine as a predictive factor for hip fracture in older persons. *N Engl J Med*, *350*, 2042-2049.

[114] Green, TJ; McMahon, JA; Skeaff, CM; Williams, SM; Whiting, SJ (2007). Lowering homocysteine with B vitamins has no effect on biomarkers of bone turnover in older persons: a 2-y randomized controlled trial. *Am J Clin Nutr*, *85*, 460-464.

[115] Flicker, L; Vasikaran, SD; Thomas, J; Acres, JM; Norman, P; Jamrozik, K; Hankey, GJ; Almeida, OP (2006). Efficacy of B vitamins in lowering homocysteine in older men: maximal effects for those with B12 deficiency and hyperhomocysteinemia. *Stroke*, *37*, 547-549.

[116] Sato, Y; Honda, Y; Iwamoto, J; Kanodo, T; Satoh, K (2005). Effect of folate and mecobalamin on hip fractures in patients with stroke. A randomized controlled trial. *JAMA*, *293*, 1082-1088.

[117] Nguyen, TV; Center, JR; Eisman, JA (2000). Osteoporosis in elderly men and women: Effects of dietary calcium, physical activity, and body mass index. *J Bone Miner Res*, *15*, 322-331.

[118] Uusi-Rasi, K; Sievanen, H; Pasanen, M; Oja, P; Vuori, I (2001). Maintenance of body weight, physical activity and calcium intake helps preserve bone mass in elderly women. *Osteoporos Int*, *12*, 373-379.

[119] Lau, EM; Suriwongpaisal, P; Lee, JK; Das De, S; Festin, MR; Saw, SM; Khir, A; Torralba, T; Sham, A; Sambrook, P (2001). Risk factors for hip fracture in Asian men and women: The Asian osteoporosis study. *J Bone Miner Res*, *16*, 572-580.

[120] Turner CH; Robling AG (2005). Mechanisms by which exercise improves bone strength. *J Bone Miner Metab*, *23*, 16-22.

[121] Kerr, D; Ackland, T; Maslen, B; Morton, A; Prince, R (2001). Resistance training over 2 years increases bone mass in calcium-replete postmenopausal women. *J Bone Miner Res*, *16*, 175-181.

[122] Chien, MY; Wu, YT; Hsu, AT; Yang, RS; Lai, JS (2000). Efficacy of a 24-week aerobic exercise program for osteopenic postmenopausal women. *Calcif Tissue Int*, *67*, 443-448.

[123] Welsh, L; Rutherford, OM (1996). Hip bone mineral density is improved by high-impact aerobic exercise in postmenopausal women and men over 50 years. *Eur J Appl Physiol Occup Physiol*, *74*, 511-517.

[124] Kemmler, W; Lauber, D; Weineck, J; Hensen, J; Kalender, W; Engelke, K (2004). Benefits of 2 years of intense exercise on bone density, physical fitness, and blood lipids in early postmenopausal osteopenic women; results of the Erlangen Fitness Osteoporosis Prevention Study (EFOPS). *Arch Int Med*, *164*, 1084-1091.

[125] Ryan, AS; Ivey, FM; Hurlbut, DE; Martel, GF; Lemmer, JT; Sorkin, JD; Metter, EJ; Fleg, JL; Hurley, BF (2004). Regional bone mineral density after resistive training in young and older men and women. *Scand J Med Sci Sports*, *14*, 16-23.

[126] Vincent, KR; Braith, RW (2002). Resistance exercise and bone turnover in elderly men and women. *Med Sci Sports Exerc*, *34*, 17-23.

[127] Adami, S; Gatti, D; Braga, V; Bianchini, D; Rossini, M (1999). Site-specific effects of strength training on bone structure and geometry of ultradistal radius in postmenopausal women. *J Bone Miner Res*, *14*, 120-124.

[128] Liu-Ambrose, TY; Khan, KM; Eng, JJ; Heinonen, A; McKay, HA (2004). Both resistance and agility training increase cortical bone density in 75- to 85-year-old women with low bone mass: A 6-month randomized controlled trial. *J Clin Densitom*, *7*, 390-398.

[129] Ouellette, MM; LeBrasseur, NK; Bean, JF; Philips, E; Stein, J; Frontera, WR; Fielding, RA (2004). High-intensity resistance training improves muscle strength, self-reported function, and disability in long-tern stroke survivors. *Stroke*, *35*, 1404-1409.

[130] Macko, RF; Ivey, FM; Forrester, LW; Hanley, D; Sorkin, JD; Katzel, LI; Silver, KH; Goldberg, AP (2005). Treadmill exercise rehabilitation improves ambulatory function

and cardiovascular fitness in patients with chronic stroke. A randomized, controlled trial. *Stroke*, *36*, 2206-2211.

[131] Duncan, P; Studenski, S; Richards, L; Gollub, S; Lai, SM; Reker, D; Perera, S; Yates, J; Koch, V; Rigler, S; Johnson, D (2003). Randomized clinical trial of therapeutic exercise in subacute stroke. *Stroke*, *34*, 2173-2180.

[132] Salbach, N; Mayo, NE; Wood-Dauphinee, S; Hanley, JA; Richards, CL; Cote, R (2004). A task-oriented intervention enhances walking distance and speed in the first year post stroke: a randomized controlled trial. *Clin Rehabil*, *18*, 509-519.

[133] Katz-Leurer, M; Shochina, M; Carmeli, E; Friedlander, Y (2003). The influence of early aerobic training on the functional capacity in patients with cerebrovascular accident at the subacute stage. *Arch Phys Med Rehabil*, *84*, 1609-1614.

[134] Pang, MYC; Eng, JJ; Dawson, AS; McKay, HA; Harris, JE (2005). A community-based fitness and mobility exercise program for older adults with chronic stroke: A randomized, controlled trial. *J Am Geriatr Soc*, *53*, 1667-1674.

[135] Pang, MYC; Ashe, MC; Eng, JJ; McKay, HA; Dawson, AS (2006). A 19-week exercise program for people with chronic stroke enhances bone geometry at the tibia: A peripheral quantitative computed tomography study. *Osteoporos Int*, *17*, 1615-1625.

In: Osteoporosis: Etiology, Diagnosis and Treatment
Editors: Bilar E. Mattingly and Albert C. Pillare
ISBN 978-1-60692-397-9

Chapter 6

New Perspectives in the Management of Osteoporosis: The OPG/RANK/RANKL System

Enrico M. Messalli and Cono Scaffa
Department of Gynaecology, Obstetrics and Reproductive Medicine,
Second University of Naples,
Largo Madonna delle Grazie 1, 80138 Naples, Italy

Abstract

During the last years, several medications have been used for the management of osteoporosis. Bisphosphonates are the most prescribed drugs: daily or weekly alendronate and risedronate have demonstrated their ability to reduce fracture rates at the spine and hip; ibandronate has demonstrated spine antifracture efficacy with intervals between dosings greater than weekly. New developments in this class include intravenous administration of ibandronate or zoledronate, once every three months or once yearly. Raloxifene, a selective estrogen-receptor modulator, reduces spine fractures and, in post-hoc analyses, non-spine fractures in high-risk subjects. New selective estrogen-receptor modulators, including lasofoxifene, bazedoxifene and arzoxifene, are expected to demonstrate antifracture efficacy at the hip level, whilst retaining the extra-skeletal benefits (such as in the breast). The peptides from the parathyroid hormone family are potent stimulators of bone formation: teriparatide reduces spine and non-spine fractures for up to 30 months after the withdrawal of treatment. Strontium ranelate is suggested to be the first medication to uncouple bone formation from bone resorption. New developments include: inhibitors of cathepsin K, a cysteine protease that is involved in the cleavage of collagen, and, mainly, denosumab, a monoclonal antibody against a cytokine responsible for osteoclastogenesis.

This last perspective is born from the discovery of OPG/RANK/RANKL system. Osteoprotegerin (OPG) is a protein expressed by osteoblasts that, linking the receptor activator of nuclear factor κB (RANK) ligand (RANKL), produced by osteoblasts, blocks the process of osteoclastic differentiation and modulates osteoclastic apoptosis. The importance of OPG in bone metabolism is suggested by the positive correlation between the gene production of OPG and the bone mass increase in animal models. In humans, OPG is implicated in the pathogenesis of postmenopausal osteoporosis and of other metabolic diseases, characterized by bone loss. Estrogens and other drugs used in the treatment of osteoporosis stimulate the production of OPG from osteoblasts carrying out their antiresorption activity, at least in part, as means of the OPG/RANK/RANKL system. In vitro and in vivo data demonstrate that these drugs could improve osteoporosis, also through an increase of OPG production by osteoblasts, opening further therapeutic use of OPG or anti-RANKL drugs. The fully human monoclonal antibody denosumab (formerly known as AMG 162) binds RANKL with high affinity and specificity and inhibits RANKL action. In postmenopausal women with low bone mass, subcutaneously administered denosumab increased bone mineral density and decreased bone resorption. These preliminary data suggest that denosumab might be an effective treatment for osteoporosis.

1. Introduction

The decreased estrogen circulating level during postmenopausal age represents the main cause of bone loss and osteoporosis, well-established risk factor for fracture [1,2]. However, a rapid decrease of bone mass is evident into the first 5-10 years following the menopause (Figure 1). The annual rate of bone loss is maximum about 4% per annum during the former four years [3], than it shows back to 1% [4]. In this period, the physiological bone remodelling is characterized mainly by a relevant prevalence of the resorption due to the osteoclastic activity [5].

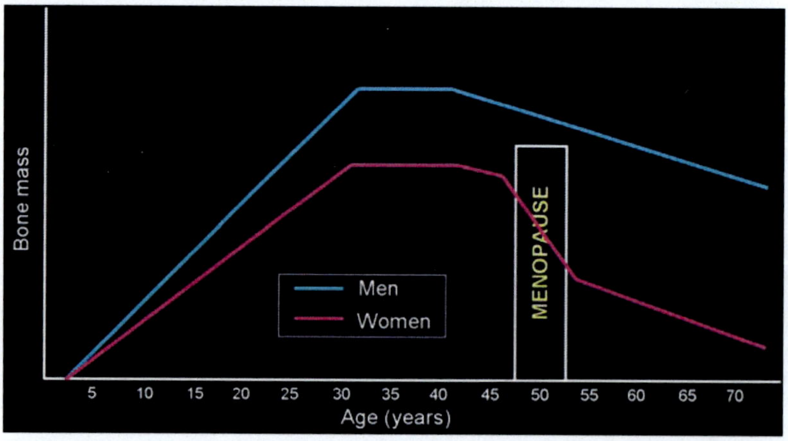

Figure 1.

During the last twenty years, many drugs have been granted a marketing license for treatment of osteoporosis. Bisphosphonates are the most widely prescribed drugs: alendronate and risedronate are given daily or weekly and have demonstrated efficacy on reduction of fracture rates at the spine and hip; ibandronate has demonstrated spine antifracture efficacy with intervals between doses greater than weekly; new developments in this class include intravenous administration of ibandronate or zoledronate, once every three months or once yearly. Strontium ranelate is suggested to be the first medication to uncouple bone formation from bone resorption; it has shown antifracture efficacy at all sites in a large number of postmenopausal women.

The peptides from the parathyroid hormone family are potent stimulators of bone formation: teriparatide (1-34 amino acid fragment of the parathyroid hormone) reduces spine and non-spine fractures, an effect that is sustained for up to 30 months after the withdrawal of treatment; the intact parathyroid hormone - PTH (1-84 amino acids) showed similar results on spine fractures, and more data are requested to evaluate its effect on non-spine or hip fractures.

Raloxifene, a selective estrogen-receptor modulator (SERM), reduces spine fractures and, in post-hoc analyses, non-spine fractures in high-risk subjects. New SERMs, including lasofoxifene, bazedoxifene and arzoxifene, are expected to demonstrate antifracture efficacy at the hip level, whilst retaining the extra-skeletal benefits (such as in the breast) that are obtained with raloxifene.

New developments on management of osteoporosis include: denosumab, a monoclonal antibody against a cytokine responsible for osteoclastogenesis, and inhibitors of cathepsin K, a cysteine protease that is involved in the cleavage of collagen [6].

Despite treatment options can reduce the risk of fracture in patients with osteoporosis, few patients fully adhere to current therapies. A recent study reported one-year adherence rates of less than 25% for all osteoporosis therapies examined [7]. This adherence rate is substantially lower than that for therapies for other asymptomatic conditions, such as hypertension (50-70% adherence) [8].

Thus, new treatment approaches that engender high adherence are needed. Besides, osteoporosis is a chronic disease requiring long-term therapy, thus, it is important to evaluate new potential therapies over several years. Aim of this chapter is to analyze the role of a new cytokine pathway of bone turnover modulators on the mechanism of action of old, recent, and investigational drugs for osteoporosis management.

2. The OPG/RANK/RANKL System

The integrity of the skeleton and the bone remodelling that occurs throughout life requires the coordinated regulation and activity of osteoblasts and osteoclasts. The number of active osteoclasts is determined by the net result of differentiation and fusion of osteoclast precursors and by the loss of osteoclasts through apoptosis. An increase in active osteoclast pool size, with increased bone resorption and decreased bone mass, occurs in many osteopathic disorders, including postmenopausal osteoporosis.

A large number of hormones, growth and inflammatory factors, and cytokines are known to regulate osteoclast formation (osteoclastogenesis) and function. Osteoclasts derive from the monocyte/macrophage lineage precursor cells and their bone resorption activity is regulated by a variety of factors such as interleukins IL-1, IL-6, IL-11, macrophage colony stimulating factor (M-CSF), PTH and calcitonin [9]. An important development in understanding of osteoclastogenesis has been achieved with the discovery that new members of the tumor necrosis factor (TNF) family of ligands and receptors play a crucial role in osteoclast formation and activity and may be the molecular mediators [10]. Recently, new perspectives in the management of osteoporosis are born from the discovery of a cytokine pathway that regulates osteoclastogenesis and modulates osteoclastic bone resorption: the OPG/RANK/RANKL system [11-16] (Figure 2).

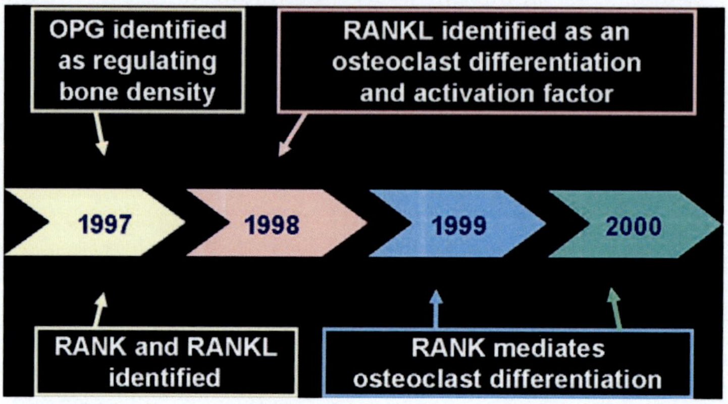

Figure 2.

The receptor activator of nuclear factor κB (RANK) ligand (RANKL), expressed by osteoblastic stromal cells, bone marrow stromal cells and activated T cells, is a member of the TNF family that is an essential mediator of osteoclast formation, differentiation, activation, function, and survival [11,12,17-19]. RANKL is a type II homotrimeric transmembrane protein (317-amino acid peptide) that is expressed as a membrane-bound and a secreted protein, which is derived from the membrane form as a result of either proteolytic cleavage or alternative splicing [20]. RANKL is highly expressed in lymph nodes, thymus and lung and at low levels in a variety of other tissues including spleen and bone marrow [21]; many factors stimulate osteoblast expression of RANKL (Figure 3).

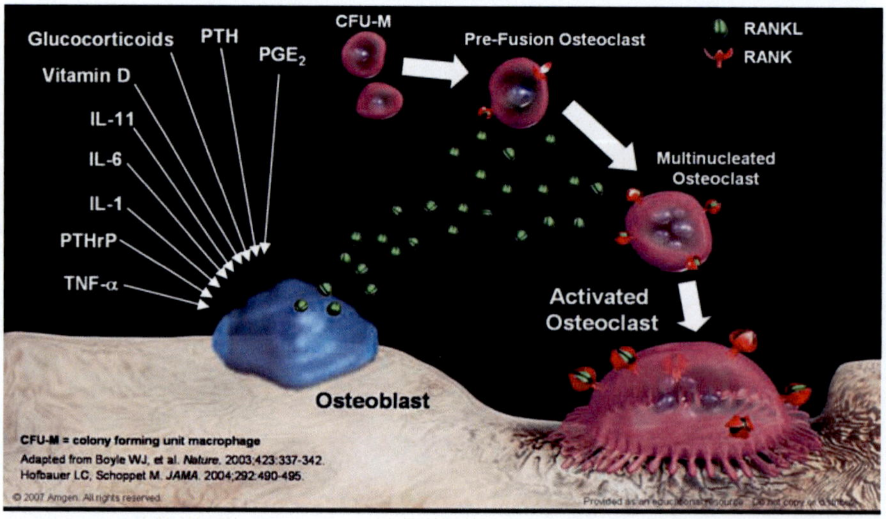

Figure 3.

RANK, a transmembrane protein that acts as the cognate receptor of RANKL, has been identified on the surface of osteoclasts at several stages of differentiation, including prefusion osteoclasts and mature osteoclasts [22,23] (Figure 4). RANK is a type I homotrimeric transmembrane protein (616-amino acid peptide) whose expression was initially detected only on osteoclast precursors, mature osteoclasts, and dendritic cells. Like RANKL, however, it is expressed widely [21].

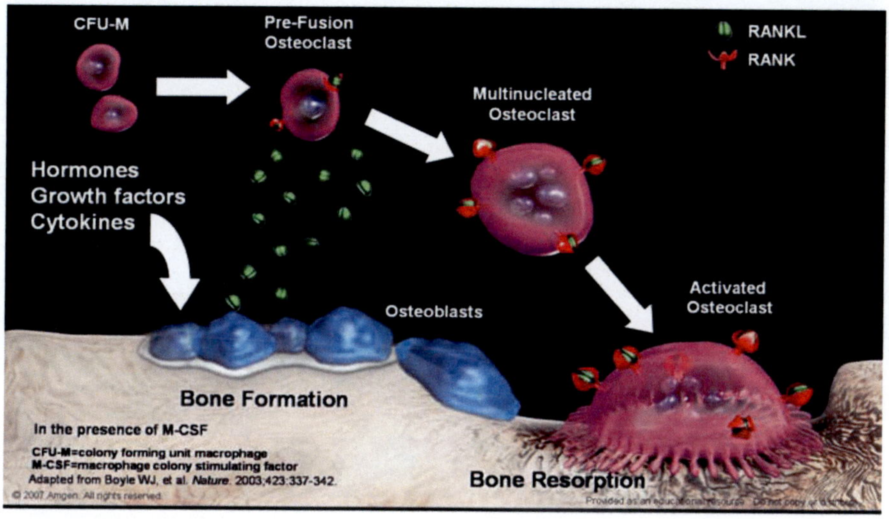

Figure 4.

The binding of RANKL to RANK on osteoclasts initiates a cascade of intracellular signalling events [24].

A key regulator of the RANK-RANKL interaction is the soluble cytokine decoy receptor, osteoprotegerin (OPG), 401 amino acid peptide, with a 21-amino acid propeptide that was cleaved, resulting in a mature protein of 380 amino acids [13]. It is a naturally occurring member of the TNF receptor family that competes with RANK to bind RANKL, thus sequestering RANKL and neutralizing its effects [11,13,18] (Figure 5). In contrast to all other TNF receptor family members, OPG lacked transmembrane and cytoplasmic domains and was secreted as a soluble protein [13]. OPG is a soluble protein expressed by osteoblasts that, linking RANKL, blocks the process of osteoclastic differentiation and modulates osteoclastic apoptosis. It acts as a decoy receptor for RANKL blocking the process of osteoclast differentiation and modulating apoptosis process in these cells [25,26] (Figure 6). On the contrary, the osteoclastic activation induces an IL-1β mediated osteoblastic production of OPG as a feed-back mechanism [27]. OPG is expressed in many tissues apart from osteoblasts, including heart, kidney, liver, spleen, and bone marrow [21]. Its expression is regulated by most of the factors that induce RANKL expression by osteoblasts. OPG is a negative regulator of osteoclast mediated bone resorption [22] and when RANKL overwhelms OPG, bone resorption can become excessive leading to osteoporosis, therefore, a healthy skeleton depends on a balanced RANKL/OPG ratio [23] (Figure 7). Although there are contradictory data, in general up-regulation of RANKL is associated with down-regulation of OPG, or at least lower induction of OPG, such that the ratio of RANKL to OPG changes in favour of osteoclastogenesis. Many reports have supported the assertion that the RANKL/OPG ratio is a major determinant of bone mass [23].

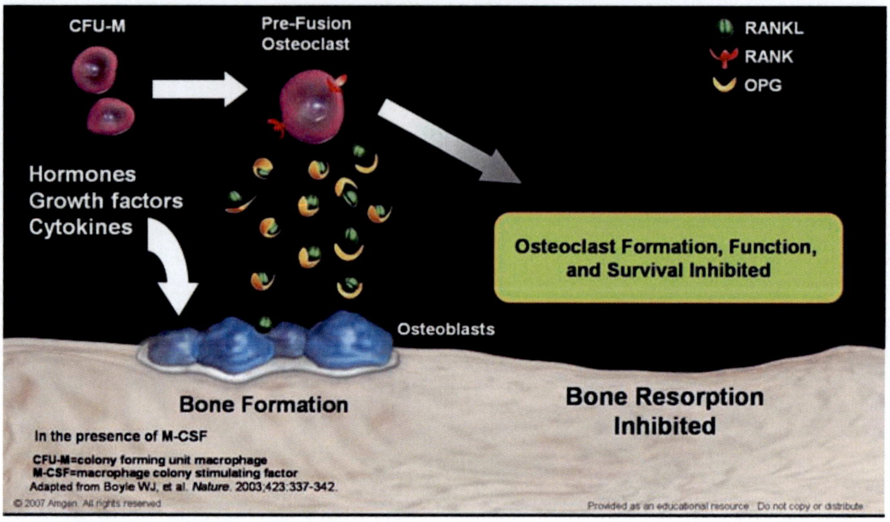

Figure 5.

Agents enhancing RANKL/OPG ratio are glucocorticoids (enhance osteoclastogenesis by OPG inhibition and OPG ligands production via cells of osteoblastic line, which leads to increased osteoresorption), some inflammatory cytokines (IL-1β, IL-4, IL-6, IL-11, IL-17, and TNF-α stimulate osteoclastogenesis by induction of OPG ligands expression), basic fibroblast growth factor 2 (inhibits OPG production and stimulates RANKL production), PTH (inhibits OPG production and promotes RANKL production), prostaglandins E2, 1,25-OH vitamin D3 [10,28-32]. The agents reducing RANKL/OPG ratio are estrogens (enhance OPG secretion by osteoblastic cells and inhibit RANKL production) and TGF-β released from matrix degradation (induces OPG secretion) [31,33,34].

Years of menopause, age, together with bone turnover markers were the main factors affecting serum concentrations of OPG and RANKL. The importance of OPG in bone metabolism is suggested by the positive correlation between the gene production of OPG [26] and the bone mass increase in animal models [2,35]. In humans, OPG is implicated in the pathogenesis of postmenopausal osteoporosis and other metabolic diseases, characterized by bone loss: in postmenopausal women OPG increases both in serum and bone [36,37] whereas RANKL is higher in bone marrow stromal cells without any difference in serum levels if compared to premenopausal values [38]. In a group of women monitored for thyroid carcinoma, postmenopausal patients showed higher levels of serum OPG and lower levels of bone mineral density (BMD) compared to premenopausal patients [39]. These data suggest that circulating OPG may reflect OPG activity on bone although this does not seem to be the case with serum RANKL. Other authors [40] state that circulating OPG levels reflect an antiresorptive activity in bone or are significantly related to BMD [41], while a negative relationship between OPG and bone turnover status have been reported [42-44].

The link between OPG levels and bone markers is also under debate. Rogers et al. hypothesize a significant positive relationship between OPG and BMD at total body, and a significant weak positive relationship between circulating OPG and serum estradiol has been showed. They also suggest that circulating levels of OPG may reflect OPG activity in bone and are related to circulating endogenous levels of estradiol [45]. Recently a weak correlation between OPG and serum markers of bone formation in healthy population has been shown, whereas others found a strong relationship between serum OPG and markers of bone turnover only in postmenopausal women [46-48]. This statement is questioned by other authors, because circulating OPG levels are depended on several factors and paracrine mechanisms involved in osteoporosis genesis [40,49] and on non-skeletal sources [42].

The elevation of serum OPG along with age might be a compensatory mechanism against the accelerated bone resorption, while the decreased level of serum RANKL might be helpful for restoring the reduced bone formation in postmenopausal women [50].

3. New perspectives in the management of osteoporosis

Since the osteoclast is the only cell in the body that is capable of resorbing bone, analysis of the differentiation, maturation, regulation, and bone resorption mechanisms of osteoclasts may point to a therapeutic approach for osteoporosis. The discovery of the OPG/RANK/RANKL system as the primary mediator of osteoclast differentiation, activation, and survival facilitated the design of molecules that specifically target this pathway for the treatment of osteoporosis.

Clinical and preclinical evidence suggest that, in many disease states, RANKL is implicated in the bone loss that leads to skeletal fragility and fracture [23,38,51,52]. Moreover, preclinical studies have shown that RANKL inhibition leads to skeletal benefits that include increases in BMD, volume, and strength [13,53-57]. The results of these studies have shown that inhibition of RANKL leads to improved bone geometry and increased BMD and strength.

Estrogens and other drugs used in the treatment of osteoporosis stimulate the production of OPG from osteoblasts carrying out their antiresorption activity, at least in part, as means of the OPG/RANK/RANKL system. In vitro and in vivo data demonstrate that these drugs could improve osteoporosis, also through an increase of OPG production by osteoblasts, opening further therapeutic use of OPG or anti-RANKL drugs.

In this chapter, we distinguish drugs blocking osteoclast differentiation or through induction of the expression of OPG from osteoblasts (OPG-inducing drugs), or mimicking the OPG action (OPG-mimicking drugs/anti-RANKL drugs) (Figure 8).

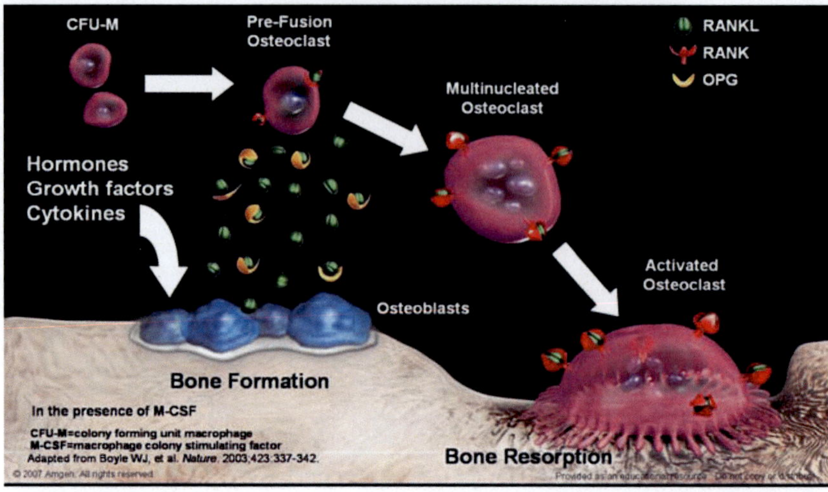

Figure 6.

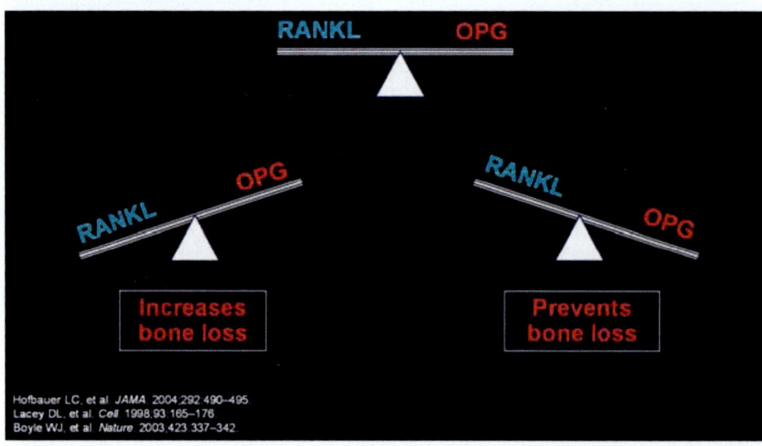

Figure 7.

OPG-inducing drugs	OPG-mimicking drugs
Estrogens	Recombinant OPG
Raloxifene	Denosumab
Bisphosphonates	
Strontium ranelate	
Teriparatide	
Genistein	

Figure 8.

3.1. OPG-inducing drugs

Estrogens act on bone with a double activity [58]: one mediated by the estrogen receptors present on the bone cell [59-61], the other, indirect and delayed, that acts through a change of calcium metabolism both at level of intestine, kidneys and parathyroids [62]. Estrogen deficiency determines an inhibition of mature osteoblasts and osteocytes, while it promotes faster osteoblastic apoptosis [63]. Estrogens prevent postmenopausal bone loss also by regulating the production of several cytokines that modulate osteoclastic bone resorption, including OPG, RANKL, IL-6, IL-1β, TNF-α and C-telopeptides of type-1 collagen (CrossLaps) by cells of the osteoblastic lineage [64-66]. Estrogens deficit interfere with the osteoclastic lineage increasing its recruitment and activation due to the stimulation of osteoblast cytokines release. Data obtained in in vitro studies have demonstrated that estrogens stimulate the OPG production by osteoblasts [25,59,60]. However, the role of OPG in physiological bone remodelling and its regulation in vivo is under investigation [40,67,68]. The interaction of pro-inflammatory cytokines mainly produced by the stromal cells/osteoblasts in bone tissue, with menopausal decrease of ovarian hormones are not entirely understood, but experimental and clinical studies support a link between the increased activity of these cytokines and postmenopausal bone loss [69,70]. After hormone replacement therapy (HRT), RANKL/OPG ratio decreased, but this changes have no association with changes in any bone marker or BMD. The OPG/RANK/RANKL system might be involved in reduced bone resorption after HRT, but does not seem to be clinically useful for predicting BMD or bone turnover status and bone response after hormone therapy [71].

On the contrary, another study demonstrates that circulating OPG decreased significantly after HRT in postmenopausal women. The decrease in serum OPG was observed in women treated with oestrogen alone as well as in those treated with a combination of oestrogen and progestin. The decrease in serum concentrations of OPG after HRT may occur to compensate for the action of estrogen in suppressing bone resorption [42].

Raloxifene is a selective estrogen receptor modulator (SERM) used to increase BMD, with a molecular mechanism, not well known [72]. An osteoblast release of OPG is stimulated by raloxifene, as well as demonstrated in vitro for estrogens [59,60]; this antiresorptive activity, at least in part, is carried out throughout the OPG/RANK/RANKL system and other cytokines, in particular IL-6. An increase of OPG levels, and on the contrary, an IL-6 fall in concentrations have been demonstrated in in vitro data [25,59,60]. Raloxifene acts on bone in a similar manner to estrogens, but its osteoblastic actions remain to be fully clarified. Studies in vitro show that raloxifene modulates the bone homeostasis inhibiting osteoclastogenesis and the bone resorption with dose-dependent activity [60]. In fact, the inhibition of osteoclastic differentiation happens only at low concentration. The mechanism, however, seems to be more complex so that it could imply direct and indirect activities on bone cells [59,62], and a down-regulation of the osteoblastic production of IL-6 and other cytokines has been suggested [25,60]. Raloxifene stimulates the production of OPG and inhibits the production of IL-6 from cultured human osteoblasts, confirming the hypothesis that raloxifene stimulant action on the osteoblastic differentiation is linked to an increased production of OPG [59]. On the contrary, raloxifene and estradiol seem to downregulate the OPG production by human osteoblasts in culture [25,73]. This effect is probably due to the lower expression of ER in cell cultured by these authors. In in vitro model, OPG protein release is higher in cells overexpressing ER-α, because raloxifene acts mainly on ER-alfa, and therefore, these effects might be the consequence of different expression of ER-α by human osteoblasts [25,31,60,61,67,74]. On 2006 in vivo data confirm in vitro results: serum OPG levels in postmenopausal women after 6 months of oral raloxifene treatment were statistically significant increased versus baseline and versus placebo [75].

Bisphosphonates, well-known bone resorption inhibitors, increase the OPG production from osteoblasts in cellular lines such as an additional mechanism of induction of osteoclasts apoptosis [76]. In a study on Paget's disease of bone treated with intravenous bisphosphonates, we found an increase in OPG levels statistically significant; a trend toward a decrease in RANKL levels after treatment was also observed. The RANKL/OPG ratio was significantly reduced after 3 and 6 months of therapy [77]. There are some reports about the effect through the osteoblast to suppress bone resorption [78-81], and an increased OPG production by normal human osteoblasts following pamidronate and zoledronate has been demonstrated in vitro [82]. Recently zoledronic acid showed to inhibit osteoclast maturation indirectly by increasing OPG secretion and decreasing transmenbrane RANKL expression in human osteoblast [83]. In a previous study on 42 Paget disease patients with polyostotic disease, Mossetti et al. found a similar increase in serum OPG after oral risedronate treatment for 120 days [84]. This results are also consistent with a recent study that demonstrated and increase in OPG at 6 and 12 months in bisphosphonates-treated osteoporotic women (oral daily doses of 10 mg alendronate or 5 mg risedronate in combination with calcium/vitamin D) and suggest a stimulatory effects of amino bisphosphonates on OPG production [85]. In this prospective, randomized controlled trial of previously untreated postmenopausal women with osteoporosis, changes in serum OPG levels are positively correlated to changes in BMD response. The changes in serum OPG levels during treatment could result from effects on osteoclastogenesis and osteoclast apoptosis as well as from a direct stimulatory effect on osteoblastic OPG production. These changes in OPG levels may be used to predict the individual response of patients to bisphosphonates treatment [85].

Strontium ranelate, a new oral drug for the treatment of postmenopausal osteoporosis, acts as an antiosteoporotic drug through its anti-resorbing and also-bone forming effects [86,87]. The dual effect of strontium ranelate in bone cells in vitro was also found in animals. [88-90]. Consistent with preclinical studies, strontium ranelate reduced the incidence of vertebral and hip fractures in two large randomized, double-blind, placebo-controlled clinical studies: the Spinal Osteoporosis Therapeutic Intervention (SOTI) trial [91] and the TReatment Of Peripheral OSteoporosis study (TROPOS) [92]. Interestingly, recent in vitro data indicate that strontium ranelate may act on bone metabolism also by regulating the expression of RANKL and OPG. It downregulates the expression of RANKL and enhances the expression of OPG in primary human osteoblastic cells in vitro, thereby decreasing the RANKL/OPG ratio [93]. This beneficial effect of strontium ranelate on the RANKL/OPG ratio was demonstrated in parallel in murine calvaria cells [94]. However, further studies are needed to investigate whether strontium ranelate can also act by modulating RANKL and OPG expression in animal models of bone loss.

Teriparatide (human recombinant PTH 1-34) therapy, potent anabolic drugs on bone, in women with postmenopausal osteoporosis results in acute increase in serum RANKL levels but does not affect serum OPG. These changes may reflect an increase in the number of active osteoblasts with therapy and might be responsible for the acceleration of bone turnover rate that characterizes teriparatide [95].

Genistein, the main soy derived phytoestrogen, play a role on RANKL/OPG ratio. By comparison with placebo, the ratio is lower in the genistein group and in HRT women and this findings suggest that also the OPG/RANK/RANKL system may mediate a beneficial effects of genistein on bone remodelling in postmenopausal women [96].

3.2. OPG-mimicking drugs (anti-RANKL drugs)

The direct application of recombinant OPG protein has many limitations: OPG protein is unstable and difficult to obtain; it undergoes rapid degradation in vivo; it involves daily injections; it is likely to cause side effects in other organs [97]. But also mimicking OPG we can inhibit the RANKL signal pathway and the formation and differentiation of osteoclasts; this concept can be utilized in osteoporosis treatment.

Denosumab is a investigational fully human monoclonal antibody (IgG_2) that binds to RANKL with high affinity and specificity and blocks the interaction of RANKL with RANK, mimicking the endogenous effects of OPG (Figure 9). Preclinical studies in cynomolgus monkeys and transgenic mice showed that denosumab and OPG had similar effects on BMD and turnover [54,57]. The mechanism of action for denosumab differs from that of bisphosphonates. Denosumab binds with high affinity and specificity to RANKL, inhibiting osteoclast-mediated bone resorption as well as osteoclast maturation and survival. In contrast, bisphosphonates bind to the mineralized surface of bone and reduce osteoclast activity [98].

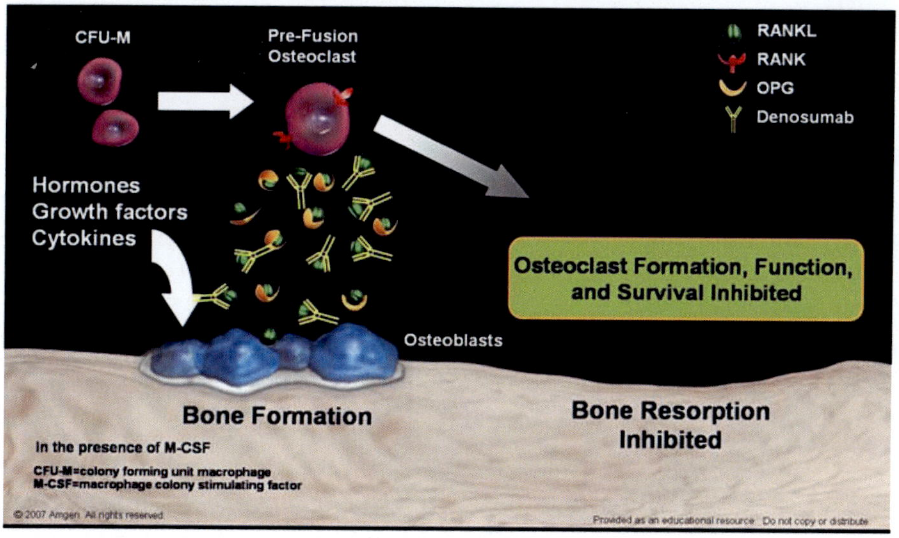

Figure 9.

The bone antiresorptive activity and safety of denosumab were evaluated in 49 postmenopausal women in a phase 1 randomized, double-blind, placebo-controlled, single-dose, dose escalation study. In this 9 months study, a single subcutaneous injection of denosumab resulted in a dose-dependent decrease in bone resorption, as measured by changes in serum and urinary N-telopeptide (NTX), markers of osteoclastic bone resorption. Denosumab was well tolerated and no related serious adverse events occurred [99].

Subsequently, the efficacy and safety of subcutaneously administered denosumab were evaluated over a period of 12 months in 412 postmenopausal women with low BMD. Subjects were randomly assigned to receive denosumab either every three months (at a dose of 6, 14, or 30 mg) or every six months (at a dose of 14, 60, 100, or 210 mg), open-label oral alendronate once weekly (at a dose of 70 mg), or placebo. Denosumab treatment for 12 months resulted in an increase in BMD at the lumbar spine of 3.0 to 6.7% (as compared with an increase of 4.6 percent with alendronate and a loss of 0.8% with placebo), at the total hip of 1.9 to 3.6% (as compared with an increase of 2.1% with alendronate and a loss of 0.6% with placebo), and at the distal third of the radius of 0.4 to 1.3% (as compared with decreases of 0.5% with alendronate and 2.0 percent with placebo). The duration of the suppression of bone turnover appeared to be dose-dependent [100].

The prespecified randomized, placebo-controlled study of 412 postmenopausal women with low BMD, evaluated with same methods the efficacy and safety of denosumab through 24 months. Denosumab increased BMD at all measured skeletal sites and decreased concentrations of bone turnover markers compared with placebo at 24 months. At the lumbar spine, BMD increases with denosumab ranged from 4.1 to 8.9%. The incidence of adverse events was similar in the placebo, denosumab, and alendronate treatment groups [101].

The phase 3 of the same study evaluated the efficacy of denosumab for increasing BMD and decreasing bone turnover in early and later postmenopausal women with low bone mass. Denosumab, 60 mg administered subcutaneously every 6 months, significantly increased BMD at all measured skeletal sites and significantly reduced markers of bone turnover compared with placebo, with reductions sustained throughout the 24 month treatment period in early and later postmenopausal women. These results confirm the findings of the phase 2 dose-ranging study with denosumab in postmenopausal women [100-101] and support the ongoing investigation of the denosumab 60 mg, 6 month dosing regimen in phase 3 trials [102].

No significant differences were observed between the profiles of adverse events in the denosumab groups and those in the placebo group and the alendronate group, with the exception of the incidence of dyspepsia, which appeared to be significantly greater in the alendronate. Upper respiratory tract infection was the most common adverse event in the denosumab group. Other adverse events that occurred with > 20% frequency in any treatment group were arthralgia, dyspepsia, and nausea. The incidences of hypertension and urinary tract infection were greater in the denosumab group than the placebo group, and the incidences of dyspepsia and osteoarthritis were greater in the open-label alendronate group. Six cases of serious adverse events of infections associated with hospitalization were observed in the denosumab group (two cases each of diverticulitis and pneumonia and one case each of atypical pneumonia and labyrinthitis successfully treated with standard antibiotics during uncomplicated hospital courses). Safety analyses identified no clinically relevant changes in either serum chemistry or haematology values. No notable differences among treatment groups in mean values, changes in toxicity grades, or individual patient trends over time were observed. As previously reported, two subjects had transient, non neutralizing, anti-denosumab-binding antibodies in the first 12 months [100]. No neutralizing antibodies to denosumab were observed during the first or second year of treatment [101].

In postmenopausal women with low bone mass, subcutaneously administered denosumab increased BMD and decreased bone resorption with a rapid onset of action and a sustained but reversible effect by means of a long plasma-circulating time after a single injection. The increase in BMD observed appeared to be superior to those with placebo and similar to or greater than those with open-label alendronate [99,100].

4. Conclusion

Adherence to osteoporosis medications is relatively poor. Approximately 20-30% of patients taking daily or weekly treatments may suspend their treatment within 6 to 12 months of initiating therapy. Patients with poor adherence increase their risk of osteoporotic fractures and hospitalisation. The majority of patients who discontinue therapy appear to do so because of drug-induced adverse effects. Fear of adverse effects or other health risks is another commonly cited reason for discontinuing therapy. For example, bisphosphonates, a common class of drugs for treating osteoporosis, have specific administration requirements (e.g. fasting, remaining upright and not ingesting other medications concomitantly) [103].

Strategies to increase adherence include reducing administration frequency to weekly or monthly, monitoring patients with bone markers and BMD testing, providing adequate instructions, practitioner feedback and support, and educational materials and sessions. Future studies are needed regarding strategies to increase adherence to osteoporosis medications [103].

The OPG/RANK/RANKL system is one of the most important discoveries in bone biology in the past decade. This system is critical for skeletal health, and disruption of it leads to or causes numerous bone diseases. In particular, identification in the mid to late 1990s of this pathway provided a major breakthrough that clarified the role played by osteoblasts in osteoclastogenesis. As with any breakthrough in basic science, the onus rapidly falls on the clinical investigator to translate the findings into a better understanding of disease as well as potentially new treatment approaches.

More and more evident in the recent study is the role of a OPG/RANK/RANKL pathway on action of old, new, and investigational drugs for osteoporosis management. In fact, the discovery of the this pathway as the primary mediator of osteoclast differentiation, activation, and survival facilitated the clarification of the mechanism of present drugs and the design of molecules that specifically target this system for the treatment of osteoporosis. Therefore, we distinguish drugs blocking osteoclast differentiation through induction of the expression of OPG from osteoblasts (OPG-inducing drugs), and drugs mimicking the OPG action (OPG-mimicking drugs/anti-RANKL drugs). Nowadays, the leader drug of the former group is raloxifene for its positive effect not only on bone mass but also on breast, while for the later group, denosumab is to be considered the most promising drug for its specific antiosteoporotic action.

Acknowledgement

- Gianni Amato, M.D. - Department of Clinical and Experimental Medicine "F. Magrassi & A. Lanzara", Second University of Naples, Naples, Italy, for text revision

- Amgen Dompé S.p.A., for iconographic supply

References

[1] NIH Consensus Development Panel on Osteoporosis Prevention, Diagnosis, and Therapy. Osteoporosis prevention, diagnosis, and therapy. *JAMA*, 2001;285,785-95.

[2] Luisetto, G; Zangari, M; Tizian, L; Nardi, A; Ramazzina, E; Adami, S; Galuppo, P. Influence of aging and menopause in determining vertebral and distal forearm bone loss in adult healthy women. *Bone Miner*, 1993;22,9-25.

[3] Wark, JD. Osteoporosis: pathogenesis, diagnosis, prevention and management. *Baillieres Clin Endocrinol Metab*, 1993;7,151-81.

[4] Hui, SL; Wiske, PS; Norton, JA; Johnston, CC Jr. A prospective study of change in bone mass with age in postmenopausal women. *J Chronic Dis*, 1982;35,715-25.

[5] Riggs, BL; Khosla, S; Melton III, LJ. A unitary model for involutional osteoporosis: estrogen deficiency causes both type I and type II osteoporosis in postmenopausal women and contributes to bone loss in aging men. *J Bone Miner Res*, 1998;13,763-73.

[6] Close, P; Neuprez, A; Reginster, JY. Developments in the pharmacotherapeutic management of osteoporosis. *Expert Opin Pharmacother*, 2006;7,1603-15.

[7] McCombs, JS; Thiebaud, P; McLaughlin-Miley, C; Shi, J. Compliance with drug therapies for the treatment and prevention of osteoporosis. *Maturitas*, 2004;48,271-87.

[8] Schroeder, K., Fahey, T., Ebrahim, S. (2004). Interventions for improving adherence to treatment in patients with high blood pressure in ambulatory settings. *Cochrane Database Syst Rev* [CD004804],2.

[9] Vega, D; Maalouf, NM; Sakhaee, K. Clinical review: the role of receptor activator of nuclear factor-kappaB (RANK)/RANK ligand/osteoprotegerin: clinical implications. *J Clin Endocrinol Metab*, 2007;92,4514-21.

[10] Aubin, JE; Bonnelye, E. Osteoprotegerin and its ligand: a new paradigm for regulation of osteoclastogenesis and bone resorption. *Osteoporos Int*, 2000;11,905-3.

[11] Lacey, DL; Timms, E; Tan, HL; Kelley, MJ; Dunstan, CR; Burgess, T; Elliott, R; Colombero, A; Elliott, G; Scully, S; Hsu, H; Sullivan, J; Hawkins, N; Davy, E; Capparelli, C; Eli, A; Qian, YX; Kaufman, S; Sarosi, I; Shalhoub, V; Senaldi, G; Guo, J; Delaney, J; Boyle, WJ. Osteoprotegerin ligand is a cytokine that regulates osteoclast differentiation and activation. *Cell*, 1998;93,165-76.

[12] Hsu, H; Lacey, DL; Dunstan, CR; Solovyev, I; Colombero, A; Timms, E; Tan, HL; Elliott, G; Kelley, MJ; Sarosi, I; Wang, L; Xia, XZ; Elliott, R; Chiu, L; Black, T; Scully, S; Capparelli, C; Morony, S; Shimamoto, G; Bass, MB; Boyle, WJ. Tumor necrosis factor receptor family member RANK mediates osteoclast differentiation and

activation induced by osteoprotegerin ligand. *Proc Natl Acad Sci USA*, 1999;96,3540-5.

[13] Simonet, WS; Lacey, DL; Dunstan, CR; Kelley, M; Chang, MS; Lüthy, R; Nguyen, HQ; Wooden, S; Bennett, L; Boone, T; Shimamoto, G; DeRose, M; Elliott, R; Colombero, A; Tan, HL; Trail, G; Sullivan, J; Davy, E; Bucay, N; Renshaw-Gegg, L; Hughes, TM; Hill, D; Pattison, W; Campbell, P; Sander, S; Van, G; Tarpley, J; Derby, P; Lee, R; Boyle, WJ. Osteoprotegerin: a novel secreted protein involved in the regulation of bone density. *Cell*, 1997;89,309-19.

[14] Anderson DM, Maraskovsky E, Billingsley WL, Dougall WC, Tometsko ME, Roux ER, Teepe MC, DuBose RF, Cosman D, Galibert L. A homologue of the TNF receptor and its ligand enhance T-cell growth and dendritic-cell function. *Nature*, 1997;390,175-9.

[15] Wong, BR; Rho, J; Arron, J; Robinson, E; Orlinick, J; Chao, M; Kalachikov, S; Cayani, E; Bartlett, FS 3rd; Frankel, WN; Lee, SY; Choi, Y. TRANCE is a novel ligand of the tumor necrosis factor receptor family that activates c-Jun N-terminal kinase in T cells. *J Biol Chem*, 1997;272,25190-4.

[16] Li, J; Sarosi I; Yan XQ; Morony S; Capparelli C; Tan HL; McCabe S; Elliott R; Scully S; Van G; Kaufman S; Juan SC; Sun Y; Tarpley J; Martin L; Christensen K; McCabe J; Kostenuik P; Hsu H; Fletcher F; Dunstan CR; Lacey DL; Boyle WJ. RANK is the intrinsic hematopoietic cell surface receptor that controls osteoclastogenesis and regulation of bone mass and calcium metabolism. *Proc Natl Acad Sci USA*, 2000;97,1566-71.

[17] Burgess, TL; Qian, Y; Kaufman, S; Ring, BD; Van, G; Capparelli, C; Kelley, M; Hsu, H; Boyle, WJ; Dunstan, CR; Hu, S; Lacey, DL. The ligand for osteoprotegerin (OPGL) directly activates mature osteoclasts. *J Cell Biol*, 1999;145,527-38.

[18] Lacey, DL; Tan, HL; Lu, J; Kaufman, S; Van, G; Qiu, W; Rattan, A; Scully, S; Fletcher, F; Juan, T; Kelley, M; Burgess, TL; Boyle, WJ; Polverino, AJ. Osteoprotegerin ligand modulates murine osteoclast survival in vitro and in vivo. *Am J Pathol*, 2000;157,435-48.

[19] Yasuda, H; Shima, N; Nakagawa, N; Yamaguchi, K; Kinosaki, M; Mochizuki, S; Tomoyasu, A; Yano, K; Goto, M; Murakami, A; Tsuda, E; Morinaga, T; Higashio, K; Udagawa, N; Takahashi, N; Suda, T. Osteoclast differentiation factor is a ligand for osteoprotegerin/osteoclastogenesis-inhibitory factor and is identical to TRANCE/RANKL. *Proc Natl Acad Sci USA*, 1998;95,3597-602.

[20] Ikeda, T; Kasai, M; Utsuyama, M; Hirokawa, K. Determination of three isoforms of the receptor activator of nuclear factor-[kappa]B ligand and their differential expression in bone and thymus. *Endocrinology*, 2001;142,1419-26.

[21] Wada, T; Nakashima, T; Hiroshi, N; Penninger, JM. RANKL-RANK signaling in osteoclastogenesis and bone disease. *Trends Mol Med*, 2006;12,17-25.

[22] Boyle, WJ; Simonet, WS; Lacey, DL. Osteoclast differentiation and activation. *Nature*, 2003;423,337-42.

[23] Hofbauer, LC; Schoppet, M. Clinical implications of the osteoprotegerin/RANKL/RANK system for bone and vascular diseases. *JAMA*, 2004;292,490-5.

[24] Feng, X. RANKing intracellular signaling in osteoclasts. *IUBMB Life*, 2005;57,389-95.

[25] Cheung, J; Mak, YT; Papaioannou, S; Evans, BAJ; Fogelman, I; Hampson, G. Interleukin-6 (IL-6), IL-1, receptor activator of nuclear factor κB ligand (RANKL) and

osteoprotegerin production by human osteoblastic cells: comparison of the effects of 17-βoestradiol and raloxifene. *J Endocrinol*, 2003;177,423-33.
[26] Liao, EY; Luo, XH; Su, X. Comparison of the effects of 17beta-E2 and progesterone on the expression of osteoprotegerin in normal human osteoblast-like cells. *J Endocrinol Invest*, 2002;25,785-90.
[27] Lambert, C; Oury, C; Dejardin, E; Chariot, A; Piette, J; Malaise, M; Merville, MP; Franchimont, N. Further insights in the mechanisms of interleukin-1beta stimulation of osteoprotegerin in osteoblast-like cells. *J Bone Miner Res*, 2007;22,1350-61.
[28] Suda, T; Takahashi, N; Udagawa, N; Jimi, E; Gillespie, MT; Martin, TJ. Modulation of osteoclast differentiation and function by the new members of the tumor necrosis factor receptor and ligand families. *Endocr Rev*, 1999;3,345-57.
[29] Yano, K; Nakagawa, N; Yasuda, H; Tsuda, E; Higashio, K. Synovial cells from a patient with rheumatoid arthritis produce osteoclastogenesis inhibitory factor/osteoprotegerin: reciprocal regulation of the production by inflammatory cytokines and basic fibroblast growth factor. *J Bone Miner Metab*, 2001;6,365-72.
[30] Ma, Y L; Cain, RL; Halladay, DL; Yang, X; Zeng, Q; Miles, RR; Chandrasekhar, S; Martin, TJ; Onyia, JE. Catabolic effects of continuous human PTH (1-38) in vivo is associated with sustained stimulation of RANKL and inhibition of osteoprotegerin and gene-associated bone formation. *Endocrinology*, 2001;142,4047-54.
[31] Hofbauer, LC; Khosla, S; Dunstan, CR; Lacey, DL; Spelsberg, TC; Riggs, BL. Estrogen stimulates gene expression and protein production of osteoprotegerin in human osteoblastic cells. *Endocrinology*, 1999;140,4367-70.
[32] Hofbauer, LC; Heufelder, AE. Role of receptor activator of nuclear factor-kappaB ligand and osteoprotegerin in bone cell biology. *J Mol Med*, 2001;79,243-53.
[33] Thirunavukkarasu, K; Miles, RR; Halladay, DL; Yang, X; Galvin, RJ; Chandrasekhar, S; Martin, TJ; Onyia, JE. Stimulation of osteoprotegerin (OPG) gene expression by transforming growth factor-beta (TGF-beta). Mapping of the OPG promoter region that mediates TGF-beta effects. *J Biol Chem*, 2001;276,36241-50.
[34] Browner, WB; Li-Yang, L; Cummings, SR. Associations of Serum Osteoprotegerin Levels With Diabetes, Stroke, Bone density, fractures and mortality in Elderly Women. *J Clin Endocrinol Metab*, 2001;86,631-7.
[35] Mizuno, A; Amizuka, N; Irie, K; Murakami, A; Fujise, N; Kanno, T; Sato, Y; Nakagawa, N; Yasuda, H; Mochizuki, S; Gomibuchi, T; Yano, K; Shima, N; Washida, N; Tsuda, E; Morinaga, T; Higashio, K; Ozawa, H. Severe osteoporosis in mice lacking osteoclastogenesis inhibitory factor/osteoprotegerin. *Biochem Biophys Res Commun*, 1998;247,610-5.
[36] Yano, K; Tsuda, E; Washida, N; Kobayashi, F; Goto, M; Harada, A; Ikeda, K; Higashio, K; Yamada, Y. Immunological characterization of circulating osteoprotegerin/osteoclastogenesis inhibitory factor: increased serum concentrations in postmenopausal women with osteoporosis. *J Bone Miner Res*, 1999;14,518-27.
[37] Ueland, T; Bollerslev, J; Godang, K; Muller, F; Froland, SS; Aukrust, P. Increased serum osteoprotegerin in disorders characterized by persistent immune activation or glucocorticoid excess-possible role in bone homeostasis. *Eur J Endocrinol*, 2001;145,685-90.
[38] Eghbali-Fatourechi, G; Khosla, S; Sanyal, A; Boyle, WJ; Lacey, DL; Riggs, BL. Role of RANK ligand in mediating increased bone resorption in early postmenopausal women. *J Clin Invest*, 2003;111,1221-30.

[39] Mazziotti, G; Sorvillo, F; Piscopo, M; Cioffi, M; Pilla, P; Biondi, B; Iorio, S; Giustina, A; Amato, G; Carella, C. Recombinant human TSH modulates in vivo C-telopeptides of type-1 collagen and bone alkaline phosphatase, but not osteoprotegerin production in postmenopausal women monitored for differentiated thyroid carcinoma. *J Bone Miner Res*, 2005;20,480-6.

[40] Oh, KW; Rhee, EJ; Lee, WY; Kim, SW; Oh, ES; Baek, KH; Kang, MI; Choi, MG; Yoo, HJ; Park, SW. The relationship between circulating osteoprotegerin levels and bone mineral metabolism in healthy women. *Clin Endocrinol (Oxf)*, 2004;61,244-9.

[41] Mezquita-Raya, P; de la Higuera, M; García, DF; Alonso, G; Ruiz-Requena, ME; de Dios Luna, J; Escobar-Jiménez, F; Muñoz-Torres, M. The contribution of serum osteoprotegerin to bone mass and vertebral fractures in postmenopausal women. *Osteoporos Int*, 2005 Nov;16,1368-74.

[42] Han, KO; Choi, JT; Choi, HA; Moon, IG; Yim, CH; Park, WK; Yoon, HK; Han, IK. The changes in circulating osteoprotegerin after hormone therapy in postmenopausal women and their relationship with oestrogen responsiveness on bone. *Clin Endocrinol (Oxf)*, 2005;62,349-53.

[43] Hegedus, D; Ferencz, V; Lakatos, PL; Meszaros, S; Lakatos, P; Horvath, C; Szalay, F. Decreased bone density; elevated serum osteoprotegerin, and beta-cross-laps in Wilson disease. *J Bone Miner Res*, 2002;17,1961-7.

[44] Delmas, PD; Eastell, R; Garnero, P; Seibel, J. The use of biochemical markers of bone turnover in osteoporosis. *Osteoporos Int*, 2000;(Suppl 6),S2-S17.

[45] Rogers, A; Saleh, G; Hannon, RA; Greenfield, D, Eastell, R. Circulating estradiol and osteoprotegerin as determinants of bone turnover and bone density in postmenopausal women. *J Clin Endocrinol Metab*, 2002;87,4470-5.

[46] Grigorie, D; Neacsu, E; Marinescu, M; Popa, O. Circulating osteoprotegerin and leptin levels in postmenopausal women with and without osteoporosis. *Rom J Internal Med*, 2003;41,409-15.

[47] Fahrleitner-Pammer, A; Dobnig, H; Piswanger-Soelkner, C; Bonelli, C; Dimai, HP; Leb, G; Obermayer-Pietsch, B. Osteoprotegerin serum levels in women: correlation with age, bone mass, bone turnover and fracture status. *Wien Klin Wochenschr*, 2003;115,291-7.

[48] Indridason, OS; Franzson, L; Sigurdsson, G. Serum osteoprotegerin and its relationship with bone mineral density and markers of bone turnover. *Osteoporos Int*, 2005;16,417-23.

[49] Kudlacek, S; Schneider, B; Woloszczuk, W; Pietschmann, P; Willvonseder, R; Austrian Study Group on Normative Values of Bone Metabolism. Serum levels of osteoprotegerin increase with age in healthy adult population. *Bone*, 2003;32,681-6.

[50] Liu, JM; Zhao, HY; Ning, G; Zhao, YJ; Chen, Y; Zhang, LZ; Xu, MY; Chen, JL. The relationships between changes of serum osteoprotegerin, nuclear factor-kappa B ligand receptor activator, and age, menopause, bone biochemical markers and bone mineral densities in women aged 20-75. *Zhonghua Nei Ke Za Zhi*, 2004;43,447-50.

[51] Giuliani, N; Bataille, R; Mancini, C; Lazzaretti, M; Barille, S. Myeloma cells induce imbalance in the osteoprotegerin/osteoprotegerin ligand system in the human bone marrow environment. *Blood*, 2001;98,3527-33.

[52] Kong, YY; Feige, U; Sarosi, I; Bolon, B; Tafuri, A; Morony, S; Capparelli, C; Li, J; Elliott, R; McCabe, S; Wong, T; Campagnolo, G; Moran, E; Bogoch, ER; Van, G; Nguyen, LT; Ohashi, PS; Lacey, DL; Fish, E; Boyle, WJ; Penninger, JM. Activated T

cells regulate bone loss and joint destruction in adjuvant arthritis through osteoprotegerin ligand. *Nature*, 1999;402,304-9.

[53] Campagnuolo, G; Bolon, B; Feige, U. Kinetics of bone protection by recombinant osteoprotegerin therapy in Lewis rats with adjuvant arthritis. *Arthritis Rheum*, 2002;46,1926-36.

[54] Kostenuik, PJ; Bolon, B; Morony, S; Daris, M; Geng, Z; Carter, C; Sheng, J. Gene therapy with human recombinant osteoprotegerin reverses established osteopenia in ovariectomized mice. *Bone*, 2004;34,656-64.

[55] Mochizuki, S; Fujise, N; Higashio, K; Tsuda, E. Osteoclastogenesis inhibitory factor/osteoprotegerin ameliorates the decrease in both bone mineral density and bone strength in immobilized rats. *J Bone Miner Metab*, 2002;20,14-20.

[56] Capparelli, C; Morony, S; Warmington, K; Adamu, S; Lacey, D; Dunstan, CR; Stouch, B; Martin, S; Kostenuik, PJ. Sustained antiresorptive effects after a single treatment with human recombinant osteoprotegerin (OPG): A pharmacodynamic and pharmacokinetic analysis in rats. *J Bone Miner Res*, 2003;18,852-8.

[57] Ominsky, MS; Schroeder, J; Smith, SY; Farrell, DJ; Kostenuik, PJ; Atkinson, JE. Denosumab (AMG 162, a fully human RANKL antibody) increases cortical and cancellous bone mass and density in aged, ovariectomized cynomolgus monkeys. *J Bone Miner Res*, 2006;21,S1;S72.

[58] Riggs, BL; Khosla, S; Atkinson, EJ; Dunstan, CR; Melton III, LJ. Evidence that type I osteoporosis results from enhanced responsiveness of bone to estrogen deficiency. *Osteoporos Int*, 2003;14,728-33.

[59] Viereck, V; Gründker, C; Blaschke, S; Niederkleine, B; Siggelkow, H; Frosch, KH; Raddatz, D; Emons, G; Hofbauer, LC. Raloxifene concurrently stimulates osteoprotegerin and inhibits interleukin-6 production by human trabecular osteoblasts. *J Clin Endocrinol Metab*, 2003;88,4206-13.

[60] Taranta, A; Brama, M; Teti, A; De Luca, V; Scandurra, R; Spera, G; Agnusdei, D; Termine, JD; Migliaccio, S. The selective estrogen receptor modulator raloxifene regulates osteoclast and osteoblast activity in vitro. *Bone*, 2002;30,368-76.

[61] Bord, S; Ireland, DC; Beavan, SR; Compston, JE. The effects of estrogen on osteoprotegerin, RANKL, and estrogen receptor expression in human osteoblasts. *Bone*, 2003;32,136-41.

[62] Oleksik, AM; Duong, T; Pliester, N; Asma, G; Popp-Snijders, C; Lips, P. Effects of the selective estrogen receptor modulator, raloxifene on the somatotropic axis insulin-glucose homeostasis. *J Clin Endocrinol Metab*, 2001;86,2763-8.

[63] Xing, L; Boyce, BF. Regulation of apoptosis in osteoclasts and osteoblastic cells. *Biochem Biophys Res Commun*, 2005;328,709-20.

[64] Compston JE. Sex steroids and bone. *Physiol Rev*, 2001;81,419-47.

[65] Koka, S; Petro, TM; Reinhardt, RA. Estrogen inhibits interleukin-1 beta-induced interleukin-6 production by human osteoblast-like cells. *J Interferon Cytokine Res*, 1998;18,479-83.

[66] Secreto, FJ; Grover, A; Pacurari, M; Rice, MB; Kantorow, M; Bidwai ,AP; Blaha, JD; Keeting, PE. Estrogen potentiates the combined effects of transforming growth factor-beta and tumor necrosis factor-alfa on adult human osteoblast-like cell prostaglandin E2 biosynthesis. *Calcif Tissue Int*, 2003;73,565-74.

[67] Hofbauer, LC; Kuhne, CA; Viereck, V. The OPG/RANKL/RANK system in metabolic bone diseases. *J Musculoskelet Neuronal Interact* 2004;4,268-75.

[68] Bashir, A; Mak YT; Sankaralingam, S; Cheung, J; McGowan, NW; Grigoriadis, AE; Fogelman, I; Hampson, G. Changes in RANKL/OPG/RANK gene expression in peripheral mononuclear cells following treatment with estrogen or raloxifene. *Steroids*, 2005;70,847-55.

[69] Scheidt-Nave, C; Bismar, H; Leidig-Bruckner, G; Woitge, H; Seibel, MJ; Ziegler, R; Pfeilschifter, J. Serum Interleukin 6 is a major predictor of bone loss in women specific to the first decade past menopause. *J Clin Endocrinol Metab*, 2001;86,2032-42.

[70] Manolagas, SC; Jilka, RL. Bone marrow; cytokines; and bone remodelling. Emerging insights into the pathophysiology of osteoporosis. *N Engl J Med*, 1995;332,305-11.

[71] Kim, JG; Kim, JH; Lee, DO; Kim, H; Kim, JY; Suh, CS; Kim, SH; Choi, YM. Changes in the serum levels of osteoprotegerin and soluble receptor activator for nuclear factor kappaB ligand after estrogen-progestogen therapy and their relationships with changes in bone mass in postmenopausal women. *Menopause*, 2008;15,357-62.

[72] Riggs, BL; Melton, LJ. Bone turnover matters: the raloxifene treatment paradox of dramatic decreases in vertebral fractures without commensurate increases in bone density. *J Bone Miner Res*, 2002;171,11-4.

[73] Li, J; Tang, JG; Wu, HY; Wu, WK. Effect of raloxifene and estradiol on the biological function and osteoprotegerin expression of osteoblasts in vitro. *Di Yi Jun Yi Da Xue Xue Bao*, 2005;25,787-90.

[74] Lindberg, MK; Erlandsson, M; Alatalo, SL; Windahl, S; Andersson, G; Halleen, JM; Carlsten, H; Gustafsson, JA; Ohlsson, C. Estrogen receptor alpha; but not estrogen receptor beta, is involved in the regulation if the OPG/RANKL (osteoprotegerin/receptor activator of NF-Kappa B ligand) ratio and serum interleukin-6 in male mice. *J Endocrinol*, 2001;171,425-33.

[75] Messalli, EM; Mainini, G; Scaffa, C; Cafiero, A; Cobellis, L; Salzillo, PL; Ragucci, A. Raloxifene therapy interacts with serum osteoprotegerin in postmenopausal women. *Maturitas*, 2007;56,38-44.

[76] Biskobing, DM; Novy, AM; Downs Jr, R. Novel therapeutic options for osteoporosis. *Curr Opin Rheumatol*, 2002;14,447-52.

[77] Martini, G; Gennari, L; Merlotti, D; Salvadori, S; Franci, MB; Campagna, S; Avanzati, A; De Paola, V; Valleggi, F; Nuti, R. Serum OPG and RANKL levels before and after intravenous bisphosphonate treatment in Paget's disease of bone. *Bone*, 2007;40,457-63.

[78] Reinholz, GG; Getz, B; Pederson, L; Sanders, ES; Subramaniam, M; Ingle, JN; Spelsberg, TC. Bisphosphonates directly regulate cell proliferation, differentiation, and gene expression in human osteoblasts. *Cancer Res*, 2000;60, 6001-7.

[79] Plotkin, LI; Weinstein, RS; Parfitt, AM; Roberson, PK; Manolagas, SC; Bellido, T. Prevention of osteocyte and osteoblast apoptosis by bisphosphonates and calcitonin. *J Clin Invest*, 1999;104,1363-74.

[80] Giuliani, N; Pedrazzoni, M; Negri, G; Passeri, G; Impicciatore, M; Girasole, G. Bisphosphonates stimulate formation of osteoblast precursors and mineralized nodules in murine and human bone marrow cultures in vitro and promote early osteoblastogenesis in young and aged mice in vivo. *Bone*, 1998;22,455-61.

[81] Giuliani, N; Pedrazzoni, M; Passeri, G; Girasole, G. Bisphosphonates inhibit IL-6 production by human osteoblast-like cells. *Scand J Rheumatol*, 1998; 27,38-41.

[82] Viereck, V; Emons, G; Lauck, V; Frosch, KH; Blaschke, S; Gründker, C; Hofbauer, LC. Bisphosphonates pamidronate and zoledronic acid stimulate osteoprotegerin

production by primary human osteoblasts. *Biochem Biophys Res Commun*, 2002;291,680-6.

[83] Pan, B; Farrugia, AN; To, LB; Findlay, DM; Green, J; Lynch, K; Zannettino, AC. The nitrogen-containing bisphosphonates, zoledronic acid, influences RANKL expression in human osteoblast-like cells by activating TNF-alpha converting enzyme (TACE). *J Bone Miner Res*, 2004;19,147-54.

[84] Rendina, D; Mossetti, G; Viceconti, R; Sorrentino, M; Nunziata, V. Risedronate and pamidronate treatment in the clinical management of patients with severe Paget's disease of bone and acquired resistance to bisphosphonates. *Calcif Tissue Int*, 2004;75,189-96.

[85] Dobnig, H; Hofbauer, LC; Viereck, V; Obermayer-Pietsch, B; Fahrleitner-Pammer, A. Changes in the RANK ligand/osteoprotegerin system are correlated to changes in bone mineral density in bisphosphonate-treated osteoporotic patients. *Osteoporos Int*, 2006;17,693-703.

[86] Marie, PJ; Ammann, P; Boivin, G; Rey ,C. Mechanisms of action and therapeutic potential of strontium in bone. *Calcif Tissue Int*, 2001;69,121-9.

[87] Marie, PJ. Strontium ranelate: a dual mode of action rebalancing bone turnover in favour of bone formation. *Curr Opin Rheumatol*, 2006;18,S11-5.

[88] Ammann, P; Shen, V; Robin, B; Mauras, Y; Bonjour, JP; Rizzoli, R. Strontium ranelate improves bone resistance by increasing bone mass and improving architecture in intact female rats. *J Bone Miner Res*, 2004;19,2012-20.

[89] Buehler, J; Chappuis, P; Saffar, JL; Foos, E; Vignery, A. Strontium ranelate inhibits bone resorption whilst maintaining bone formation in alveolar bone in monkeys. *Bone*, 2001;29,176-9.

[90] Geoffroy, V; Marty, C; Lalande, A; De Vernejoul, MC. Strontium ranelate reduces new vertebral fractures in a severe osteoporotic mice model with spontaneous fractures by improving bone microarchitecture. *Calcif Tissue Int*, 2006;78(Suppl 1),S38.

[91] Meunier, PJ; Roux, C; Seeman, E; Ortolani, S; Badurski, JE; Spector, TD; Cannata, J; Balogh, A; Lemmel, EM; Pors-Nielsen, S; Rizzoli, R; Genant, HK; Reginster, JY. The effects of strontium ranelate on the risk of vertebral fracture in women with postmenopausal osteoporosis. *N Engl J Med*, 2004;350,459-68.

[92] Reginster, JY; Seeman, E; De Vernejoul, MC; Adami, S; Compston, J; Phenekos, C; Devogelaer, JP; Curiel, MD; Sawicki, A; Goemaere, S; Sorensen, OH; Felsenberg, D; Meunier, PJ. Strontium ranelate reduces the risk of nonvertebral fractures in postmenopausal women with osteoporosis: Treatment of peripheral osteoporosis (TROPOS) study. *J Clin Endocrinol Metab*, 2005;90,2816-22.

[93] Brennan, T; Rybchyn, MS; Conigrave, AD; Mason, RS. Strontium ranelate effect on proliferation and OPG expression in osteoblasts. *Calcif Tissue Int*, 2006;78(Suppl 1),129.

[94] Bonnelye, E; Lalande, A; Judric, P. Strontium ranelate stimulates murine osteoblast differentiation while decreasing their osteoclastogenic abilities. *J Bone Miner Res*, 2006;21(Suppl 1),S426.

[95] Anastasilakis, AD; Goulis, DG; Polyzos, SA; Gerou, S; Pavlidou, V; Koukoulis, G; Avramidis, A. Acute changes in serum osteoprotegerin and receptor activator for nuclear factor-kappaB ligand levels in women with established osteoporosis treated with teriparatide. *Eur J Endocrinol*, 2008;158,411-5.

[96] Crisafulli, A; Altavilla, D; Squadrito, G; Romeo, A; Adamo, EB; Marini, R; Inferrera, MA; Marini, H; Bitto, A; D'Anna, R; Corrado, F; Bartolone, S; Frisina, N; Squadrito,

F. Effects of the phytoestrogen genistein on the circulating soluble receptor activator of nuclear factor kappaB ligand-osteoprotegerin system in early postmenopausal women. *J Clin Endocrinol Metab*, 2004;89,188-92.

[97] Kostenuik, PJ. Osteoprotegerin and RANKL regulate bone resorption, density, geometry and strength. *Curr Opin Pharmacol*, 2005;5,618-25.

[98] Miller ,PD; Bolognese, MA; Lewiecki, EM; McClung, MR; Ding, B; Austin, M; Liu, Y; San Martin, J. Effect of denosumab on bone density and turnover in postmenopausal women with low bone mass after long-term continued, discontinued, and restarting of therapy: A randomized blinded phase 2 clinical trial. *Bone*, 2008;43,222-29.

[99] Bekker, PJ; Holloway, DL; Rasmussen, AS; Murphy, R; Martin, SW; Leese, PT; Holmes, GB; Dunstan, CR; DePaoli, AM. A single-dose placebo-controlled study of AMG 162, a fully human monoclonal antibody to RANKL, in postmenopausal women. *J Bone Miner Res*, 2004;19,1059-66.

[100] McClung, MR; Lewiecki, EM; Cohen, SB; Bolognese, MA; Woodson, GC; Moffett, AH; Peacock, M; Miller, PD; Lederman, SN; Chesnut, CH; Lain, D; Kivitz, AJ; Holloway, DL; Zhang, C; Peterson, MC; Bekker, PJ; AMG 162 Bone Loss Study Group. Denosumab in postmenopausal women with low bone mineral density. *N Engl J Med*, 2006;354,821-31.

[101] Lewiecki, EM; Miller, PD; McClung, MR; Cohen, SB; Bolognese, MA; Liu, Y; Wang, A; Siddhanti, S; Fitzpatrick, LA; AMG 162 Bone Loss Study Group. Two-year treatment with denosumab (AMG 162) in a randomized phase 2 study of postmenopausal women with low BMD. *J Bone Miner Res*, 2007;22,1832-41.

[102] Bone, HG; Bolognese, MA; Yuen, CK; Kendler, DL; Wang, H; Liu, Y; San Martin, J. Effects of denosumab on bone mineral density and bone turnover in postmenopausal women. J *Clin Endocrinol Metab*, 2008;93,2149-57.

[103] Papaioannou, A; Kennedy, CC; Dolovich, L; Lau, E; Adachi, JD. Patient adherence to osteoporosis medications: problems, consequences and management strategies. *Drugs Aging*, 2007;24,37-55.

Reviewed by: Gianni Amato, M.D. - Department of Clinical and Experimental Medicine "F. Magrassi & A. Lanzara", Second University of Naples, Naples, Italy

In: Osteoporosis: Etiology, Diagnosis and Treatment
Editors: Bilar E. Mattingly and Albert C. Pillare
ISBN 978-1-60692-397-9

Chapter 7

Intermittent Dosing of Calcitriol and Calcitonin Improves Bone Quality and Strength in Previously Ovariectomized Rats

Cedo M. Bagi*[*], *Edwin Berryman, Maria Moalli and Catharine J. Andresen

World Wide Comparative Medicine, Global Science & Technology, PGRD, Pfizer Inc, Groton, CT 06340, U.S.A.

Abstract

Calcitonin (CT), through its action via a specific receptor, is a powerful inhibitor of osteoclast activity. Unlike the bisphosphonates, CT has only a transitory action and is quickly eliminated from the skeleton. Calcitriol (Vt.D_3; 1α,25-$(OH)_2D_3$) has been reported to increase lumbar BMD in postmenopausal and senile osteoporoses, but its clinical use is limited due to considerable calcemic activity, particularly after higher doses or prolonged use. Recent data showing that another calciotropic hormone, PTH, when used intermittently reduces fracture risk through considerable bone forming activity, led us to investigate the action of a combination treatment paradigm using Vt.D_3 and CT. Utilization of Vt.D_3 and calcitonin treatment in combination intuitively makes sense from a therapeutic perspective since these two hormones act on different cellular targets and could potentially create an additive beneficial effect on bone structure and strength.

Experiments were carried out in Ovx female S-D rats that had surgery at 8 weeks. Four weeks post surgery the rats were allocated to one of the following groups: 1. Sham vehicle; 2. Ovx vehicle; 3. Ovx + CT; 4. Ovx + Vt.D_3; 5. Ovx+Vt.D_3 + CT and 6.

* Correspondence concerning this article should be addressed to: Cedo M. Bagi, M.D., Ph.D., PGRD, Comparative Medicine. Pfizer Inc, Eastern Point Road 8274-1312, Groton, CT 06340. Phone: (860)-715-6465; FAX: (860)-715-3577; e-mail: cedo.bagi@pfizer.com.

Ovx+Vt.D_3 + CT. Both CT (2μg/kg, sc) and Vt.D_3 (2μg/kg, PO) were administered once per day, 5 days/week. Rats in group 3 received calcitonin every week throughout the study. Rats in group 4 received Vt.D_3 only one week every month. Rats in group 5 received Vt.D_3 during the first week, followed by 3 weeks of calcitonin, while rats in group 6 received simultaneous dosing with Vt.D_3 and calcitonin during the first week, followed by 3 weeks of calcitonin treatment. The 4-week dosing cycle was repeated 3 times with a monthly evaluation of bone metabolism and structure.

In vivo m-CT revealed that ovariectomy resulted in deterioration in bone mass, reduced trabecular number and thickness and impaired connectivity of cancellous bone. *Ex vivo* m-CT data paralleled *in vivo* findings at the tibial metaphysis. Unlike metaphisis, epiphyseal cancellous bone was only moderately affected by ovariectomy. Intermittent dosing with calcitriol and calcitonin improved bone mass and structure at both epiphysis and metaphysis, with group 5 being particularly effective. Cortical bone was more affected with calcitonin treatment due to low endocortical resoprtion and periosteal modeling due to ovariectomy. Our data demonstrate that uncoupling of bone resorption and formation can be achieved by intermittent treatment with two calciotropic hormones that separately target bone formation (Vt.D_3) and bone resorption (calcitonin).

Keywords: Ovariectomized rats, Calcitriol, Calcitonin, Bone quality, Bone strength.

INTRODUCTION

Results from epidemiological studies suggest that prolonged vitamin D deficiency leads to low bone mineral density and muscle weakness, which if left untreated results in osteoporosis and eventually fractures [1-3]. The majority of clinicians recommend supplementation with calcium and vitamin D for women at increased risk for osteoporosis and also for those who have already developed osteoporosis [4]. Clinical data shows that supplementation with vitamin D and calcium is most effective in osteoporotic patients if given orally either daily or quarterly, and if daily, the dose should be in excess of 700-800 IU per day [5]. Calcitriol (1α,25-$(OH)_2D_3$) is known for its stimulation of intestinal calcium absorption, enhancement of calcium reabsorption, inhibition of PTH synthesis and secretion and regulation of bone resorption and bone formation [6]. Analogs of 1α,25-$(OH)_2D_3$ are known to improve survival of osteoblasts which is postulated to be the main mechanism underlying the anabolic bone effects of calcitriol independent of dietary calcium supplementation [7-9]. Undesirable calcemic activity has limited the use of natural vitamin D metabolites for both mineral-related and novel indications and has prompted a search for synthetic vitamin D analogues lacking this side effect [10].

Deficiency of calcitonin, another calciotropic hormone, following menopause has been hypothesized as the causative factor in osteoporosis even though very low levels of human calcitonin and diurnal variations in humans made this hypothesis difficult to demonstrate [11]. Use of calcitonin in osteoporotic patients positively effected bone micro-architecture resulting in fewer fragility fractures and exhibited an analgesic effect in patients with vertebral crush syndromes. Calcitonin also prevented immobilization induced bone loss, improved remobilization, decreased morbidity and thereby improved the quality of life [12-14]. Calcitonin is a powerful inhibitor of osteoclast activity but unlike bisphosphonates, calcitonin has only a transitory action and is quickly eliminated from the skeleton allowing normal remodeling to take place. Lastly, calcitonin could also have mild anabolic properties as a result of cross-reactivity among bone cell receptors for calcitonin, calcitonin -gene related peptide and amylin [15].

There is a great medical need for anabolic therapies to treat osteoporoses of various etiologies because, particularly in elderly patients with severe bone loss, antiresorptive therapy with estrogens, selective estrogen receptor modulators, bisphosphonates or calcitonin cannot return bone mass and structure to normal. Utilization of calcitriol and calcitonin in combination is intuitive from a therapeutic perspective since these two hormones act on different cellular targets and could potentially have an additive beneficial effect on bone structure and strength when used in combination. The goal of this study was to explore a combination treatment paradigm using intermittent dosing with calcitriol and calcitonin.

MATERIAL AND METHODS

Animals

Experiments were carried out in female Sprague-Dawley (CD) rats that were either ovariectomized (Ovx) or sham operated (Sham) at Charles River (Wilmington MA) when 8 weeks old. Three weeks later rats were shipped to Pfizer and were maintained in an Association for Assessment and Accreditation of Laboratory Animal Care International (AAALAC) accredited research facility. All animal procedures were approved by the Institutional Animal Care and Use Committee and conformed to NIH standards established in the "Guidelines for the Care and use of Laboratory Animals" [16]. Rats were acclimatized for one week before start of the experiment. All rats were single-housed in polycarbonate cages in a room maintained at 23 ± 1°C, 55 ± 5% humidity with a 12-hour light/dark cycle; water and standard rat chow containing 0.80 % Ca, 0.60 % P and 2.2 IU/gm of vitamin D were provided *ad libitum*. Body weights were recorded once per week throughout the study.

Methods

Salmon thyrocalcitonin (Sigma, St. Louis, MO) was prepared in sterile saline at a concentration of 2.0 μg/ml and dosed at 1 ml/kg by subcutaneous injection. Calcitriol, 1,25-dihydroxyvitamin D_3 (1α,25-$(OH)_2D_3$, Calbiochem, Germany) was prepared daily in corn oil (Sigma, St. Louis, MO) at a concentration of 2.0 μg/ml and dosed orally at 1 ml/kg.

Study Design

Four weeks post surgery rats were assigned to one of the following groups: 1. Sham vehicle; 2. Ovx vehicle; 3. Ovx + CT; 4. Ovx + Vt.D_3; 5. Ovx+Vt.D_3 + CT and 6. Ovx+Vt.D_3 + CT. Both CT (2μg/kg, sc) and Vt.D_3 (2μg/kg, PO) were administered once per day, 5 days/week. Rats in group 3 received CT every week throughout the study. Rats in group 4 received Vt.D_3 only one week every month. Rats in group 5 received Vt.D_3 during the first week, followed by 3 weeks of CT, while rats in group 6 received simultaneous dosing with Vt.D_3 and CT during the first week, followed by 3 weeks of CT treatment. The 4-week dosing cycle was repeated 3 times with a monthly evaluation of bone metabolism and structure (Figure 1). Rats were sacrificed at the end of the study by CO_2 inhalation; femurs and tibias were dissected and either snap-frozen in liquid N_2 and stored at -80^0 C for radiological analyses and mechanical testing or fixed in 10% formalin for histological analyses.

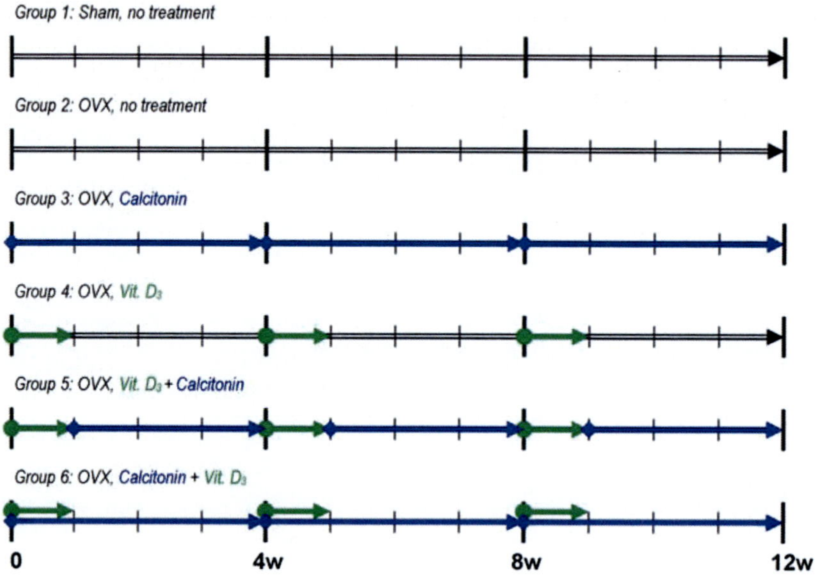

Figure 1. Schematic representation of the study protocol showing experimental groups 1 to 6. *In vivo* m-CT scans on proximal tibial metaphysis and blood collected for assessment of chemistry biomarkers and biomarkers of bone formation (OC) and bone resorption (CTX) were performed at time point 0, 4, 8 and 12. Blue arrow indicates CT administration, green arrow indicates Vt.D3 administration.

Serum Chemistry and Bone Biomarkers

Blood samples were obtained prior to start of treatment (week 0) and then 4, 8 and 12 weeks (end-point) following initiation of dosing. At each time point, 0.5 ml of blood was collected by retro-orbital bleed; animals were lightly anesthetized during the bleed procedure with CO_2/O_2. Determination of serum chemistry parameters was done using a Hitachi 917 auto analyzer (Roche, Indianapolis, IN); the standard core chemistry panel included: aspartate aminotransferase (AST), alanine aminotransferase (ALT), alkaline phosphatase, blood urea nitrogen (BUN), glucose, cholesterol, bilirubin, total protein, albumin, globulin, sodium, phosphorus and chloride. Commercially available ELISA kits were utilized for determination of serum biomarkers: osteocalcin (OC; Nordic Bioscience, Denmark) and specific epitope of collagen type l alpha 1 (CTX; Nordic Bioscience, Denmark).

Micro-Computed Tomography (m-CT)

In vivo m-CT analysis was performed using a Viva m-CT-40® computed tomography system (Scanco Medical, Bassersdorf, Switzerland). Evaluation of bone structure was performed on rats at baseline, and than at 4, 8 and 12 weeks following treatment initiation. The rats were maintained on 2.5% isoflurane anesthesia for the duration of the scan utilizing an IMPAC6 (VetEquip Inc., Pleasanton, CA) anesthesia system. Animal was laid on its back in scanner bed with right leg extended distally and foot secured by leg holder. Care was taken to avoid unnatural strain on the joints. The proximal tibial metaphysis containing secondary spongiosa was identified as scan area of interest. Samples were scanned at medium resolution with a source energy kVp of 70 and mA of 85. Sample scan time was 10 minutes with a 2.5 mm scan area. Upon completion, rats were allowed to recover in their home cages. 2-D and 3-D analysis was performed on cancellous bone compartment with a region of interest (ROI) manually defined to eliminate sub-cortical bone areas. A ROI for the metaphysis was drawn on 238 slices from 1.5 to 5.5 mm distal to the growth plate and defined to eliminate cortical bone. The following parameters were measured: bone volume (BV), bone surface (BS), bone volume/tissue volume (BV/TV), bone surface/bone volume (BS/BV), trabecular number (Tb.N), trabecular thickness (Tb.Th), trabecular separation (Tb.Sp), connective density (Conn.D) and structure model index for shape (SMI).

Ex Vivo Assessment of Cancellous Bone by m-CT

In addition to assessing cortical bone of the femur, cancellous bone of the proximal tibial metaphysis and epiphysis and distal femoral metaphysis were analyzed using m-CT methods previously described [17]. Briefly, the right tibia and femur were cleaned of soft tissue, and the frontal aspect of the proximal tibial metaphysis or distal femoral metaphysis shaved using a scalpel blade. Samples were scanned at high resolution with a source voltage of 55 kV and I mA of 145. Three-dimensional histomorphometric analysis was performed on the metaphyseal cancellous bone area 1 to 5 mm distal to the growth plate and on the entire epiphysis. These measurements were used to confirm bone effects of ovariectomy or treatment modalities.

Cortical Bone Assessment by m-CT

The m-CT images were segmented into bone and marrow regions by applying a visually chosen, fixed threshold for all samples (305 of maximal grey-scale value), after smoothing the image with a 3D gaussian low-pass filter (sigma 0.7 voxels). The outer contour of the bone was found automatically with the built-in Scanco iterative contouring tool (steepest edge finder). Total area (TA) was calculated by counting all voxels within the contour, bone area (BA) by counting all voxels that were segmented as bone, and marrow area (MA) was calculated as TA-BA. This calculation was performed on all 20 slices (1 slice = 12.5 mm), using average for the final calculation. The outer and inner perimeter of the cortical mid-shaft was determined by a 3D triangulation of the bone surface (BS) of the 20 slices, and cortical thickness was calculated by the formula C.Th = ½ *BS/BV. In 2D analyses, the average areal moment of inertia was calculated in x and y direction as well as the polar moment of inertia (I_P). An Eigen-value analysis of the MOI [please define MOI] tensor gave the principal directions and minimal and maximal I values (I_{MIN} and I_{MAX}). Maximal radial extents in the directions perpendicular to I_{MAX} and I_{MIN} were calculated (C_{MIN} and C_{MAX}, short for 'C_{MIN} for I_{MIN}' and 'C_{MAX} for I_{MAX}'). Section modul, I_{MAX} /C_{MAX} and I_{MIN} /C_{MIN} , were determined and they were used as determinants of bending strength. The polar moment of inertia (I_P; mm^4) was calculated as I_{MAX} + I_{MIN}. The moment of inertia calculations were performed in 2D mode, thus it was assumed that the bones were aligned with the axis of the scanner [18].

Mechanical Testing

Femurs were mechanically tested in three-point bending. They were positioned cranial side up across the lower contacts of a custom-built three-point bending rig on a Materials Testing System (Alliance RT/5; MTS Systems Corporation, Cary, NC). The lower contacts had a span width of 15.0 mm, and the upper contact was centered between the lower contacts. A static preload of 0.5 N was used to fix the bone between the contacts. The bone was subsequently broken in three-point bending using a crosshead speed of 20.0 mm/min. During testing, force and displacement data were collected every 0.1 seconds (at a frequency of 10 Hz) using TestWorks 4 software (Version 4.08A; MTS Systems Corporation, Eden Prairie, MN). Force versus displacement curves were visually inspected, and ultimate force (N), force at yield (N), stiffness (N/mm), energy to fracture (N.mm; how much energy the bone absorbs before it breaks), elongation (mm; how far the bone bends before it brakes), and post yield displacement (mm; how much the bone bends between the time it starts to crack until it brakes) were recorded.

Statistical Analysis

Data from biochemical bone measurement analyses are presented as Mean ± SD. Statistical analysis of the data was performed by unpaired Student's t-test. Differences were considered to be statistically significant when a p-value <0.05 was found.

Results

All animals originally enrolled in the study completed study as scheduled and demonstrated no overt clinical signs. Body weights were recorded once per week throughout the study. All Ovx rats were significantly heavier than Sham controls at both baseline (319.0 ± 25.5 vs. 262.4 ± 8.1; 21.6% difference) and at the end of the study (414.0 ± 25.2 vs. 336.1 ± 19.2.; 23.2% difference). There was no difference in body weight between Ovx groups regardless of dosing regimen.

Serum chemistry endpoints including creatinine, calcium, phosphorus, and Ca/P ratio were measured and analyzed but no significant differences between control and treated rats were noted. Serum biomarkers of bone metabolism, osteocalcin and CTX, were measured at select time points throughout the study. Before initiation of dosing (time 0) and 4 weeks after

Ovx surgery all Ovx rats had significantly higher osteocalcin relative to Sham controls (Figure 2). After one week of dosing, osteocalcin value in Ovx control rats remained elevated compared to sham controls; Ovx rats receiving CT exhibited significantly lower osteocalcin values compared to Ovx controls, while rats receiving Vt.D_3 showed significantly increased osteocalcin (Figure 2). As expected, rats in group 5 that were intermittently dosed with Vt.D_3 and CT exhibited osteocalcin values similar to group 4 at 1 week time point, while osteocalcin values in rats from group 6 that received simultaneous administration of CT and Vt. D_3 remained similar to Ovx controls (Figure 2). At the end of study (week 12) osteocalcin in Ovx control rats were still elevated relative to sham controls, however, absolute osteocalcin values were much lower compared to values recorded for Ovx controls at week 0. Rats receiving Vt.D_3 showed elevated osteocalcin, while rats in group 5 that were intermittently dosed with Vt.D_3 and CT exhibited osteocalcin values that were similar to values recorded for Ovx controls. Rats in group 6 that were simultaneously dosed with Vt.D_3 and CT had lower osteocalcin compared to Ovx controls (Figure 2 and 3).

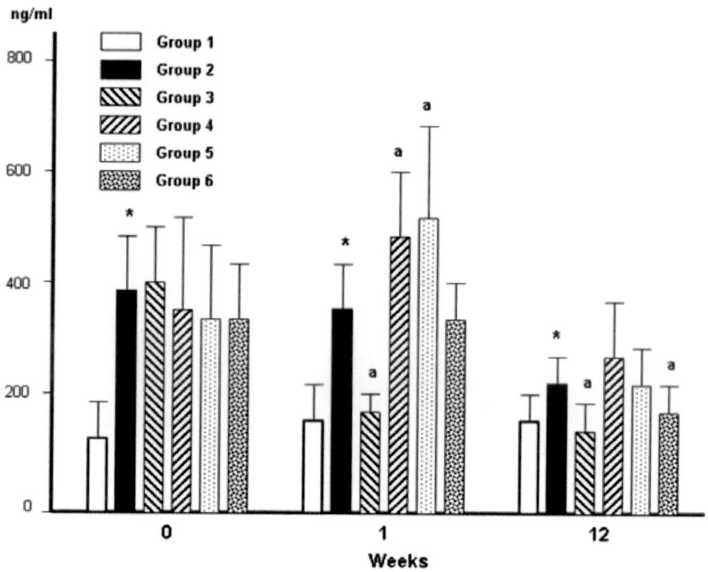

Figure 2. Serum osteocalcin was measured at several time-points throughout the study; before initiation of dosing (week 0), after first week of dosing (week 1) and at end of study (week 12). There were 8 rats in each experimental group. Data expressed as mean $\pm$ SD. Significance at $^*p<0.05$ relative to Sham controls and at $^ap<0.05$ compared to Ovx control.

Serum CTX was elevated in all Ovx rats relative to Sham controls at time 0 (Figures 3 and 4). After one week of dosing (week 1), all Ovx groups except group 3 still exhibited increased CTX values relative to Sham controls, however, rats in group 3 receiving CT showed somewhat lower values relative to Ovx controls. At the end of 12-week study bone resorption in Ovx control rats and rats receiving Vt.D_3 was still significantly elevated relative to Sham controls, while rats receiving CT alone or in combination with Vt.D_3 showed somewhat lower CTX values relative to Ovx controls, although these values were still elevated compared to Sham controls (Figure 4).

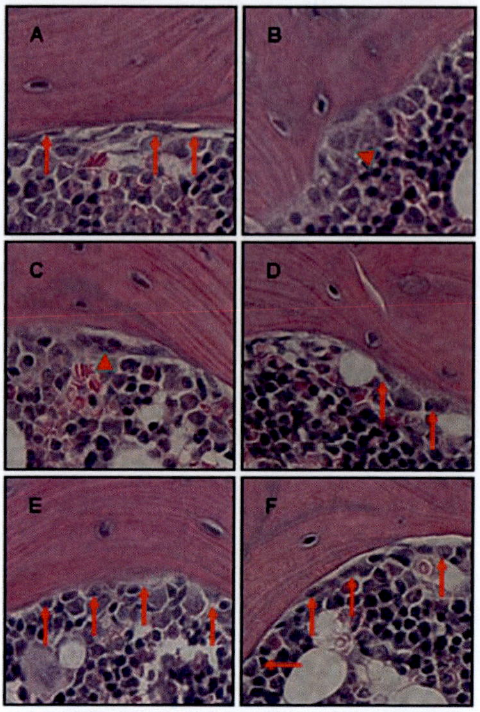

Figures 3A – 3F. Depicts H & E images of trabecular bone from Sham control rat (A), Ovx control rat (B), rat treated with CT (C), rat treated with Vt.D_3 (D), rat treated with Vt.D_3 followed by CT (E) and rat simultaneously treated with Vt.D_3 and CT (F). Epiphyses of the long bones in rats are characterized by low turnover rate with most of the cells adjacent to bone surfaces showing morphological characteristics of bone lining cells indicated by arrows (A). Ovariectomy resulted in increased bone resorption carried out by osteoclasts indicated by arrowhead (B). Treatment with CT curbed bone resorption (arrowhead indicates an inactive osteoclast; C). Treatment with Vt.D_3 resulted in increased bone formation (arrows indicate osteoblasts, D), while combination therapy (E and F) regardless of treatment regimen, resulted in fewer active osteoclasts and larger areas of bone formation indicated by arrows.

In vivo m-CT scans performed at proximal tibial metaphysis at time 0 showed significant differences between Sham and Ovx rats in bone volume, bone surface, trabecular number, trabecular thickness, trabecular separation and connectivity index (Table 1). Similar changes in bone structural parameters between Sham controls and Ovx control rats was also seen at the end of 12 weeks with the only exception being trabecular thickness (Table 1). Treatment with CT prevented further deterioration of bone mass and structure but failed to restore bone (Table 1). Administration of Vt.D_3 improved bone volume by increasing trabecular number and preservation of trabecular thickness (Table 1). Uncoupled administration of Vt.D_3 and CT (group 5) elicited significant improvement in bone volume, bone surface, trabecular number and connectivity index compared to Ovx control rats (Table 1). Simultaneous administration of Vt.D_3 and CT (group 6) showed a significant improvement in bone volume and trabecular connectivity parameters compared to Ovx controls, and a positive overall trend toward improving bone structure after 12 weeks of dosing (Table 1), although measured changes were less substantial compared to those observed in group 5.

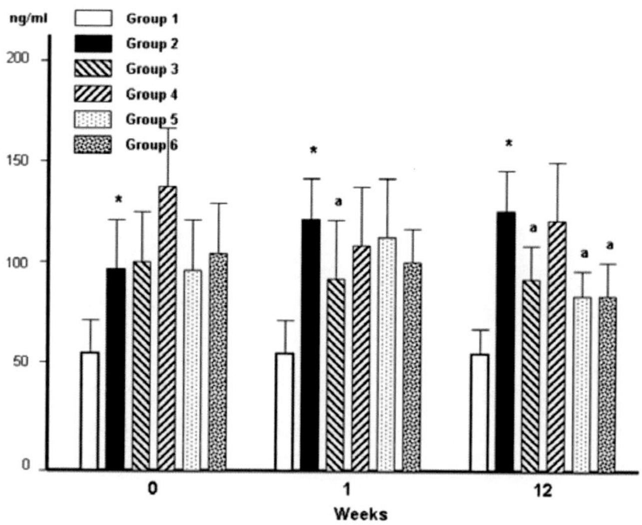

Figure 4. Serum CTX was measured at several time-points throughout the study; before initiation of dosing (week 0), after first week of dosing (week 1) and at necropsy (week 12). There were 8 rats in each experimental group. Data expressed as mean ± SD. Significance at *p<0.05 relative to Sham controls and at [a]p<0.05 compared to Ovx control.

Table 1. Structural 3-dimensional cancellous bone parameters evaluated *in vivo* at proximal tibial metaphysis (secondary spongiosa) at time 0 and time 12 (italic) using *Viva* µCT-40® system. Data expressed as mean ± SD; n = 8 rats/group

Parameters	*Time (week)*	TREATMENT GROUPS					
		Sham Control (Group 1)	*Ovx Control (Group 2)*	*Ovx + CT (Group 3)*	*Ovx + Vt.D3 (Group 4)*	*Ovx + CT+ Vt.D3 (Group 5)*	*Ovx + Vt.D3+CT (Group 6)*
BV (mm³)	0	1.14±0.71	0.12±0.07*	0.20±0.16	0.12±0.08	0.16±0.06	0.20±0.15
	12	*1.36±0.69*	*0.13±0.11**	*0.20±0.09*	*0.23±0.19*	*0.49±0.26*[a]	*0.32±0.16*[a]
BV/TV (1)	0	0.07±0.04	0.007±0.01	0.01±0.01	0.006±0.00	0.009±0.00	0.009±0.01
	12	*0.10±0.06*	*0.01±0.01*	*0.01±0.06*	*0.02±0.01*	*0.04±0.02*[a]	*0.02±0.01*
BS (mm²)	0	65.77±32.04	10.71±5.89*	15.65±11.97	10.19±6.56	12.75±4.09	14.69±9.85
	12	*71.40±29.31*	*6.81±5.66**	*11.37±6.32*	*12.82±10.64*	*24.71±11.54*[a]	*17.58±9.33*
BS/BV (1/mm)	*0*	62.21±8.73	86.34±5.01*	80.38±8.75	84.77±6.01	82.53±7.64	78.39±7.19
	12	*55.66±7.86*	*53.67±7.87*	*56.65±9.21*	*55.17±6.31*	*52.72±6.44*	*53.48±5.29*
Tb.N (1/mm)	0	2.02±0.88	0.28±0.14*	0.29±0.25	0.25±0.15	0.34±0.13	0.35±0.19
	12	*2.67±1.15*	*0.26±0.19**	*0.41±0.17*	*0.43±0.25*	*0.87±0.32*[a]	*0.54±0.21*
Tb.Th (mm)	0	0.033±0.01	0.023±0.00*	0.025±0.00	0.024±0.00	0.024±0.00	0.026±0.00
	12	*0.037±0.01*	*0.038±0.01*	*0.036±0.01*	*0.037±0.01*	*0.038±0.01*	*0.038±0.00*
Tb.Sp (mm)	0	0.55±0.23	4.55±2.53*	3.65±2.89	6.13±4.82	3.33±1.40	3.99±2.59
	12	*0.41±0.22*	*5.65±1.56**	*2.97±1.66*	3.94±2.68	*1.35±0.62*[a]	*2.14±1.02*[a]
Conn.D (1/mm³)	0	48.51±31.45	0.06±0.01*	1.19±2.30	0.12±0.20	0.17±0.33	1.21±2.25
	12	*62.43±51.13*	*2.62±0.36**	*3.23±1.52*	*4.13±4.57*	*11.76±8.83*[a]	*4.46±3.16*[a]
SMI (1)	0	3.14±0.37	3.85±0.17	3.75±0.19	3.88±0.22	3.75±0.13	3.72±0.17
	12	2.90±0.42	*3.17±0.36*	*3.18±0.29*	*3.23±0.32*	*3.08±0.27*	*3.08±0.24*

The differences between Sham control and Ovx control group are statistically significant at *p<0.05 and between Ovx control group and treatment groups at [a]p<0.05.

Table 2. Structural 3-dimensional cancellous bone parameters evaluated *ex vivo* at proximal tibial metaphysis (secondary spongiosa) using μCT-40® system. All data expressed as mean ± SD; n = 8 rats/group

Parameters	TREATMENT GROUPS					
	Sham Control (Group 1)	*Ovx Control (Group 2)*	*Ovx + CT (Group 3)*	*Ovx + Vt.D3 (Group 4)*	*Ovx + CT Vt.D3 (Group 5)*	*Ovx + Vt.D3 +CT (Group 6)*
BV (mm^3)	1.88±0.61	0.54±0.21*	0.70±0.31	0.66±0.29	1.03±0.41[a]	0.86±0.23
BV/TV (1)	0.29±0.09	0.09±0.03*	0.11±0.04	0.11±0.05	0.16±0.07[a]	0.13±0.03
BS (mm^2)	65.62±11.82	19.09±6.99*	25.67±9.97	20.67±7.06	31.83±9.12[a]	28.73±6.45[a]
BS/BV (1/mm)	36.15±4.65	35.52±5.60	36.45±3.29	31.94±2.30	31.65±3.20	33.36±2.09
Tb.N (1/mm)	5.16±1.05	1.50±0.44*	2.06±0.68	1.67±0.55	2.65±0.59[a]	2.38±0.32
Tb.Th (mm)	0.056±0.01	0.058±0.01	0.055±0.01	0.063±0.00	0.064±0.01[a]	0.060±0.00
Tb.Sp (mm)	0.15±0.05	0.69±0.16*	0.49±0.18	0.51±0.15	0.40±0.14[a]	0.41±0.08[a]
Conn.D ($1/mm^3$)	184.94±64.46	24.48±13.47*	39.72±25.25	24.55±11.67	44.22±19.99	37.84±12.33
SMI (1)	1.15±0.79	2.24±0.21*	2.32±0.22	2.20±0.16	2.04±0.31	2.11±0.11

The differences between Sham control and Ovx control group are statistically significant at *p<0.05 and between Ovx control group and treatment groups at [a]p<0.05.

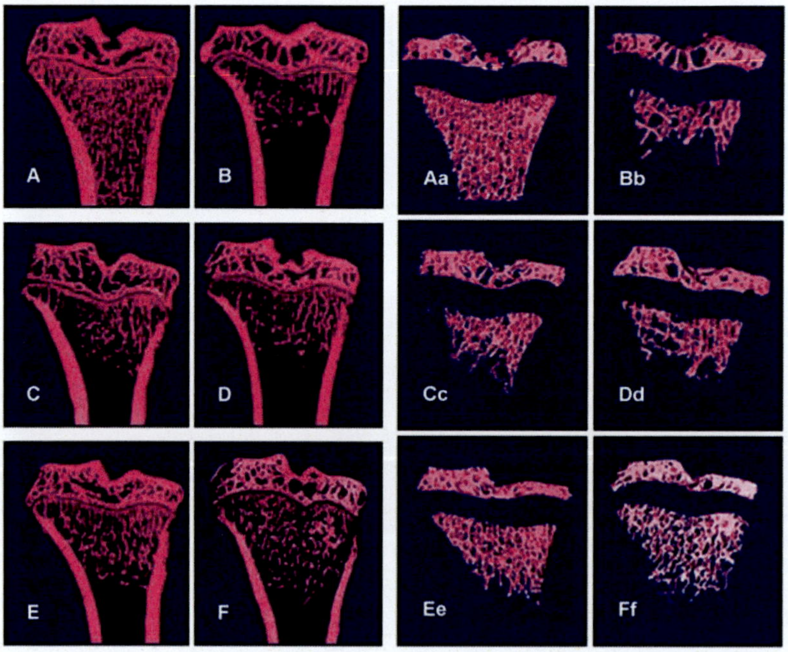

Figures 5A - 5F and 5Aa - 5Ff show 2D and 3D μCT images of cancellous bone at the proximal tibial metaphysis (secondary spongiosa) and epiphysis at the end of the12-week study. Note significant bone loss in Ovx control rats (B, Bb) compared to sham controls (A, Aa). Treatment with CT (C, Cc) prevented to some extent Ovx-induced bone loss. Rats treated with Vt.D3 (D, Dd) had more bone in secondary spongiosa relative to Ovx controls, while the most effective treatment appeared to be intermittent combination of Vt.D3 and CT (E, Ee). Rats that received simultaneous treatment of CT and Vt.D3 (F, Ff) also exhibited substantially more cancellous bone compared to Ovx controls.

Ex vivo m-CT scans performed at proximal tibial metaphysis at the end of 12 weeks of dosing showed significant difference in cancellous bone volume and structure between Ovx controls and Sham rats (Table 2, Figures 5A, 5Aa and 5B, 5Bb). Treatment with CT showed a trend toward preventing the deterioration of bone mass and structure caused by ovariectomy, but the effect did not reach statistical significance (Table 2; Figures 5C, 5Cc). Treatment with Vt.D_3 also showed a positive trend (non-significant) toward improving bone mass and structure relative to Ovx controls (Table 2; Figures 5D, 5Dd). Uncoupled administration of Vt.D_3 and CT (group 5) elicited significant improvement in bone volume, bone surface, trabecular number and connectivity index compared to Ovx control rats (Table 2; Figures 5E, 5Ee). Even though changes in bone volume and surface, as well as in trabecular number and thickness did not reach statistical significance, simultaneous administration of Vt.D_3 and CT (group 6) improved bone parameters compared to Ovx controls after 12 weeks of dosing to a greater degree than either CT or Vt.D_3 alone (Table 2; Figures 5F and 5Ff).

Ex vivo m-CT scans performed at the proximal tibial epiphysis at the end of 12 weeks of dosing showed no significant difference in measured bone parameters between Ovx controls and Sham rats (Table 3, Figures 5A, 5Aa and 5B, 5Bb). No change in bone volume and structure at tibial epiphysis was observed in rats treated with CT (Table 3; Figures 5C, 5Cc). Administration of Vt.D_3 alone had no significant effect on bone mass at epiphysis, but increased trabecular thickness relative to Ovx controls (Table 3; Figures 5D, 5Dd). Uncoupled administration of Vt.D_3 and CT (group 5) significantly increased trabecular thickness when compared to Ovx control rats (Table 3; Figures 5E, 5Ee). Simultaneous administration of Vt.D_3 and CT (group 6) increased some structural parameters of the cancellous bone at tibial epiphysis including, bone volume, trabecular number and connectivity, however the change was too small to reach statistical significance (Table 3; Figures 5F and 5Ff).

Table 3. Structural 3-dimensional cancellous bone parameters evaluated *ex vivo* at proximal tibial epiphysis using μCT-40®. All data expressed as mean ± SD; n = 8 rats/group

Parameters	TREATMENT GROUPS					
	Sham Control (Group 1)	*Ovx Control (Group 2)*	*Ovx + CT (Group 3)*	*Ovx + Vt.D3 (Group 4)*	*Ovx + CT+Vt.D3 (Group 5)*	*Ovx + Vt.D3 +CT (Group 6)*
BV (mm^3)	1.08±0.13	1.06±0.17	1.13±0.23	1.22±0.19	1.42±0.25	1.34±0.15
BV/TV (1)	0.42±0.05	0.39±0.04	0.38±0.05	0.48±0.07	0.54±0.06[a]	0.49±0.04[a]
BS (mm^2)	22.94±3.21	22.12±3.51	22.63±4.36	20.69±2.76	22.09±3.26	24.12±3.13
BS/BV (1/mm)	21.28±1.54	20.95±1.42	20.24±2.55	17.05±1.37	15.65±1.12[a]	17.97±1.57
Tb.N (1/mm)	4.49±0.51	4.04±0.30	3.87±0.38	4.06±0.49	4.18±0.42	4.42±0.44
Tb.Th (mm)	0.094±0.01	0.096±0.01	0.100±0.01	0.118±0.01[a]	0.128±0.01[a]	0.112±0.01[a]
Tb.Sp (mm)	0.13±0.02	0.15±0.02	0.14±0.03	0.13±0.03	0.13±0.02	0.12±0.02
Conn.D ($1/mm^3$)	65.83±18.41	54.91±13.07	54.66±10.25	47.04±11.79	49.49±7.31	63.87±13.95
SMI (1)	-0.25±0.44	-0.01±0.34	0.04±0.35	-0.47±0.50	-0.90±0.65	-0.56±0.39

The differences between Sham control and Ovx control group are statistically significant at *p<0.05 and between Ovx control group and treatment groups at [a]p<0.05.

Table 4. Structural 3-dimensional cancellous bone parameters evaluated *ex vivo* at distal femoral metaphysis using a μCT-40®. All data expressed as mean ± SD; n = 8 rats/group

Parameters	TREATMENT GROUPS					
	Sham Control (Group 1)	*Ovx Control (Group 2)*	*Ovx + CT (Group 3)*	*Ovx + Vt.D3 (Group 4)*	*Ovx + CT + Vt.D3 (Group 5)*	*Ovx + Vt.D3 + CT (Group 6)*
BV (mm^3)	2.99±1.34	0.17±0.12*	0.50±0.37	0.85±0.34	1.65±0.42[a]	1.09±0.37[a]
BV/TV (1)	0.24±0.09	0.01±0.01*	0.04±0.03	0.06±0.05	0.11±0.05[a]	0.07±0.04[a]
BS (mm^2)	96.42±31.83	6.66±4.44*	19.57±13.35	25.12±20.11	45.45±20.67[a]	35.07±21.12[a]
BS/BV (1/mm)	33.95±5.26	41.09±6.22	39.73±3.02	31.26±4.74	29.71±4.48	34.15±3.31
Tb.N (1/mm)	3.88±1.04	0.25±0.17*	0.70±0.35[a]	0.81±0.33[a]	1.47±0.53[a]	1.10±0.52[a]
Tb.Th (mm)	0.06±0.01	0.05±0.01	0.05±0.00	0.07±0.01	0.07±0.01[a]	0.06±0.01
Tb.Sp (mm)	0.21±0.07	9.56±3.12*	2.07±1.41[a]	4.87±2.24[a]	0.78±0.43[a]	1.41±0.67[a]
Conn.D ($1/mm^3$)	90.62±37.74	1.51±1.47*	8.33±5.63	10.04±6.62	20.47±8.51[a]	15.86±7.08[a]
SMI (1)	1.64±0.65	2.91±0.26*	2.68±0.24	2.37±0.47	1.98±0.47[a]	2.27±0.33

The differences between Sham control and Ovx control group are statistically significant at *$p<0.05$ and between Ovx control group and treatment groups at [a]$p<0.05$.

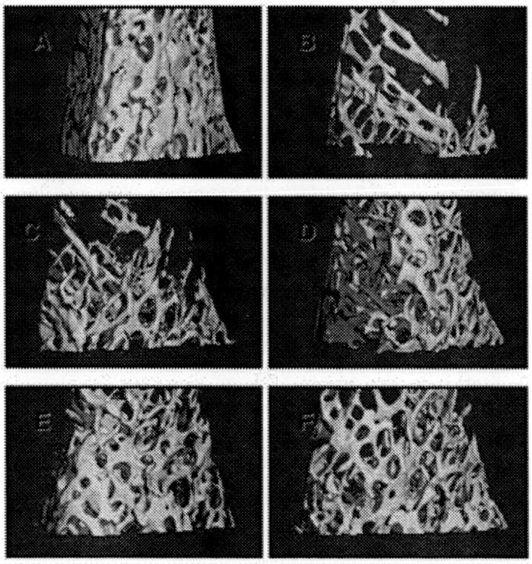

Figures 6A to 6F. Depict structural 3D (A-F) images of cancellous bone at distal femoral metaphysis (secondary spongiosa) at the end of 12-week study using μCT-40® system. Note significant bone loss in Ovx control rats (B) compared to sham controls (A). Treatment with CT (C) prevented to some extent bone loss induced by ovariectomy. Rats treated with $Vt.D_3$ (D) had more bone in secondary spongiosa relative to Ovx controls, while the most effective treatment seems to be intermittent combination of $Vt.D_3$ and CT (F). Rats that received simultaneous treatment of CT and $Vt.D_3$ (E) exhibited substantially more cancellous bone compared to Ovx controls.

Ex vivo m-CT measurements performed at distal femoral metaphysis showed highly significant differences in all measured bone parameters between Ovx controls and Sham rats (Table 4, Figures 6A and 6B, 7A, 7Aa and 7B, 7Bb). Treatment with CT ameliorated deterioration of bone volume and surface, trabecular number, trabecular space and connectivity but failed to improve trabecular thickness (Table 4; Figures 6C, 7C and 7Cc). Treatment with $Vt.D_3$ had a positive effect on bone volume and surface, trabecular number, thickness, space and connectivity however most of these changes did not reach statistical significance (Table 4; Figures 6D, 7D and 7Dd). Uncoupled administration of Vt.D_3 and CT (group 5) elicited significant improvement in bone volume, bone surface, trabecular number, space and connectivity index compared to Ovx control rats (Table 4; Figures 6E, 7E and 7Ee). Although, the changes in bone volume and surface, as well as in trabecular number and thickness in rats receiving simultaneous administration of Vt.D_3 and CT (group 6) were milder relative to group 5, significant improvements in bone parameters compared to Ovx controls were evident in this group (Table 4; Figures 6F, 7F and 7Ff).

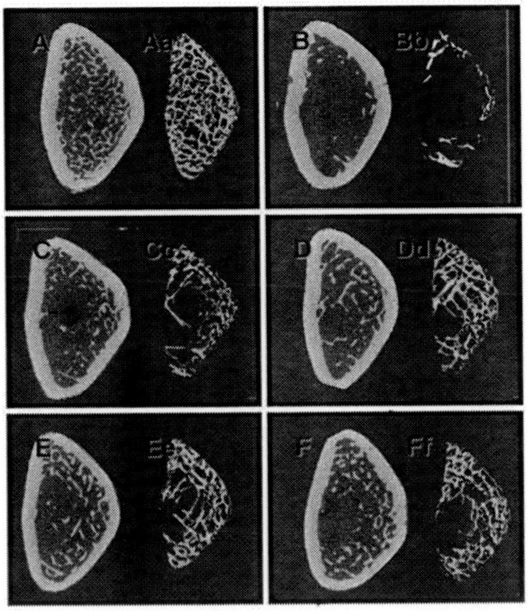

Figures 7A to7F. Depict structural 2D (A-F) and 3D (a-f) images of cancellous bone at distal femoral metaphysis (secondary spongiosa) at the end of 12-week study using μCT-40® system. Note significant bone loss in Ovx control rats (B, Bb) compared to sham controls (A, Aa). Treatment with CT (C, Cc) prevented to some extent bone loss induced by ovariectomy. Rats treated with Vt.D_3 (D, Dd) had more bone in secondary spongiosa relative to Ovx controls, while the most effective treatment seems to be intermittent combination of Vt.D_3 and CT (F, Ff). Rats that received simultaneous treatment of CT and Vt.D_3 (E, Ee) exhibited substantially more cancellous bone compared to Ovx controls.

There were only mild, insignificant changes in cortical bone geometry between Sham and Ovx rats (Table 5; Figures 8A and 8B). Treatment with CT caused slight increases in cortical thickness, I_{MIN} and I_{MAX} and in polar moment of inertia relative to Ovx controls (Table 5; Figure 8C). Similarly, administration of Vt.D_3 caused slight increases in cortical thickness, I_{MIN} and I_{MAX} and in polar moment of inertia relative to Ovx controls (Table 5; Figure 8D). Uncoupled administration of Vt.D_3 and CT (group 5) demonstrated an insignificant, but positive trend toward improving cortical bone parameters when compared to Ovx control rats (Table 5; Figure 8E). Similarly, non-significant improvements in some parameters of cortical bone geometry were observed following coupled (group 6) administration of CT and Vt.D_3 (Table 5; Figure 8F).

Table 5. Cross-sectional structural geometric properties were measured at femoral diaphysis using *ex vivo* µCT-40® system. All data expressed as mean ± SD; n = 8 rats/group

Parameters	TREATMENT GROUPS					
	Sham Control (Group 1)	*Ovx Control (Group 2)*	*Ovx + CT (Group 3)*	*Ovx + Vt.D3 (Group 4)*	*Ovx + CT + Vt.D3 (Group 5)*	*Ovx + Vt.D3 + CT (Group 6)*
TV (mm^3)	0.16±0.03	0.15±0.01	0.16±0.01	0.16±0.01	0.16±0.01	0.16±0.01
BV (mm^3)	0.07±0.00	0.07±0.00	0.07±0.00	0.08±0.01	0.08±0.00	0.08±0.00
BA (mm^2)	3.24±0.16	3.23±0.14	3.49±10.17	3.67±0.27	3.56±0.19	3.57±0.21
MA (mm^2)	0.08±0.03	0.09±0.01	0.08±0.01	0.09±0.01	0.08±0.01	0.08±0.01
Ct.Th (mm)	0.98±0.03	0.94±0.06	0.99±0.09	0.99±0.09	0.98±0.05	1.02±0.04
I_{MIN} (mm^4)	5.09±0.74	5.66±0.61	6.13±0.86	6.53±1.18	6.31±0.76	5.96±0.95
I_{MAX} (mm^4)	9.26±1.70	9.97±0.99	11.16±1.61	11.69±2.19	11.08±1.07	10.62±0.91
Ip (mm^4)	14.36±2.41	15.63±1.45	17.29±2.41	18.23±3.24	17.39±1.71	16.58±1.72
I_{MAX}/C_{MAX} (mm^4)	5.65±0.81	5.78±0.39	6.51±0.68	6.70±1.10	6.53±0.57	6.26±0.42

Mechanical testing data obtained by 3-point bending method showed that femurs from Ovx control rats had a significantly increased ultimate load parameter compared to Sham controls (Table 6). Treatment with CT significantly improved ultimate load, energy to failure and stiffness of the cortical bone relative to Ovx controls. Treatment with Vt.D3 also showed improved mechanical properties of cortical bone however measured changes didn't reach statistical significance. Both treatment modalities with Vt.D3 and CT showed higher (non-significant change) values for ultimate load, energy to failure and stiffness of the cortical bone relative to Ovx controls (Table 6).

Table 6. shows results of mechanical testing performed by 3-point bending method on right femurs (diaphysis). All data expressed as mean ± SD; n = 8 rats/group

Parameters	TREATMENT GROUPS					
	Sham Control (Group 1)	*Ovx Control (Group 2)*	*Ovx + CT (Group 3)*	*Ovx + Vt.D3 (Group 4)*	*Ovx + CT + Vt.D3 (Group 5)*	*Ovx + Vt.D3 + CT (Group 6)*
Ultimate Load (N)	128.9±22.8	159.8±10.7*	186.8±13.9[b]	184.6±30.2[a]	170.3±18.4	172.2±27.5
Elongation (mm)	0.58±0.10	0.62±0.09	0.63±0.07	0.62±0.11	0.66±0.09	0.61±0.04
Energy to Failure (N*mm)	48.07±18.6	59.78±10.4	74.43±9.4[b]	71.17±15.8	73.76±21.6	67.91±14.9
Stiffness (N/mm)	304.8±62.6	369.8±67.3	481.8±79.9[b]	451.7±96.5	423.9±81.2	442.2±90.3

The differences between Sham control and Ovx control group are statistically significant at $*p<0.05$ and between Ovx control group and treatment groups at $^{a}p<0.05$ and $^{b}p<0.005$.

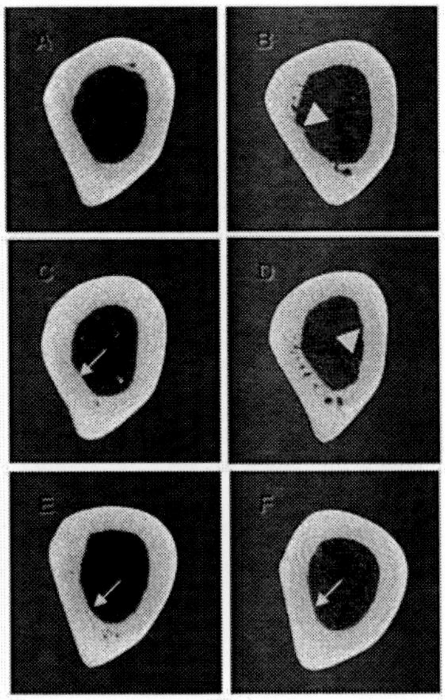

Figures 8A to 8F. Depict 2-dimensional (A-F) images of cortical bone at femoral diaphysis (midshaft) at the end of 12-week study using µCT-40® system. Note scalloped endocortical surfaces indicating bone resorption (arrowheads) in Ovx control rats (B) and rats receiving Vt.D3 therapy (D). Treatment with CT (C) prevented endocortical bone resorption induced by ovariectomy as indicated by smooth endocortical surfaces (arrow). Rats treated with $Vt.D_3$ and CT combo also seems to have reduced endocortical resorption (arrows; E and F).

Discussion

There is convincing preclinical and clinical evidence that intermittent administration of PTH leads to an increase in bone mass. Forteo® is a potent bone forming agent with demonstrated ability to increase vertebral, femoral, and total-body bone mineral density [19-21]. Clinical data indicate that after one year of treatment with PTH (1-84) bone mineral density gains will quickly disappear if treatment with PTH is not followed by an antiresorptive maintenance therapy [22]. Recent studies have also found that concurrent treatment with bisphosphonates may blunt the anabolic action of PTH, suggesting that maintenance of active bone remodeling may be critical for PTH to have an anabolic effect [23-25]. In addition, concurrent treatment with PTH and antiresorptive agents did not affect bone quality or strength to a greater or lesser extent than PTH alone [26, 27]. Therefore, it is possible that due to a long half-life of bisphosphonates in the skeleton, consecutive treatment with PTH in patients that have taken bisphosphonates may not be as effective as expected because of impaired bone remodeling. Calcitonin, unlike the bisphosphonates, has only a transitory action and is quickly eliminated from the skeleton allowing CT-treated osteoclasts to regain their bone resorption capacity [28-30]. Work by Davey and Morris [31] demonstrated that in addition to slowing bone resorption, treatment with CT induced hypocalcemia and secondary hyperparathyroidism with the effect being more pronounced in Ovx rats relative to intact rats, a finding that is consistent with actions of CT in states of increased bone turnover induced by estrogen deficiency in humans.

Clinical application of the bone forming potential of both PTH and calcitriol is limited by their relatively narrow therapeutic indices and limits on treatment duration, as well as the need to use follow-up antiresorptive therapy to preserve newly formed bone. For example, long-term administration of the synthetic PTH (1-34) was associated with adverse events that are somewhat similar to those reported for $1{,}25(OH)_2D_3$ [32]. Sato et al., [33] reported that the daily administration of as little as 8 μg/kg of PTH (1-34) for 1 year in Ovx rats led to an 11% increase in brittleness of cortical bone at diaphysis and 48% reduction in diaphyseal marrow space. In addition to these adverse skeletal effects, exogenous PTH therapy has been associated with hypercalcemia in both preclinical studies and in clinical trials [19]. Therefore, we hypothesized that a reduction in the dosing frequency with $1\alpha{,}25\text{-}(OH)_2D_3$ at a relatively high dose could circumvent some of safety hurdles associated with prolonged treatment with $1\alpha{,}25\text{-}(OH)_2D_3$ and that an intermittent dosing paradigm followed by an anti-resorptive drug should still be sufficient to correct the negative calcium balance often seen in osteoporotic patients [34, 35].

Serum chemistry data from our study showed no significant difference in serum creatinine, calcium, phosphorus and Ca/P ratio between control and treated rats at all time points measured. Serum osteocalcin and CTX values collected before initiation of dosing clearly demonstrated effect of ovariectomy on bone remodeling events. After first week, dosing with CT alone reduced bone remodeling by lowering bone resorption (CTX) and through coupled mechanism also reduced bone formation (osteocalcin). Treatment with calcitriol increased bone formation and had no effect on bone resorption, while rats in group 6 showed increased bone formation and decreased bone resorption after first week of simultaneous dosing with calcitriol and CT relative to Ovx controls.

After 3 dosing cycle (12-week time point) Ovx rats still showed elevated bone remodeling compared to Sham controls resulting in significantly lower bone volume, trabecular number and reduced connectivity at tibial cancellous bone. Treatment with CT decreased bone remodeling relative to Ovx rats, but bone resorption remained somewhat elevated relative to Shams, perhaps due to "escape" phenomenon, an event that is defined as an increase in resorption in bones stimulated by CT, despite the continued presence of CT in concentrations that are known to inhibit bone resorption [36, 37]. Micro-CT data paralleled serum findings showing only marginal improvement in cancellous bone volume, trabecular number and connectivity in CT treated rats relative to Ovx controls. One week per month dosing with calcitriol had limited effect on bone biomarkers at the end of study, but showed positive trend toward improving cancellous bone mass, trabecular number and connectivity compared to Ovx controls. Groups 5 and 6 that received the dual therapy with calcitonin and calcitriol showed decreased bone resorption relative to Ovx controls, while bone formation remained similar to Ovx control values and m-CT results showed significant improvement in metaphyseal cancellous bone parameters relative to Ovx controls, although sequential treatment with calcitriol followed by CT (group 5) showed some advantage relative to simultaneous treatment (group 6).

Radiological data obtained *ex vivo* by m-CT on tibial metaphysis and epiphysis showed loss of cancellous bone mass and altered structure following Ovx surgery on metaphyseal cancellous bone, but not on cancellous bone at epiphysis. Cancellous bone at these two skeletal compartments is known to have different metabolic and mechanical properties. While metaphyseal bone in rats has high turn over rate and serves predominantly to store calcium and phosphorus (metabolic role), cancellous bone at epiphysis has low turnover rate and relevant mechanical function [38-41]. Treatment with calcitriol as a single agent one week per month had marginal effect on cancellous bone at metaphysis, although improvement in thickness of existing trabeculae was recorded by m-CT. Treatment with calcitonin had a protective effect on cancellous bone properties preserving trabecualar number at tibial metaphysis but had no effect on epiphyseal cancellous bone. Combination of calcitonin and calcitriol had additive beneficial effect on bone mass and structural properties of cancellous bone at both metaphysis and epiphysis with slightly better results obtained when calcitriol was dosed first followed by calcitonin treatment (group 5). Similar results were also seen at distal femoral metaphysis confirming that combination therapy seems to have additive effect on cancellous bone mass and structure where calcitonin seems to act mostly by preventing excessive bone resorption and preservation of trabeculae that can be used as a template for depositing newly formed bone matrix under influence of calcitriol. In our study ovariectomy had mild effect on cortical bone resulting in increased endocortical resorption and periosteal modeling driven bone formation, resulting in change of cortical bone geometry [42, 43]. As a result of described changes, cortical bone in Ovx rats showed higher ultimate load, elongation, energy to failure and stiffness parameters compared to sham controls. Treatment with calcitonin inhibited endocortical bone resorption but did not change the ovariectomy driven periosteal modeling that improved cortical thickness and inertia thus resulting in significantly higher ultimate load, energy to failure and stiffness. Intermittent treatment with calcitriol was sufficient to improve mechanical properties of cortical bone mainly through enabling periosteal modeling and changing of bone geometry. Both combination treatment paradigms elicited response at cortical envelopes similar to one observed in calcitonin group, resulting in mild improvement in cortical area and thickness, as well as in moment of inertia parameter. Even though ultimate load, energy to failure and cortical bone stiffness was improved in both combination treatment groups relative to Ovx controls, obtained results didn't reach statistical significance. Although one should generally be cautious when extrapolating animal experimental findings to humans, in particular data obtained on cortical bone that is largely influenced by bone modeling events [42-44], collectively results from this study would suggest that intermittent treatment of osteoporotic patients using higher doses of calcitriol provides a solid therapeutic strategy that could be safe, yet more efficacious in restoring bone properties compared to standard treatment paradigms in which vitamin D_3 is used only to ensure availability of calcium. Even though there is a great deal of correlation between m-CT data obtained *in vivo* and *ex vivo*, we feel that deployment of high resolution mode in *ex vivo* studies allows for more precise measurements of bone structure, as well as accurate delineation of regions of interest with distinct metabolic and mechanical properties (metaphysis vs. epiphysis).

Within the constraints imposed by the study design, we conclude that intermittent dosing with calcitriol and calcitonin is robust enough to improve cancellous bone mass and structure through controlled bone remodeling process. The beneficial effect of this combined treatment comes from calcitriol's ability to increase bone formation and by calcitonin's potential to prevent accelerated bone resorption, yet not impair the bone formation segment of bone remodeling. Obviously, there are numerous options on how to combine treatment with the two hormones calcitonin and calcitriol in terms of dose, duration, optimal time to initiate therapy and in what order to dose the hormones. Our data provides initial evidence that a combination therapy with calcitriol and calcitonin can be devised to ameliorate the skeletal defects associated with established or developing osteoporosis. This intermittent dosing approach may also be applied to allow full therapeutic utilization of vitamin D_3 or new analogs in treating immunological diseases [45] in addition to osteoporoses of various etiologies.

Acknowledgement

The authors thank Charles Turner for providing mechanical testing data and Rich Pero for providing excellent technical assistance during the study conduct.

References

[1] Bischoff-Ferrari HA, Dietrich T, Orav EJ, Dawson-Hughes B. 2004. Positive association between 25-hydroxivitamin D levels and bone mineral density: a population-based study of younger and older adults. *Am J Med 116*:634-639.

[2] Visser M, Deeg DJH, Lips P. 2003. Low vitamin D and high parathyroid hormone levels as determinants of loss of muscle strength and muscle mass (sarcopenia): the Longitudinal Aging Study Amsterdam. *J Clin Endocrinol Metab 88*:5766-5772.

[3] Lips P. 2001. Vitamin D deficiency and secondary hyperparathyroidism in the elderly: consequences for bone loss and fractures and therapeutic implications. *Endocrin Rev 22*;477-501.

[4] Rizzoli R, Boonen S, Brandi ML, Burlet N, Delmas P, Reginster JY. 2008. The role of calcium and vitamin D in the management of osteoporosis. *Bone 42*:246-249.

[5] Bischoff-Ferrari HA. 2007. How to select the dose of vitamin D in the management of osteoporosis. *Osteoporosis Int 22*:401-407.

[6] Holick MF. 2006. Resurrection of vitamin D deficiency and rickets. *J Clin Invest 116*:2062-2072.

[7] Narbaitz R, Stumpf WE, Sar M, Huang S, DeLuca HF. 1983. Autoradiographic localization of target cells for 1α,25-dihydroxyvitamin D_3 in bones from fetal rats. *Calcif Tissue Int 35*: 177-182.

[8] Erben RG, Bromm S, Stangassinger M. 1998. Therapeutic efficacy of 1α,25-dihydroxyvitamin D_3 and calcium in osteopenic ovariectomized rats: Evidence for a direct anabolic effect of 1α,25-dihydroxyvitamin D_3 on bone. *Endocrinology 139*:4319-4328.

[9] Montero-Odasso M, Duque G. 2005. Vitamin D in the aging musculoskeletal system: An authentic strength preserving hormone. *Mol Aspects Med 26*:203-219.

[10]Pike WJ. 2006. New steroidal vitamin D receptor modulators: Are these ligands the real deal? *BoneKey-Osteovision 3*:14-18.

[11]Chesnut CH III, Silverman S, Andriano K, Genant H, Gimona A, Harris S, Kiel D, LeBoff M, Maricic M, Miller P, Moniz C, Peacock M, Richardson P, Watts N, Baylink D. 2000. A randomized trial of nasal spray salmon calcitonin in postmenopausal women with established osteoporosis: The prevent recurrence of osteoporotic fractures study. PROOF Study group. *Am J Med 109*:267-276.

[12]McDermott MT, Kidd GS. 1987. The role of calcitonin in the development and treatment of osteoporosis. *Endocrine Reviews 8*:377-3390.

[13]Body J-J. 2002. Calcitonin for the long-term prevention and treatment of postmenopausal osteoporosis. *Bone 30*:75S-79S.

[14]Kanis JA. 2002. Calcitonin in osteoporosis. *Bone 30*:65S-66S.

[15]Wallach S, Roussau G, Martin L, Azria M. 1999. Effects of calcitonin on animal and *in vitro* models of skeletal metabolism. *Bone 25*:509-516.

[16]Food and Drug Administration. 1994. *Guidelines for preclinical and clinical evaluation of agents used in the prevention or treatment of postmenopausal osteoporosis*. Washington, DC: FDA Division of Metabolism and Endocrine Drug Products.

[17]Hanson N, Bagi CM. 2004. Alternative approach to assessment of bone quality using micro computed tomography. *Bone 35*:326-333.

[18]Bagi CM, Hanson N, Andresen C, Pero R, Lariviere R, Turner CH, Laib A. 2006. The use of μCT to assess cortical bone strength – correlation with mechanical testing. *Bone 38*:136-144.

[19]Dempster DW, Cosman F, Parisien M, Shen V, Lindsay R. 1993. Anabolic actions of parathyroid hormone on bone. *Endocrine Rev 14*:690-709.

[20]Kimmel DB, Bozzato RP, Kronis KA, Coble T, Sindrey D, Kwong P, Recker RR. 1993. The effect of recombinant human (1-84) or synthetic human (1-34) parathyroid hormone on the skeleton of adult osteopenic ovariectomized rats. *Endocrinology 132*:1577-1584.

[21]Crandall C. 2002. Parathyroid hormone for treatment of osteoporosis. *Arch Intern Med 16*:2297-2309.

[22]Black DM, Bilezikian JP, Ensrud KE, Greenspan SL, Palermo L, Hue T, Lang TF, McGowan JA, Rosen CJ. 2005. One year of alendronate after one year of parathyroid hormone (1-84) for osteoporosis. *N Engl J Med 353*:555-565.

[23]Black DM, Greenspan SL, Ensrud KE, Palermo L, McGowen JA, Lang TF, Garnero P, Bouxsein ML, Bilezikian JP, Rosen CJ. 2003. The effects of parathyroid hormone and alendronate alone or in combination in postemenopausal osteoporosis. *N Engl J Med 25*:1207-1215.

[24]Finkelstein JS, Hayes A, Hunzelman JL, Wyland JJ, Lee H, Neer RM. 2003. The effects of parathyroid hormone, alendronate, or both in men with osteoporosis. *N Engl J Med 25*:1216-1226.

[25]Delmas PD, Vergnaud P, Arlot ME, Pastoureau P, Meunier PJ, Nilssen MH. 1995. The anabolic effect of human PTH (1-34) on bone formation is blunted when bone resorption is inhibited by the bisphosphonate tiludronate – is activated resorption a prerequisite for the *in vivo* effect of PTH on formation in a remodeling system? *Bone 16*:603-610.

[26]Li M, Mosekilde Li, SØgaard CH, Thomsen JS, Wronski TJ. 1995. Parathyroid hormone monotherapy and cotherapy with antiresorptive agents restore vertebral bone mass and strength in aged ovariectomized rats. *Bone 16*:629-635.

[27]Baumann BD, Wronski TJ. 1995. Response of cortical bone to antiresorptive agents and parathyroid hormone in aged ovariectomized rats. *Bone 16*:247-253.

[28]Wada S, Udagawa N, Nagata N et al. 1996. Calcitonin receptor down-regulation relates to calcitonin resistance in mature mouse osteoclasts. *Endocrinology 137*:1042-1048.

[29]Zaidi m, Inzerillo AM, Moonga BS, Bevis PJR, Huang CL-H. 2002. Forty years of calcitonin-Where are we now? A tribute to the work of Iain Macintyre, FRS. *Bone 30*:655-663.

[30]Martin TJ. 1999. Calcitonin, an update. *Bone 24 (Suppl.)*:63S-65S.

[31]Davey RA, Morris HA. 2005. The effects of salmon calcitonin-induced hypocalcemia on bone metabolism in ovariectomized rats. *J Bone Min Metab 23*:359-365.

[32]Vahle JL, Sato M, Long GG, Young JK, Francis PC, Engelhardt JA, Westmore MS, Linda Y, Nold JB. 2002. Skeletal changes in rats given daily subcutaneous injections of recombinant human parathyroid hormone (1-34) for 2 years and relevance to human safety. *Toxicol Pathol 30*:312-321.

[33]Sato M, Ma YL, Hock JM, Westmore MS, Vahle J, Villanueva A, Turner CH. 2002. Skeletal efficacy with parathyroid hormone in rats was not entirely beneficial with long-term treatment. *J Pharmacol Exp Ther 302*:304-313.

[34]Lau KHW, Baylink D. 1999. Vitamin D therapy of osteoporosis: Plain vitamin D therapy versus active vitamin D analog (D-hormone) therapy. *Calcify Tissue Int 65*:295-306.

[35]Andersen CJ, Moalli M, Turner CH, Berryman E, Pero R, Bagi CM. 2008. Bone parameters are improved with intermittent dosing of vitamin D3 and calcitonin. *Calcif Tissue Int* 83:393-403.

[36]Raisz LG, Wener JA, Trummel CL, et al. 1972. Induction, inhibition and escape as phenomenon in bone resorption. *Excerpta Medica Int Congress Series 243*:446-453.

[37]Messer HH, Copp DH. 1974. Changes in response to calcitonin following prolonged administration to intact rats. *Proc Soc Exp Biol Med 146*:643-647.

[38]Wronski TJ, Dann LM, Scott KS, Cintron M. 1989b. Long-term effects of ovariectomy and aging on the rat skeleton. *Calcif Tissue Int 45*:360-366.

[39]Frost HM. 1990. Structural adaptation to mechanical usage (SATMU). 1. Redefining Wolff's law: The bone remodeling problem. *Anat Rec 226*:414-422.

[40]Miller SC, Wronski TJ. 1993. Long-term osteopenic changes in cancellous bone structure in ovariectomized rats. *Anat Rec 236*:433-441.

[41]Bagi CM, Miller SC. 1994. Comparison of osteopenic changes in cancellous bone induced by ovariectomy and/or immobilization in adult rats. *Anat Rec 239*:243-254.

[42]Miller Sc, Bowman BM, Miller, MA, Bagi CM. 1991. Calcium absorption and osseous organ-, tissue-, and envelope-specific changes following ovariectomy in rats. *Bone 12*:4390446.

[43]Bagi CM, Mecham M, Weiss J, Miller SC. 1993. Comparative morphometric changes in rat cortical bone following ovariectomy and/or immobilization. *Bone 14*:877-883

[44]Kalu ND. 1991. The ovariectomized rat model of postmenopausal bone loss. *Bone Mineral 15*:175-192.

[45]Andresen CJ, Olson E, Nduaka CI, Pero R, Bagi CM. 2006. Action of calciotropic hormones on bone metabolism – Role of vitamin D_3 in bone remodeling events. *Am J Immunol 2*:40-51.

In: Osteoporosis: Etiology, Diagnosis and Treatment
Editors: Bilar E. Mattingly and Albert C. Pillare
ISBN 978-1-60692-397-9

Chapter 8

The Role of B cells in Physiological and Pathological Bone Turnover

*M. Neale Weitzman**

Division of Endocrinology & Metabolism & Lipids
Emory University School of Medicine
101 Woodruff Circle, 1305 WMRB
Atlanta, Georgia 30322
and
The Atlanta Veterans Affairs Medical Center
1670 Clairmont Road, Decatur, Georgia 30033

Abstract

It has been accepted for decades that osteoclasts, the cells responsible for bone breakdown, are derived from precursors that circulate among the monocyte/macrophage population, cells more commonly associated with immune surveillance and defense. However, it is only relatively recently that the depth of integration and interaction between components of the immune and skeletal systems has begun to be appreciated. A large body of evidence has begun to accumulate implicating T cells in the bone destruction commonly associated with inflammatory and autoimmune conditions such as rheumatoid arthritis, periodontitis, Crohn's disease, and infection. Compelling data from animal models, [1] supported by recent human studies [2,3] now suggest that T cells may also play a critical role in exacerbating bone destruction in postmenopausal osteoporosis, the archetypal osteoporotic condition.

In contrast to T cells, the role of B cells in physiological and pathological bone turnover is more obscure. However, recent animal studies demonstrate that B cells may be a critical component of the mechanism by which peak bone mass is achieved and maintained. Bone homeostasis is regulated by a delicate balance between bone formation by osteoblasts and bone resorption by osteoclasts. Physiological osteoclast renewal is

* Tel: (404) 727-1389, Fax (404) 727-1300, E-Mail: MWeitzm@Emory.EDU

controlled primarily by the ratio of the key osteoclastogenic cytokine, Receptor Activator of NF-kappaB Ligand (RANKL), relative to that of its physiological inhibitor, osteoprotegerin (OPG), a RANKL decoy receptor. Historically, the predominant source of both RANKL and OPG under physiological conditions has been attributed to osteoblasts and their precursors, the bone marrow stromal cells. Human B cells have long been known to make OPG especially in response to CD40 costimulation in vitro [4]. Recently, studies from our laboratory have found that in mice, B cell precursors, immature and mature B cells, and plasma cells together account for up to 64% of total bone marrow OPG production, with 45% derived from mature B cells alone [5]. Consequently B cells are essential to the attainment and maintenance of peak bone mineral density (BMD) and bone structure in the mouse. Interestingly, B cell OPG production is regulated, in part, through interactions with T cells, via the costimulatory molecule CD40 ligand (CD40L), suggesting a critical role of lymphocytes in the regulation of basal bone mass.

This chapter will review the current knowledge base concerning the potential role of B cells and their precursors in the regulation of physiological and pathological bone turnover.

INTRODUCTION

Bone Growth, Homeostasis and Decline

The skeleton is a highly dynamic organ that constantly regenerates throughout life. Osteoblasts are the unique bone building cells of the body and differentiate from pluripotent bone marrow stromal cells, a product of the mesenchymal stem cell lineage. Osteoblasts layer down bone matrix comprising predominantly type I collagen fibers oriented into linear bundles and cross-linked together. Osteoblasts further coat the matrix with bone mineral, predominantly calcium phosphate crystals in the form of hydroxyapatite. The processes of bone formation and renewal are extremely complex and have been the subject of numerous excellent reviews [6-11]. Consequently, only the basic principles are summarized below to provide context to the central topic.

In the young growing skeleton, bone accretion and growth occurs by the process of bone modeling, whereby bone is removed (resorbed) from one area, and new bone synthesized at another [7]. In modeling the rate of new bone formation exceeds that of bone resorption leading to a net gain of bone tissue. Bone growth reaches completion during early adulthood, and modeling converts to a bone renewal function termed remodeling. Unlike modeling which results in net bone gain, bone remodeling is homeostatic, and bone resorption is exactly balanced by new bone formation. Consequently, there is no net gain or loss of bone mass. As the body ages changes in factors such as the levels of numerous hormones and cytokines, lead to a slow increase in bone resorption that ultimately outpaces bone formation, causing a breakdown in skeletal homeostasis, and promoting net bone loss [9]. Numerous age associated changes in immunology, biochemistry and metabolism speed this decline in bone mass [1,10], however, a central step that accelerates the demise of the skeleton is the decline in estrogen levels following menopause in women, and a slower persistent declining of free testosterone in men [7,12,13]. Furthermore, an impressive assortment of pathological conditions can assert themselves on bone turnover leading the development of osteoporosis. Such conditions include inflammatory and autoimmune disorders such as rheumatoid arthritis [14] and periodontitis [15], Crohn's disease [16], several solid tumor and hematological cancers including breast and prostate cancer [17] and multiple myeloma [18]. Adding insult to injury numerous therapeutic agents and procedures use to treat cancer, inflammatory, and other diseases can themselves induce osteoporosis. These include adjuvant chemotherapies and hormonal therapy, such as androgen and estrogen ablation, and radiation therapy [19,20], glucocorticoids [21-23] and immunosuppressive agents used in organ transplantation [24].

Osteoclasts and Bone Resorption

Bone resorption is accomplished by specialist cells known as osteoclasts. Osteoclast precursors circulate among the monocyte/macrophage population and may be distinguished from regular monocytes and macrophages by the presence of Receptor Activator of NF-κB (RANK) on their cell membranes. In the presence of permissive concentrations of Macrophage-Colony Stimulating Factor (M-CSF), a survival and growth factor for all cells of the monocytic-linage, osteoclast precursors differentiate into mononucleated preosteoclasts under the direct action of the key osteoclastogenic cytokine, RANKL, which binds to the RANK receptor. Preosteoclasts fuse together into giant multinucleated mature bone resorbing osteoclasts. Under basal conditions RANKL is generally considered to be produced predominantly by cells of the osteoblast lineage [25,26], however under inflammatory or other pathological conditions numerous other cell types are capable of acting as additional sources of RANKL. These cell types include T cells [2,27,28], B cells [2,29], fibroblasts, and synoviocytes [30,31]. RANKL activity is moderated by its physiological decoy receptor OPG, and osteoclast formation and activity is consequently a function of the ratio of RANKL with respect to OPG in the bone microenvironment [11]. Overexpression of OPG in mice results in a high bone mass phenotype, driven by low osteoclast number and/or activity [32]. While not required for embryonic bone formation, OPG is essential for the maintenance of postnatal bone mass [33,34]. Consequently, OPG Knock Out (KO) mice are born with identical bone mass as their wild type (WT) littermates but display decreased BMD by one month of age. Heterozygous OPG KO mice display a slower loss of BMD, achieving statistical significance over a period of several months [33] suggesting that even a partial loss of OPG has a severe impact on bone homeostasis.

In conditions predisposing bone loss the levels of RANKL exceed those of OPG leading to elevated osteoclastogenesis and bone resorption. Although many cell types are endowed with the capacity to make OPG [8], historically the dominant source of this factor in the bone microenvironment has generally been attributed to osteoblasts and/or their precursors, the bone marrow stromal cells [25,26,35-38].

Centralization of B cell and skeletal regulatory factors

The development of a number of genetic knockout models has opened a window into the complex interactions between B cell regulatory factors and the skeletal system. A surprising discovery was that ablation of the critical B lymphocyte developmental transcription factor O/E-1 (Ebf1) causes an enhancement in osteoblastogenesis, leading to a striking increase in osteoblast number and in bone formation indices. These mice also display a dramatic increase in adipocyte number in the bone marrow. Interestingly, the number of osteoclasts in bone is normal in younger (4 wk old) Ebf1-/- mice but increased in older (12 wk old) Ebf1-/- mice [39,40].

Equally unexpected was the identification of severe osteopetrosis, a high bone mass phenotype, in Brutons tyrosine kinase (Btk) and Tec kinase Double-KO mice. These two characteristic B cell non-receptor tyrosine kinases were also found to be highly expressed in osteoclasts, and led to defective osteoclastogenesis and bone resorption when deleted [41].

By contrast, the deletion of Pax5, a critical B cell developmental factor that encodes the B cell-specific activator protein (BSAP), causes severe osteopenia due to a significant elevation in the number of osteoclasts. Pax5 KO mice have a developmental arrest in the B cell lineage at the pro-B cell stage however, enhanced osteoclastogenesis was attributed to a direct effect of Pax5 deficiency on osteoclast precursors, rather than as an indirect consequence of B cell depletion [39]. As these mice typically die by 18 days of age, it is presently unknown whether other effects of Pax5 on postnatal bone turnover, mediated directly though B cells may emerge over time. While the mechanisms of Pax5 action on osteoclasts remain incompletely defined, the loss of Pax5 has been reported to result in the expression of c-fms, the M-CSF receptor, on $B220^{+}CD19^{-}$ pro-B cells, while restoration of Pax5 activity represses this lineage-promiscuous transcription [42]. M-CSF is a critical survival factor for cells of the monocytic-lineage, including osteoclasts [11], and c-fms repression by Pax5 may thus play an essential role in suppressing alternative lineage choices such as commitment of early pluripotent B cell precursors along the monocytic pathway. Interestingly, stimulation with appropriate cytokines induces Pax5-/- pro-B cells to differentiate into functional macrophages, osteoclasts, dendritic cells, granulocytes and natural killer cells [42].

Further evidence of this close association between B cell precursors and osteoclast precursors is provided by studies demonstrating that $B220^{+}$ cells isolated from bone marrow differentiate into bone resorbing osteoclasts when cocultured with vitamin D3-stimulated ST2 stromal cells as a source of RANKL [45]. We [43] and others [44] have further demonstrated that a subset of $B220^{+}$ cells can be differentiated into osteoclasts in direct response to RANKL in vitro. In addition, cells coexpressing both Tartrate-Resistant Acid Phosphatase (TRAP), a specific osteoclast marker, and B220, a B-lineage marker, in freshly isolated unfractionated bone cells [45] provides tantalizing evidence that this unusual pathway to osteoclast formation may function in vivo. The frequency of osteoclast formation from these B cell precursors in vivo under basal conditions however remains unclear, and this pathway may or may not ultimately be a significant contributor to osteoclast formation under physiological conditions.

This emerging evidence of centralization of critical B cell transcription factors and functional regulators with elements of skeletal generation and regeneration that has only recently begun to be appreciated is unexpected and may suggest a co-evolution of B lymphocytes and bone cells.

THE ROLE OF B CELLS IN PHYSIOLOGICAL BONE TURNOVER

B cells are an essential component of the adaptive immune system and play a critical role in humoral immune responses. The principal function of B cells is to make antibodies against soluble antigens. Recent advances in the bone biology field suggest that B cells also play critical roles in physiological bone turnover.

A decade ago experiments in our laboratory identified an anti-osteoclastogenic activity mediated by human peripheral blood B cells, and the B cell line RAJI in vitro [46]. However, the role of B cells in the regulation of basal bone turnover in vivo has only recently been delineated following the development of the μMT/μMT B cell KO mouse, a model that produces no functional immature B cells, mature B cells, or plasma cells as a result of targeted disruption of the immunoglobulin mu chain gene [47].

A detailed phenotypic analysis of the bone structure of B cell KO mice reveled a striking decrease in BMD at multiple anatomic positions including total body, lumbar spine and femurs (Figure 1A), in 4 month old μMT/μMT mice relative to WT controls. Micro-Computed Tomography (μCT) confirmed a significant deficit in both trabecular and cortical bone compartments in B cell KO mice [5] (Figure 1B). As peak BMD is achieved by 4 months of age in C57BL/6 mice, [48] and peak bone strength is achieved at 5 months [49], this data suggested that B cells have a significant impact on the processes of bone accretion and modeling.

Serum C-Terminal Telopeptide of collagen (CTx), a specific and sensitive marker of in vivo bone resorption revealed a significantly elevated rate of osteoclastic resorption in B cell KO mice while serum osteocalcin, a sensitive and specific marker of bone formation showed no change [5]. These data suggested that aberrant bone turnover in B cell KO mice was a sole consequence of stimulated bone resorption.

As RANKL and OPG are the primary regulators of basal bone turnover, these factors were further examined and revealed that the increase in bone resorption was a consequence of a significant deficit (>40%) in total OPG mRNA and protein concentration in the bone marrow of B cell KO mice [5]. As RANKL concentrations were not significantly impacted by B cell deficiency the osteoporotic phenotype was accounted for by a decline in the OPG concentration leading to an increase in the RANKL/OPG ratio. B cell KO mice were rescued by reconstitution of B cells by adoptive transfer into 1 month old mice, which restored OPG concentrations to WT levels, and prevented the development of osteoporosis.

Taken together these studies provided the first in vivo evidence that B cells directly regulate basal BMD and indices of bone structure, by either secreting OPG or by indirectly regulating its production [5].

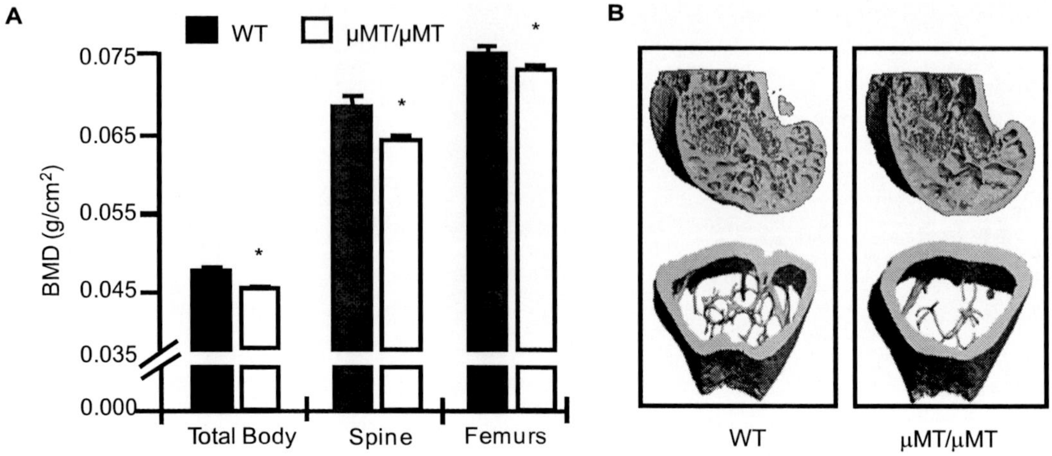

Figure 1. B cell KO mice are osteopenic. A) BMD was determined by Dual-energy X-ray Absorptiometry (DXA) in WT and B cell KO (μMT/μMT) mice, at total body, lumbar spine (spine) and femurs. B) Representative 3D reconstructions of WT and B cell KO (μMT/μMT) femurs. Originally published in Blood. Li Y, Toraldo G, Li A, Yang X, Zhang H, Qian WP, Weitzmann MN; B cells and T cells are critical for the preservation of bone homeostasis and attainment of peak bone mass *in vivo*. Blood. 2007;109(9):3839–3848.© the American Society of Hematology.

B cells are a major source of OPG in the bone micro-environment

OPG mRNA has been reported to be expressed in a number of tissues, including lung, heart, kidney, liver, stomach, intestine, brain and spinal cord, thyroid gland, bone marrow stromal cells and osteoblasts [8]. B cells, have also been implicated as OPG producers and studies have demonstrated that human B cell OPG production is significantly upregulated when stimulated by CD40 antibodies in vitro [50]. However, historically osteoblasts and their precursors have been regarded as the primary source of OPG during the process of physiological bone renewal [8]. Interestingly, purification of B cells from whole nucleated WT mouse bone marrow revealed that B cell mRNA expression and secreted protein concentrations account for over 40% of the total OPG produced in bone marrow under basal conditions (Figure 2). These data demonstrated that B cells are responsible for a significant proportion of OPG in the bone microenvironment [5].

OPG Production by cells of the B-lineage

In adults, B-lymphopoiesis occurs in the bone marrow. B lymphocytes are derived from hemopoietic stem cells (HSC) in the medullary cavity of the bone marrow and progress through a series of distinct developmental stages defined by various phenotypic markers and the rearrangement and expression of immunoglobulin genes [51]. Cells at multiple different stages of development and maturation are found in bone marrow. Interestingly, not only do mature B cells make OPG, but $B220^{+}IgM^{-}$ B cell precursors, immature B cells ($B220^{+}$ IgM^{+} IgD^{-}), and small numbers of plasma cells ($B220^{-}$ $CD138^{+}$) that home back to the bone marrow also secrete OPG, contributing additional concentrations to the total levels. The B-lineage cells producing the highest OPG levels on a cell by cell basis are plasma cells, followed by mature B cells, immature B cells, and finally B cell precursors. However, after normalization for the proportion of each population in the bone marrow, mature B cells are found to be the dominant source, responsible for 45% of total bone marrow OPG, while B cell precursors, immature B cells and plasma cells contribute an additional 19%. Overall the entire B-lineage is responsible for 64% of total mouse bone marrow OPG [5].

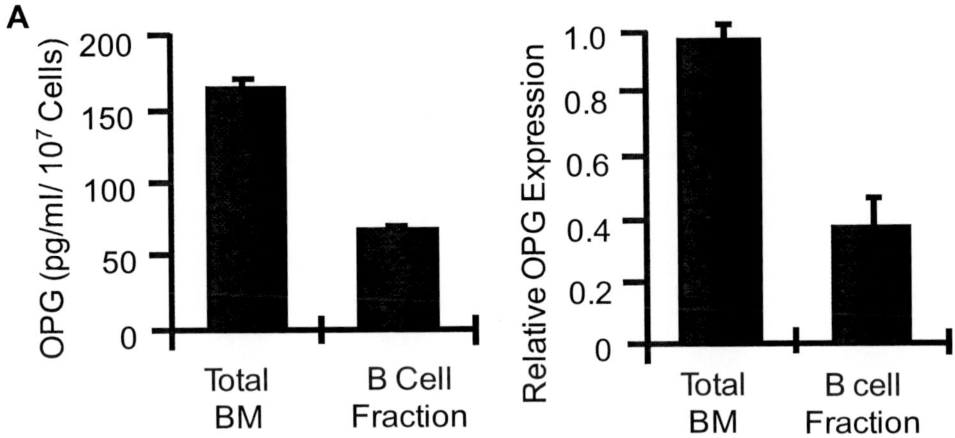

Figure 2. B cells Account for over 40% of total bone marrow OPG. A) OPG protein production in total bone marrow (BM) relative to B cell component thereof, quantitated by ELISA. B) OPG mRNA expression in total bone marrow (BM) relative to the B cell component thereof. Originally published in Blood. Li Y, Toraldo G, Li A, Yang X, Zhang H, Qian WP, Weitzmann MN; B cells and T cells are critical for the preservation of bone homeostasis and attainment of peak bone mass *in vivo*. Blood. 2007;109(9):3839–3848.© the American Society of Hematology.

Recent preliminary studies using an elegant transgenic mouse model in which osteoblasts and their immediate progenitors are specifically ablated further supports the contention that osteoblasts are not the dominant source of OPG in bone, as OPG transcript levels and osteoclast number remained unaffected following osteoblast ablation [52].

B cell production by B cells in peripheral organs

Large numbers of B cells exist outside of the bone marrow in peripheral organs. Fifty percent of the mouse spleen is composed of B cells [53] and lymph nodes and the peripheral circulation are additional rich sources of B cells. Not only do bone marrow derived B cells express OPG, but mature B cells irrespective of their origin (peripheral blood, lymph nodes and spleen) also express OPG, although concentrations produced are site specific, with bone marrow and peripheral blood derived B cells producing almost 3 times as much OPG as equivalent numbers of B cells derived from lymph nodes and spleens [5].

As a consequence of its immediate proximity to sites of osteoclastogenesis OPG production in the bone microenvironment is undoubtedly relevant to osteoclast formation, and bone resorption in vivo. However, OPG injected subcutaneously or intravenously in humans [54], monkeys [55] and rodents [56] effectively enters the circulation, localizes to the bone microenvironment and leads to significant reductions in bone resorption. Subcutaneous injection of OPG lead to delayed tooth eruption in mice [57]. Thus, sources of OPG external to the bone marrow are thus also likely to be highly relevant to bone remodeling, and B cells though out the body likely contribute to total OPG levels.

T cell-B cell interactions and the regulation of basal bone mass and B cell OPG production

Infection and inflammatory processes lead to significant T cell activation, and RANKL and TNFα production, driving osteoclastogenesis and bone loss in pathological conditions such as rheumatoid arthritis, periodontitis and in animal models of postmenopausal osteoporosis [1]. However, under basal conditions T cells have been reported to be a significantly source of RANKL, and T cell deficient nude mice do not show evidence of diminished or elevated RANKL mRNA in their bone marrow [5]. Nonetheless, even under physiological conditions in otherwise healthy humans and animals, a constant barrage of self- and foreign-antigens, many of them of bacterial origin physiologically absorbed in the gut, lead to a local and systemic low grade T cell activation. A moderate immune response is thus constantly in place [1]. This response by autoreactive T cells is thought to be essential for immune cell survival and renewal [58]. CD40L is a costimulatory molecule that is transiently upregulated on the surface of activated T cells and binds to its counterpart, CD40, a receptor expressed by professional antigen presenting cells (APC) such as macrophages, dendritic cells and B cells. It has been demonstrated that antibody induced activation of the CD40 costimulatory molecule stimulates OPG production by human tonsil B cells [50]. Consistent with these data CD40 ligation to its physiological ligand, induces a 2 fold stimulation of OPG production by mouse splenic B cells in vitro [5].

In vivo CD40 is activated by its ligand expressed on T cells. In line with these data both CD40 and CD40L KO mice display an osteoporotic phenotype and a significant deficiency in bone marrow OPG concentrations. These deficiencies in total OPG further correlate with a B cell specific deficiency in OPG production. Consistently, basal bone turnover is significantly disrupted in T cell-deficient nude mice, where diminished B cell OPG production leads to an enhanced rate of basal bone resorption leading to low bone mass [5]. Likewise, T cell depletion of mice using CD4 and CD8 antibodies have similarly led to a complete suppression of OPG expression in bone marrow cultures ex vivo [59].

The contribution of human bone marrow B cells to total OPG production and the role of CD40 to CD40L costimulation remain to be investigated, although osteoporosis and fractures are common in humans with the inherited disease, X-linked hyper-IgM syndrome, caused by mutations in the CD40L gene. These patients have significantly lower BMD than sex- and age-matched control subjects and exhibit elevated levels of N-terminal telopeptides of type I collagen (NTX), a urinary marker indicative of osteoclast activity [60]. Activated $CD4^+$ CD40L null T cells from humans or mice express normal levels of RANKL, but promoted marked osteoclastogenesis in vitro, in part due to a severe deficiency in IFN-gamma production, an in vitro inhibitor of osteoclast formation [60]. In addition, polymorphisms in the Kozak sequence of the CD40 gene are reported to be associated with low bone mass in postmenopausal women [61]. Whether increased basal bone resorption in X-linked hyper-IgM patients or low bone mass in postmenopausal women carrying specific polymorphisms in CD40 are also associated with diminished B cell OPG production remains to be examined.

The emerging data now suggests that the B lineage is a major source of OPG in the bone microenvironment and that T cell signaling to B cells, through the costimulatory molecules CD40L and CD40, play an important role in regulating basal osteoclast formation and in regulating bone homeostasis. This model is summarized in Figure 3.

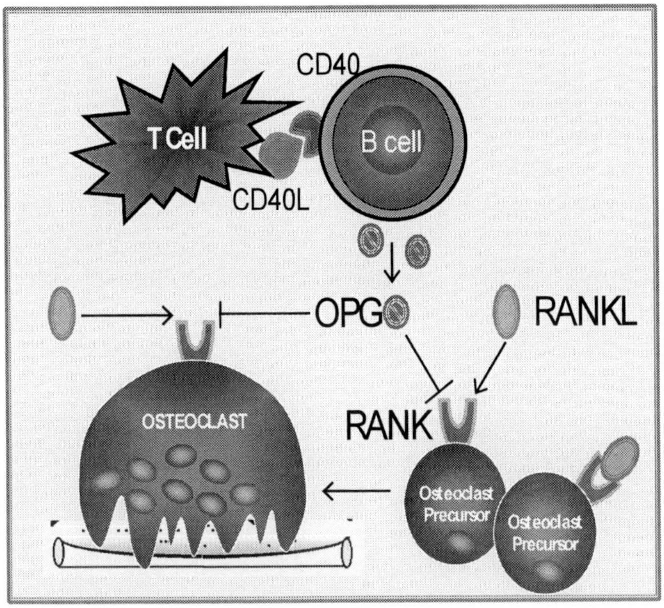

Figure 3. Model: B cells and T cells are critical regulators of basal osteoclastogenesis. Under the influence of CD40 costimulation by CD40L on activated T cells, B cells upregulate OPG production antagonizing RANKL association with its receptor RANK on osteoclast precursors and mature osteoclasts. OPG thus lowers the rate of RANKL induced osteoclast differentiation and fusion into mature osteoclasts, and reduces their resorptive activity and lifespan. Alterations in either T cell or B cell function lower B cell OPG production leading to increased osteoclastic bone resorption and decreased bone mass.

These findings remain to be translated into the human system, and if relevant may provide in part novel potential explanations for the propensity for osteopenia and osteoporosis development in numerous pathological conditions in which altered immune function or immunodeficiency in B cells and/or T cells results. Such conditions include HIV infection, solid organ and bone marrow transplantation, multiple myeloma in which normal B cells are significantly depleted, and patients treated with immunosuppressive agents such as glucocorticoids.

The role of B cells in Pathological Bone Turnover

B cells and postmenopausal osteoporosis

It has long been suspected that cells of the B-lineage may play important roles in the bone loss associated with a number of disease states. One such state is postmenopausal osteoporosis, a disease characterized by increased osteoclastic bone resorption following estrogen decline associated with the menopause. Over a decade ago surgical depletion of estrogen by means of ovariectomy in mice, an animal model of postmenopausal osteoporosis, was observed to significantly stimulate B-lymphopoiesis leading to an accumulation of $B220^+$ IgM^- early B cell precursors, although more mature IgM^+ B cell populations were not found to be significantly elevated [62]. Consistent with these observations estrogen treatment is reported to down-regulate B lymphopoiesis [62], although under these conditions immunoglobulin production is upregulated [63]. Interestingly, the lymphopoietic cytokine IL-7 has been shown to closely mimic some of the effects of estrogen deficiency in mice including upregulating B-lymphopoiesis and stimulating osteoclastic bone resorption. These findings suggested that the perturbations in B-lymphopoiesis observed in the bone marrow of ovariectomized mice were somehow linked to the loss of bone mass [64]. IL-7 action however turns out to be extremely complex and more recent studies have revealed that the primary osteoclastogenic action of IL-7 in vivo is directed through T cells rather than through B-lineage cells. IL-7 has been shown to potently stimulate T cell production of the osteoclastogenic cytokines RANKL and TNFα, upregulating osteoclastogenesis and inducing bone loss [43,65-67]. IL-7 also promotes bone loss in part by suppressing bone formation [66,68]. IL-7 action however is pleiotropic and when added to RANKL and M-CSF stimulated osteoclast cultures in vitro it lowers osteoclast formation [69]. While the mechanism remains unclear IL-7 may channel the differentiation of early B cell precursors, capable of acting as osteoclast precursors [43,45,69] into more mature B cell populations, thus reducing the concentrations of available osteoclast precursors. Alternatively IL-7 may promote T cell IFNγ production, a cytokine that inhibits osteoclast formation in vitro [70], while stimulating it in vivo through antigen-driven T cell activation [71]. IL-7 KO mice have been reported to have both decreased [64] and increased [40] bone mass. Similarly, while global transgenic IL-7 expression leads to a considerably expanded bone marrow cavity and focal osteolysis of the cortices [72], targeted overexpression of IL-7 specifically in osteoblasts led to increased trabecular bone mass suggesting that IL-7 actions on bone cells are dependent on whether IL-7 is delivered systemically or locally [40].

A role for mature B cells in estrogen deficiency-induced bone loss in mice has been excluded by recent experiments involving ovariectomy of μMT/μMT B cell KO mice. Estrogen deprivation induces bone loss of equivalent magnitude in B cell KO mice as that of WT control mice [73]. Although these studies suggest that mature B cells are likely not central mediators of ovariectomy-induced bone loss in vivo, at least in mice, a role for the early $B220^+$ precursors, which still exist in μMT/μMT mice, cannot be excluded. As described earlier, a number of studies have now shown that B cell precursors which expand during estrogen deficiency may have the capacity to differentiate along an osteoclastic lineage [43,45,69]. Consequently, it has been hypothesized that estrogen deficiency may augment osteoclastogenesis, in part by increasing the population of osteoclast precursors

[45]. Despite these intriguing speculations as to whether B cell precursors may facilitate bone loss during estrogen deficiency, definitive data demonstrating a direct cause-effect relationship between B cell precursors and ovariectomy-induced bone loss remains absent.

Other studies have suggested that B cell precursors may have the capacity to make RANKL, and that most $B220^+$ cells in the bone marrow are positive for RANKL, when analyzed by flow cytometry [74]. Studies from our laboratory however, have failed to detect soluble RANKL production by ELISA in cultures of unstimulated murine $B220^+$ IgM^- B cell precursors ex vivo [5], and recent human studies have reported that less than 20% of B cells in the gingival tissues of healthy subjects express RANKL [29]. Despite these data, some of the most compelling evidence for a role of B cells in the elevated RANKL production associated with estrogen deficiency comes from a human clinical study where a 3 fold increase in B cell RANKL production was observed in B cells derived from postmenopausal women relative to premenopausal women. Acute estrogen replacement significantly reduced B cell RANKL production [2]. The contribution of B cell RANKL to total RANKL concentrations, in the face of elevated RANKL production by T cells, bone marrow stromal cells and other cell types remains unclear.

B cells and postmenopausal osteoporosis in aged humans

Ovariectomy in the mouse or rat is an excellent model of postmenopausal osteoporosis and recapitulates many of the features associated with the acute phase of bone loss sustained by postmenopausal women immediately following the menopause. Nonetheless, there are some significant differences that have to be considered when extrapolating conclusions drawn from animal studies into human disease. One such confounder is that rodent models typically involve young animals due to the ease of availability, reduced costs, and due to the fact that osteoclastic responses to estrogen ablation are extremely robust in younger animals, mimicking within weeks events that occur over a decade in humans. Nonetheless, aging itself is one of the most important risk factors for osteoporosis and bone fracture and leads to an immunological microenvironment that is significantly different to that of young humans and animals.

Aging is established to lead to significant perturbations in immune function. The aged immune system is characterized by a progressive decline in responsiveness to antigens and tumors, and a paradoxical increase in autoimmunity [75], driven in part by a contraction in diversity of the T cell and B cell repertoires, and the accumulation of autoreactive T and B cells [76,77]. Autoimmunity in the aged further contributes to the development of a chronic inflammatory state, known as "Inflamm-aging" and is characterized by elevated cytokines in plasma and tissues such as bone marrow, including the osteoclastogenic factors IL-1, IL-6, TNFα, RANKL, M-CSF and Reactive Oxygen Species (ROS) [78-80]. Consequently, the T cells and B cells present in aging humans may function very differently in older humans relative to those present in their younger counterparts and in young mice.

Estrogen has been found to stimulate OPG production by osteoblasts [37] and pre-osteoblastic cell lines such as ST2 [81]. Consequently, under conditions of estrogen deficiency, OPG levels would be anticipated to decline, consistent with the increased osteoclastic bone loss associated with estrogen deficiency. Surprisingly, contrary to this expectation the serum level of OPG is in fact not diminished in postmenopausal women with either normal BMD, or with osteoporosis and displaying increased bone turnover [82]. Indeed, clinical studies confirm a significant elevation in serum OPG levels in both men and women with aging [83,84]. Such increases in OPG have been suggested to act as a homeostatic mechanism limiting even more rapid bone loss [8,83]. Given the apparent decline in osteoblastic OPG production during aging, the source of elevated serum OPG becomes an interesting question. Preliminary studies from our laboratory suggest that B cell OPG production is dramatically upregulated in aged mice, relative to young mice, and that B cells may account for these elevated total OPG concentrations characteristic of aging. Interestingly, T cells also undergo significant immunesenescence with aging leading to diminished CD40L expression and B cell costimulation [75]. Nonetheless, despite the loss of this stimulatory signal, B cell OPG production appears to be greatly enhanced. The relevant mechanisms involved in OPG regulation during aging are still under investigation.

Conclusion

The involvement of B cells in the regulation of bone turnover under physiological and pathological conditions is a topic that has been under investigation for a decade or more, however only recently has the importance of these cells in the maintenance of bone homeostasis begun to be appreciated. While significant progress has been made in our understanding of the mechanisms of bone regulation by B cells in vitro and in vivo much still remains to be clarified. Most of our current understanding of B cell regulation of bone turnover is based on animal studies in particular rodents, and for the most part these findings remain to be validated in humans. Translation of lessons learned in animal studies into humans, although difficult, will be essential for defining the role of B cells in the stabilization of basal bone turnover in young and adult humans and the protective effects of B cell derived OPG on the aged skeleton. The role of B cells in the etiology of bone loss in genetic diseases such as X-linked hyper-IgM syndrome and polymorphisms in the CD40 gene remain to be examined, as does the impact of B cell active agents such as Rituximab, an anti-CD20 antibody now used therapeutically to treat rheumatoid arthritis and B cell non-Hodgkin's lymphoma. If the lessons learned in mice hold true for humans these patients may be at additional risk for development of osteoporosis and bone fracture. Numerous diseases and therapeutic agents associated with osteoporosis affect the immune system, in particular lymphocytes. It is likely that B cell OPG production is impacted in many if not all of these conditions. Finally, long term studies may identify novel mechanisms to manipulate B cells to produce higher levels of OPG to elevate peak BMD and stave off bone loss in osteoporotic diseases.

Acknowledgments

M. Neale Weitzmann is supported by grants from the National Institute of Arthritis and Musculoskeletal and Skin Diseases (AR053607 and AR056090), the National Cancer Institute (U54CA119338) and by Award Number 1I01BX000105 from the Biomedical

Laboratory Research & Development Service of the VA Office of Research and Development.

REFERENCES

[1] Weitzmann MN & Pacifici R (2006). Estrogen deficiency and bone loss: an inflammatory tale. *J Clin Invest. 116,* 1186-1194.

[2] Eghbali-Fatourechi G; Khosla S; Sanyal A; Boyle WJ; Lacey DL & Riggs BL (2003). Role of RANK ligand in mediating increased bone resorption in early postmenopausal women. *J Clin Invest. 111,* 1221-1230.

[3] D'Amelio P; Grimaldi A; Di Bella S; Brianza SZ; Cristofaro MA; Tamone C; Giribaldi G; Ulliers D; Pescarmona GP & Isaia G (2008). Estrogen deficiency increases osteoclastogenesis up-regulating T cells activity: A key mechanism in osteoporosis. *Bone. 43,* 92-100.

[4] Yun TJ; Tallquist MD; Aicher A; Rafferty KL; Marshall AJ; Moon JJ; Ewings ME; Mohaupt M; Herring SW & Clark EA (2001). Osteoprotegerin, a crucial regulator of bone metabolism, also regulates B cell development and function. *J Immunol. 166,* 1482-1491.

[5] Li Y; Toraldo G; Li A; Yang X; Zhang H; Qian WP & Weitzmann MN (2007). B cells and T cells are critical for the preservation of bone homeostasis and attainment of peak bone mass in vivo. *Blood. 109,* 3839-3848.

[6] Manolagas SC & Jilka RL (1995). Bone marrow, cytokines, and bone remodeling. *N. Eng. J. Med. 332,* 305-311.

[7] Manolagas SC (2000). Birth and death of bone cells: basic regulatory mechanisms and implications for the pathogenesis and treatment of osteoporosis. *Endocr Rev. 21,* 115-137.

[8] Khosla S (2001). Minireview: the OPG/RANKL/RANK system. *Endocrinology. 142,* 5050-5055.

[9] Riggs BL; Khosla S & Melton LJ, 3rd (2002). Sex steroids and the construction and conservation of the adult skeleton. *Endocr Rev. 23,* 279-302.

[10] Clowes JA; Riggs BL & Khosla S (2005). The role of the immune system in the pathophysiology of osteoporosis. *Immunol Rev. 208,* 207-227.

[11] Teitelbaum SL (2000). Bone resorption by osteoclasts. *Science. 289,* 1504-1508.

[12] Manolagas SC; Kousteni S & Jilka RL (2002). Sex steroids and bone. *Recent Prog Horm Res. 57,* 385-409.

[13] Khosla S; Amin S & Orwoll E (2008). Osteoporosis in Men. *Endocr Rev.*

[14] Feldmann M; Brennan FM & Maini R (1996). Rheumatoid arthritis. *Cell. 85,* 307-310.

[15] Teng YT (2003). The role of acquired immunity and periodontal disease progression. *Crit Rev Oral Biol Med. 14,* 237-252.

[16] Abitbol V; Roux C; Chaussade S; Guillemant S; Kolta S; Dougados M; Couturier D & Amor B (1995). Metabolic bone assessment in patients with inflammatory bowel disease. *Gastroenterology. 108,* 417-422.

[17] Hu MI; Gagel RF & Jimenez C (2007). Bone loss in patients with breast or prostate cancer. *Curr Osteoporos Rep. 5,* 170-178.

[18] Alsina M; Boyce B; Devlin RD; Anderson JL; Craig F; Mundy GR & Roodman GD (1996). Development of an in vivo model of human multiple myeloma bone disease. *Blood. 87,* 1495-1501.

[19] Hirbe A; Morgan EA; Uluckan O & Weilbaecher K (2006). Skeletal complications of breast cancer therapies. *Clin Cancer Res. 12,* 6309s-6314s.

[20] Brufsky AM (2008). Cancer treatment-induced bone loss: pathophysiology and clinical perspectives. *Oncologist. 13,* 187-195.

[21] O'Brien CA; Jia D; Plotkin LI; Bellido T; Powers CC; Stewart SA; Manolagas SC & Weinstein RS (2004). Glucocorticoids act directly on osteoblasts and osteocytes to induce their apoptosis and reduce bone formation and strength. *Endocrinology. 145,* 1835-1841.

[22] Jia D; O'Brien CA; Stewart SA; Manolagas SC & Weinstein RS (2006). Glucocorticoids act directly on osteoclasts to increase their life span and reduce bone density. *Endocrinology. 147,* 5592-5599.

[23] Bernstein CN; Seeger LL; Sayre JW; Anton PA; Artinian L & Shanahan F (1995). Decreased bone density in inflammatory bowel disease is related to corticosteroid use and not disease diagnosis. *J Bone Miner Res. 10,* 250-256.

[24] Epstein S; Shane E & Bilezikian JP (1995). Organ transplantation and osteoporosis. *Curr Opin Rheumatol. 7,* 255-261.

[25] Gori F; Hofbauer LC; Dunstan CR; Spelsberg TC; Khosla S & Riggs BL (2000). The expression of osteoprotegerin and RANK ligand and the support of osteoclast formation by stromal-osteoblast lineage cells is developmentally regulated. *Endocrinology. 141,* 4768-4776.

[26] Suda T; Takahashi N; Udagawa N; Jimi E; Gillespie MT & Martin TJ (1999). Modulation of osteoclast differentiation and function by the new members of the tumor necrosis factor receptor and ligand families. *Endocr Rev. 20,* 345-357.

[27] Horwood NJ; Kartsogiannis V; Quinn JM; Romas E; Martin TJ & Gillespie MT (1999). Activated T Lymphocytes Support Osteoclast Formation in Vitro. *Biochem Biophys Res Commun. 265,* 144-150.

[28] Weitzmann MN; Cenci S; Rifas L; Haug J; Dipersio J & Pacifici R (2001). T cell activation induces human osteoclast formation via receptor activator of nuclear factor kappaB ligand-dependent and -independent mechanisms. *J Bone Miner Res. 16,* 328-337.

[29] Kawai T; Matsuyama T; Hosokawa Y; Makihira S; Seki M; Karimbux NY; Goncalves RB; Valverde P; Dibart S; Li YP; Miranda LA; Ernst CW; Izumi Y & Taubman MA (2006). B and T lymphocytes are the primary sources of RANKL in the bone resorptive lesion of periodontal disease. *Am J Pathol. 169,* 987-998.

[30] Romas E; Gillespie MT & Martin TJ (2002). Involvement of receptor activator of NFkappaB ligand and tumor necrosis factor-alpha in bone destruction in rheumatoid arthritis. *Bone. 30,* 340-346.

[31] Colucci S; Brunetti G; Cantatore F; Oranger A; Mori G; Quarta L; Cirulli N; Mancini L; Corrado A; Grassi F & Grano M (2007). Lymphocytes and synovial fluid fibroblasts

support osteoclastogenesis through RANKL, TNFalpha, and IL-7 in an in vitro model derived from human psoriatic arthritis. *J Pathol.*

[32] Simonet WS; Lacey DL; Dunstan CR; Kelley M; Chang MS; Luthy R; Nguyen HQ; Wooden S; Bennett L; Boone T; Shimamoto G; DeRose M; Elliott R; Colombero A; Tan HL; Trail G; Sullivan J; Davy E; Bucay N; Renshaw-Gegg L; Hughes TM; Hill D; Pattison W; Campbell P; Boyle WJ & et al. (1997). Osteoprotegerin: a novel secreted protein involved in the regulation of bone density. *Cell. 89,* 309-319.

[33] Bucay N; Sarosi I; Dunstan CR; Morony S; Tarpley J; Capparelli C; Scully S; Tan HL; Xu W; Lacey DL; Boyle WJ & Simonet WS (1998). osteoprotegerin-deficient mice develop early onset osteoporosis and arterial calcification. *Genes Dev. 12,* 1260-1268.

[34] Mizuno A; Amizuka N; Irie K; Murakami A; Fujise N; Kanno T; Sato Y; Nakagawa N; Yasuda H; Mochizuki S; Gomibuchi T; Yano K; Shima N; Washida N; Tsuda E; Morinaga T; Higashio K & Ozawa H (1998). Severe osteoporosis in mice lacking osteoclastogenesis inhibitory factor/osteoprotegerin. *Biochem Biophys Res Commun. 247,* 610-615.

[35] Takai H; Kanematsu M; Yano K; Tsuda E; Higashio K; Ikeda K; Watanabe K & Yamada Y (1998). Transforming growth factor-beta stimulates the production of osteoprotegerin/osteoclastogenesis inhibitory factor by bone marrow stromal cells. *J Biol Chem. 273,* 27091-27096.

[36] Rifas L; Arackal S & Weitzmann MN (2003). Inflammatory T cells rapidly induce differentiation of human bone marrow stromal cells into mature osteoblasts. *J Cell Biochem. 88,* 650-659.

[37] Hofbauer LC; Khosla S; Dunstan CR; Lacey DL; Spelsberg TC & Riggs BL (1999). Estrogen stimulates gene expression and protein production of osteoprotegerin in human osteoblastic cells. *Endocrinology. 140,* 4367-4370.

[38] Hofbauer LC; Khosla S; Dunstan CR; Lacey DL; Boyle WJ & Riggs BL (2000). The roles of osteoprotegerin and osteoprotegerin ligand in the paracrine regulation of bone resorption. *J Bone Miner Res. 15,* 2-12.

[39] Horowitz M (2007). B Lymphocytes and the Skeleton. *Ann N Y Acad Sci.*

[40] Lorenzo J; Horowitz M & Choi Y (2008). Osteoimmunology: interactions of the bone and immune system. *Endocr Rev. 29,* 403-440.

[41] Shinohara M; Koga T; Okamoto K; Sakaguchi S; Arai K; Yasuda H; Takai T; Kodama T; Morio T; Geha RS; Kitamura D; Kurosaki T; Ellmeier W & Takayanagi H (2008). Tyrosine kinases Btk and Tec regulate osteoclast differentiation by linking RANK and ITAM signals. *Cell. 132,* 794-806.

[42] Nutt SL; Heavey B; Rolink AG & Busslinger M (1999). Commitment to the B-lymphoid lineage depends on the transcription factor Pax5. *Nature. 401,* 556-562.

[43] Toraldo G; Roggia C; Qian WP; Pacifici R & Weitzmann MN (2003). IL-7 induces bone loss in vivo by induction of receptor activator of nuclear factor kappa B ligand and tumor necrosis factor alpha from T cells. *Proc Natl Acad Sci U S A. 100,* 125-130.

[44] Lee SK; Kalinowski JF; Jacquin C; Adams DJ; Gronowicz G & Lorenzo JA (2006). Interleukin-7 influences osteoclast function in vivo but is not a critical factor in ovariectomy-induced bone loss. *J Bone Miner Res. 10.1359/JBMR.060117.*

[45] Sato T; Shibata T; Ikeda K & Watanabe K (2001). Generation of bone-resorbing osteoclasts from B220+ cells: its role in accelerated osteoclastogenesis due to estrogen deficiency. *J Bone Miner Res. 16,* 2215-2221.

[46] Weitzmann MN; Cenci S; Haug J; Brown C; DiPersio J & Pacifici R (2000). B lymphocytes inhibit human osteoclastogenesis by secretion of TGFbeta. *J Cell Biochem. 78,* 318-324.

[47] Kitamura D; Roes J; Kuhn R & Rajewsky K (1991). A B cell-deficient mouse by targeted disruption of the membrane exon of the immunoglobulin mu chain gene. *Nature. 350,* 423-426.

[48] Beamer WG; Donahue LR; Rosen CJ & Baylink DJ (1996). Genetic variability in adult bone density among inbred strains of mice. *Bone. 18,* 397-403.

[49] Brodt MD; Ellis CB & Silva MJ (1999). Growing C57Bl/6 mice increase whole bone mechanical properties by increasing geometric and material properties. *J Bone Miner Res. 14,* 2159-2166.

[50] Yun TJ; Chaudhary PM; Shu GL; Frazer JK; Ewings MK; Schwartz SM; Pascual V; Hood LE & Clark EA (1998). OPG/FDCR-1, a TNF receptor family member, is expressed in lymphoid cells and is up-regulated by ligating CD40. *J Immunol. 161,* 6113-6121.

[51] Min H; Montecino-Rodriguez E & Dorshkind K (2006). Effects of aging on the common lymphoid progenitor to pro-B cell transition. *J Immunol. 176,* 1007-1012.

[52] O'Brien CA; Fu Q; Mommsen L; Dusevich V; Bonewald L; Manolagas SC & Jilka RL (2006). Osteoblasts are not the source of RANKL and OPG in bone but are required for maintenance of osteoclast function [Abstract]. *J Bone Miner Res. 21,* S31.

[53] Uchida J; Lee Y; Hasegawa M; Liang Y; Bradney A; Oliver JA; Bowen K; Steeber DA; Haas KM; Poe JC & Tedder TF (2004). Mouse CD20 expression and function. *Int Immunol. 16,* 119-129.

[54] Bekker PJ; Holloway D; Nakanishi A; Arrighi M; Leese PT & Dunstan CR (2001). The effect of a single dose of osteoprotegerin in postmenopausal women. *J Bone Miner Res. 16,* 348-360.

[55] Ominsky MS; Kostenuik PJ; Cranmer P; Smith SY & Atkinson JE (2007). The RANKL inhibitor OPG-Fc increases cortical and trabecular bone mass in young gonad-intact cynomolgus monkeys. *Osteoporos Int. 18,* 1073-1082.

[56] Capparelli C; Morony S; Warmington K; Adamu S; Lacey D; Dunstan CR; Stouch B; Martin S & Kostenuik PJ (2003). Sustained antiresorptive effects after a single treatment with human recombinant osteoprotegerin (OPG): a pharmacodynamic and pharmacokinetic analysis in rats. *J Bone Miner Res. 18,* 852-858.

[57] Wise GE; Yao S & Liu D (2006). Injections of osteoprotegerin and PMA delay tooth eruption. *Clin Anat. 19,* 19-24.

[58] Tanchot C; Lemonnier FA; Perarnau B; Freitas AA & Rocha B (1997). Differential requirements for survival and proliferation of CD8 naive or memory T cells. *Science. 276,* 2057-2062.

[59] Grcevic D; Lee SK; Marusic A & Lorenzo JA (2000). Depletion of CD4 and CD8 T lymphocytes in mice In vivo enhances 1, 25- dihydroxyvitamin D(3)-stimulated

osteoclast-like cell formation In vitro by a mechanism that is dependent on prostaglandin synthesis. *J Immunol. 165,* 4231-4238.

[60] Lopez-Granados E; Temmerman ST; Wu L; Reynolds JC; Follmann D; Liu S; Nelson DL; Rauch F & Jain A (2007). Osteopenia in X-linked hyper-IgM syndrome reveals a regulatory role for CD40 ligand in osteoclastogenesis. *Proc Natl Acad Sci U S A. 104,* 5056-5061.

[61] Pineda B; Laporta P; Hermenegildo C; Cano A & Garcia-Perez MA (2007). A C >T polymorphism located at position -1 of the Kozak sequence of CD40 gene is associated with low bone mass in Spanish postmenopausal women. *Osteoporos Int.*

[62] Masuzawa T; Miyaura C; Onoe Y; Kusano K; Ohta H; Nozawa S & Suda T (1994). Estrogen deficiency stimulates B lymphopoiesis in mouse bone marrow. *J Clin Invest. 94,* 1090-1097.

[63] Erlandsson MC; Jonsson CA; Islander U; Ohlsson C & Carlsten H (2003). Oestrogen receptor specificity in oestradiol-mediated effects on B lymphopoiesis and immunoglobulin production in male mice. *Immunology. 108,* 346-351.

[64] Miyaura C; Onoe Y; Inada M; Maki K; Ikuta K; Ito M & Suda T (1997). Increased B-lymphopoiesis by interleukin 7 induces bone loss in mice with intact ovarian function: similarity to estrogen deficiency. *Proc Natl Acad Sci U S A. 94,* 9360-9365.

[65] Ryan MR; Shepherd R; Leavey JK; Gao Y; Grassi F; Schnell FJ; Qian WP; Kersh GJ; Weitzmann MN & Pacifici R (2005). An IL-7-dependent rebound in thymic T cell output contributes to the bone loss induced by estrogen deficiency. *Proc Natl Acad Sci U S A. 102,* 16735-16740.

[66] Weitzmann MN; Cenci S; Roggia C; Toraldo G; Weitzmann L & Pacifici R (2002). Increased production of IL-7 uncouples bone formation from bone resorption during estrogen deficiency. *J Clin Invest. 110,* 1643-1650.

[67] Weitzmann MN; Cenci S; Rifas L; Brown C & Pacifici R (2000). Interleukin-7 stimulates osteoclast formation by up-regulating the T- cell production of soluble osteoclastogenic cytokines. *Blood. 96,* 1873-1878.

[68] Giuliani N; Colla S; Morandi F; Lazzaretti M; Sala R; Bonomini S; Grano M; Colucci S; Svaldi M & Rizzoli V (2005). Myeloma cells block RUNX2/CBFA1 activity in human bone marrow osteoblast progenitors and inhibit osteoblast formation and differentiation. *Blood. 106,* 2472-2483.

[69] Lee SK; Kalinowski JF; Jastrzebski SL; Puddington L & Lorenzo JA (2003). Interleukin-7 is a direct inhibitor of in vitro osteoclastogenesis. *Endocrinology. 144,* 3524-3531.

[70] Takayanagi H; Ogasawara K; Hida S; Chiba T; Murata S; Sato K; Takaoka A; Yokochi T; Oda H; Tanaka K; Nakamura K & Taniguchi T (2000). T-cell-mediated regulation of osteoclastogenesis by signalling cross-talk between RANKL and IFN-gamma. *Nature. 408,* 600-605.

[71] Gao Y; Grassi F; Ryan MR; Terauchi M; Page K; Yang X; Weitzmann MN & Pacifici R (2007). IFN-gamma stimulates osteoclast formation and bone loss in vivo via antigen-driven T cell activation. *J Clin Invest. 117,* 122-132.

[72] Valenzona HO; Pointer R; Ceredig R & Osmond DG (1996). Prelymphomatous B cell hyperplasia in the bone marrow of interleukin-7 transgenic mice: precursor B cell

dynamics, microenvironmental organization and osteolysis. *Exp Hematol. 24,* 1521-1529.

[73] Li Y; Li A; Yang X & Weitzmann MN (2006). Ovariectomy-induced bone loss occurs independently of B cells. *J Cell Biochem. 100,* 1370-1375.

[74] Kanematsu M; Sato T; Takai H; Watanabe K; Ikeda K & Yamada Y (2000). Prostaglandin E2 induces expression of receptor activator of nuclear factor-kappa B ligand/osteoprotegrin ligand on pre-B cells: implications for accelerated osteoclastogenesis in estrogen deficiency. *J Bone Miner Res. 15,* 1321-1329.

[75] Weyand CM; Brandes JC; Schmidt D; Fulbright JW & Goronzy JJ (1998). Functional properties of CD4+ CD28- T cells in the aging immune system. *Mech Ageing Dev. 102,* 131-147.

[76] Goronzy JJ & Weyand CM (2003). Aging, autoimmunity and arthritis: T-cell senescence and contraction of T-cell repertoire diversity - catalysts of autoimmunity and chronic inflammation. *Arthritis Res Ther. 5,* 225-234.

[77] Weksler ME (2000). Changes in the B-cell repertoire with age. *Vaccine. 18,* 1624-1628.

[78] Salvioli S; Capri M; Valensin S; Tieri P; Monti D; Ottaviani E & Franceschi C (2006). Inflamm-aging, cytokines and aging: state of the art, new hypotheses on the role of mitochondria and new perspectives from systems biology. *Curr Pharm Des. 12,* 3161-3171.

[79] Grimble RF (2003). Inflammatory response in the elderly. *Curr Opin Clin Nutr Metab Care. 6,* 21-29.

[80] Cao J; Venton L; Sakata T & Halloran BP (2003). Expression of RANKL and OPG correlates with age-related bone loss in male C57BL/6 mice. *J Bone Miner Res. 18,* 270-277.

[81] Saika M; Inoue D; Kido S & Matsumoto T (2001). 17beta-estradiol stimulates expression of osteoprotegerin by a mouse stromal cell line, ST-2, via estrogen receptor-alpha. *Endocrinology. 142,* 2205-2212.

[82] Yano K; Tsuda E; Washida N; Kobayashi F; Goto M; Harada A; Ikeda K; Higashio K & Yamada Y (1999). Immunological characterization of circulating osteoprotegerin/osteoclastogenesis inhibitory factor: increased serum concentrations in postmenopausal women with osteoporosis. *J Bone Miner Res. 14,* 518-527.

[83] Khosla S; Arrighi HM; Melton LJ, 3rd; Atkinson EJ; O'Fallon WM; Dunstan C & Riggs BL (2002). Correlates of osteoprotegerin levels in women and men. *Osteoporos Int. 13,* 394-399.

[84] Indridason OS; Franzson L & Sigurdsson G (2005). Serum osteoprotegerin and its relationship with bone mineral density and markers of bone turnover. *Osteoporos Int. 16,* 417-423.

In: Osteoporosis: Etiology, Diagnosis and Treatment
Editors: Bilar E. Mattingly and Albert C. Pillare
ISBN 978-1-60692-397-9

Chapter 9

ANABOLIC AGENTS IN THE CURRENT MANAGEMENT OF OSTEOPOROSIS

Jean-Yves Reginster* and Audrey Neuprez
University of Liège, Liège, Belgium.

ABSTRACT

Since the mid-eighties, several medications, aiming at the inhibition of bone resorption, have consistently shown their ability to reduce fracture rates, at various skeletal locations, in osteoporotic post-menopausal women. Unfortunately, the diagnosis of osteoporosis is frequently made after the first fracture occurs. At this stage, bone strength has significantly decreased, as a result of low bone mineral density and disrupted bone micro architecture. Medications have now been developed to specifically stimulate bone formation, with the ultimate goal to restore the affected skeleton and to bring back bone biomechanical resistance to a normal level. The peptides from the parathyroid hormone family (1-34 human recombinant fragment or teriparatide and the 1-84 full length hormone) are potent stimulators of bone formation. They both have shown their ability to dramatically reduce vertebral fractures, whereas teriparatide alone has, so far, confirmed this effect on non-spinal events. These peptides were shown to have a carry-over effect, with their anti-fracture efficacy (teriparatide) maintained up to 30 months after treatment has been interrupted. However, the prescription of an anti-resorptive agent after withdrawal of teriparatide prevents further bone loss. Strontium ranelate is characterized by a dual mechanism of action, combining an inhibition of bone resorption and a simulation of bone formation. This new chemical entity has been tested in long-term studies which have shown, after 5 years, a reduction of fracture rates at the spine, at non vertebral locations and at the hip (in patients above 74 years old with prevalent low bone density at the femoral neck). Strontium ranelate reduces fractures in patients with or without prevalent vertebral fractures, in osteoporotic patients, in osteopenia and in

* Correspondence concerning this article should be addressed to: Jean-Yves Reginster, Unité d'exploration de l'os et du cartilage, CHU Centre Ville, 45 Quai Godefroid Kurth, 4020 Liège, Belgium. Fax : +32-4-270.32.53 / mail: jyreginster@ulg.ac.be.

subjects above the age of 80 years. Development of medications aiming at the restoration of normal bone strength and resistance is one of the most exciting perspectives in the management of post-menopausal osteoporosis.

Keywords: Osteoporosis treatment, anabolic agents, teriparatide, Strontium ranelate.

Peptides from the Parathyroid Hormone Family

Peptides from the parathyroid hormone (PTH) family have been investigated in the management of osteoporosis for > 30 years [1]. A continuous endogenous production or exogenous administration of PTH, as is the case in primary or secondary hyperparathyroidism, can lead to deleterious consequences on the skeleton, particularly on cortical bone. However, intermittent administration of PTH (e.g, through daily subcutaneous injections) results in an increase of the number and activity of osteoblasts, leading to an increase in bone mass and an improvement in skeletal architecture, at both the trabecular and cortical skeleton. This treatment also increases cortical bone width.

The full length (1-84) molecule and the 1-34 N-terminal fragment are currently used for the management of osteoporosis. Based on their respective molecular weights, equivalent dose of 1-34 fragment, relative to 1-84 molecule, is 40% (e.g. 20 and 40 μg of 1-34 PTH is equivalent to 50 and 100 μg of 1-84 PTH, respectively).

In order to assess the effects of the 1–34 N-terminal fragment of PTH on fractures, 1637 postmenopausal women with prior spine fractures were randomly assigned to receive 20 or 40 μg of 1–34 PTH or placebo, subcutaneously self-administered daily. Spine radiographs were obtained at baseline and at the end of the study (median duration of observation, 21 months), and serial measurements of bone mass were performed by dual-energy X-ray absorptiometry.

New spine fractures occurred in 14% of the women in the placebo group and in 5% and 4% of the women in the 20- and 40-μg dose groups, respectively. The relative risk of fracture, as compared with the placebo group, was 0.35 and 0.31 (95% CI, 0.22–0.55 and 0.19–0.50), respectively. New non-spine fractures occurred in 6% of the women in the placebo group and 3% of those in each PTH (RR, 0.47 and 0.46, 95% CI, 0.25–0.88 and 0.25–0.86, respectively). PTH had only minor side effects (occasional nausea and headache) [2].

The anti-fracture efficacy of PTH on spine fracture was not modulated by the age of the subjects (< 65 years of age, 65–75 years of age or > 75 years of age), prevalent spinal BMD values (T -score <-2.5 or >-2.5) or number of prevalent fractures (one or two or more fractures) [3].

At the end of this trial, patients were followed for an additional 18-month period without PTH, during which they were allowed to use any antiosteoporotic medication considered appropriate by their caregiver. Although the proportion of patients having received an inhibitor of bone resorption was slightly higher in patients previously in the placebo group than in the patients having received 20 PTH μg/day, the reduction of spine fractures observed in this particular group during the initial trial was confirmed during this 18-month period

(RR, 0.59; 95% CI, 0.42–0.85) [4]. A follow up in 1262 women was conducted up to 30 months after discontinuation of treatment. The hazard ratio for combined teriparatide groups (20 and 40 μg) for the 50-month period after baseline was 0.57 (95% CI; 0.40-0.82), suggesting a sustained effect in reducing the risk of non-spine fragility fracture [5].

Teriparatide-mediated relative fracture risk reduction was shown to be independent of pre-treatment bone turnover, demonstrating that this therapy offers clinical benefit to patients across a range of disease severity [6].

Full-length recombinant human PTH (1-84) has also been investigated in the management of postmenopausal osteoporosis. It has been postulated that the C-terminal region of PTH, which teriparatide lacks, also has biological functions in the bone that are mediated by a novel receptor, specific for this region of the hormone. Teriparatide, for instance, has been associated with osteosarcoma in rats, treated with massive doses during most of their lifespan, possibly related to its anti-apoptotic effects in bone cells and decrease in production of C-terminal PTH fragments. In contrast, researchers suggest that PTH (1-84) is likely to not have such effect due to the pro-apoptotic effects of C-terminal PTH fragments that maintain normal bone cell turnover [7,8]. In a Phase II study, women self-administered PTH (50, 75 or 100 μg) or placebo by daily subcutaneous injection for 12 months. The 100-μg dose increased BMD significantly at 3 months and 12 months (+7.8%). Bone area also significantly increased (+2.0%). Non significant decrease (-0.9%) in total hip BMD occurred during the first six months with the 100 μg dose, but this trend reversed (+1.6%) during the second six months. Bone turnover markers increased during the first half of the study and were maintained at elevated levels during the second six months. Dose-related incidences of transient hypercalcemia occurred but only 1 patient (100-μg group) was withdrawn because of repeated hypercalcemia [8,9]. Results from the pivotal Phase III studies have not yet been published as full papers. Evidence from the TOP (Treatment of Osteoporosis with Parathyroid Hormone) study, including women with low BMD (with or without previous fracture) suggest that PTH (1-84) reduced the incidence of vertebral fractures in all patients and prevented the incidence of first vertebral fracture in women with postmenopausal osteoporosis [8]. Reduction of non-vertebral or hip fractures does not clearly appear from the currently available data [9,10,11].

STRONTIUM RANELATE

Strontium ranelate is composed of an organic moiety (ranelic acid) and two atoms of strontium. Its chemical name is 5-[bis(carboxymethyl)amino]-2-carboxy-4-cyano-3-thiophenacetic acid distrontium salt. Ranelic acid was chosen among 26 strontium salts and was the compound simultaneously presenting the best physicochemical characteristics (eg, high percentage of strontium with two atoms of strontium linked to the molecule, solubility, no chelating properties, chirality, stability), the best pharmacokinetic characteristics (eg, bioavailabilty, exposure to strontium), and good safety. It has been shown to have specific action on bone cells. Strontium ranelate, developed by Laboratoires Servier, was recently demonstrated to significantly reduce the vertebral and hip fracture risk in women with postmenopausal osteoporosis, and to have a good tolerability profile [12].

Strontium ranelate was administered to 160 postmenopausal women in a 24-month double blind placebo controlled prospective randomized study. Doses of 0.125, 0.5, 1 g/day p.o. of strontium ranelate were compared with placebo. All patients received 500 mg of elemental calcium daily. The main characteristics of the study population were: mean age: 54 years; duration of menopause: 3 years, lumbar BMD (as measured by dual-energy X-ray [DXA] on Hologic densitometers): 0.931 +/-0.135 g/cm² (mean ± standard deviation [SD]) corresponding to a mean lumbar T-score =-1.4+/-1.4. At the conclusion of the study, the lumbar BMD increased in a dose-dependent manner with strontium ranelate. The percentage variation of lumbar BMD from baseline was significantly different in the group receiving strontium ranelate 1 g/day as compared with placebo: +5.53% versus –0.75% respectively (95% confidence interval [CI]: 3.90, 8.67, respectively; $p<0.001$). Increase in total hip and neck BMD averages are 3.2 % and 2.5%, respectively. The percentage variation of total hip and femoral neck BMD were significantly different in the group receiving strontium ranelate 1 g/day as compared to placebo (+3.21% versus –0.88%; 95% CI : 1.86, 6.31, respectively +2.46% versus –0.87%, 95% CI: 0.69, 5.96 respectively, both $p<0.001$). The overall percentage of study withdrawals due to adverse reaction was 15% in the placebo group and 11% in strontium ranelate-treated patients. In conclusion, while significantly increasing bone mineral density of the spine and femur in early postmenopausal women, over 24-month period, compared to a placebo, strontium ranelate 1 g/day p.o. does not induce any significant adverse reaction compared to those observed in women receiving a placebo for the same duration [13]. The 1 g/day dose was therefore retained as the dose for preventive treatment of bone loss after menopause.

The effects of strontium ranelate in postmenopausal women with vertebral osteoporotic fractures were assessed during a double-blind, placebo-controlled trial. Either strontium ranelate (0.5 g, 1 g or 2 g/day) or placebo were given to 353 Caucasian women (age: 66 years; lumbar BMD by DXA: 0.699+/-0.098g/cm² corresponding to mean lumbar T-score= -3.9+/-1.0, mean number of prevalent vertebral fracture per patient= 2.7+/-2.5, mean menopausal duration 18+/-8 years and mean body-mass index [BMI] = 25 +/-3 kg/m^2).

All patients were also given a daily supplement of calcium (0.5 g) and vitamin D_3 (800 international units [I.U.]. At the conclusion of this 2-year study, strontium ranelate dose-dependently increased the lumbar BMD values by comparison with baseline: +5.9% for 0.5 g; +8.3% for 1 g and + 13.6% for 2 g. The annual increase in lumbar BMD in the group receiving 2 g of strontium ranelate was +7.3% ($p<0.001$) and significantly different when compared to placebo. A significant increase in bone alkaline phosphatase was associated with a simultaneous and significant decrease in N-telopeptide crosslinks (NTX) throughout the 2-year period in the group receiving strontium ranelate 2 g. During the second year of treatment, the dose of 2 g was associated with a 44% reduction in the number of patients experiencing a new vertebral deformity. Bone histomorphometry showed no mineralisation defects. The same percentage of withdrawals following an adverse effect (10%) was observed for patients receiving placebo and for those receiving strontium ranelate 2 g [14]. Further analysis of this trial investigated strontium ranelate interactions with bone mineral. Transiliac bone biopsies were quantified by X-ray microanalysis for strontium ranelate uptake and the distribution in bone mineral. Changes in the mean and distribution of the degrees of mineralisation of bone (MDMB) were measured by quantitative microradiography. In strontium ranelate-treated women, strontium ranelate was dose dependently deposited into compact and cancellous bone, with significantly higher contents in new bone than in old bone. Measurement of strontium concentration in iliac crest bone biopsies from patients treated up to 60 months in the phase III studies with strontium ranelate 2g/day indicate that the strontium content in total bone (expressed as the ratio Sr/(Sr+Ca)mmol%) reaches a plateau from month 36. Strontium ranelate was mainly deposited on new bone. MDMB was not significantly different in strontium ranelate and placebo groups at either compact or cancellous bone levels [15].

Strontium ranelate has been investigated in a large Phase III program, initiated in 1996 which includes two extensive clinical trials for the treatment of established osteoporosis. The Spinal Osteoporosis Therapeutic Intervention (SOTI) study was aimed at assessing strontium ranelate's effect on the risk of vertebral fractures. TRreatment Of Peripheral Osteoporosis (TROPOS) trial aimed to evaluate the effect of strontium ranelate on peripheral (non spinal) fractures. All patients included in these two studies had previously participated in a run-in study Fracture International Run-in strontium Ranelate Trials (FIRST) aimed at starting the normalisation of calcium and Vitamin D. The patients received a calcium/vitamin D supplement throughout the studies, which were individually adapted according to their deficiencies (500 or 1000 mg of calcium, and 400 or 800 IU of vitamin D_3) [16]. Both studies are multinational, randomized, double-blind and placebo-controlled with two parallel groups (strontium ranelate 2 g/day versus placebo) involving 75 clinical centers in 12 countries in Europe and Australia. The study duration is 5 years, with main statistical analysis planned after 3 years of follow-up. From > 9000 osteoporotic postmenopausal women having taken part in FIRST, 1649 patients were included in SOTI with a mean age of 70 years, and 5091 patients were included in TROPOS with a mean age of 77 [17]. In these two studies, the main statistical analysis has been performed in the intention-to-treat (ITT) population, which means in patients who took at least one sachet of study treatment and with baseline and post baseline evaluation of the main criteria. The primary analysis of the SOTI study, evaluating the effect of 2 g of strontium ranelate on vertebral fracture rates, revealed a 41% reduction in relative risk (RR) of experiencing a first new vertebral fracture (semi-quantitative assessment) with strontium ranelate throughout the 3-year study compared with placebo, 139 patients with vertebral fracture versus 222 respectively (RR = 0.59, 95% CI: 0.48; 0.73; $p < 0.001$) in the ITT population. The RR of experiencing a new vertebral fracture was significantly reduced in the strontium ranelate group as compared with the placebo group for the first year: over the 0 – 12-month period the RR reduction was of 49% (RR: 0.51, 95% CI: 0.36; 0.74, respectively Cox model: $p < 0.001$). These results have also been confirmed when combining both diagnostic methods (semi-quantitative plus quantitative) for incident vertebral fracture. Semi-quantitative assessment was performed according to the semi-quantitative visual grading of vertebral deformities recommended by H.K Genant [18]. Bone specific alkaline phosphatase increased in the strontium ranelate group while serum type I collagen C-telopeptides crosslinks (CTX) decreased. The lumbar BMD increased in the treated group when compared to the placebo group (+11.4% versus –1.3% respectively, $p < 0.001$). Strontium ranelate was well tolerated without any specific adverse event [19,20,21].

The primary analysis of the TROPOS Study, evaluating the effect of strontium ranelate 2 g/day on non-vertebral fracture, showed reduction in RR of 16% in all vertebral fractures over a 3-year follow-up period (RR = 0.84; 95% CI (0.702;0.995); P = 0.04). Strontium ranelate treatment was associated with a 19% reduction in risk of major non-vertebral osteoporotic fractures (RR = 0.81; 95% CI:0.66; 0.98; P = 0.031). In the high risk fracture subgroup (women with age ≥74 years and with femoral-neck BMD T-score ≤-2.4 according to NHANES normative value), treatment was associated with a 36% reduction in risk of hip fracture (RR = 0.64; 95% CI (0.412; 0.997); P = 0.046) (Figure 1).

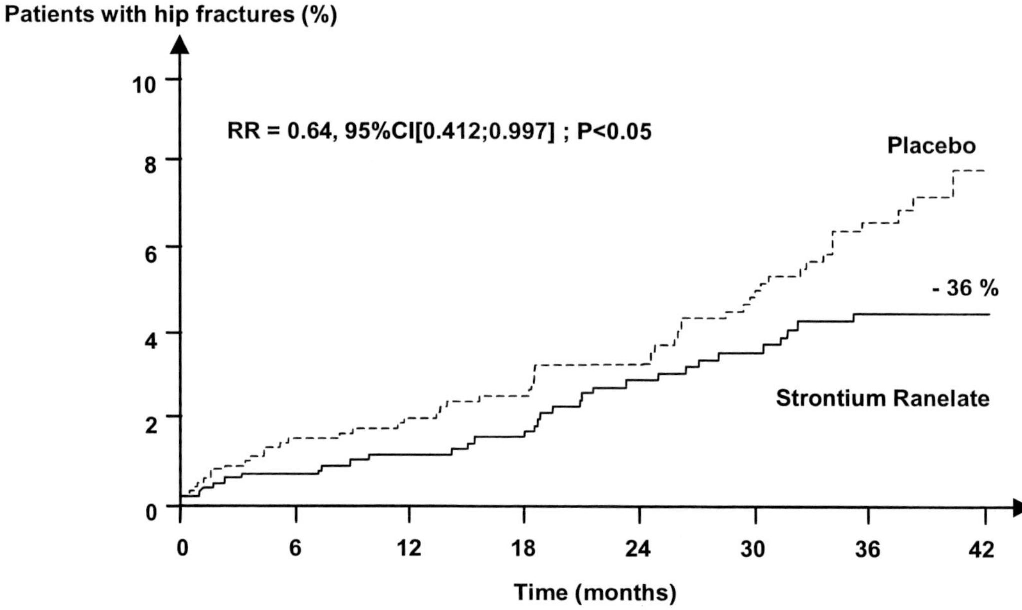

Figure 1. Proportion of patients who had one and more hip fractures over 3 years in the intention-to-treat population.

In order to assess the efficacy of strontium ranelate according to the main determinants of vertebral fracture risk: age, baseline BMD, prevalent fractures, family history of osteoporosis, baseline BMI, and addiction to smoking, data of two large multinational randomized double-blind studies were pooled, with a population of 5082 (2536 receiving strontium ranelate 2 g/day and 2546 receiving a placebo), 74 years of age on average, and a 3-year follow-up.

The treatment decreased the risk of both vertebral (relative risk [RR] = 0.60 [0.53-0.69] p < 0.001) and non-vertebral (RR = 0.85 [0.74-0.99] p = 0.03) fractures. The decrease in risk of vertebral fractures was 37% (p = 0.003) in women <70 years, 42% (p < 0.001) for those 70-80 years of age, and 32% (p = 0.013) for those > or = 80 years. The RR of vertebral fracture was 0.28 (0.07-0.99) in osteopenic and 0.61 (0.53-0.70) in osteoporotic women, and baseline BMD was not a determinant of efficacy. The incidence of vertebral fractures in the placebo group increased with the number of prevalent vertebral fractures, but this was not a determinant of the effect of strontium ranelate. In 2605 patients, the risk of experiencing a first vertebral fracture was reduced by 48% (p < 0.001). The risk of experiencing a second vertebral fracture was reduced by 45% (p < 0.001; 1100 patients). Moreover, the risk of experiencing more than two vertebral fractures was reduced by 33% (p < 0.001; 1365 patients). Family history of osteoporosis, baseline BMI, and addiction to smoking were not determinants of efficacy. This study showed that a 3-year treatment with strontium ranelate leads to anti-vertebral fracture efficacy in postmenopausal women independently of baseline osteoporotic risk factors [22].

Women ≥80 years of age comprise ~8% of the postmenopausal population but contribute >30% of all fragility fractures and 60% of hip fractures because of the high prevalence of osteoporosis and high incidence of falls [23]. Because this group of women constitutes the fastest growing segment of the population, the number of elderly individuals with osteoporosis will increase markedly in the coming years [24].

Despite the important contribution to the public health burden of fractures made by fractures in this group, few studies of fracture prevention have focused on the elderly.

To determine whether strontium ranelate also reduces fractures in the elderly, an analysis based on preplanned pooling of data from the SOTI and TROPOS trials included 1488 women between 80 and 100 years of age followed for 3 years. Yearly spinal X-rays were performed in 895 patients. Only radiographically confirmed non-vertebral fractures were included.

Baseline characteristics did not differ in placebo and treatment arms. In the intent-to-treat analysis, the risk of vertebral, non-vertebral, and clinical (symptomatic vertebral and non-vertebral) fractures was reduced within 1 year by 59% (p = 0.002), 41% (p = 0.027), and 37% (p = 0.012), respectively. At the end of 3 years, vertebral, non-vertebral, and clinical fracture risks were reduced by 32% (p = 0.013), 31% (p = 0.011), and 22% (p = 0.040), respectively. The medication was well tolerated, and the safety profile was similar to that in younger patients. The authors concluded that treatment with strontium ranelate safely reduces the risk of vertebral and non-vertebral fractures in women with osteoporosis ≥80 years of age [25].

Many fractures occur in women with moderate fracture risk due to osteopenia. Strontium ranelate was studied in 1431 postmenopausal women with osteopenia. In women with lumbar spine osteopenia, strontium ranelate decreased the risk of vertebral fracture by 41% (RR=0.59;IC95:0.43;0.82, p=0.002), by 59% in women with no prevalent fractures (RR=0.41;IC95:0.17;0.99, p=0.039) and by 38% in women with prevalent fractures (RR=0.62;IC95:0.44;0.88, p=0.008). In women with osteopenia both at the lumbar spine and the femoral neck, strontium ranelate reduced the risk of fracture by 52% (RR=0.48; IC95:0.24;0.96; p=0.034) [26].

To assess the capacity of strontium ranelate to restore normal bone mineral density (WHO definition: T-score >or=-1) in post-menopausal osteopenic women (T-score between -1 and -2.5) at baseline, a post-hoc analysis from SOTI and TROPOS studies of 1428 patients randomly assigned them to receive either 2 g of strontium ranelate a day or placebo for three years. Bone mineral density was measured at baseline and each year for three years. Results were analyzed on an intention-to-treat basis. At lumbar spine, after one, two and three years of treatment with strontium ranelate, 26.4, 42.1 and 58.2% respectively of osteopenic patients normalized their bone mineral density, compared with 6.6, 8.9 and 11.9% in the placebo group (all p<0.001). At total hip, the percentage of patients normalizing their bone mineral density was 5.4, 10.0 and 19.6% in the strontium ranelate group and 1.8, 1.4 and 1.6% in the placebo one (all p<0.001). Strontium ranelate is able to normalize bone mineral density in a significant proportion of osteopenic patients after one, two and three years of treatment [27].

Significant increases in lumbar spine, femoral neck, and total hip BMD have been consistently reported in all populations exposed to strontium ranelate [14,20,21,28].

To analyze the relationship between bone mineral density (BMD) changes and fracture incidence during 3-yr treatment with strontium ranelate, women from the strontium ranelate arm of the SOTI and TROPOS trials were evaluated, the outcome measures included BMD at the lumbar spine, femoral neck, and total proximal femur assessed at baseline and after a follow-up of 1 and 3 yr; semi-quantitative visual assessment of vertebral fractures; and non-vertebral fractures based on written documentation. After 3 year of strontium ranelate treatment, each percentage point increase in femoral neck and total proximal femur BMD was associated with a 3% (95% adjusted confidence interval, 1-5%) and 2% (1-4%) reduction in risk of a new vertebral fracture, respectively. The 3-yr changes in femoral neck and total proximal femur BMD explained 76% and 74%, respectively, of the reduction in vertebral fractures observed during the treatment. Three-year changes in spine BMD were not statistically associated with the incidence of new vertebral fracture (P = 0.10). No significant associations were found between 3-yr changes in BMD and incidence of new non-vertebral fractures, but a trend was found for femoral neck BMD (P = 0.09) and for total proximal femur BMD (P = 0.07). An increase in femoral neck BMD after 1 yr was significantly associated with the reduction in incidence of new vertebral fractures observed after 3 year (P = 0.04). The authors concluded that, during 3-year strontium ranelate treatment, an increase in femoral neck BMD was associated with a proportional reduction in vertebral fracture incidence [29].

In a post-hoc analysis of 465 women aged over 74 years with low BMD at the femoral neck (T-score < or = -2.4 according to NHANES normative values), selected from the population of the TROPOS trial, BMD was assessed at the femoral neck at baseline and after a follow-up of 3 years. Hip fractures were reported by board in hospital reports. After adjusting for age, body mass index, femoral neck BMD at baseline and number of prevalent vertebral fractures, for each 1% increase in femoral neck BMD observed after 3 years, the risk to experience a hip fracture after 3 years decreased by 7% (95% CI: 1-14%) (p = 0.04). In patients experiencing a hip fracture over 3 years of treatment with SR, femoral neck BMD increased by (mean [SE]) 3.41 (1.02) % compared to 7.23 (0.81)% in patients without hip fracture (p = 0.02) [30].

The safety of strontium ranelate on bone was investigated through the analysis of 141 transiliac bone biopsies performed in a subset of women enrolled in the STRATOS, SOTI or TROPOS trials. Histomorphometry provided a 2D demonstration of the bone safety of strontium ranelate, with significantly higher mineral apposition rate (MAR) in cancellous bone (+9% versus control, p = 0.019). Osteoblast surfaces were significantly higher (+38% versus control, p = 0.047). 3D analysis of 3-year biopsies with strontium ranelate (20 biopsies) and placebo (21 biopsies) using microcomputed tomography showed significant changes in microarchitecture with, in the strontium ranelate group, higher cortical thickness (+18%, p = 0.008) and trabecular number (+14%, p = 0.05), and lower structure model index (-22%, p = 0.01) and trabecular separation (-16%, p = 0.04), with no change in cortical porosity. These analysis have provided evidence of the good bone safety of strontium ranelate in the treatment of postmenopausal osteoporosis and are fully consistent with the mode of action of strontium ranelate involving dissociation between bone formation and bone resorption. The change in 3D trabecular and cortical microarchitecture may improve bone biomechanical competence and explain the decreased fracture rate after strontium ranelate treatment [31].

Quality of life was a secondary endpoint in the strontium ranelate phase 3 studies using QUALIOST®, a dedicated questionnaire for vertebral osteoporosis [32]. QUALIOST® was used to assess quality of life in 1240 patients from the SOTI trial who completed the questionnaire at baseline and every 6 months [33]. After 3 years of treatment, strontium ranelate had a beneficial effect on quality of life compared with placebo (P=0.016 for global score; P=0.019 and P=0.032 for emotional and physical scores, respectively) [33]. The improvement in the emotional score was related to fewer negative feelings and concerns regarding the disease, while the improvement in the physical score was associated with reduced pain and increased mobility.

In the SOTI and TROPOS trials, the incidence of adverse events, serious adverse events, and withdrawals due to adverse events was similar in the strontium ranelate and placebo groups [34,35]. During the first 3 months of treatment, nausea, diarrhea, headache, dermatitis, and eczema were more frequently associated with strontium ranelate compared with placebo but, thereafter, there was no difference in incidence between the strontium ranelate and placebo groups concerning nausea and diarrhea. Importantly, there were no age-associated increases in adverse events when the safety of strontium ranelate was assessed in a pre-specified analysis in individuals aged 80 years or more [25].

In the SOTI and TROPOS trials, small changes in homeostasis parameters were observed (decrease in calcium and parathyroid hormone serum levels, increase in blood phosphorus). The levels were transient and not associated with any clinical sequelae. It has been suggested that these observations may be linked to the activation of the calcium-sensing receptors by strontium. A slight transcient increase in serum creatine phosphokinase concentrations was observed in strontium ranelate-treated patients [20,21]. This was not associated with an increase in muscular symptoms and, in the majority of patients, values returned to normal during the trial without any change in treatment.

In pooled data from the SOTI and TROPOS trials, there was an apparent increased risk of venous thromboembolism (VTE) in the strontium ranelate group (0.6% vs 0.9% per year), although the annual incidence was similar in the strontium ranelate and placebo groups in the individual trials. It has been suggested that the reason for the initial finding may have been an imbalance in the number of people with previous VTE in the active treatments arms. When treatment arms were corrected for this, there was no significant increase in VTE risk in the strontium ranelate arm.

Recently, the post-marketing experience of patients treated with strontium ranelate reported cases of the DRESS (Drug Reaction with Eosinophilia and Systemic Symptoms) syndrome (less than 20 for a total of 570.000 patient-year of exposure) [35]. This incidence is in the vicinity of what has been previously reported, as severe skin reactions, with most of the other currently marketed anti-osteoporosis medications.

A causative link has not been firmly established as strontium is a trace element naturally present in human body and ranelic acid is poorly absorbed. However, due to the possible fatality linked to this syndrome, it seems reasonable to discontinue immediately strontium ranelate and other concomitant treatment known to induce such syndrome in case of suspicious major skin disorders, occurring within 2 months of treatment initiation [36] and to introduce adapted treatment and follow up to avoid systemic symptoms.

Conclusion

Women consult often, for the first time, after the diagnosis of osteoporosis has already been made. Therefore, medications have been developed in order to stimulate bone formation, with the ultimate goal to restore bone quantity and quality and to reduce spinal and peripheral fractures to a greater extend than what is obtained with inhibitors of bone resorption. Peptides from the parathyroid hormone family when given intermittently, increase the number and activity of osteoblasts leading to an increase in bone mass and in an improvement in skeletal architecture. Teriparatide (1-34 parathyroid hormone[PTH]) reduces vertebral and non-vertebral fractures at the dose of 20 μg/day given in subcutaneous daily injections. 1-84 PTH reduces vertebral fractures but results on non-vertebral fractures are missing. Strontium ranelate, suggested to uncouple bone formation from bone resorption, reduces vertebral, non-vertebral and hip fractures (above 74 years) in osteoporotic patients.

References

[1] Reginster, JY; Taquet, AN; Fraikin, G; Gosset, C: Zegels B. Parathyroid hormone in the treatment of involutional osteoporosis: back to the future. *Osteoporos Int,* 1997;7:S163–167.

[2] Neer, RM; Arnaud, CD; Zanchetta, JR; Prince, R; Gaich, GA; Reginster, JY; Hodsman, AB; Eriksen, EF; Ish-Shalom, S; Genant, HK; Wang, O; Mitlak, BH. Effect of parathyroid hormone (1–34) on fractures and bone mineral density in postmenopausal women with osteoporosis. *N Engl J Med*, 2001;344:1434–1441.

[3] Marcus, R; Wang, O; Satterwhite, J; Mitlak, B. The skeletal response to teriparatide is largely independent of age, initial bone mineral density, and prevalent vertebral fractures in postmenopausal women with osteoporosis. *J Bone Min Res*, 2003;18:18–23.

[4] Lindsay, R; Scheels, WH; Neer, R; Pohl, G; Adami, S; Mautalen, C; Reginster, JY; Stepan, JJ; Myers, SL; Mitlak, BH. Sustained vertebral fracture risk reduction after withdrawal of teriparatide (recombinant human parathyroid hormone (1–34)) in postmenopausal women with osteoporosis. *Arch Int Med*, 2004;164:2024–2030.

[5] Prince, R; Sipos, A; Hossain, A; Syversen, U; Ish-Shalom, S; Marcinowska, E; Halse, J; Lindsay, R; Dalsky, GP; Mitlak, BH. Sustained nonvertebral fragility fracture risk reduction after discontinuation of teriparatide treatment. *J Bone Miner Res,* 2005;20:1507-1513.

[6] Delmas PD, Licata AA, Reginster JY, Crans, GG; Chen, P; Misurski, DA; Wagman, RB; Mitlak, BH. Fracture Risk reduction during treatment with teriparatide is independent of pre-treatment bone turnover. *Bone*, 2006;39:237-243.

[7] Jilka, RL; Weinstein, RS; Bellido, T; Roberson, P; Parfitt, AM; Manolagas, SC. Increased bone formation by prevention of osteoblast apoptosis with parathyroid hormone. *J Clin Invest*, 1999;104:371-373.

[8] Greenspan, SL; Bone, HG; Ettinger, MP; Hanley, DA; Lindsay, R; Zanchetta, JR; Blosch, CM; Mathisen, AL; Morris, SA; Marriott, TB; Treatment of Osteoporosis with Parathyroid Hormone Study Group. Effect of recombinant human parathyroid hormone (1-84) on vertebral fracture and bone mineral density in postmenopausal women with osteoporosis: a randomized trial. *Ann Intern Med,* 2007;146:326-339.

[9] Shrader, SP; Raggucci, KR. Parathyroid hormone (1-84) and treatment of osteoporosis. *Ann Pharmacother,* 2005;39:1511-1516.

[10]Hodsman, AB; Hanley, DA; Ettinger, MP; Bolognese, MA; Fox, J; Metcalfe, AJ; Lindsay, R. Efficacy and safety of human parathyroid hormone (1-84) in increasing bone mineral density in postmenopausal osteoporosis. *J Clin Endocrinol Metab*, 2003; 88:5212-5220.

[11]Hodsman, AB; Bauer; DC; Dempster, DW; Dian, L; Hanley, DA; Harris, ST; Kendler, DL; McClung, MR; Miller, PD; Olszynski, WP; Orwoll, E; Yuen, CK. Parathyroid hormone and teriparatide for the treatment of osteoporosis: a review of the evidence and suggested guidelines for its use. *Endocr Rev*, 2005;26:688-703.

[12]Reginster, JY; Sarlet, N; Lejeune, E; Leonori, L. Strontium ranelate: a new treatment for postmenopausal osteoporosis with a dual mode of action. *Curr Osteoporos Rep*, 2005;3:30-34.

[13]Reginster, JY; Deroisy, R; Dougados, M; Jupsin, I; Colette, J; Roux, C. Prevention of early postmenopausal bone loss by strontium ranelate: a randomized, two-year, double-blind, dose-ranging, placebo-controlled trial. *Osteoporos Int*, 2002;13,925-931.

[14]Meunier, PJ; Slosman, DO; Delmas, PD; Sebertn, JL; Brandin, ML; Albanese, C; Lorenc, R; Pors-Nielsen, S; De Vernejoul, MC; Roces, A; Reginster, JY. Strontium ranelate: dose-dependent effects in established postmenopausal vertebral osteoporosis: a 2-year randomized placebo controlled trial. *J Clin Endocrinol Metabolism*, 2002;87,2060-2066.

[15]Boivin, G; Foos, E; Tupinon-Mathieu, I; Meunier, PJ. Strontium deposition in bone is dose dependent and does not alter the degree of mineralization of bone in osteoporotic patients treated with strontium ranelate. *J Bone Miner Res,* 2000;15(S1),305.

[16]Reginster, JY; Diez-Perez, A; Ortolani, S; Pors-Nielsen, S; Meunier, PJ. Calcium-vitamin D supplementation in clinical trials of osteoporosis should be titrated on the basis of pre-study assessments. *Osteoporos Int*, 2002;13(S1),S24.

[17]Reginster, JY; Spector, T; Badurski, J; Ortolani, S; Martin, TJ; Diez-Perez, A; Lemmel, E; Balogh, A; Pors-Nielsen, S; Phenekos, C; Meunier, PJ. A short-term run-in study can significantly contribute to increasing the quality of long-term osteoporosis trials. The strontium ranelate Phase III program. *Osteoporos Int*, 2002;13(S1),S30.

[18]Genant, HK; WU, CY; Van Kuijk, C; Newit, MC. Vertebral semi quantitative assessment using a semi-quantitative technique. *J Bone Miner Res*, 1993;8,1137-1148.

[19]Meunier, PJ; Roux, C; Ortolani, S; Badurski, J; Kaufman, JM; Spector, T; Diez-Perez, A; Seeman, E; Lemmel, E; Balogh, A; Pors-Nielsen, S; Phenekos, C; Rizzoli, R; Slosman,

D; Tupinon-Mathieu; I; Reginster, JY. Strontium ranelate reduces the vertebral fracture risk in women with postmenopausal osteoporosis. *Osteoporos Int*, 2002;13(S1),O45.

[20]Meunier, PJ; Roux, C; Seeman, E; Ortolani, S; Badurski, JE; Spector, TD; Cannata, J; Balogh, A; Lemmel, EM; Pors-Nielsen, S; Rizzoli, R; Genant, HK; Reginster, JY. The effect of strontium ranelate on the risk of vertebral fracture in Women with Post Menopausal Osteoporosis. *N Eng J Med*, 2004;350,459-468.

[21]Reginster, JY; Seeman, E; De Vernejoul, MC; Adami, S; Compston, J; Phenekos, C; Devogelaer, JP; Curiel, MD; Sawicki, A; Goemaere, S; Sorensen, OH; Felsenberg, D; Meunier, PJ. Strontium ranelate reduces the risk of nonvertebral fractures in postmenopausal women with osteoporosis: treatment of peripheral osteoporosis (TROPOS) study. *J Clin Endocrinol Metabolism,* 2005;90,2816-2822.

[22]Roux, C; Reginster, JY; Fechtenbaum, J; Kolta, S; Sawicki, A; Tulassay, Z; Luisetto, G; Padrino, JM; Doyle, D; Prince, R; Fardellone, P; Sorensen, OH; Meunier, PJ. Vertebral fracture risk reduction with strontium ranelate in women with postmenopausal osteoporosis is independent of baseline risk factors. *J Bone Miner Res*, 2006;21:536-542.

[23]Population Division of the Department of Economic and Social Affairs of the Nations Secretariat 2002 World Population Prospects: The 2002 Revision and World Urban Prospects. Available online at http://esa.un.org/unpp

[24]Ettinger, MP; Aging bone and osteoporosis: Strategies for preventing fractures in the elderly. *Arch Intern Med*, 2003;163:2237–2246.

[25]Seeman, E; Vellas, B; Benhamou, C; Aquino, JP; Semler, J; Kaufman, JM; Hoszowski, K; Varela, AR; Fiore, C; Brixen, K; Reginster, JY; Boonen, S. Strontium ranelate reduces the risk of vertebral and nonvertebral fractures in women eighty years of age and older. *J Bone Miner Res*, 2006;21:1113-1120.

[26]Seeman, E; Devogelaer, J; Lorenc, R; Spector, T; Brixen, K; Balogh, A; Stucki, G; Reginster, JY. Strontium ranelate reduces the risk of vertebral fractures in patients with osteopenia. *J Bone Miner Res*, 2008,23:433-438.

[27]Malaise, O; Bruyere, O; Reginster, JY. Strontium ranelate normalizes bone mineral density in osteopenic patients. *Aging Clin Exp Res*, 2007;19:330-333.

[28]Reginster, JY; Meunier, PJ. Strontium ranelate phase 2 dose-ranging studies: PREVOS and STRATOS studies. *Osteoporos Int*, 2003;14:S56-S65.

[29]Bruyere, O; Roux, C; Detilleux, J; Slosman, DO; Spector, TD; Fardellone, P; Brixen, K; Devogelaer, JP; Diaz-Curiel, M; Albanese, C; Kaufman, JM; Pors-Nielsen, S; Reginster, JY. Relationship between bone mineral density changes and fracture risk reduction in patients treated with strontium ranelate. *J Clin Endocrinol Metab,* 2007;92:3076-3081.

[30]Bruyere, O; Roux, C; Badurski, J; Isaia, G; de Vernejoul, MC; Cannata, J; Ortolani, S; Slosman, D; Detilleux, J; Reginster, JY. Relationship between change in femoral neck bone mineral density and hip fracture incidence during treatment with strontium ranelate. *Curr Med Res Opin*, 2007;23:3041-3045.

[31]Arlot, ME; Jiang, Y; Genant, HK; Zhao, J; Burt-Pichat, B; Roux, JP; Delmas, PD; Meunier, PJ. Histomorphometric and μ-CT Analysis of Bone Biopsies from Postmenopausal Osteoporotic Women Treated with Strontium Ranelate. *J Bone Miner Res*, 2008;23:215-222.

[32]De la Loge, C; Sullivan, K; Pinkney, R; Marquis, P; Roux, C; Meunier, PJ. Cross-cultural validation and analysis of responsiveness of the QUALIOST®: QUAlity of Life questionnaire In OSTeoporosis. *Health Qual Life Outcomes*, 2005;3:69.

[33]Marquis, P; De la Loge, C; Diaz-Curiel, M; Spector, T; Meunier, PJ. Beneficial effects of strontium ranelate on the quality of life in patients with vertebral osteoporosis (SOTI study). *Osteoporos Int*, 2005;16:S54.

[34]Shea, B; Wells, G; Cranney, A; Zytaruk, N; Robinson, V; Griffith, L; Hamel, C; Ortiz, Z; Peterson, J; Adachi, J; Tugwell, P; Guyatt, G. Osteoporosis Methodology Group; Osteoporosis Research Advisory Group. Calcium supplementation on bone loss in postmenopausal women. *Cochrane Database Syst Rev*, 2004;1:CD004526.

[35]Question and answers on the safety of PROTELOS/OSSEOR. Doc. Ref. EMEA/534613/2007 www.emea.europa.eu/humandocs/PDFs/EPAR/protelos/Protelos_ Q&A_ 53461307en.pdf-2007-11-16.

[36]Tas, S; Simonart, T. Management of drug rash with eosinophilia and systemic symptoms (DRESS syndrome): an update. *Dermatology,* 2003;206:353-356.

In: Osteoporosis: Etiology, Diagnosis and Treatment
Editors: Bilar E. Mattingly and Albert C. Pillare
ISBN 978-1-60692-397-9

Chapter 10

PHYSICAL EXERCISE AND REHABILITATION IN THE PREVENTION AND TREATMENT OF OSTEOPOROSIS

APR Lirani-Galvao, LDF Moreira-Pfrimer, RV Marin, ML Oliveira, MAC Pedrosa-Castro and M Lazaretti-Castro
Federal University of Sao Paulo, Sao Paulo, Brazil.

ABSTRACT

Background: Osteoporosis is a skeletal disorder characterized by reduced bone mass and deterioration of bone microarchitecture, predisposing it to an increased risk of fracture (NIH Consensus, 2001). There are many strategies to prevent osteoporosis and maintain (or gain) bone mineral density, and physical exercises are among the most important ones. Bone is constantly built and rebuilt through remodeling, which is controlled by endogenous hormones and external mechanical forces which result from physical activity, for example.

Purposes: To update the specific physical exercise and rehabilitation protocols that show significant effects on the treatment and prevention of osteoporosis and to review the mechanisms through which exercise can maintain (or augment) bone mass and strength.

Methods: Research studies published until March 2008 were identified through a review of the literature available on the NLM PubMed and Elsevier-Science Direct databases.

Results: Most of the physical exercise and rehabilitation programs elaborated for osteoporotic patients showed that weight-bearing exercises, high-impact activities and strength training were able to maintain or increase bone mineral density. Balance and coordination exercises could decrease the fall risk, and aerobic exercises could also benefit osteoporotic patients, since they provide them more disposition to perform their activities of daily living, leading to a more active life style.

Conclusion: Recent evidences confirm that certain physical exercises are not only important to maintain or increase bone mass, but also to reduce fall risk and to improve the quality of life of osteoporotic patients.

INTRODUCTION

Bone Biology and Biomechanics

The past two decades testify the development of new and efficient pharmacological therapies to enhance bone mineral density (BMD) as well as to reduce the risk of fractures in osteoporotic patients. The same has happened to non-pharmacological treatments in the past years, with an increasing sum of researchers committed to studying the possible mechanisms that make physical exercises act on bone structure.

In 1892, a scientist called Julius Wolff demonstrated the importance of mechanical load to bone health and established the Wolff's law (Wolff, 1892), which affirms that bone responds to mechanical loads by adapting its internal architecture, so that the normal structure of a specific bone would have a close relation to the mechanical demand required from that bone. Consequently, the living bone reacts and adapts itself to the mechanical load applied upon it. And, in order to do so, these environmental loads must be detected and converted into biochemical and/or bioelectrical signals in the cellular level, a process nominated mechanotransduction (Burger & Klein-Nulend, 1999; Liedert et al., 2006). Later on, Fukada and Yasuda (1957) demonstrated the phenomenon of piezoelectricity of bone tissue, which means that this material is able to transform mechanical load, which is applied to it, into electrical signs. Since then, a new field of investigation has started to study the role of mechanical and electrical signs in bone remodeling.

Mechanotransduction refers to many mechanisms by which cells convert a mechanic stimulus into chemical and electrical activity. To better understand how this process happens, we can compare the bone structure to a fluid-filled sponge. When compressed in a loading condition, the sponge's channels and pores (lacunar-canalicular network) release its fluid contents (interstitial fluid). When relaxed in an unloaded condition, the sponge is free to reabsorb this fluid (Burger & Klein-Nulend, 1999). This fluid flow transports the nutrients required to keep osteocytes (cells in charge of perceiving the mechanical stimulus) alive and also allows the other mechanisms to load detection.

Mechanotransduction of bone tissue can be separated into four different phases:

a- Mechanocoupling – initiated by environmental mechanical load applied to bone followed by the detection of these loads by sensory cells;

b- Biochemical coupling – conversion of the local mechanical signal into biochemical signal;

c- Transmission of signal from the sensory cells to the effector cells (osteoblasts and osteoclasts);

d- Effector cells response (bone formation) (Turner et al., 1995).

Since the establishment of Wolff's law, strain magnitude has been considered the main osteogenic stimulus (Vainionpaa et al., 2007; Rubin & Lanyon, 1985; Turner et al., 1994b;

Mosley et al., 1997). Nevertheless, the current comprehension of bone metabolism has extended the perspective to several tissue-level mechanical parameters also including components such as strain rate, strain frequency, cycle numbers, bout intervals and strain directions (Turner et al., 1995; Turner et al., 1998; Warner et al., 2006).

Studies show that strain magnitude is highly related to new bone formation (Rubin & Lanyon, 1985; Turner et al., 1994b; Mosley et al., 1997; Cullen et al., 2001), so that the larger the generated deformation on bone matrix, the larger the overall bone response.

Another component found to be very important to bone formation is the strain rate. If we analyze studies proposing programs including isometric exercise we can clearly notice that even when exercise is done with extremely high intensity loads, it is not always osteogenic. This happens because it lacks a high rate of stimulus, which means that dynamic loads are required to osteogenic response. The theory of fluid flow during mechanotransduction explains this phenomenon. Static loads, even at high intensities, do not create any hydrostatic pressure gradients to initiate fluid flow in the bone lacuno-canalicular network, so they produce a state similar to disuse that has been found to result in bone resorption (Lanyon & Rubin, 1984) and suppression of normal appositional growth in bone (Robling & Turner, 2002).

Some studies have shown that a higher strain rate is more important to provide a greater osteogenic stimulus for bone formation than strain magnitude (Mosley & Lanyon, 1998). This deduction was made after finding that increasing the frequency of loading with a constant strain magnitude, a significant increase on bone formation rate occurs (at frequencies of 0.5–2.0 Hz) (Turner et al., 1994a; Turner et al., 1995). These phenomena have been described with loading frequencies of 2 Hz or less, which include most of the physiologic loading frequencies (Vainionpää et al., 2007; Hsieh & Turner, 2001), and also with small loads associated to high frequencies, culminating in a higher number of loading cycles, which can be very osteogenic (Vainionpää et al., 2007; Rubin et al., 2001; Rubin et al., 2002).

Although most of the results presented above emerged from studies in animal models, they can guide us to the understanding of what an exercise program should have in order to enhance bone formation in humans. Based on the mechanotransduction theory, it is possible to suggest that one viable way through which physical exercise can stimulate bone formation is impact exercises. Another mechanism is through resistive exercises, since the muscle insertion causes stress locally on bone and this stimulus may be spread via fluid flow (Hingorjo et al., 2008). Bone mechanical loading via ground reaction forces and/or muscle pulling on bone are generally accepted as necessary stimuli to attain peak BMD and maintain bone homeostasis (Warner et al., 2006). In the next topics we are going to discuss studies on the prescription of exercise programs for osteoporotic patients.

PHYSICAL EXERCISES AND BONE HEALTH

It is well known that physical activity brings many benefits to our health. Many studies have shown the relevance of physical activity to improve or maintain bone mass in all ages.

Bailey et al. (1999) studied the relationship between bone mass and physical activity in boys and girls and demonstrated that bone mass increased respectively 9 and 17%, when compared to children that did not practice any physical activities. Pre-pubertal active gymnasts submitted to physical training showed an increase of 30-85% in areal BMD of total body, spine and legs, when compared to controls (Bass et al., 1998).

Creighton et al. (2001) evaluated BMD and bone formation and resorption markers in young athletes, and divided them into four groups: control, exercises of high impact (volleyball and basketball), medium impact (soccer and short distance running) and no impact (swimming). They verified that high impact subjects presented the higher values of spine and femoral neck BMD, when compared to other groups, and that swimming, a no impact exercise, presented the lowest BMD, and also lower bone formation and resorption markers values when compared to high and medium impact activities. These findings reinforce the theory of positive effects of physical exercise with loading on bone mineral content and density of children and adolescents, involved in high impact activities (gymnastics, volleyball) and rapid multidirectional activities (tennis).

Besides, many studies emphasize physical training in order to preserve or improve bone mass in postmenopausal women with low BMD (Bergström et al., 2008; Kemmler et al., 2002). Post-menopausal women, when submitted to an exercise program based on stretching, balance, resisted exercises and impacts exercises associated to hormone therapy, showed a higher BMD of femoral neck, when compared to women only submitted to hormone therapy (Going et al., 2003).

Short periods of loading are able to induce adaptative responses. The organization of bone tissue is probably driven by low magnitude strains, which are performed during natural daily activities (Fritton et al., 2000); that means that our daily activities are responsible for the maintenance of bone. However, when osteoporotic patients are concerned, these daily life stimulus are not enough to preserve or improve their bone mass.

Physical Exercises Recommended to Osteoporotic Patients

Recent studies in bone biology have established that exercise in the form of short, repetitive mechanical loading and in different directions, leads to greatest gains in bone strength. Physical exercise, to be osteogenic, must produce an environment of loads which differs from the habitual, where bone architecture would be already adapted. A load that would be initially osteogenic, has no longer this potential when bone is already adapted to it. Bone formation will only happen if a certain threshold is achieved, and this process is influenced by intensity, frequency, amplitude and duration of stimulus intercalated with resting periods (Bono & Einhorn, 2003; Ehrlich & Lanyon, 2002). Beyond this point, exercise may be deleterious (Bakker, 2003).

According to the recommendations of the American College of Sports Medicine (Kohrt et al., 2004), a program of physical exercises for osteoporotic people should include, besides strength exercises, weight bearing and impact exercises, and also flexibility, coordination and balance activities and cardiovascular conditioning. These factors are important because they contribute directly to a better quality of life of osteoporotic patients, decreasing the fall risk and providing them to have a more active life style, avoiding, then, a greater bone loss caused by inactivity. These recommendations indicate that not only highly osteogenic exercises (eg. strength training and running) are indicated in the treatment and prevention of osteoporosis. The development of balance and coordination leads the subject to have more body consciousness, with a reduced fall risk. Aerobic exercises also benefit osteoporotic patients because they give them more disposition to daily activities, allowing them to develop the habit of a more active lifestyle.

Studies have shown that exercises that stimulate bone formation usually present the following characteristics: dynamism, high intensity and short duration of stimulus (Turner, 1998; Notomi et al., 2000). Resistance exercises performed in a very dynamic way (resistance + velocity = power training) with high loads and few repetitions, involve vigorous muscle contractions and demand fiber type II action, and it seems that these fibers are the most capable of stimulating bone formation (Turner, 2007).

In this context, Stengel et al. (2007) conducted a randomized trial in which 53 pre-trained women (mean age 58.2 years) were randomly assigned to a strength training (ST) or power training (PT) group. The difference between the two groups was the movement velocity during the resistance training: ST - 4 seconds for concentric and 4 seconds for eccentric contraction; PT – explosive concentric and 4 seconds for eccentric contraction). Otherwise both groups carried out progressively planned resistance training (10–12 exercises, 2–4 sets, 4–12 repetitions at 70–92.5% of the one-repetition maximum (2/week) for 2 years. After 2 years of training, women submitted to PT lost only 0.3% of lumbar spine BMD, while ST lost 2.4%. These results led the authors to the conclusion that power training may be superior to maintain BMD in postmenopausal women than strength training. In addition, power training was safe as it did not lead to increased injury or pain.

Besides the recognized relevance of physical activity on bone health, it is extremely important to perform exercises carefully and safely, in order to avoid muscular pain, inadequate posture and fractures in places that are more fragile due to osteoporosis. It is recommended to avoid movements with greater stress potential to the spine such as spine flexion, rotation and lateral flexion, as well as to carry weight inadequately. Since 1966, Nachemson has shown in experimental studies that high pressure gradients are present in vertebral body when spine is performing movements such as flexion positions (Nachemsom, 1966). Sinaki & Mikkelsen (1984) demonstrated that there is a greater incidence of compression vertebral fractures in osteoporotic patients who perform trunk flexion during training.

Thus, besides the precautions of prescribing an exercise program, the osteoporotic patients benefit a lot from physical exercise. Exercises with rapid and slow alternate movements, impact exercises such as walking, jogging and aerobic exercises (which exceed 70% of cardiac frequency) and programs that involve important muscle groups and displacement in various directions, may be used with the aim of reducing bone loss (Bloomfield, 2001).

The main objective of any therapy on osteoporosis is to avoid fractures. Besides promoting bone mass maintenance, exercise may lead to other benefits, such as:

- Preserve and increase muscle strength

- Alleviate pain and maintain flexibility
- Avoid deformities and postural alterations
- Improve physical conditioning
- Improve balance and gait
- Maintain the quality of daily life activities

Preserving and Improving Muscle Strength

It is known that muscle strength presents its peak on the second and third decade of life, stays stable or slightly decreases on the next 20 years and diminishes considerably in the elderly. Besides muscle strength loss, the muscle ability to produce force rapidly (muscle power) decreases with aging, and its consequence is a reduced capacity to perform daily life activities such as climbing stairs or carrying weight, since these activities require a degree of power to be performed. Strength training exercises have many benefits not only directly to improve muscle strength, but also to improve balance and maintain BMD (Fleck & Kraemer, 1999).

Hughes et al (1995) suggest that the magnitude of muscle contraction may have impact in their origins and insertions on bone, since BMD and muscle strength are related. A study with male tennis players, age average 30 years old, showed through computed tomography (CT), that the dominant arm had a higher bone mineral content (BMC) when compared to controls, showing that the osteogenic stimulus acts locally where the load is applied (Kannus et al., 1995).

Some studies demonstrate the relevance of resisted physical exercise to improve bone mass in osteoporotic patients. Sinaki et al. (2002) evaluated the effects of strength training exercises on extensor lumbar muscles in post-menopausal women, and demonstrated a reduced incidence of vertebral fractures, showing that resistive exercise helps to prevent the loss and or to maintain bone mass, improving balance and reducing falls, one of the greatest factor risk in this population.

Strength training exercises of extensor back muscles, and respiratory exercises, are indicated, as well as abdominal exercises, which should be done with some precautions. Abdominal strengthening is very important to maintain posture and proper ventilatory mechanics, but these exercises performed with trunk flexion, are not indicated to individuals who show augmented risk to spine fractures. So when prescribing an exercise program to osteoporotic patients, some strategies may be used to work abdominal muscles without increasing the risk of vertebral fractures. Some different exercises may be included with the principle of hip flexion with stabilized trunk, instead of spine flexion.

Strength training exercises and a more active lifestyle may help post-menopausal women to maintain BMD, and osteopenic and osteoporotic women to improve spine and hip BMD (Zehnacker & Bemis-Dougherty, 2007). In this systematic review, it was found that BMD increment is site specific and requires training between 70% to 90% of 1 maximal repetition, 8 to 12 repetitions, 2 to 3 sessions per week, in a period of 1 year.

Back-extensor-strengthening exercises can significantly reduce the incidence of new fractures in patients submitted to vertebroplasty (Huntoon et al., 2008). An investigation with post-menopausal osteoporotic women, who had had at least one vertebral fracture, showed an improvement of quality of life of the participants after an exercise program. This program included stretching exercises, strength training and walking for 1 hour, 3 times a week (Papaioannou et al., 2003).

The strength of certain muscles was recently found to correlate with BMD. Monaco et al. (2000) demonstrated that hand grip may correlate with femoral ($r= 0.37$ $p<. 01$), lumbar spine ($r= 0.44$ $p<. 01$) and total body ($r= 0.37$ $p<.01$) BMDs. Besides, Lindsey et al. (2005) also associated physical performance measures and BMD in old post-menopausal women. Variables such as static balance and hand grip were associated to total body, lumbar spine, hip and forearm BMDs. These items should, then, be considered by clinicians, when evaluating osteoporotic patients.

Are Aquatic Exercises Recommended to Osteoporotic Patients?

Aquatic activities, such as hidrogymnastics and swimming, allow the subject immersed into the water to perform exercises without being the direct responsible for their own body sustenance, since there is fluctuation in water. It is very important to point out that exercise in water may be very useful when it comes to enhance muscle strength. This idea goes in the opposite direction of what many health professionals still think of aquatic exercise: that in water there is no gravity force, no impact exercises and very little possibilities to develop muscle strength because fluctuation force helps movements to happen in the vertical direction - so it would not bring any benefits to osteoporotic patients. The scientific truth is that someone exercising in water in the vertical position does suffer the action of gravity (Harrison, Hillman & Bulstrode,1992), can perform impact exercises if feet touch and lose contact with the pool floor (Harrison, Hillman & Bulstrode,1992) (although gravity and impact are diminished compared to ground exercises because of the fluctuation action), and can also perform strength exercises by using fluctuation force as resistance and not as assistance (Poyhonen et al., 2002).

Cardoso et al. (2004) studied 34 women, mean age of 55 years, who exercised for 12 weeks, twice a week, doing deep water exercises with emphasis in muscle strength. Subjects performed movements using lower and upper limbs, from 70 to 90% of maximum intensity, with and without resistive equipment. Results demonstrated that both training with bare limbs and with equipment significantly improved muscle strength of subjects in the study, showing that water workout with emphasis in muscle strength can enhance this neuromuscular variable. In another trial, Kruel et al. (2005) analyzed the effects of a water workout muscle strength program in 17 women (mean age of 52.5 years), training for 11 weeks, and concluded that strength training performed in water is an efficient way to improve muscle strength of upper and lower limb muscles.

It is clear that there are significant gains of muscle strength and resistance in subjects submitted to aquatic exercise programs (Ruoti et al., 1994; Sanders & Rippee, 2001). Thus, evidences show that, even with reduced articular impact into the water, it is possible to develop some osteogenic potential through specific muscle strength training in the aquatic environment.

Considering bone mineral density and aquatic exercises, one study did not find differences in BMD when comparing swimming athletes and sedentary subjects (Taaffe, 1999), while others compared athletes of a variety of modalities and aquatic sports individuals showed the lowest BMD (Creighton et al., 2001; Andreoli et al., 2001). However, these athletes were kept into the water training 3 to 5 hours a day, 5 to 6 times a week, which is a totally different reality of the aquatic activities proposed to the elderly in order to maintain health and quality of life.

In a study with 77 post-menopausal women, who practiced hidrogymnastics for 12 months, lumbar BMD (L2-L4) declined 1% and femoral neck BMD was maintained, indicating that the aquatic exercises used in this study did not improve bone mass in this population (Bravo et al., 1997). However, recent research has indicated a different perspective about bone health and aquatic exercises. A study in the University of Sao Paulo, Brazil, (Pinto et al., 2003) compared 30 caucasian girls (14.3 ± 1.8 years) swimming athletes with a control group. Results showed that BMD was higher in athletes for total body, lumbar spine and similar for femoral neck, when compared to controls, showing that swimming, apart from being a non weight bearing exercise against gravity, may have a positive effect on BMD of these adolescents.

Tsukahara et al., (1994), in a 36-month study with 75 post-menopausal women, in sessions of 30 minutes of hidrogymnastics plus 10 minutes of swimming, reported a significant increase of lumbar (L1-L4) BMD. Women who already practiced this activity before the study showed an increase of 1,55% and the recent sedentary participants increased 2,16% lumbar BMD, and control group showed a loss of 0,92% in BMD.

Aye Yurtkuran (2003) found an anabolic effect of aquatic exercises on bone of post-menopausal women which was evidenced by hormonal markers (insuline-like growth factor-1 and growth hormone) and calcaneous ultrasound measurements. The authors suggest that aquatic exercises should be included in training programs for sedentary post-menopausal women.

Independently of where physical exercise will be performed, ground or water, it is very important to include in every program developed to osteoporotic patients: muscle strengthening of back extensors, hip flexors and knee extensors, since these muscles are directly involved in gait and consequently in the prevention of osteoporotic fractures (Miyakoshi et al. ,2007).

PHYSICAL THERAPY AND OSTEOPOROSIS

Posture and Pain Relief

Since osteoporosis is an asymptomatic illness, pain only appears in the presence of fractures, associated osteoarthritis (Dai Ly, 1998) and postural alterations. Individuals with severe osteoporosis present a postural alteration which is characterized by an augmentation of dorsal kyphosis, which alters the normal biomechanics of respiratory muscles, tending to cause a hypotrophy of intercostals muscles and reduced pulmonary complacence, which results in a greater rest energy expense (Lombardi Júnior et al., 2004). Pulmonary function and aerobic capacity are significantly diminished in patients with osteoporosis, so ventilatory muscle training and aerobic exercises may offer a therapeutic potential adjunct to current osteoporosis therapies (Gokkaya et al., 2008).

Besides the augmentation of dorsal kyphosis, the osteoporotic patient may present lumbar rectification, knee flexion and narrow feet base. Individuals with osteoporosis and hyper-kyphosis present decreased strength of lower limb and spine back extensor muscles, slower gait, diminished balance and a greater postural oscillation on orthostatic position, resulting on predisposition to falls (Sinaki, 2007).

Stretching and flexibility exercises help to prevent muscle shortenings, decrease excessive muscular tensions on articulations, preserve normal amplitude of movement and decrease pain (Figure 1). Pain can also be locally managed with some physical agents, such as ultrasound, laser therapy and TENS (transcutaneous electrical nerve stimulation) (Allen R, 2006).

Stretching exercises with eccentric contractions contribute to decrease excessive loads on articulations, relief pain, improve balance, physical conditioning, muscle and articular proprioception, maintain good posture or correct vicious and antialgic postures (Pascal, 2000). Individuals with postural alterations present a deficit on balance, because their body oscillation is increased in standing positions. So, in an exercise program, balance should also be trained.

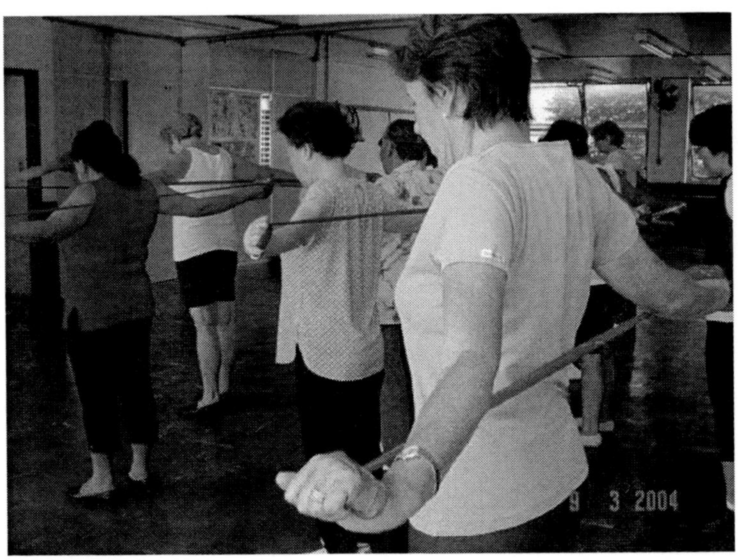

Figure 1. Pectoralis muscle stretching (Rehabilitation and Physical Exercise Program Developed for Osteoporotic Patients - PRADO, Federal University of Sao Paulo, UNFESP, Brazil).

Balance

Falls are among the most important risk factors for fractures, and that is why it is so important to prevent them when a patient is diagnosed with osteoporosis (Madureira et al., 2007). Before starting physical therapy with an elderly osteoporotic patient it is important to verify the serum vitamin D (25-hydroxivitamin D or 25OHD) levels of this subject. Scientific literature has already observed that many of these individuals present low levels (< 50 nmol/L) of serum 25OHD (Saraiva et al., 2007). Besides being responsible for calcium absorption, vitamin D has some specific receptors identified in human muscle tissue. Cross-sectional studies show that elderly people with higher vitamin D serum levels have increased muscle strength and a lower number of falls, which can be explained by the improvement in musculoskeletal function (Bischoff et al., 2003). So, if necessary, along with physical therapy, the patient should see a physician to consider vitamin D supplementation.

Muscle strength and balance have been pointed as determinant factors for fall risk, and consequently, fracture risk (Bergström et al., 2008; Kemmler et al., 2002; Cussler et al., 2003. Exercise to improve balance and, thus, prevent falls, should focus on training of protection reactions, proprioception, motor coordination, gait and improving posture.

A 12-month balance training program was effective in improving functional and static balance, mobility and falling frequency in elderly women with osteoporosis (Madureira et al., 2007). The intervention consisted of 1 hour of exercises once a week, with a total of 40 classes, supervised by an experienced physiotherapist. Training included 15 minutes of warm up and stretching exercises, consisting of head rotation, shoulder rotation and stretching of upper and lower limbs; 15 minutes walking with associated exercises for the upper limbs throughout the walk and balance exercises for 30 minutes. Some activities used to improve balance were:

- Walking backwards and sideways;
- Walking on the tips of the toes and on the heels;
- Walking in the tandem position (one foot right in front of the other);
- Raise arm and contra-lateral leg while walking;
- Alternate elevating arms and legs while walking (this also improves motor coordination);
- Standing on one leg;
- Standing in the tandem position, while increasing the period of permanence in these last two static positions (Madureira et al., 2007);
-

Besides, other exercises can be performed such as:

- Weight transference in non stable superficies such as balance boards and elastic bed, with one or two feet on the floor, with or without support, depending on individual conditions;
- Jumping exercises are recommended only to patients without augmented risk to fracture, after 6 months of the program;
- Carefully throwing medicine balls one to the other, in order to practice protection reactions, dissociation of scapular and pelvic waists, coordination and proprioception.

Data from our group of research (PRADO-UNIFESP) demonstrated that a specific rehabilitation program to osteoporotic patients can improve motor coordination and dynamic balance in osteoporotic women, with only one session per week in a period of one year. The program included upper and lower limb stretching (Figure 1), strength training mainly for lower limb, coordination, static and dynamic balance exercises (Figure 2) and orientation in order to prevent falls as well as to correct postures to perform daily life activities (Lirani-Galvao et al., 2007).

A physiotherapy program of 12 sessions (2 per week) of balance, coordination and ambulation exercises as well as cognitive tasks was able to improve balance, assessed by up-and-go and one-leg balance tests in 68 osteoporotic patients older than 70 years of age. The program included: sensory awareness exercises (massaging the soles of the feet, self-mobilizing the feet); stretching exercises for the lower limb muscles; muscle-strengthening exercises; proprioceptive awareness training of the lower limbs, trunk and cervical spine; eye-neck coordination exercises; balance coordination, and agility exercises (ball games) exercises; functional exercises (walking forward, backward, and sidewalks); and exercises to minimize the adverse consequences of falls (getting up from the floor). In addition, patients were given a home-exercise program that included massaging the feet with a ball, games to develop upper and lower limb coordination, and balance exercises (Vaillant et al., 2006).

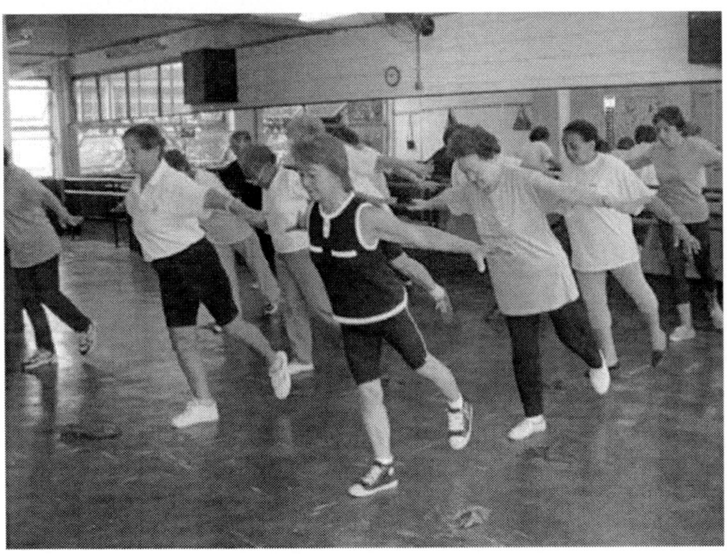

Figure 2. Exercise to improve balance (Rehabilitation and Physical Exercise Program Developed for Osteoporotic Patients - PRADO, Federal University of Sao Paulo, UNIFESP, Brazil).

These activities may be performed individually or in groups, in a playful and pleasant way, such as in dancing, hidrogymnastics, and through techniques such as *Tai Chi Chuan*, which can decrease the risk of falls in elderly population up to 47% after 4 months of once-a-week practice (Wolf et al., 1996). *Tai Chi* may also improve neuromuscular coordination and quality of life of these patients (Wang, 2004).

Beside these exercises, some physical agents have been investigated aiming to prevent and treat osteoporosis in humans. Based on bone piezoelectricity, vibrating platforms have demonstrated to maintain BMD of postmenopausal women (Rubin et al., 2004), augment bone and muscle mass in young women with low BMD (Gilsanz et al., 2006), and improve postural control and muscle strength (Verschueren et al., 2004). Pulsed electrical magnetic fields (PEMF) have also shown positive effects on bone of postmenopausal osteoporotic women. Bone formation markers were augmented when submitted to PEMF, as shown by the increase on osteocalcin and pro-collagen type I C-terminal peptide levels (Giordano et al., 2001).

Even with so many investigations showing the positive effects of physiotherapy for osteoporotic patients, these professionals are still concerned about treating this population. A cross-sectional study that interviewed 171 physiotherapists in British Columbia, Canada, showed that 97% of them reported to use only strength exercises and postural reeducation, and 45% of them reported to practice manual therapy for osteoporotic patients. Most of them have concerns about the risk of fractures during the physical rehabilitation using these techniques in this population (Sran & Khan, 2005), and that is why it is so important to disseminate information on how to safely treat osteoporotic patients among physiotherapists.

It is relevant to accentuate that when an osteoporotic fracture occurs, a multidisciplinary rehabilitation program should be emphasized, including early mobilization, noninvasive surgical procedures, use of orthoses and fall prevention information (Schwab & Klein, 2008) followed by strength training, balance and coordination exercises. The objective of this treatment is to offer this patient the possibility of recovery in order to perform his/her activities of daily living as soon and safe as possible. After this acute rehabilitation, the patient should be included in a specific physical therapy program with all the recommendations cited above.

Conclusions

No matter what physical activity is selected to each patient, when balance, motor coordination, muscle strength and posture are improved, there are significant direct and indirect contributions to keep the osteoporotic patients more active and independent, giving them conditions to perform their daily life activities with more comfort and safety (Schwab & Klein, 2008). Besides, these benefits may last even one year after the cessation of exercises (Liu-Ambrose et al., 2005).

The best training program to an osteoporotic patient involves more than one type of exercise and, considering limitations of each one, it may match walking + strength training+ balance training or hidrogymnastics + weight training + balance training. Many exercises are recommended, such as walking, jogging, strength training, *Tai Chi Chuan*, dance, hidrogymnastics and swimming. However, some sports are not indicated due to the risk of falls and fractures (volleyball, basketball, soccer, football, handball, skiing, climbing etc).

To choose the type of exercise, frequency, intensity, number of series repetitions and interval between them, it will all depend on the objectives and limits of each patient, age, physical limitations, anterior practice of physical exercises, among many other factors obtained in the physical evaluation. Exercises are normally performed two to three times a week, in order to promote rest, according to the load applied. Shorter periods of rest are indicated when loads are lighter and recovery is faster (Bloomfield, 2001).

As for any kind of physical exercise, it is important to perform a warm up and stretching of the muscles which will be involved during that specific training session. While prescribing strength training it is important to remember that load must be progressively augmented, so that the stimulus continues to be osteogenic. When the same load is continuously applied, an adaptation occurs on bone, which stops responding to the stimulus. A 2-year study showed that progressive increase of load during a strength training program (until 3 series of 8 maximum repetitions) in post-menopausal women had a better effect on lumbar, femoral neck and radius BMDs, when compared to a group that performed the same exercises with a lower load and no progression (Kerr et al., 2001).

A correct posture should not only be stimulated during daily life activities but also during exercises practice. A physical exercise program should cause well being and should respect the physiological limits of each patient. Physiotherapists and physical education professionals should be constantly aware of the osteoporotic patient situation, and change the exercise or rehabilitation programs whenever needed, mainly focusing on the objectives of a better quality of life, promoting safe osteogenic stimulus and gains in mobility and independent lifestyle.

References

Allen, R. Physical Agents Used in the Management of Chronic Pain by Physical Therapists. *Phys Med and Rehab Clinics Am.*, 2006, 17(2): 315 – 345.

Andreoli, A; Monteleone, M; Van Loan, M; Promenzio, L; Tarantino, U; De Lorenzo, A. Effects of different sports on bone density and muscle mass in highly trained athletes. *Med Sci Sports Exerc*, 2001, Apr., 33(4): 507-511.

Ay, A.; Yurtkuran, M. Evaluation of hormonal response and ultrasonic changes in the heel bone by aquatic exercise in sedentary postmenopausal women. *Am J Phys Med Rehabil*, 2003, 82: 942-949.

Bailey, DA; McKay, HA; Mirwald, RL; Crocker, PR; Faulkner, RA. A six-year longitudinal study of the relationship of physical activity to bone mineral accrual in growing children: the university of Saskatchewan bone mineral accrual study. *J Bone Miner Res*, 1999, 14:1672-1679.

Bass, S; Pearce, G; Bradney, M; Hendrich, E; Delmas, PD; Harding, A; Seeman, E. Exercise before puberty may confer residual benefits in bone density in adulthood: studies in active prepurberal and retire female gymnasts. *J Bone Miner Res*, 1998,13:500-507.

Bergström, I; Landgren, BM; Brinck, J; Freyschuss, B. Physical training preserves bone mineral density in postmenopausal women with forearm fractures and low bone mineral density. *Osteoporosis Int.*, 2008, 19(2): 177-183.

Bischoff, HA; Stähelin, HB; Dick, W; Akos, R; Knecht, M; Salis, C; Nebiker, M; Theiler, R; Pfeifer, M; Begerow, B; Lew, RA; Conzelmann, M. Effects of Vitamin D and Calcium Supplementation on Falls: A Randomized Controlled Trial. *Journal of Bone and Mineral Research*, 2003, Feb.,18:343-351.

Bloomfield, SA. Optimizing bone health: impact of nutrition, exercise, and hormones. *Sports Science Exchange* [serial online] 2001 [cited 2004 Mar 10]; 14(3):1-6.

Bono, CM; Einhorn, TA. Overview of osteoporosis: pathophysiology and determinants of bone strength. *Eur Spine J*, 2003, 12 (Suppl 2): S90-S96.

Bravo, G; Gauthier, P; Roy, PM; Payette, H; Gaulin, P. A weight-bearing, water-based exercise program for osteopenic women: Its impact on bone, functional fitnees, and well-bering. *Arch Phys Med Rehabil*, 1997, 78:1375-1380.

Burger, EH; Klein-Nulend, J. Mechanotransduction in bone – role of the lacuno-canalicular network. *FASEB J*, 1999, 13 (8 Suppl): S101-S112.

Cardoso, AS; Tartaruga, LP; Barella, RE; Brentano, MA; Kruel, LFM. Effects of a deep water training program on women's muscle strength. *Journal of the Internation Federation of Physical Education*, 2004, 74, Special Edition; 590-592.

Creighton, DL; Morgan, AL; Boardley, D; Brolinson, PG. Weight-bearing exercises and markers of bone turnover in female athletes. *J Appl Physiol*, 2001, 90: 565-570.

Cullen, DM; Smith, RT; Akhter, MP; Cullen, DM; Smith, RT; Akhter MP. Bone-loading response varies with strain magnitude and cycle number. *J Appl Physiol*, 2001, 91: 1971-1976.

Cussler, EC; Lohman, TG; Going, SB; Houtkooper, LB; Metcalfe, LL; Flint-Wagner, HG; Harris, RB; Teixeira, PJ. Weight Lifted in Strength Training Predicts Bone Change in Postmenopausal Women. *Med. Sci. Sports Exerc*., 2003, 35(1):10-17.

Dai LY. The relationship between osteoarthrits and osteoporosis in the spine, *Clin Rheumatol*., 1998,16:44-46.

Ehrlich, PJ; Lanyon, LE. Mechanical strain and bone cell function: A review. *Osteoporos Int*, 2002, 13: 688-700.

Fleck, SJ; Kraemer, WJ. Treinamento de força para idosos. In: Fleck, SJ; Kraemer, WJ. (Eds.) *Fundamentos do treinamento de força muscular*. 2.ed. Porto Alegre: Artmed, 1999, 200-211.

Fritton, SP; McLeod, KJ; Rubin, CT. Quantifying the strain history of bone spatial uniformity and self-similarity of low-magnitude strains. *J Biomech*, 2000, 33: 317-325.

Fukada, E; Yasuda, I. On the Piezoelectric effect of bone. *Journal of the Physical Society Of Japan*, 1957, 12:1158-1162.

Gilsanz, V; Wren, TA; Sanchez, M; Dorey, F; Judex, S; Rubin, C. Low-level, high-frequency mechanical signals enhance musculoskeletal development of young women with low BMD. *J Bone Miner Res*., 2006, Sep;21(9):1464-74.

Giordano, N; Battisti, E; Geraci, S; Fortunato, M; Santacroce, C; Rigato, M; Luigi Gennari, L; Gennari, C. Effect of electromagnetic fields on bone mineral density and biochemical markers of bone turnover in osteoporosis: a single-blind, randomized pilot study. *Current Therapeutic Research*, 2001, 62(3): 187-193.

Going, S; Lohman, T; Houtkooper, L; Metcalfe, L; Flint-Wagner, H; Blew, R; Stanford, V; Cussler, E; Martin, J; Teixeira, P; Harris, M; Milliken, L; Figueroa-Galvez, A; Weber, J. Effects of exercise on bone mineral density in calcium-replete postmenopausal women with and without hormone replacement therapy. *Osteoporos Int*,, 2003, 14: 637-643.

Gokkaya, NKO; Koseoglu, F; Albayrak, N. Reduced aerobic capacity in patients with severe osteoporosis: a cross sectional study. *Eur J Phys Rehabil Med*., 2008, Jun; 44(2):141-147.

Harrison, RA; Hillman, M; Bulstrode, S. Loading of the lower limb when walking partially immersed: Implicatons for Clinical Practice. *Physiotherapy*, 1992, 78(3):164-166.

Hingorjo, MR; Syed, S; Qureshi, MA. Role of exercise in osteoporosis prevention--current concepts. *J Pak Med Assoc.*, 2008, Feb, 58(2):78-81.

Hsieh, YF; Turner, CH. Effects of loading frequency on mechanically induced bone formation. *J Bone Miner Res.*, 2001, 16: 918-924.

Hughes, VA; Frontera, WR; Dallal, GE; Lutz, KJ; Fisher, EC; Evans, WJ. Muscle strength and body composition: associations with bone density in older subjects. *Med Sci Sports Exerc*, 1995, 27: 967-74.

Huntoon, EA; Schmidt, CK; Sinaki, M. Significantly fewer refractures after vertebroplasty in patients who engage in back-extensor-strengthening exercises. *Mayo Clin Proc.*, 2008, 83(1):54-57.

Kannus, P; Haapasalo, H; Sankelo, M; Sievänen, H; Pasanen, M; Heinonen, A; Oja, P; Vuori, I. Effect of starting age of physical activity on bone mass in the dominant arm of tennis and squash players. *Ann Intern Med*, 1995, 123: 27-31.

Kemmler, W; Engelke, K; Lauber, D; Weineck, J; Hensen, J; Kalender, WA. Exercise effects on fitness and bone mineral density in early postmenopausal women: 1-year EFOPS results. *Med Sci Sports Exerc.*, 2002, 34:2115-23.

Kerr, D; Ackland, T; Maslen, B; Morton, A; Prince, R. Resistance training over 2 years increase bone mass in calcium-replete postmenopausal women. *J Bone Miner Res.*, 2001, 16: 175-181.

Kohrt, WM; Bloomfield, SA; Little, KD; Nelson, ME; Yingling, VR. American College of Sports Medicine Position Stand: physical activity and bone health. *Med Sci Sports Exerc.*, 2004, 36(11):1985-1996.

Kruel, LFM; Barella, RE; Graef, F; Brentano, MA; Figueiredo, PP; Cardoso, AS; Severo, CR. Effects of resistance training in women engaged in hydrogymnastics programs. *Revista Brasileira de Fisiologia do Exercício*, 2005, 4, (1): 32-38.

Lanyon, LE; Rubin, CT. Static vs dynamic loads as an influence on bone remodelling. *J Biomech*, 1984, 17: 897-905.

Liedert, A; Kaspar, D; Blakytny, R; Claes, L; Ignatius, A. Signal transduction pathways involved in mechanotransduction in bone cells. *Biochemical and Biophysical Research Communications*, 2006, 349 (1): 1-5.

Lindsey, C; Brownbill, RA; Bohannon, RA; Ilich, JZ. Association of Physical Performance Measures with Bone Mineral Density in Postmenopausal Women. *Arch Phys Med Rehabil.,* 2005, 86: 1102 - 1107.

Lirani-Galvão, APR; Oliveira, ML; Marin, RV; Moreira-Pfrimer, LDF; Lazaretti-Castro, M. Programa de reabilitação melhora coordenação motora e equilíbrio dinâmico em mulheres osteoporóticas. In: *XVII Congresso Brasileiro de Fisioterapia*, 2007, São Paulo - SP. Revista Brasileira de Fisioterapia., 2007, Out; 11:738. Abstract in Portuguese.

Liu-Ambrose, TYL; Khan, KM; McKay, JJHA; Gillies, GL; Stephen, R. Lord The Beneficial Effects of Group-Based Exercises on Fall Risk Profile and Physical Activity Persist 1 Year Postintervention in Older Women with Low Bone Mass: Follow-Up After Withdrawal of Exercise. *J. AM Geriatr Soc.*, 2005, 53(10): 1767-1773.

Lombardi Jr., I; Oliveira, LM; Monteiro, CR; Confessor, YQ; Barros, TL; Natour, J. Evaluation of physical capacity and quality of life in osteoporotic women. *Osteoporos Int.*, 2004, 15: 80-85.

Madureira, MM; Takayama, L; Gallinaro, AL; Caparbo, VF; Costa, RA; Pereira, RM. Balance training program is highly effective in improving functional status and reducing the risk of falls in elderly women with osteoporosis: a randomized controlled trial. *Osteoporos Int.*, 2007, 18: 419-25.

Miyakoshi, N; Hongo, M; Maekawa, S; Ishikawa, Y; Shimada, Y; Itoi E. Back extensor strength and lumbar spinal mobility are predictors of quality of life in patients with postmenopausal osteoporosis. *Osteoporos Int.*, 2007, Oct, 18(10):1397-403.

Monaco, Mdi; Monaco, Rdi; Manca, M; Cavanna, A. Handgrip Strength is a Independent Predictor of Distal Radius Bone Mineral Density in Postmenopausal Women. *Clinical Rheumatology*, 2000, 19: 473-476.

Mosley, JR; Lanyon, LE. Strain rate as a controlling influence on adaptive modeling in response to dynamic loading of the ulna in growing male rats. *Bone*, 1998, 23: 313-318.

Mosley, JR; March, BM; Lynch, J; Lanyon, LE. Strain magnitude related changes in whole bone architecture in growing rats. *Bone*, 1997, 20: 191-198.

Nachemson A. The load on lumbar discs in different positions of the body. *Clin Orthop.*, 1966, 45:107-122.

Notomi, T; Lee, SJ; Okimoto, N; Okazaki, Y; Takamoto, T; Nakamura, T; Suzuki, M. Effects of resistance exercise training on mass, strength, and turnover of bone in growing rats. Eur *J Appl Physiol.*, 2000, Jul, 82(4):268-274.

Papaioannou, A; Adachi, JD; Winegard, K; Ferko, N; Parkinson, W; Cook, RJ; Webber, C; McCartney, N. Efficacy of home-based exercise for improving quality of life among elderly women with symptomatic osteoporosis-related vertebral fractures. *Osteoporos Int.*, 2003, 14(8): 677-682.

Pascal, AM. *Cadeias Musculares: Um programa para ensinar avaliação fisioterapêutica global*. São Paulo: Manole, (2000).

Pinto, ALS; Takayama, L; Carazzato, JG.; Pereira, RMR; Lima, F. The beneficial effect of swimming on bone mass. *Medicine & Science in Sports & Exercise*, 2003, 35(5): (Supp 1).

Poyhonen, T; Sipila, S; Kar, ILK; Arto H; Jukka, S; Esko M. Effects of aquatic resistance training on neuromuscular performance in healthy women. *Medicine & Science in Sports & Exercise*, 2002, Dec, 34(12):2103-2109.

Robling AG; Turner CH. Mechanotransduction in bone: genetic effects on mechanosensitivity in mice. *Bone*, 2002, 31: 562-569.

Rubin, C; Recker, R; Cullen, D; Ryaby, J; McCabe, J; McLeod, K. Prevention of postmenopausal bone loss by a low-magnitude, high-frequency mechanical stimuli: a clinical trial assessing compliance, efficacy, and safety. *J Bone Miner Res.*, 2004, 19: 343–51.

Rubin, C; Turner, AS; Bain, S; Mallinckrodt, C; McLeod, K. Anabolism. Low mechanical signals strengthen long bones. *Nature*, 2001, 412: 603-604.

Rubin, C; Turner, AS; Mallinckrodt, C; Jerome, C; McLeod, K; Bain, S. Mechanical strain, induced noninvasively in the high-frequency domain, is anabolic to cancellous bone, but not cortical bone. *Bone*, 2002, 30: 445-452.

Rubin, CT; Lanyon, LE. Regulation of bone mass by mechanical strain magnitude. *Calcif Tissue Int.*, 1985, 37: 411-417.

Ruoti, RG; Toup, JT; Berger, RA. The effects of nonswimming water exerciseon olders adults. *J Orthop Sports Phys Ther*, 1994, 19:140-145.

Sanders, ME; Rippee, NE. Fitness Acuático. *Manual de Instructor*. Volumen I. Agua poco profunda. Madrid: Gymnos, (2001).

Saraiva, GL; Cendoroglo, MS; Ramos, LR; Araújo, LMQ; Vieira, JGH; Maeda, SS; Borba, VZC; Kunii, I; Hayashi, LF; Lazaretti-Castro, M Prevalence of vitamin D deficiency, insufficiency and secondary hyperparathyroidism in the elderly inpatients and living in the community of the city of São Paulo, Brazil. *Arq Bras Endocrinol Metab.*, 2007, Apr., 51(3): 437-442.

Schwab, P; Klein, RF. Nonpharmacological approaches to improve bone health and reduce osteoporosis. *Current Opinion Rheumatol.*, 2008, 20(2): 213-217.

Sinaki M. The role of physical activity in bone health: a new hypothesis to reduce risk of vertebral fracture. *Phys Med Rehabil Clin N Am.*, 2007, Aug, 18(3):593-608, xi-xii.

Sinaki, M; Itoi, E; Wahner, HW; Wollan, P; Gelzcer, R; Mullan, BP; Collins, DA; Hodgson, SF.Stronger back muscles reduce the incidence of vertebral fractures: A prospective 10 year follow-up of postmenopausal women. *Bone*, 2002, 6: 836-841.

Sinaki, M; Mikkelsen, BA. Postmenopausal spinal osteoporosis: Flexion versus extension exercises. *Archives of Physical Medicine and Rehab*ilitation, 1984, 65(10):593–596.

Sran, MM; Khan, KM. Physiotherapy and osteoporosis: practice behaviors and clinicians' perceptions-a survey. *Man Ther.*, 2005, Feb; 10(1):21-7.

Stengel, SV; Kemmler, W; Kalender, WA; Engelke, K; Lauber, D. Differential effects of strength versus power training on bone mineral density in postmenopausal women: a 2-year longitudinal study. *British Journal of Sports Medicine*, 2007, 41:649-655.

Taafee, DR; Marcus, R. Regional and total body bone mineral density in elite collegiate male swimmers. *J Sports Med Phys Fitness*, 1999, Jun., 39(2):154-159.

Tsukahara, N; Toda, A; Goto, J; Ezawa, I. Cross-sectional and longitudinal studies on the effect of water exercise in controlling bone loss in Japanese postmenopausal women. *J Nutr Sci Vitaminol*, (1994), 40: 37-47.

Turner CH. Three rules for bone adaptation to mechanical stimuli. *Bone*, 1998, 23: 399-407.

Turner, CH. Aging and fragility of bone. *J Musculoskelet Neuronal Interact.*, 2007, Oct-Dec, 7(4):342-343.

Turner, CH; Forwood, MR; Otter, MW. Mechanotransduction in bone: do bone cells act as sensors of fluid flow? *FASEB J*, 1994a, 8: 875-878.

Turner, CH; Forwood, MR; Rho, JY; Yoshikawa, T. Mechanical loading thresholds for lamellar and woven bone formation. *J Bone Miner Res.*, 1994b, 9: 87-97.

Turner, CH; Owan, I; Takano, Y. Mechanotransduction in bone: role of strain rate. American *Journal of Physiology*, 1995, 269: E438-E442.

Vaillant, J; Vuillerme, N; Martigné, P; Caillat-Miousse, JL; Parisot, J; Nougier, V; Juvin, R. Balance, aging, and osteoporosis: effects of cognitive exercises combined with physiotherapy. *Joint Bone Spine*, 2006, Jul; 73(4):414-418.

Vainionpää, A; Korpelainen, R; Sievänen, H; Vihriälä, E; Leppäluoto, J; Jämsä, T. Effect of impact exercise and its intensity on bone geometry at weight-bearing tibia and femur. *Bone*, 2007, Mar; 40(3):604-11.

Wang, C; Collet, PJ; Lau, J. The Effect of Tai Chi on Health Outcomes in Patients With Chronic Conditions A Systematic Review. *Arch Intern Med.*, 2004, 164:493-501.

Warner, SE; Shea, JE; Miller, SC; Shaw, JM. Adaptations in Cortical and Trabecular Bone in Response to Mechanical Loading with and without Weight Bearing. *Calcif Tissue Int.*, 2006, 79:395-403.

Wolf, SL; Barnhart, HX; Kutner, NG; McNeely, E; Coogler, C; Xu, T; Atlanta FICSIT Group. Reducing frailty and falls in older persons: an investigation of tai chi and computerized balance training. *J Am Geriatr Soc.*, 1996, 44: 489-497.

Wolff, J. (1892). Das Gesetz der Transformation der Knochen. Translation by Maquet, P & Furlong, R: *The law of bone remodelling*. Berlin, 1986: Springer-Verlag.

Zehnacker, CH; Bemis-Dougherty, A. Effect of weighted exercises on bone mineral density in post menopausal women a systematic review. *J Geriatr Phys Ther.*, 2007, 30(2):79-88.

In: Osteoporosis: Etiology, Diagnosis and Treatment
Editors: Bilar E. Mattingly and Albert C. Pillare

ISBN 978-1-60692-397-9

Chapter 11

The Role of Periosteum: A Neglected Aspect of Osteoporosis

***Yin Xiao*[1], *Wei Fan*[2], *Stefan AW Bouwense*[3] *and Ross Crawford*[4]**
Queensland University of Technology, Brisbane, Queensland, Australia.

Abstract

Most current studies on the pathogenesis of osteoporosis emphasize the bone metabolic activities occurring on endosteal surfaces, whereas the periosteal aspect is somewhat neglected. In terms of bone physiology, periosteum plays a determining role in *de novo* cortical bone formation and cortical bone expansion through periosteum is the most efficient way of increasing bone strength against fractures. Despite the important role of periosteum in the pathogenesis and treatment of osteoporosis, little is known about the structural and cellular features of periosteum in osteoporosis. This chapter will focus on the major changes occurring in the periosteum of osteoporosis and the possible implications of these changes in the pathogenesis of osteoporosis. The changes identified in the periosteum of osteoporosis are mainly located in the metaphyseal compartment, which include: (a) much thicker and more cellular cambial layer; (b) increased number of $TRAP^+$ (tartrate resistant acid phosphatase), $VEGF^+$ (vascular endothelial growth factor) cells and the degree of vascularization; and (c) enhanced expression of sympathetic nerve fibers. The structural and cellular changes of osteoporotic periosteum indicate that

[1] Yin Xiao, Ph.D., M.D.Sc., B.D.Sc., Associate Professor, Institute of Health and Biomedical Innovation, Queensland University of Technology, Brisbane, Queensland, Australia. Email: yin.xiao@qut.edu.au; Tel: +61-7-31386240; Fax: +61-7-31396030.

[2] Wei Fan, D.D.S., M.D.Sc., B.D.Sc., Institute of Health and Biomedical Innovation, Queensland University of Technology, Brisbane, Queensland, Australia. Email: w3.fan@student.qut.edu.au; Tel: +61-7-31386405; Fax: +61-7-31396030.

[3] Stefan AW Bouwense, B.Sc. UMC St Radboud, Nijmegen, the Netherlands. Email: S.Bouwense@gmail.com

[4] Ross Crawford, D.Phil, M.D., Professor, Institute of Health and Biomedical Innovation, Queensland University of Technology, Brisbane, Queensland, Australia. Email: r.crawford@qut.edu.au. Tel: +61-7-31394481; Fax: +61-7-31396030

periosteum plays an important role in the cortical bone resorption in metaphyseal areas and this pathological process may be regulated by the sympathetic nervous system.

Introduction

The mineralization and development of bone tissue is a dynamic process determined by the balance between bone formation and resorption occurring on periosteal and endosteal surfaces [1-3]. This modeling and remodeling process will alter the size, shape, internal structure, total mass and, subsequently, the mechanical strength of bone. The thickness of cortical bone, a crucial feature in determining bending strength of the whole bone, is defined by both periosteal and endosteal bone apposition and resorption [4]. Osteoporosis is a metabolic disorder of bone tissue whereby the balance between bone formation and resorption has shifted such that the rate of bone resorption exceeds bone formation, resulting in net bone loss, trabecular and cortical thinning and porosity [5]. Bone fractures, especially of the hip, is the most serious consequence of osteoporosis, and significantly threatens the independence and, indeed, survival of those affected [6]. Cervical (intracapsular) and trochanteric (extracapsular) fractures of the hip both involve the cortical and cancellous bone compartments, requiring sophisticated surgical treatment, thus accounting for the greater portion of treatment costs for osteoporosis in the Western hemisphere [7].

The periosteum is a dense connective tissue membrane covering the surface of a majority of bones. In both physiological and pathological processes, periosteum plays a determining role in both bone formation and fracture healing, in addition to the involvement of other important factors such as growth factors and mechanical loading [4,8,9]. Periosteum is a highly vascularized tissue which contains both osteogenic and chondrogenic progenitor cells, as well as other related bioactive factors [8,10,11]. The osteogenic function of periosteum determines the amount of *de novo* postnatal periosteal bone formation defining the thickness and strength of cortical bone [4]. Previous researchers have revealed an age related structural and cellular degeneration in periosteum [12-15]. However, in osteoporosis, which is characterized by decreased bone strength and a high incidence of fractures, the changes occurring in the periosteum along the bone surface require further investigation [16,17]. Although estrogen deficiency is believed to be an intrinsic cause of osteoporosis, the process and mechanism of bone loss in osteoporosis remain unclear. Most researchers emphasized the bone resorption activity happening in the endocortical or intramedullary area; however, the structural and cellular changes in periosteum and their synergistic roles in the pathogenesis of osteoporosis have been somewhat neglected. Therefore, this chapter will focus on the periosteum and major periosteal changes occurring in osteoporosis. The possible implications of these changes in the pathogenesis of osteoporosis will also be discussed.

Periosteal Apposition and Resorption: Key Factors in Maintaining Bone Strength

The net bone loss or decrease in bone mineral density (BMD) associated with ageing in general, and osteoporosis in particular, is caused by an imbalance between bone formation and resorption. The majority of bone resorption or remodeling activities in both the osteoporosis and ageing process is thought to take place in the following areas: endocortical surfaces, intracortical surfaces of the haversian canals, and surfaces of trabecular struts. Resorption occurring on endocortical surfaces tends to decrease the thickness of bone cortex, whereas the remodeling in haversian canals or on surfaces of trabecular struts leads to increased bone porosity. Recently, the periosteal remodeling activities on femur neck surfaces in osteoporosis have been reported, although their pathogenic implications and mechanisms are not fully understood. On the other hand, the major physiological role of periosteum, during the bone development and fracture healing, is still thought to be new bone deposition. For the body to maintain enough bone strength against accidental fractures, new bone formation and bone remodeling activity on periosteal surfaces is maintained throughout life. In bone development occurring during infancy, new bone deposition on periosteal surfaces is dominant compared to bone resorption, although the resorption process is indispensable for controlling the bone growth pattern, which results in the thickening of cortical bone and increases bone strength. During adulthood new bone formation slows down and in the elderly the balance between the formation and resorption starts to tilt; in osteoporotic patients, in particular, resorption overtakes formation at an accelerated rate. Cortical bone thickness is a determining factor of mechanical bone strength, so that the shift in balance finally leads to decreased bone strength and an increased incidence of fractures.

The basis for understanding the function of tissues and organs lie in their anatomical and histological structures. The structure of periosteum has been investigated in great details by a number of researches in order to better understand how and why the periosteum alters function both in normal physiological and pathological processes. However, the histological changes taking place on the bone surfaces, and the implication of such changes in the pathogenesis of osteoporosis and the general ageing process, has tended to be overlooked by researchers. Knowledge of bone surface changes is very likely to improve our understanding of osteoporosis and assist in the development of new treatment methods for this condition.

The Histological Structure and Age-related Changes in Periosteum

The periosteum, as well as the endosteum, is a type of connective tissue which emerges from the mesoderm during embryonic development. It attaches tightly to various bone surfaces through Sharpy's fibers, forming a thin but tough membrane. The Sharpy's fibers represent a direct continuation of the periosteal collagen fibers around which the cortical lamellae has grown [8]. Histologically the periosteum is thought to consist of two or three distinct layers, depending on what model is applied [13,17] (Figure 1). In the classical "two layers" theory, the periosteum consists of an outer fibrous layer which contains fibroblasts, blood vessels, sensory and sympathetic nerve fibers, collagen fibers and extracellular substances [18]. The inner layer, referred to as the cambium layer, serves as a reservoir of undifferentiated pluripotent mesenchymal cells capable of differentiating into chondrogenic and osteoblastic lineages [11,19,20]. Cells from the periosteal cambium layer may be first in line, together with osteoblasts, to drive the cell differentiation process during bone reparation, characterized by the development of the initial fracture callus and subsequent remodeling [21]. Periosteum can be described as an *osteoprogenitor cell-containing bone envelope*, capable of being activated to proliferate by trauma, retroviruses, tumors, and lymphocyte mitogens [22].

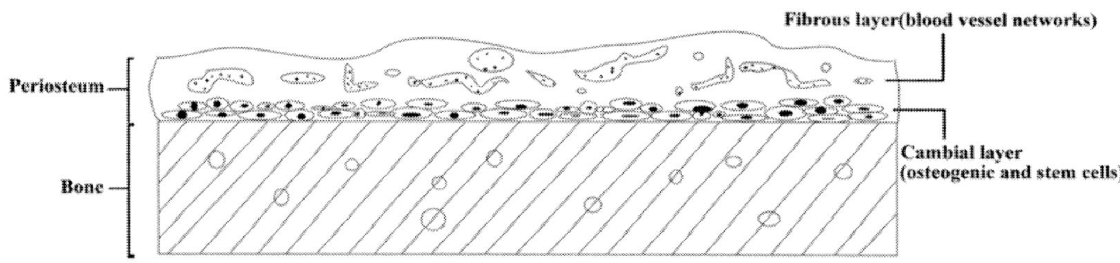

Figure 1. An illustration for the dual-layered structure of periosteum.

Study of the periosteum ultrastructure suggests it is made up of three discrete zones (layers) [13]. Zone I has an average thickness of 10 to 20 μm, consisting predominantly of osteoblasts representing 90% of the cell population, whereas collagen fibrils occupy 15% of the volume. In zone II fibroblasts and collagen make up half the volume in roughly equal proportions of 25% each, whereas capillary networks make up 15% of the volume. Zone III has the highest volume of collagen fibrils and fibroblasts compared to zones I and II. Fibroblasts account for more than 90% of all cells present in zone III. Although slightly different, the "two layers" and "three layers" periosteum theories have one feature in common, namely that the periosteum consists of an inner cambium layer and an outer vascularized and innervated fibrous layer.

The periosteum has been described as a "well vascularized osteogenic and/or chondrogenic organ" [8], providing blood circulation to bone, especially the cortical bone [23]. Stripping periosteum off the diaphysis typically destroys the arterial nutrient supply to the bone [9]; therefore, in some sense, periosteum can be thought of as the "umbilical cord" of bone. The vasculature system of periosteum was first studied in detail by Zucman and later by Eyre-Brook [9]. Eyre-Brook was able to demonstrate that the capillaries supplying blood to bone resides within the cortex that links the medullary and periosteal vessels. His study of the link between the blood vessels of muscle and bone showed that the intrinsic periosteal vessels can limit the extent of ischemia in a muscle that has had its other vascular supply removed. Some authors argue that the blood supply of periosteum has a number of features analogous to the blood supply of skin by pointing out that in skin the blood vessels in the dermal area provide nutritients and oxygen, and remove metabolic wastes from dermis and epidermis [10].

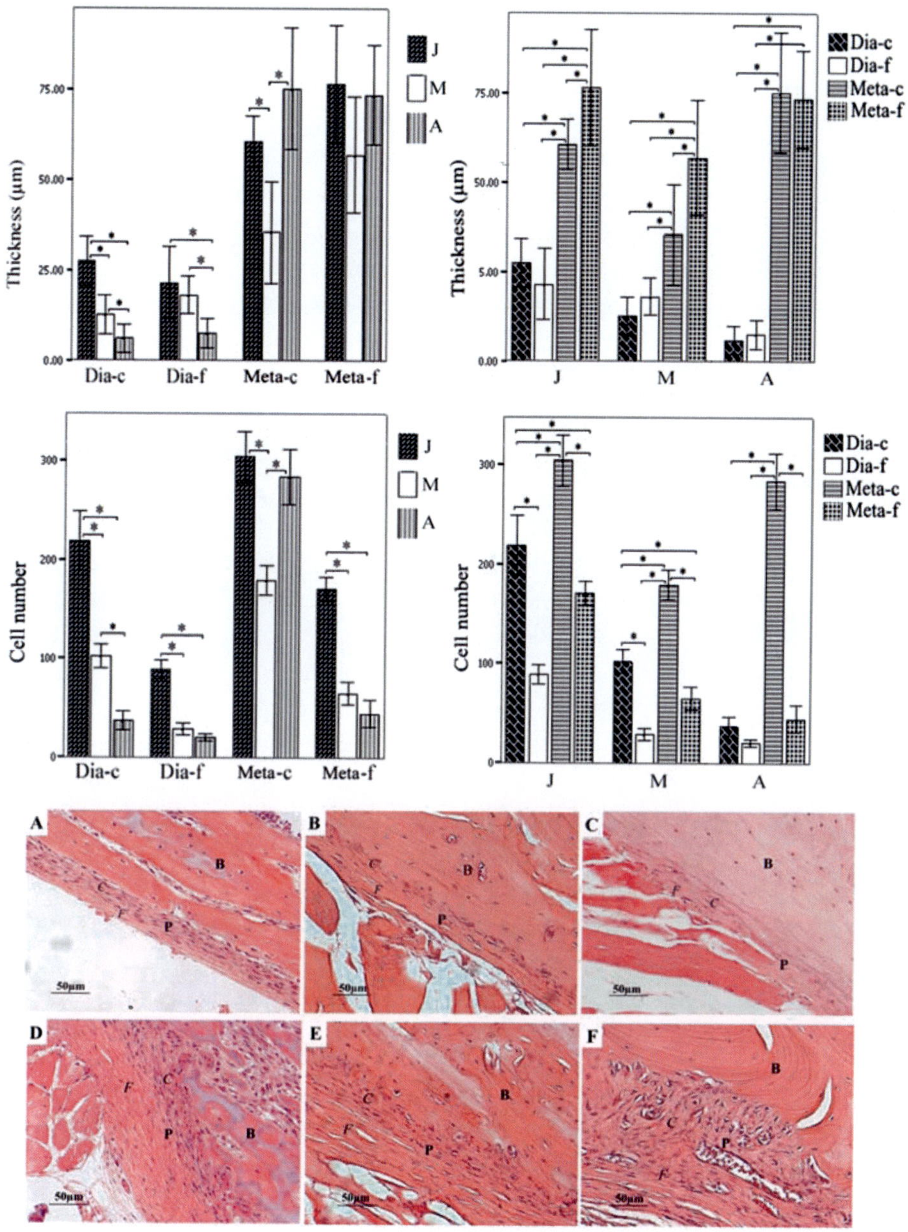

Figure 2. Diagrams and pictures (×200) of H&E observation of diaphyseal and metaphyseal periostea from different-aged rat groups. A: diaphyseal periosteum from the juvenile group; B: diaphyseal periosteum from the mature group; C: diaphyseal periosteum from the aged group; D: metaphyseal periosteum from the juvenile group; E: metaphyseal periosteum from the mature group; F: metaphyseal periosteum from the aged group. J: juvenile; M: mature; A: aged; Dia-c: cambium layer of diaphyseal periosteum; Dia-f: fibrous layer of diaphyseal periosteum; Meta-c: cambial layer of metaphyseal periosteum; Meta-f: fibrous layer of metaphyseal periosteum; *: $p<0.05$. (In pictures, B: bone tissue; P: periosteum; C: cambial layer; F: fibrous layer).

Some researchers have studied the neurological aspects of bone biology [24-26]. For example, it has been reported that sympathetic and sensory nerves are prominent in the periosteum of mammalian bones and present among blood vessels and osteogenic cells in these areas. However, the exact role of sympathetic nerve fibers in bone metabolism is still not fully understood [27-29]. Sensory nerves appear to be important in normal bone metabolism and in bone fracture repair. Increased sensory and sympathetic innervation of fracture calluses has been reported in animal experiments.

The structure of periosteum varies with age; during infancy and adolescense it is thicker, more vascularized, active and loosely attached, whereas in adulthood, it is relatively thinner, inactive and more firmly attached to bone [8,9]. Recent studies conducted in our laboratory on female rats divided into juvenile, mature and aged cohorts, have revealed that the structure and cell populations in periosteum are both age and site specific [30]. An age-related degeneration (shown as decrease in thickness and cell number) was observed in the diaphyseal periosteum; in the aged cohort this was especially prominent as a decrease in cell numbers in both the cambial and fibrous layers. However, it was noteworthy that in the metaphyseal areas, the aged rats had thicker and more cellular cambial layers than the rats from the mature group, although they were similar in the fibrous layer (Figure 2). There was also a noticeable change in cell populations within these areas, in particular an increased fractional number of osteoclasts (Figure 3). The metaphyseal periosteum in aged rats seems more destructive and vascularized than diaphyseal area. In comparison to juvenile and mature rats, aged rat has also displayed the similar destructive changes in metaphyseal periosteum (Figure 4).

Periosteal Changes and their Implications in Osteoporosis

Osteoporosis is characterized by a negative balance of bone metabolism which leads to an overall decrease of bone mass with subsequent thinning of the trabecular and cortical bone, and a significantly increased risk of bone fractures. The cortical bone expansion through periosteum is the most efficient way for the body to increase bone strength and protect against fractures. To date, basic concept within pharmacological treatment regimes of osteoporosis have tended to focus on increasing the thickness of cortical bone, by suppressing resorption and remodeling and seeking to promote periosteal bone formation [17]. Knowledge of periosteal structural and cellular characteristics is bound to enhance our understanding of this disorder and aid in the future development of more specific and effective treatment.

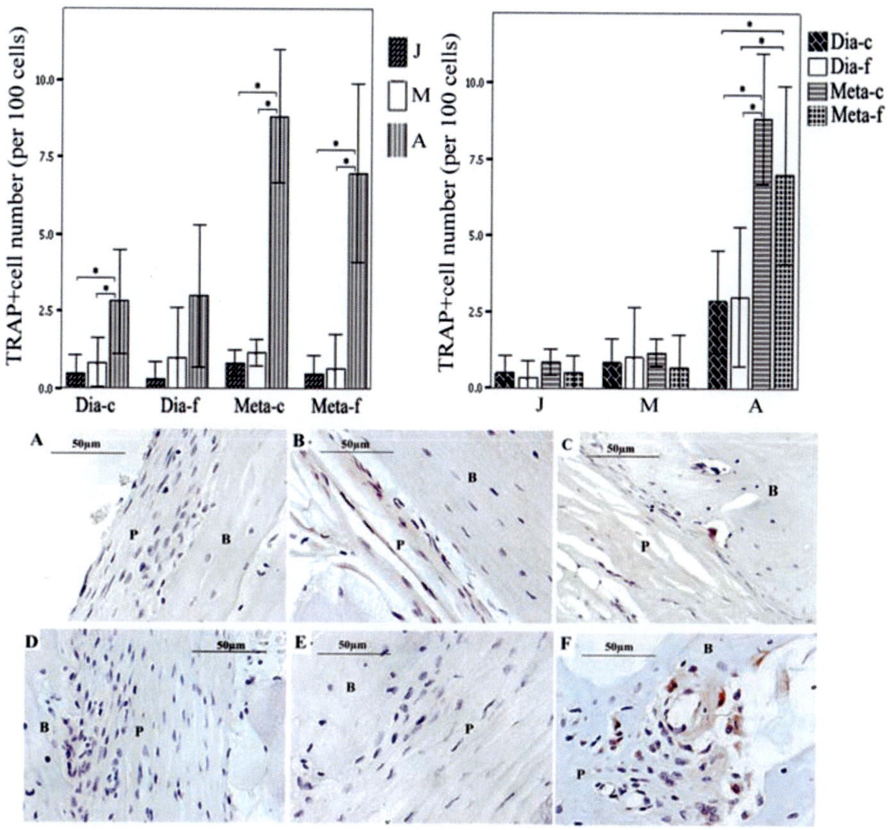

Figure 3. Osteoclasts (immunohistological staining with TRAP antibody, ×400) distribution in different periosteal areas and age rat groups. A: diaphyseal periosteum from the juvenile group; B: diaphyseal periosteum from the mature group; C: diaphyseal periosteum from the aged group; D: metaphyseal periosteum from the juvenile group; E: metaphyseal periosteum from the mature group; F: metaphyseal periosteum from the aged group. J: juvenile; M: mature; A: aged; Dia-c: cambium layer of diaphyseal periosteum; Dia-f: fibrous layer of diaphyseal periosteum; Meta-c: cambial layer of metaphyseal periosteum; Meta-f: fibrous layer of metaphyseal periosteum; *: $p<0.05$. (In pictures, B: bone tissue; P: periosteum).

Osteoporosis patients are at a greater risk of bone fractures, and the fracture pattern is quite different from "normal" fractures [7]. Most fall related fractures in osteoporotic and elderly patients begin in the cortex of the metaphyses or former epiphyses, intertrochanteric, and femoral neck cortices. They rarely, if ever, begin in the metaphyseal spongiosa or in the diaphyseal cortex [7]. This phenomenon is an evidence of a fundamental difference in the bone strength along bone axis. It is known that endosteal or intramedullary bone resorption activity is greater in osteoporotic bone compared to normal bone, and thought to be the main cause of the net bone loss suffered in osteoporosis [31]. Since the synergistic role of the periosteum in osteoporosis is so poorly understood, particularly with respect to the function of periosteum at different periosteal sites in osteoporosis, we investigated the basic structure and related cell populations in the diaphyseal and metaphyseal periosteum of osteoporotic rats.

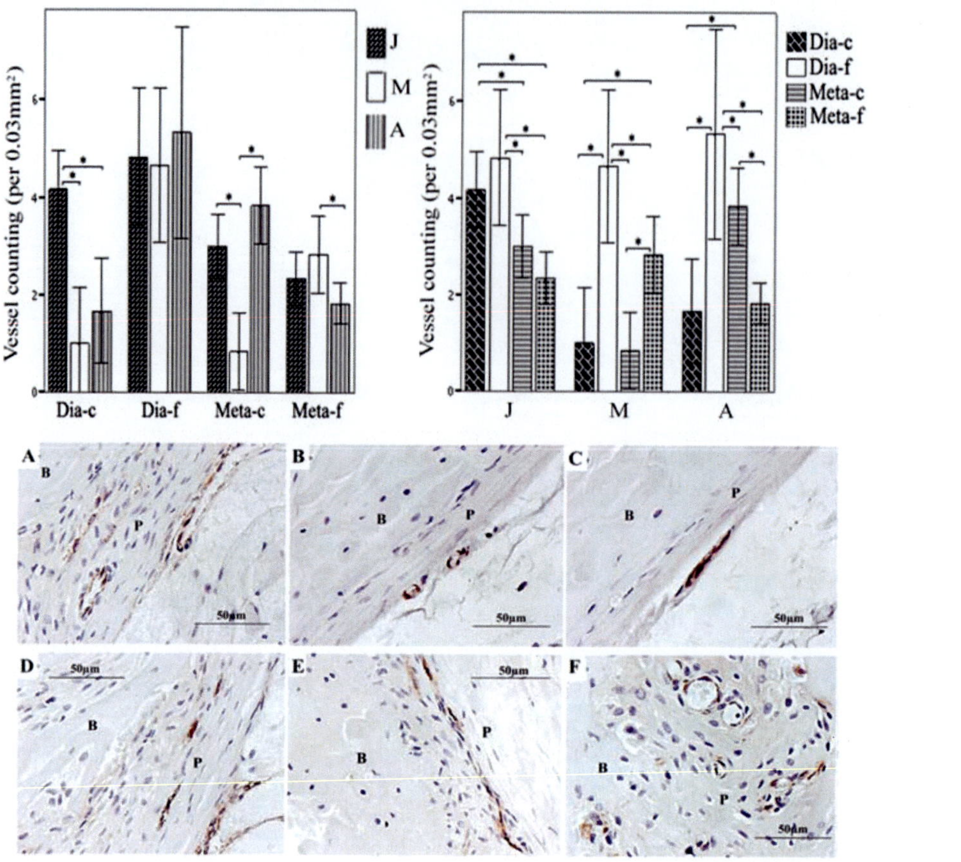

Figure 4. Blood vessel (immunohistological staining with vWF antibody, ×400) distribution in different periosteal areas and age rat groups. A: diaphyseal periosteum from the juvenile group; B: diaphyseal periosteum from the mature group; C: diaphyseal periosteum from the aged group; D: metaphyseal periosteum from the juvenile group; E: metaphyseal periosteum from the mature group; F: metaphyseal periosteum from the aged group. J: juvenile; M: mature; A: aged; Dia-c: cambium layer of diaphyseal periosteum; Dia-f: fibrous layer of diaphyseal periosteum; Meta-c: cambial layer of metaphyseal periosteum; Meta-f: fibrous layer of metaphyseal periosteum; *: $p<0.05$. (In pictures, B: bone tissue; P: periosteum).

Structural Differences between Osteoporotic and Normal Rats

In the haematoxylin and eosin stain and histomorphometry observations, the thickness and cell numbers in the cambial layer of metaphyseal periosteum from osteoporotic rats were found to be much greater compared to normal rats, despite both groups being of similar age (7 months). No statistically significant difference was found in the thickness and cell numbers between osteoporotic and normal rats of the diaphyseal periosteum, except for the thickness of the fibrous layer (Figure 5). In osteoporotic rats the metaphyseal periosteum was significantly thicker and more cellular than in the diaphyseal periosteum or normal rats, especially the cambial layer of metaphyseal periosteum (Figure 5). Although there was no significant difference between the two cohorts in the thickness of the fibrous layer in metaphyseal periosteum, the number of cells in the fibrous layers of osteoporotic rats was higher compared with normal rats. This structural difference appears to be closely related to the different cell populations found in the two cohorts, an observation confirmed by the immunohistochemical staining.

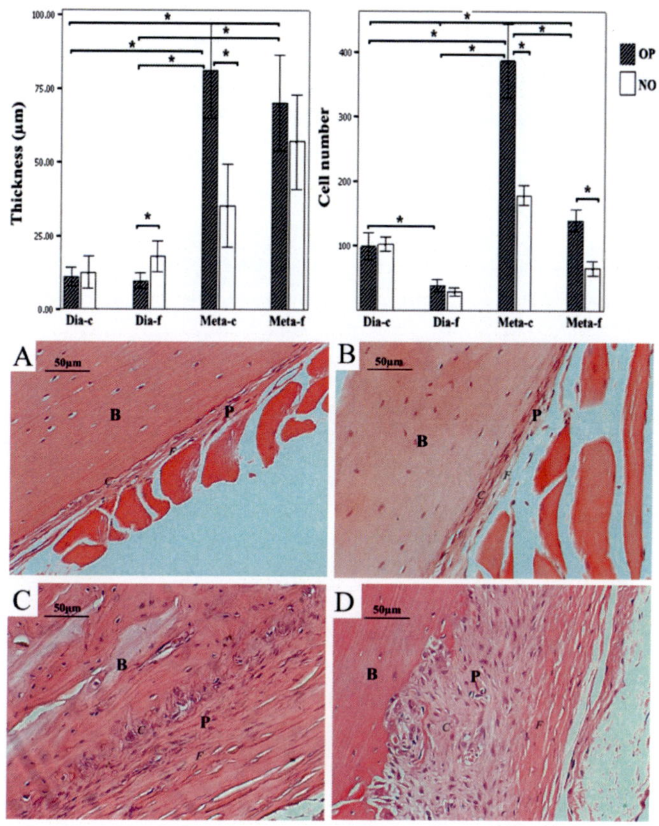

Figure 5. Diagrams and pictures (×200) of H&E observation of diaphyseal and metaphyseal periostea from normal and osteoporotic rats. A: diaphyseal periosteum from normal rats; B: diaphyseal periosteum from osteoporotic rats; C: metaphyseal periosteum from normal rats; D: metaphyseal periosteum from osteoporotic rats. NO: normal rats; OP: osteoporotic rats; Dia-c: cambium layer of diaphyseal periosteum; Dia-f: fibrous layer of diaphyseal periosteum; Meta-c: cambial layer of metaphyseal periosteum; Meta-f: fibrous layer of metaphyseal periosteum; *: $p<0.05$ (In pictures, B: bone tissue; P: periosteum).

TRAP Expression in Periosteum

To our knowledge no previous studies have documented the distribution of osteoclasts in the periosteum covering osteoporotic bones, although periosteal bone turnover activity and osteoclast distribution have recently been documented in the femoral neck of adult rhesus and Japanese macaque monkeys [32]. In our study periosteal osteoclasts were identified using TRAP specific cell markers. The osteoporotic rats had significantly more $TRAP^+$ cells in the cambial layer of both diaphyseal and metaphyseal periosteum compared to normal rats, especially in the metaphyseal area (Figure 6, 7). No statistical difference was found in the other periosteal areas. In osteoporotic rats, the cambial layer of metaphyseal periosteum had more positive cells than the cambial layer of diaphyseal periosteum (Figure 6). These immunohistochemical observations indicate a noticeable increased fraction of osteoclasts in the cambial layer of both diaphyseal and metaphyseal periostea from osteoporotic rats, especially in the metaphyseal area, which suggest greater resorptive activity on metaphyseal cortical bone surface compared to diaphyseal area in osteoporotic rats and also compared to metaphyseal cortical bone surface in normal rats. These observations have potential clinical relevance since more fractures are reported to occur in the metaphyseal areas compared to the diaphyseal areas in osteoporotic patients. Similar findings have been reported in a recent study on primates by Bliziotes *et al.*, who found an increased number of osteoclasts and eroded cortical bone surfaces, more pronounced at the femoral neck than at the shaft, especially in the castrated female animals [32]. Many researchers believe that periosteal apposition continues, even after menopause, and may partly offset the bone resorption on the endosteal surface [33]. However, the findings in our study suggest that bone resorption activity in the periosteum is greater in osteoporotic rats compared to normal rats and that the behavior of the osteoclasts may be destructive, particuarly in metaphyseal periosteum.

Osteogenic Activity in Periosteum

Osteogenic activity was demonstrated by the alkaline phosphatase (ALP) expression in periosteum. No significant difference was found in the ALP expression in either diaphyseal or metaphyseal periosteum of osteoporotic rats compared to normal rats. No difference was detected between the cambial and fibrous layers in diaphyseal and metaphyseal periosteum respectively. Nor was there any significant difference to the ALP expression between different periosteal sites in osteoporotic rats (Figures 6 and 7). Given there are an increased number of $TRAP^{+}$ osteoclasts found in the periosteum of osteoporotic rats, the relatively stable osteogenic activity may therefore be inadequate to offset bone resorption, which would consequently incur the net bone loss. The failure of periosteal apposition to compensate for increased endocortical resorption has also been reported in postmenopausal women [34].

Blood Supply in Periosteum

Vascular endothelial growth factor (VEGF) is an important growth factor reported to be involved in angiogenic, osteogenic and osteoclastogenic processes [35-37]. In osteoporotic rats, significantly more $VEGF^{+}$ cells were found in the cambial layer of the metaphyseal periosteum compared to normal rats (Figure 6, 7). No significant difference was found in other periosteal areas. In osteoporotic rats the cambial layer of both the metaphyseal and diaphyseal periosteum had more VEGF positive cells than the fibrous layers in both periosteal areas, whilst the number of VEGF positive cells in the cambial layer of metaphyseal periosteum was greater than that in the cambial layer of diaphyseal periosteum (Figure 6).

Blood vessels revealed by Von Willebrand factor (vWF) staining showed that osteoporotic rats had greater degree of vascularization in the cambial layers of both the diaphyseal and metaphyseal periosteum compared to normal rats, especially in the metaphyseal periosteum (Figure 6, 7). No significant difference was found in the fibrous layer of either periosteal area between the two groups. In osteoporotic rats, the cambial layer of metaphyseal periosteum had a greater degree of vascularization than the fibrous layer (Figure 6, 7).

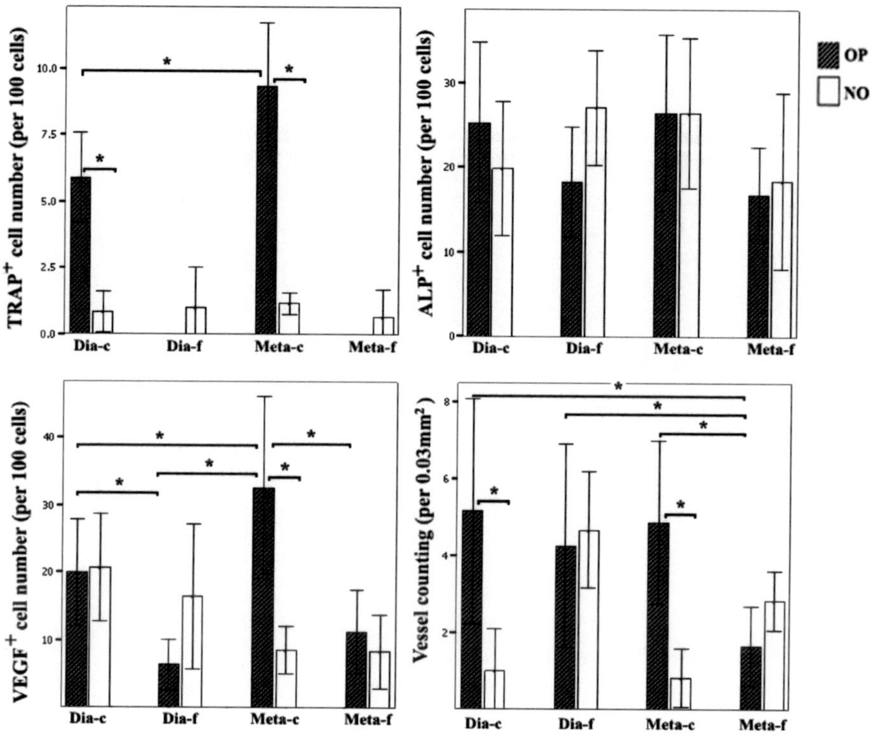

Figure 6. Diagrams of cellular differences in diaphyseal and metaphyseal periostea from normal and osteoporotic rats. NO: normal rats; OP: osteoporotic rats; Dia-c: cambium layer of diaphyseal periosteum; Dia-f: fibrous layer of diaphyseal periosteum; Meta-c: cambial layer of metaphyseal periosteum; Meta-f: fibrous layer of metaphyseal periosteum; *: $p<0.05$.

Bone development, angiogenesis, bone formation and bone resorption are all closely related processes in which VEGF is known to stimulate osteoclast activity [35-37]. It is therefore reasonable to assume that both osteoclast activity and angiogenesis are regulated by a common mediator such as VEGF. Indeed, data from our study seems to support this view since a significantly greater expression of VEGF, as well as more vWF^+ blood vessels, were found in the vicinity of $TRAP^+$ osteoclasts in the cambial layer of the metaphyseal periosteum of osteoporotic rats compared to normal rats (Figure 6 and 7). The increase of VEGF expression and periosteal vascularization in the metaphyseal periosteum of the osteoporotic rats may be related to increased bone resorptive activity in this periosteal area.

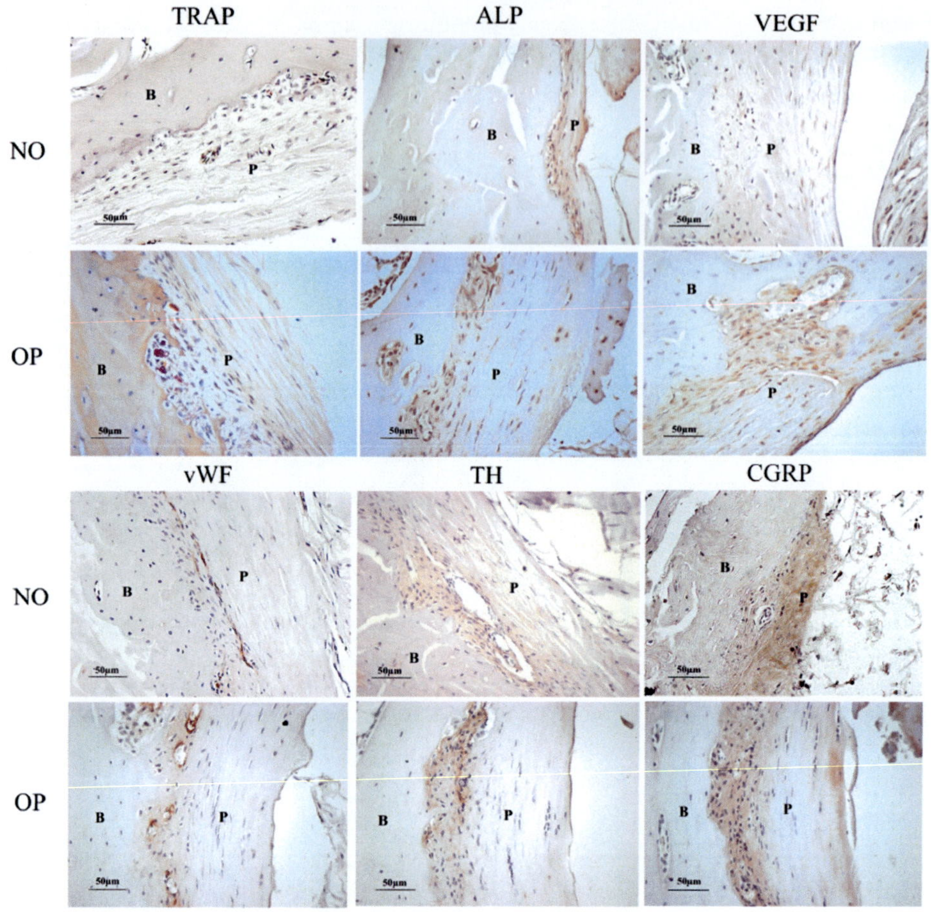

Figure 7. Immunohistological staining pictures (×200) of metaphyseal periostea from normal and osteoporotic rats. NO: normal rats; OP: osteoporotic rats (In pictures, B: bone tissue; P: periosteum).

Sympathetic and Sensory Nerves in Periosteum

The sympathetic nerve fibers revealed by tyrosine hydroxylase (TH) staining were mainly present in osteoporotic rats, predominantly in the cambial layer of metaphyseal periosteum (Figure 7). A slight TH expression was observed in the cambial layer of metaphyseal area of normal rat. No obvious staining was detected in the fibrous layer or diaphyseal area.

Sensory nerve fibers identified by calcitonin gene-related peptide (CGRP) antibodies were found in both osteoporotic and normal rats (Figure 7). There was no discernible difference in the expression of CGRP between the two groups in the different periosteal areas. However, in normal rats $CGRP^{+}$ nerve fibers appeared to be distributed in both fibrous and cambial layers, whereas in osteoporotic rats most $CGFP^{+}$ nerve fibers were present in the cambial layer of the metaphyseal area.

The reason for the increased expression of sympathetic nerve fibers in the periosteum in osteoporosis is unclear, although it is well documented that sympathetic nerve fibers are present in both the periosteum and bone [25,26]. Sympathetic innervation of periosteum and bone contributes to regulation of bone cell activity and, therefore, the equilibrium between bone modeling and remodeling [38]. It is known that both surgical and chemical sympathectomy can modulate bone cell function; however, the sympathetic nervous system (SNS) can give rise to both anabolic and catabolic effects [27-29,39], its role in regulating bone remodeling is therefore controversial. In our study, the distribution of sympathetic nerve fibers was demonstrated by applying an antibody against the SNS specific marker, tyrosine hydroxylase, which is expressed in adrenergic fibers. This revealed that there were more sympathetic nerve fibers in the cambial layer of periosteum of osteoporotic rats compared to normal rats, particularly in the metaphyseal area, a finding in accordance with the distribution of $TRAP^+$, ALP^+, $VEGF^+$ cells and blood vessels (Figure 7). The co-existence of nerve fibers and various cell populations indicates that sympathetic nerves in the periosteum are involved in the pathogenesis of osteoporosis by interacting with, and possibly regulating, osteogenic, osteoclastogenic and angiogenic factors. Sensory nerve fibers, identified by calcitonin gene related peptide (CGRP) antibodies, were found to be expressed at roughly equal rates in both osteoporotic and normal rats, although the distribution differs slightly (Figure 7). It is generally accepted that CGRP can promote osteogenesis and retard bone resorption [40,41] and it has also been shown to inhibit osteoclastic resorption like calcitonin [41]. The similar expression of CGRP seen in both osteoporotic and normal rats suggests a similar osteogenesis-related role played by CGRP in both cohorts. The observation in osteoporotic rats, where most $CGRP^+$ sensory nerve fibers were distributed in the cambial layer of the periosteum, suggests CGRP's involvement here is in response to the active bone resorption taking place in this area.

Conclusion

The net amount of bone lost in osteoporosis is *ipso facto* the result of an imbalance between two parallel, but opposing processes: bone resorption and formation. The periosteum is normally the site for new bone tissues production, whereas most bone resorption activities happens at the endosteal or intermedullary surfaces. The periosteum in osteoporosis differs both in terms of structure and cell populations, which is especially evident in the cambial layer of metaphyseal area. Bone resorption appears to be more severe in the periosteum of osteoporosis, whereas bone forming activity is relatively normal. This dysregulation of bone homeostasis in the periosteum, characteristic of the pathogenesis of osteoporosis, may therefore be the effect of the interaction between various neural pathways and the cell populations residing within it.

Acknowledgments

We would like to thank Ms. Wei Shi for her technique support in immunohistochemical work and Mr. Thor Friis for his proof reading of the entire manuscript.

REFERENCES

[1] Seeman E (2003) Reduced bone formation and increased bone resorption: rational targets for the treatment of osteoporosis. *Osteoporos Int 14 Suppl 3*:S2-8.

[2] Rauch F, Travers R, Glorieux FH (2007) Intracortical remodeling during human bone development--a histomorphometric study. *Bone 40*:274-280.

[3] Pogoda P, Priemel M, Rueger JM, Amling M (2005) Bone remodeling: new aspects of a key process that controls skeletal maintenance and repair. *Osteoporos Int 16 Suppl 2*:S18-24.

[4] Seeman E (2003) Periosteal bone formation--a neglected determinant of bone strength. N *Engl J Med 349*:320-323.

[5] Seeman E (2003) Invited Review: Pathogenesis of osteoporosis. *J Appl Physiol 95*:2142-2151.

[6] Bagi CM, Wilkie D, Georgelos K, Williams D, Bertolini D (1997) Morphological and structural characteristics of the proximal femur in human and rat. *Bone 21*:261-267.

[7] Ferretti JL, Frost HM, Gasser JA, High WB, Jee WS, Jerome C, Mosekilde L, Thompson DD (1995) Perspectives on osteoporosis research: its focus and some insights from a new paradigm. *Calcif Tissue Int 57*:399-404.

[8] Malizos KN, Papatheodorou LK (2005) The healing potential of the periosteum molecular aspects. *Injury 36 Suppl 3*:S13-19.

[9] Eyre-Brook AL (1984) The periosteum: its function reassessed. *Clin Orthop Relat Res*: 300-307.

[10]Simpson AH (1985) The blood supply of the periosteum. *J Anat 140 (Pt 4)*:697-704.

[11]Nakahara H, Bruder SP, Haynesworth SE, Holecek JJ, Baber MA, Goldberg VM, Caplan AI (1990) Bone and cartilage formation in diffusion chambers by subcultured cells derived from the periosteum. *Bone 11*:181-188.

[12]Tonna EA (1978) Electron microscopic study of bone surface changes during aging. The loss of cellular control and biofeedback. *J Gerontol 33*:163-177.

[13]Squier CA, Ghoneim S, Kremenak CR (1990) Ultrastructure of the periosteum from membrane bone. *J Anat 171*:233-239.

[14]O'Driscoll SW, Saris DB, Ito Y, Fitzimmons JS (2001) The chondrogenic potential of periosteum decreases with age. *J Orthop Res 19*:95-103.

[15]De Bari C, Dell'Accio F, Luyten FP (2001) Human periosteum-derived cells maintain phenotypic stability and chondrogenic potential throughout expansion regardless of donor age. *Arthritis Rheum 44*:85-95.

[16]Augustin G, Antabak A, Davila S (2007) The periosteum. Part 1: anatomy, histology and molecular biology. *Injury 38*:1115-1130.

[17]Allen MR, Hock JM, Burr DB (2004) Periosteum: biology, regulation, and response to osteoporosis therapies. *Bone 35*:1003-1012.

[18]Asaumi K, Nakanishi T, Asahara H, Inoue H, Takigawa M (2000) Expression of neurotrophins and their receptors (TRK) during fracture healing. *Bone 26*:625-633.

[19]Ito Y, Fitzsimmons JS, Sanyal A, Mello MA, Mukherjee N, O'Driscoll SW (2001) Localization of chondrocyte precursors in periosteum. *Osteoarthritis Cartilage 9*:215-223.

[20]Fang J, Hall BK (1997) Chondrogenic cell differentiation from membrane bone periostea. *Anat Embryol (Berl) 196*:349-362.

[21]Muramatsu K, Bishop AT (2002) Cell repopulation in vascularized bone grafts. *J Orthop Res 20*:772-778.

[22]Tran Van PT, Vignery A, Baron R (1982) Cellular kinetics of the bone remodeling sequence in the rat. *Anat Rec 202*:445-451.

[23]Hutmacher DW, Sittinger M (2003) Periosteal cells in bone tissue engineering. *Tissue Eng 9 Suppl 1*:S45-64.

[24]Bjurholm A, Kreicbergs A, Terenius L, Goldstein M, Schultzberg M (1988) Neuropeptide Y-, tyrosine hydroxylase- and vasoactive intestinal polypeptide-immunoreactive nerves in bone and surrounding tissues. *J Auton Nerv Syst 25*:119-125.

[25]Hill EL, Elde R (1991) Distribution of CGRP-, VIP-, D beta H-, SP-, and NPY-immunoreactive nerves in the periosteum of the rat. *Cell Tissue Res 264*:469-480.

[26]Hohmann EL, Elde RP, Rysavy JA, Einzig S, Gebhard RL (1986) Innervation of periosteum and bone by sympathetic vasoactive intestinal peptide-containing nerve fibers. *Science 232*:868-871.

[27]Cherruau M, Facchinetti P, Baroukh B, Saffar JL (1999) Chemical sympathectomy impairs bone resorption in rats: a role for the sympathetic system on bone metabolism. *Bone 25*:545-551.

[28]Hill EL, Turner R, Elde R (1991) Effects of neonatal sympathectomy and capsaicin treatment on bone remodeling in rats. *Neuroscience 44*:747-755.

[29]Haug SR, Brudvik P, Fristad I, Heyeraas KJ (2003) Sympathectomy causes increased root resorption after orthodontic tooth movement in rats: immunohistochemical study. *Cell Tissue Res 313*:167-175.

[30]Fan W, Crawford R, Xiao Y (2008) Structural and cellular differences between metaphyseal and diaphyseal periosteum in different aged rats. *Bone 42*:81-89.

[31]Parfitt AM (2002) Size of bone in the aged endocortical resorption. *J Bone Miner Res 17*:1306; author reply 1307-1308.

[32]Bliziotes M, Sibonga JD, Turner RT, Orwoll E (2006) Periosteal remodeling at the femoral neck in nonhuman primates. *J Bone Miner Res 21*:1060-1067.

[33]Ahlborg HG, Johnell O, Turner CH, Rannevik G, Karlsson MK (2003) Bone loss and bone size after menopause. *N Engl J Med 349*:327-334.

[34]Szulc P, Seeman E, Duboeuf F, Sornay-Rendu E, Delmas PD (2006) Bone fragility: failure of periosteal apposition to compensate for increased endocortical resorption in postmenopausal women. *J Bone Miner Res 21*:1856-1863.

[35]Cho SW, Lim SH, Kim IK, Hong YS, Kim SS, Yoo KJ, Park HY, Jang Y, Chang BC, Choi CY, Hwang KC, Kim BS (2005) Small-diameter blood vessels engineered with bone marrow-derived cells. *Ann Surg 241*:506-515.

[36]Nakagawa M, Kaneda T, Arakawa T, Morita S, Sato T, Yomada T, Hanada K, Kumegawa M, Hakeda Y (2000) Vascular endothelial growth factor (VEGF) directly enhances osteoclastic bone resorption and survival of mature osteoclasts. *FEBS Lett 473*:161-164.

[37]Peng H, Usas A, Olshanski A, Ho AM, Gearhart B, Cooper GM, Huard J (2005) VEGF improves, whereas sFlt1 inhibits, BMP2-induced bone formation and bone healing through modulation of angiogenesis. *J Bone Miner Res 20*:2017-2027.

[38]de Souza RL, Pitsillides AA, Lanyon LE, Skerry TM, Chenu C (2005) Sympathetic nervous system does not mediate the load-induced cortical new bone formation. *J Bone Miner Res 20*:2159-2168.

[39]Sherman BE, Chole RA (2000) Sympathectomy, which induces membranous bone remodeling, has no effect on endochondral long bone remodeling in vivo. *J Bone Miner Res 15*:1354-1360.

[40]Cherruau M, Morvan FO, Schirar A, Saffar JL (2003) Chemical sympathectomy-induced changes in TH-, VIP-, and CGRP-immunoreactive fibers in the rat mandible periosteum: influence on bone resorption. *J Cell Physiol 194*:341-348.

[41]Imai S, Matsusue Y (2002) Neuronal regulation of bone metabolism and anabolism: calcitonin gene-related peptide-, substance P-, and tyrosine hydroxylase-containing nerves and the bone. *Microsc Res Tech 58*:61-69.

In: Osteoporosis: Etiology, Diagnosis and Treatment
Editors: Bilar E. Mattingly and Albert C. Pillare
ISBN 978-1-60692-397-9

Chapter 12

Bone Quality: Where Should We Be Looking?

***Oran D. Kennedy*[1,2] *and Fergal J. O'Brien*[1,2,*]**
[1]Royal College of Surgeons in Ireland, Dublin 2, Ireland;
[2]Trinity College Dublin, Dublin 2, Ireland.

Abstract

Osteoporosis is known as the 'silent epidemic' due to the asymptomatic nature of the disease, prior to fracture. It is estimated that by 2020, half of all US citizens over the age of 50 will be at risk of fracture from osteoporosis if no immediate action is taken by individuals at risk, healthcare professionals, health systems and policy makers. In the US, caring for individuals with osteoporotic bone fractures costs $18 billion per annum in direct medical costs. With the global population aging rapidly, these costs will affect increasing numbers of people. Early diagnosis has the potential to substantially reduce the social and economic costs associated with this disease.

The current clinical gold standard in non-invasive bone evaluation is dual energy X-ray absorptiometry (DEXA) scanning. This technique measures areal bone mineral density (aBMD) which is a 2D parameter, whereas in reality BMD is a 3D phenomenon. This, obviously, leads to limitations in the usefulness of this measurement with respect to fracture prediction. Some have gone so far as to say that DEXA-measured in vivo BMD methodologies are intrinsically flawed and represent a misleading indicator of bone mineral status and is an erroneous gauge of relative fracture risk (Bolotin, 2007).

The mechanical properties of bone are in fact determined not only by bone mass but also by bone quality, the parameters of which include the overall shape, internal microarchitecture, mineralization and microdamage within the tissue. Bone turnover is the metabolic process which underlies all of these parameters and is important in several ways to the understanding of osteoporosis. It mediates the effects of all of the skeletal

* Correspondence concerning this article should be addressed to: Prof. Fergal J. O'Brien, Department of Anatomy, Royal College of Surgeons, 123, St Stephen's Green, Dublin 2, Ireland. Phone: +353 1 4022149; Fax: +353 1 4022355; E-mail: fjobrien@rcsi.ie.

stimuli; endocrine, nutritional and mechanical. Although turnover is a key aspect of bone physiology, very little is known about it, particularly in terms of how site-specific variations can affect local mechanical properties and overall fracture risk.

This paper addresses some of the issues relating to parameters of bone quality, specifically bone turnover and microdamage and their relationship to local mechanical properties. The clinical relevance of these issues is also addressed, particularly in relation to the use of bisphosphonates in osteoporosis therapy.

Introduction

Bone is an extraordinary dynamically adaptable material which is in a continual state of remodelling in order to conform to its function. It is this 'form-function' relationship that is the key to understanding the material properties and behaviour of bone (Katz, 1980). Human beings tend to remodel their skeleton to a greater extent than most other mammals and, unlike in other animals, remodelling activity increases with age (Currey, 1984).

Humans are unique among mammals in a more obvious way, in that we walk on our extended hind limbs. No other mammalian species, save our immediate ancestors, has experimented with this method of locomotion. Modern humans have, obviously, gained many advantages over other species since we began to walk upright. However, associated with the transition to bipedality are a host of musculoskeletal injuries and ailments that do not plague other mammals as often, such as; fractured hips and vertebrae, stress fractures, fallen arches, hernias, torn menisci, shin splints, spondylolysis, scoliosis and kyphosis – to name but a few (Latimer, 2005). It is possible that the uniquely high level of remodelling found in humans is a compensatory mechanism related to the uniquely different, and demanding, loading environment to which we subject our skeleton.

Bone Types

Bone tissue can be categorised morphologically into two distinct groups; compact and trabecular. Compact bone is, as the name suggests, a compacted and stiff material with a relatively low porosity. Trabecular bone is a more porous structure comprised of small struts and plates called trabeculae. These two types can be classified on the basis of porosity and the unit microstructure. Cortical bone has a porosity ranging between 5% and 10% while the porosity of trabecular bone ranges from 50% to 90%. The unit microstructure of these tissue types are the osteon and trabeculum, respectively. At the tissue level, it is thought that the two bone types are identical.

Compact bone forms the shaft of long bones and the cortices or outer shell of other bones. The outer surface is called the periosteal surface while the inner is called the endosteal. The predominant microstructural features of mature compact bone are Haversian systems, which were first identified by Clopton Havers in 1691 (Cohen & Harris, 1958). They contain blood vessels which are surrounded by concentric layers (or lamellae) of well organised bone tissue. The structure, including the central blood vessel and surrounding concentric bone tissue, is called an osteon. Typically, an osteon has a diameter of 150-200μm.

Trabecular bone (also known as cancellous or spongy bone) has a porous structure consisting of 'rod' or 'plate-like' struts called trabeculae each strut and plate is composed primarily of lamellar bone and occasionally trabecular plates made up of osteonal bone can be found. Trabecular bone is found in the medullary cavity of flat and short bones, and in the epiphysis and metaphysis of long bones. The microarchitecture of trabecular bone appears random, however the connections and orientation of trabeculae are found to have precise patterns which are thought to be related to the specific mechanical properties of the bone. The structure of the trabecular bone network in the femoral head and neck is classically put forward as an example of the correlation between the orientation of the trabeculae and the distribution of the principal forces during load bearing; this is known as the stress trajectoral theory.

REMODELLING

The fundamental ideas on which much orthopaedic research is based date back to the early scientists. One of the recurring arguments of Aristotle, the Greek philosopher who lived in the 4th century BC, was that the form (of, for instance, an animal) is determined by its ultimate function or 'telos'. Julius Wolff and Wilhelm Roux further developed this idea in the area of bone mechanics in the late 19th century. The law that describes the relationship between the structure and function of bone is named after the former and is known as Wolff's Law (Wolff, 1892).

Wolff's Law states that 'every change in the form and the function of a bone, or in its function alone, is followed by certain definite changes in its internal architecture and secondary alterations in its external conformation'. In simple terms, the law states that mechanical stress is responsible for determining the internal architecture of bone (Forwood et al., 1995). This law outlines what is arguably the most important factor in bone mechanics – the phenomenon of remodelling (Figure 1). Remodelling of bone occurs in response to physical stresses, or lack of them – in that bone is deposited at sites which are subjected to stress and resorbed from sites where there is little stress (Salter R, 1970). Examples of the phenomenon of remodelling can be found in everyday life, in particular in the sporting field. Young soccer players have been found to have a larger bone mass compared with non-players, the soccer players had significantly higher BMD of the total body (2.7%), lumbar spine (6.1%), and the dominant and nondominant hip. The largest increases were found in the femoral greater trochanter on both sides (dominant, 16.5%, nondominant, 14.8%) (Soderman et al., 2000). It was also shown that the playing arm in adult tennis players had thickened trabeculae compared to non-players (Ashizawa et al., 1999). At the opposite end of the scale remodelling is also at work, studies on space flights lasting more than 12 months have shown that due to weightlessness, astronauts on long missions may lose as much as 20% of their bone mass (Turner et al., 1995).

Osteoporosis and Bone Quality

Osteoporosis can be defined as 'a skeletal disorder characterized by compromised bone strength predisposing a person to an increased risk of fractures. Bone strength primarily reflects the integration of bone mineral density (BMD) and bone quality (Klibanski A, 2001). In clinical practice, dual energy X-ray absorptiometry (DEXA) scanning is the most common way of measuring BMD levels and is the current gold standard for diagnosing and monitoring osteoporosis. 'Normal' bone density is considered to be that of a healthy young adult. In DEXA scanning terms the method of comparing individual BMD measurements to the normal is called the 'T-score' system. A T-score is a measurement expressed in standard deviation units from a given mean, equal to a patient's bone mineral density measurement by DEXA minus the value in a young healthy person, divided by the standard deviation of the measurement in the population. A T-score of –1.0 or higher is considered to be in the normal healthy range. A score between –1.0 and –2.5 means that BMD is borderline for osteoporosis, this condition is called osteopenia. A score of –2.5 or more indicates osteoporosis and is associated with increased fracture risk. BMD is calculated as the mass of mineral per unit area and is normally quoted as 'areal density', this is a 2-D measurement of a 3-D property and as such it is thought to be a limiting factor for this technique. Currently, there is no accurate clinical measurement of overall bone strength *in vivo*. A study by Rice et al (1988) carried out statistical analyses of pooled data from a number of experiments, which had examined the Young's moduli and strength of cancellous bone tissue, and concluded that BMD accounts for approximately 60-70% of strength, and thus can be considered a proxy measurement. Bone quality is thought to account for the remainder.

The term osteoporosis was first used by the French pathologist Lobstein in the 1820s but it was not until 1940s when the American endocrinologist Fuller Albright defined the clinical syndrome of the disease (Reifenstein & Albright, 1947). Since then, and particularly in the last 15 years, there have been major developments in our understanding of the etiology and pathophysiology of osteoporosis. Estimates were made in the mid 1990s of the prevalence of osteoporosis based on measurements using DEXA and the World Health Organisation (WHO) classification criteria. Results suggested that 30% of postmenopausal Caucasian women have osteoporosis at the hip lumbar spine or mid-radius (Melton, 1995). This number is set to rise with the world's increasing elderly population. In the year 2000 there were an estimated 9 million osteoporotic fractures globally, of which 1.6 million were at the hip, 1.7 million at the forearm and 1.4 million were clinical vertebral fractures. The greatest number of osteoporotic fractures occurred in Europe (34.8%). World-wide, osteoporotic fractures accounted for 0.83% of the global burden of non-communicable disease and were 1.75% of the global burden in Europe (Johnell & Kanis, 2006). Thus, it is clear that a better understanding of the pathophysiology of osteoporosis, specifically the parameters that affect bone quality, is essential on order to develop better tools for diagnosis and treatment of the disease.

Bone quality is a primary contributor to bone strength. Although a precise definition of bone quality remains elusive, characteristics other than BMD such as bone turnover, microarchitecture and mineralisation of the bone matrix are important factors in the pathophysiology of osteoporosis and the mechanisms that underlie fracture (Bouxsein, 2003).

Clinical trials have shown that the risk of fracture in a 75 year old woman is 4-7 times that of a 45 year old woman with an identical bone mass (Hui et al., 1988).

It has also been shown, that after therapeutic intervention, the resulting changes in BMD explain only a small proportion of the variance in fracture risk. Often in these cases the reductions in fracture risk are evident long before changes in BMD are observed (Bouxsein, 2003). The most common clinical treatment for osteoporosis is the use of a group of anti-resorptive agents (also known as anti-catabolic agents) called bisphosphonates. These act by reducing the osteoclast's ability to adhere to the bone surface, which suppresses the resorption phase of the remodelling cycle, thus preserving bone mass. Recent observations have shown that different bisphosphonates can have up to a 7-fold difference in their effect on maintaining BMD and yet have about the same fracture prevention efficacy (Burr, 2004); further discussion on this topic is presented later in this chapter. The importance of bone quality in determining fracture risk is such that some researchers believe that bone fragility is the disease and osteoporosis is just one risk factor (Riggs & Parfitt, 2005).

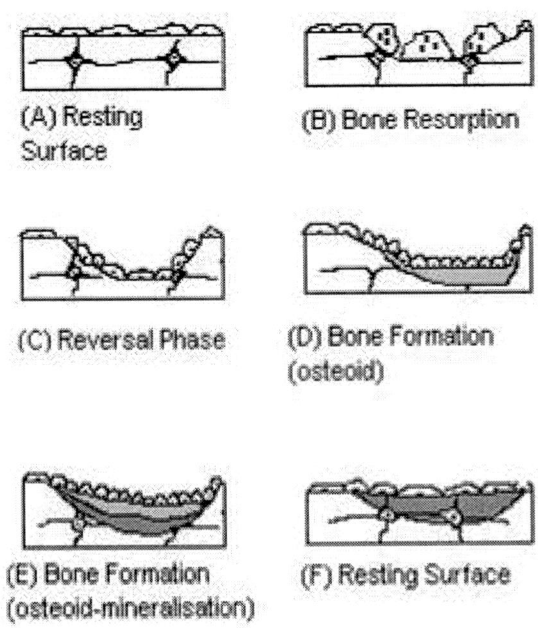

Figure 1. Schematic of the 6 major steps in the bone remodelling cycle. Each remodelling process is initiated by activation at a resting surface (A) by which osteoblastic lineage cells start to secrete collagenase which removes the thin layer of unmineralised bone typical of a resting bone surface. This exposes the mineralised bone underneath to the multinucleated mobile, osteoclasts. During osteoclastic bone resorption (B), Howship's lacunae are excavated to a maximum depth of 50-60 μm. A short reversal phase, where the cement line is formed (C). Then bone formation begins (D). Osteoblasts produce osteoid at a rate of 0.5-1.0 μm per day. When the osteoid thickness has reached approximately 12-15 μm, mineralisation begins from the bottom (mineralisation front) (E). At the termination of each remodelling process, the bone surface is again covered by an extremely thin layer of non-mineralised bone and a layer of flat lining cells. The bone is again converted into a resting surface (F). Adapted from reference (Moskilde, 1999).

BONE TURNOVER

The rate of bone turnover is one important parameter which can affect bone quality. The bone turnover cycle begins with activation of osteoclasts and their precursors to carry out bone resorption (Figure 1). Matrix components such as Transformation Growth Factor (TGF)-beta, Insulin-like Growth Factor (IGF)-I, collagen, osteocalcin and other protein and mineral components, are then released into the micro-environment. Growth factors released by resorption contribute to the recruitment of new osteoblasts to the bone surface, which begin the process of collagen synthesis and biomineralisation. In healthy adults, as many as two million remodelling sites may be active at any given time, and it is estimated that nearly one quarter of all trabecular bone is remodelled each year (Rosen, 2000). In general, resorption takes only 10-13 days, while formation is much slower and can take up to three months. Under ideal circumstances, the amount of bone resorbed equals the amount reformed, however in the case of osteoporosis more bone is resorbed than formed, resulting in a net loss of bone.

Previous studies have shown that bone turnover has a direct influence on fracture risk (Riggs & Melton, 2002). Increased bone turnover accelerates osteoclast resorption i.e. removal of old or damaged bone. Theoretical and experimental evidence has shown that the microdamage caused by repetitive stresses can stimulate bone remodelling (Martin & Burr, 1982; Martin, 2000; Lee et al., 2002). The exact mechanism by which microcracks could influence remodelling is still unknown; however, as far back as 1973, Frost proposed that the disruption of canalicular connections by microcracks crossing them may provide the stimulus to initiate remodelling. In more recent times, there is evidence to suggest that microcrack growth may lead to osteocyte apoptosis and that this is one of the targeting mechanisms for remodelling (Noble et al., 1997; Verborgt et al., 2000; Hazenberg et al., 2007).

In trabecular bone, increased osteoclastic resorption on the surface of the trabeculae can reduce their resistance to buckling and increase the risk of failure. It has been shown that a 50% reduction in bone turnover can result in a 4-fold reduction in trabecular perforation (Parfitt, 2002). In compact bone, accelerated turnover affects bone quality in a number of ways. Firstly, highly mineralised bone is removed and replaced with younger bone which contains less mineral, and so reduces the material stiffness (Kennedy et al, 2009). Secondly, the presence of more resorption sites creates more potential stress concentrations that predispose bone to microdamage. Thirdly, increased remodelling impairs isomerisation and maturation of collagen, which increases the fragility of bone (Garnero et al., 2002); Seeman & Delmas, 2006). There are still aspects of bone turnover which are not well understood. For example, it is not known how bone strength changes in relation to the rate of bone turnover, or how high bone turnover affects microdamage behaviour, some of these issues will be addressed later in this chapter. In summary, the biomechanical link into the bone turnover paradigm is still unclear.

The microarchitecture of bone tissue has a substantial impact on the quality of bone, and thus its strength. Trabecular bone that is more 'plate-like', with thicker and more trabeculae, enhances strength. Trabecular architecture that is more isotropic i.e. having similar mechanical properties in all directions may lower fracture risk further (Burr, 2004). Similarly, in cortical bone when porosity in the cortex is increased via longitudinal tunnelling of osteoclasts, the structural integrity is compromised (Hirano et al., 1999) (Burr et al., 2001). Clinical studies have shown that postmenopausal osteoporosis is characterised by loss of trabecular bone mass and connectivity as well as thinning of the cortical bone (Mosekilde, 1989).

Trabecular bone strength and stiffness are related to the connectivity and orientation of the trabeculae (Goulet et al., 1994). An equivalent amount of bone distributed as widely separated, disconnected thick trabeculae is biomechanically less competent than when arranged as more numerous, better connected, thinner trabeculae. Increased connectivity reduces the unsupported length of trabecular struts; increasing connectivity is crucial as strut strength is related inversely to the square of the unsupported length (Carter & Hayes, 1977). Euler's theorem states that, in general terms, the strength of a vertical trabeculum is inversely proportional to the square of its effective length. In a study of the effect of mass changes on trabecular bone, it was found that bone loss due to reduced trabecular number had a substantially larger impact on strength than an equal mass loss due to trabecular thinning (Guo & Kim, 2002). Therefore, for preventative therapies to be most effective they should not only possess attributes that will preserve bone mass, but also preserve trabecular connectivity.

In cortical bone, the primary structural feature which affects bone strength is the porosity. Small increases in porosity lead to disproportionately large reductions in bone strength (Turner, 2002). The distribution of pores is also an important factor in determining the effect on strength. In long bones, pores in the endocortex have less of an impact on strength than pores near the outer surface due to the higher stresses, particularly in bending, which can be present at the periosteal surface. In humans younger than 60 years, pore number and size were observed to increase with age, whereas in people over the age of 60 there continues to be increase in pore size but a decrease in pore number as the pores begin to coalesce. This is the case in osteoporosis.

In a study carried out by Waarsing et al (2004), micro computed tomography (μ-CT) technology was used to monitor spatial and temporal bone loss due to aging and ovariectomy (OVX) in the tibiae of rats. During the first year post-OVX, the tibiae of the animals were scanned at various time points using an *in vivo* μ-CT scanner. Volume fraction (BV/TV), direct trabecular thickness (TbTh), structural model index (SMI) and connectivity density (CD) were measured in an attempt to assess the effect of microarchitecture on bone quality. After 14 weeks BV/TV had decreased by 53% in OVX animals. Trabecular number was also reduced as a result of OVX, however, the remaining trabeculae increased in thickness from 139 to 153μm and in some cases complete new trabecular structures were formed. This is thought to occur so that the remaining trabeculae, that are not lost due to the disease, are optimally designed to withstand the habitual loading environment, however they would not respond well to non-habitual loading such as those produced during impact. Thus it is clear that assessing the microarchitecture of bone is an important consideration in terms of the strength of the structure.

In a study by the authors (Kennedy et al, 2009), the effects of increased bone turnover on compact bone mechanical and material properties were studied in an OVX sheep model. High turnover was modelled using OVX to induce surgical menopause in sheep. This study monitored intracortical remodelling, resorption cavity number and porosity, and measured any associated changes in bone biomechanical properties. Intravenous fluorochrome dyes were injected intravenously at five time-points over 12 months post-OVX to label sites of bone turnover. Bone turnover, as measured by labelled osteon density, was increased in the OVX group relative to normal sheep at 6, 9 and 12 months ($p<0.05$) (Figure 2). Resorption was also higher in the OVX group at 12 months ($p<0.05$). Furthermore, porosity was significantly increased in the OVX group at 12 months ($p<0.05$). While ultimate compressive strength and work to fracture did not differ between groups, stiffness and yield strength were reduced in the OVX group compared to controls ($p=0.05$). These findings provided new insights into the role that bone turnover plays in the progression of osteoporosis and the effect that is has on material and microstructural properties.

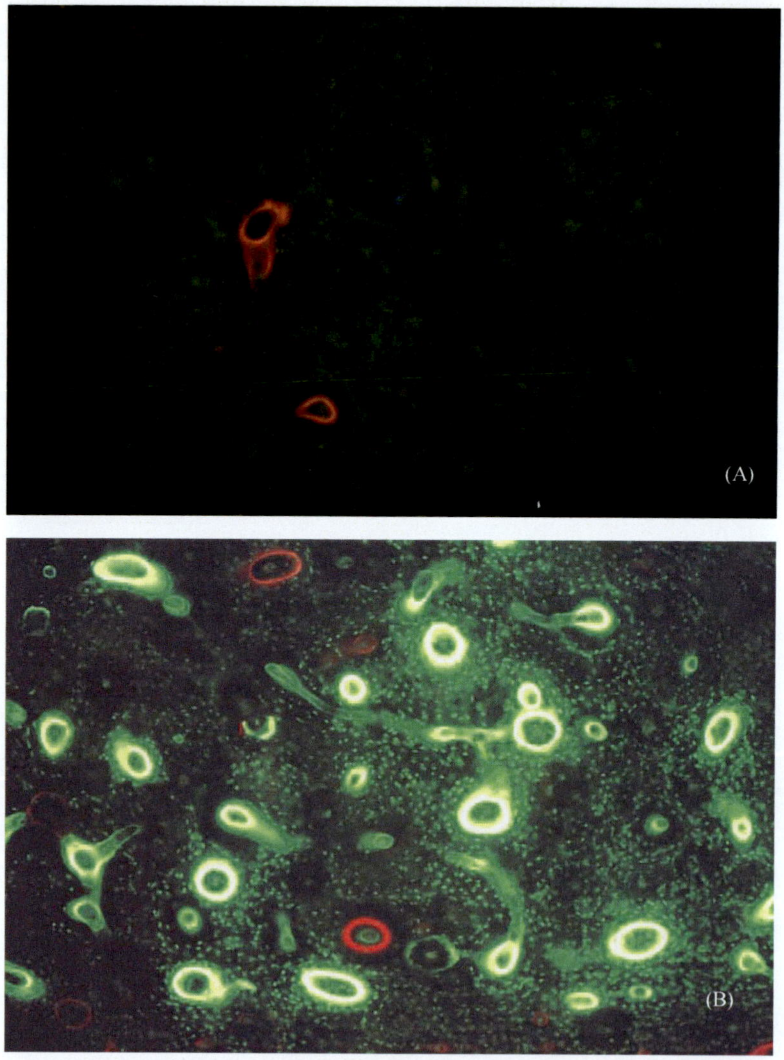

Figure 2. Histological images of bone with (A) low intracortical turnover and (B) high intracortical turnover, induced by OVX. The fluorochrome dyes which were injected intravenously to label newly formed osteons which can then be detected using UV epifluorescence microscopy.

MICRODAMAGE

It has been shown that microdamage accumulates in athletes and military recruits who experience increased rates and magnitudes of loading (Meurman & Elfving, 1980) and that microdamage accumulation reduces bone strength, stiffness and toughness (Burr, 1997). The balance between damage and repair is an important one and can be upset by increased damage creation or deficient repair. An imbalance in remodelling may cause microdamage to accumulate in the elderly (Schaffler et al., 1995; Norman & Wang, 1997; Zioupos, 2001) and could contribute to osteoporotic fractures. While no direct clinical data are available at present on microdamage accumulation in osteoporosis, recent research has shown an association between low BMD and aging in bisphosphonate-treated patients. The association between bisphosphonates and microdamage is an important one, and is discussed in more detail later in this chapter.

Microcracks have also been observed in bone *in vitro* due to fatigue loading (Figure 3). They can be classified as either individual cracks which are approximately 100μm in length, or diffuse damage which consists of a collection of small cracks which are between 2-10μm long and are oriented roughly along the loading direction (O'Brien et al., 2005). It has been shown in many studies that the majority of microcracks are found in interstitial bone (Frost, 1960; Burr et al., 1997; Lee et al., 1998). Interstitial bone tends to have a higher microdamage burden because it is comparatively older than the surrounding bone. Also, the degree of mineralisation in interstitial bone is normally relatively high, which allows microcracks to propagate easily. Histological measurements of microcracks have shown that when viewed along the longitudinal axis of the bone cracks are significantly longer than when they are viewed transversely in the bone (O'Brien et al., 2003). This is intuitively correct as the cracks in any material will preferentially travel along the path of least resistance with the 'grain' of the material (O'Brien et al., 2005).

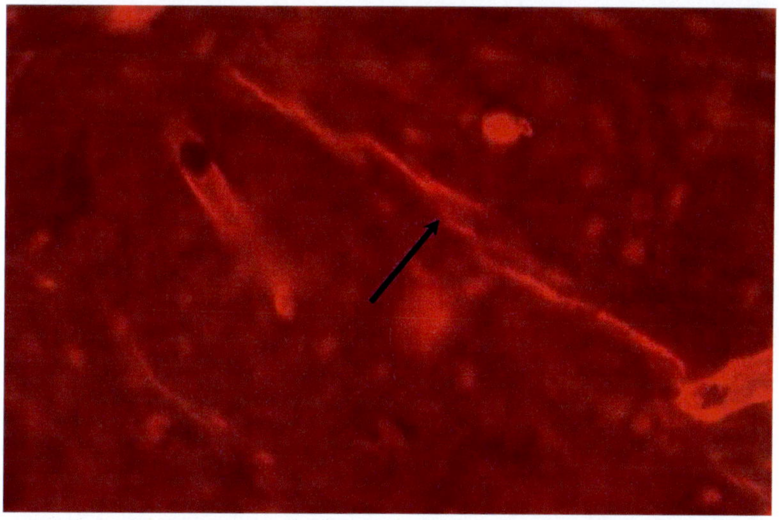

Figure 3. Histological image of a microcrack in ovine compact bone, which was induced by fatigue loading. Microdamage was analysed using UV epifluorescence microscopy by the authors.

Dai et al (2004) investigated microdamage in rats and attempted to evaluate the potential of microcracks as a measure of bone quality. Ninety rats were ovariectomised and drug treated with 17β–estradiol (EST) at 10μm/kg per day, or sham operated (sham). Compressive mechanical tests were performed on the L5 vertebral body and the maximum load required for failure (ML) and the elastic modulus of the specimen (EM) were determined. Microcrack density (CrDn; which is the number of cracks found per area measured), and microcrack surface density (CrSDn; which is the total crack length per area measured) of the adjacent L4 vertebra were determined from histological analyses. At week 21 post surgery the OVX rats showed greater CrDn and CrSDn and lower ML and EM values than both EST and sham rats. CrDn values in sham, EST and OVX rats were 0.55±0.10, 0.69±0.11 and 1.32±0.27 (#/mm^2), while CrSDn values were 26.55±4.7, 33.69±5.7 and 61.28±11.73 (μm/mm^2), respectively. Their findings showed a positive correlation between microcrack accumulation and reduction in elastic modulus and bone strength.

The behaviour of microdamage in relation to microstructural features is an important issue in relation to tissue structural properties. Recently, a study by Kennedy et al (2008) investigated how crack behaviour in areas of increased intracortical remodeling in ovine OVX and normal bone. It was hypothesized that osteon age would influence microcrack behaviour during propagation. Five fluorochrome dyes were used in this study to label sites of bone turnover. Compact bone samples were cyclically loaded to failure and then histological analyses were carried out. Figure 3 shows an example of a microcrack from this study. While numerical crack density (Cr.Dn) was not different between normal and OVX sheep, the former displayed a higher crack surface density (Cr.S.Dn) compared with OVX animals ($p<0.05$). Cracks were categorized by length into three groups; short (<100μm), intermediate (100-300μm) and long (>300μm). The behaviour of short cracks did not differ between old and new osteons, but intermediate and long cracks preferentially stopped at newer osteons compared with older ones ($p<0.05$). It may be concluded from this study that recently formed secondary osteons have a unique influence on propagating microcracks compared with older osteons as they are more likely to act as barriers to microcrack propagation to critical lengths. Therefore localised remodeling levels should be considered when studying microcrack behaviour in bone.

Noble et al (1997) were among the first to show that apoptosis could occur in osteocytes due to mechanical stresses and they also proposed that osteocyte apoptosis might be involved in bone remodelling. Although experimental observations have been made of cell apoptosis near microdamage, a direct link between cracks and cell death has not been found to date (Schaffler et al., 1995; Verborgt et al., 2000). Two popular hypotheses that exist are that cracks may cause apoptosis by the rupturing of osteocytic cell processes (Hazenberg et al., 2007) or that they may serve to shield cells from local strain (Prendergast & Huiskes, 1996), limiting the exchange of nutrients and waste thus affecting cell homeostasis. Considering the above data, it can be said that microcracks, in addition to the other factors discussed in this chapter, are a useful and important parameter for assessing bone quality in osteoporosis. However, there is still much that remains unknown about microdamage such as how its behaviour changes in areas of high bone turnover and also how microcracks behave in bone which has undergone long term treatment with anti-resorptive drugs which are commonly used to treat osteoposis.

BISPHOSPHONATE THERAPY IN OSTEOPOROSIS

Bisphosphonates inhibit resorption of bone which occurs as part of the remodelling process. This action counters the loss of bone mass which is the major feature of osteoporosis. The exact relationship between the amount of mineral per unit volume of bone and its material properties are not very well characterised at present. Increasing the amount of mineral will increase stiffness but will decrease the flexibility of the bone and both of these factors play a role in fracture resistance. The amount of energy that can be absorbed by a bone before fracture is reduced by increasing the mineralisation of the bone tissue (Currey et al., 1996). Suppression of osteoclastic activity, which is the mechanism of action of bisphosphonates in the treatment of osteoporosis, has the effect of increasing tissue mineralisation by lengthening the period of time over which secondary mineralisation can occur (Meunier & Boivin, 1997; Nuzzo et al., 2002). This has two effects; firstly, it may increase the tendency for microcracks to initiate by making the material more brittle. Secondly, it increases the homogeneity of the tissue and this may make crack propagation easier. When bone turnover is high, mineralisation is lower due to the reduced mineralisation period and this also has an adverse effect on bone strength as discussed earlier in this chapter.

'First generation' bisphosphonates such as etidronate were shown to increase BMD in the spine, hip and other clinically relevant sites but were found to adversely effect bone mineralisation and cause osteomalacia over time (Sparidans et al., 1998). 'Second generation' bisphosphonates such as alendronate are approximately 1000 times more potent than etidronate and were also found to increase BMD at all sites studied and reduce clinical fractures by 36% in women with baseline osteoporosis at the femoral neck (Cummings et al., 1995).

Zoledronic acid is a 'third generation' bisphosphonate and is the most potent bisphosphonate studied in clinical trials to date (Reid et al., 2002). It has been shown to be more than four orders of magnitude more potent than earlier bisphosphonates such as clodronate or etidronate (Green, 2002). Zoledronic acid has the added advantage of its efficacy being dependent on total cumulative dose, rather than the dosage schedule. In a study by Reid et al. (2002), 351 postmenopausal women with low BMD were treated with zolendronic acid on five different dosing regimens, 0.25mg, 0.5mg or 1mg at three month intervals, a total annual dose of 4mg as a single dose and two doses of 2mg each, six months apart. There were similar increases of approximately 5% in BMD in all the zolendronic acid groups showing that the determining factor of the efficacy of this drug is the total cumulative dose. This effect was found even over relatively large dosing intervals of up to one year.

However, these results may not be as positive as they may seem. Bisphosphonates inhibit resorption of bone which occurs as part of the remodelling process. The purpose of this action is to prevent bone loss, and bisphosphonates are generally very effective in this regard. However, by inhibiting the process of remodelling it is possible that damage which would otherwise have been repaired by the remodelling process is allowed to accumulate. Hirano et al. (2000) investigated the effect of high dose etidronate on the mechanical properties of bone and microdamage accumulation. Skeletally mature beagles were injected with a saline vehicle or etidronate at 0.5 mg/kg/day or 5mg/kg/day for one year. After sacrifice bones were removed for analysis and fractures of ribs and/or thoracic spinous processes were found in 10 of 11 animals treated with the higher dose etidronate. One fracture of a spinous process was found in the low dose and none in the control group. Biomechanical testing showed reduced strength in the ribs and lumbar vertebrae in the high dose group, while histomorphometric analysis showed a significant reduction in bone turnover in the high and low treatment groups. In the high dose group, the activation frequency was reduced to zero in both compact and trabecular bone. Interestingly, the microcrack numerical density (CrDn) increased significantly in the high dose group in the lumbar vertebrae but not in the ribs or spinous processes where fractures occurred. This was most likely the result of excessive amounts of unmineralised bone, and this may explain the occurrence of spontaneous fracture and the absence of microdamage.

A study by Mashiba et al. (2001) demonstrated increased microdamage accumulation following 12 months treatment with oral bisphosphonates. Thirty-six female beagles, 1-2 years old, were divided into three groups. The control group was treated with a saline vehicle and the remaining two groups were treated daily with either risedronate (0.5 mg/kg/day) or alendronate (1.0mg/kg/day). One year of treatment with bisphosphonates significantly suppressed trabecular remodelling in vertebrae (90% risedronate, 95% alendronate) and the ilium (76% risedronate, 90% alendronate) and significantly increased microdamage accumulation in all skeletal sites measured. Trabecular bone volume and vertebral strength increased following 12 months of treatment with bisphosphonates, however, it was demonstrated that the normalised toughness was reduced by 21% in both bisphosphonate treated groups. This study showed that suppression of bone turnover by high doses of bisphosphonates may be associated with significantly increased microdamage accumulation and a reduction in the toughness of the vertebrae.

CONCLUSION

It is quite clear that osteoporosis is a growing concern in our society, as life expectancy for the world's population increases. It is also clear that in order to accurately determine fracture risk; the tools that are currently used to diagnose osteoporosis must be combined with other considerations in order to account for bone quality. Some of the other parameters which were discussed in this review were microarchitecture, mineralization and in particular bone turnover and microdamage. A broader understanding of these phenomena is necessary to provide better pre-fracture evaluations of tissue quality and to continue developing therapies that will effectively counteract the effects of musculoskeletal disease.

REFERENCES

Ashizawa N, Nonaka K, Michikami S, et al. (1999) Tomographical description of tennis-loaded radius: reciprocal relation between bone size and volumetric BMD. *J Appl Physiol 86*, 1347-51.

Bolotin HH (2007) DXA in vivo BMD methodology: an erroneous and misleading research and clinical gauge of bone mineral status, bone fragility, and bone remodelling. *Bone 41*, 138-54.

Bouxsein ML (2003) Bone quality: where do we go from here? *Osteoporos Int 14* Suppl 5, 118-27.

Burr DB (1997) Bone, exercise, and stress fractures. *Exerc Sport Sci Rev 25*, 171-94.

Burr DB (2004) Bone quality: understanding what matters. *J Musculoskelet Neuronal Interact 4*, 184-6.

Burr DB, Forwood MR, Fyhrie DP, Martin RB, Schaffler MB, Turner CH (1997) Bone microdamage and skeletal fragility in osteoporotic and stress fractures. *J Bone Miner Res 12*, 6-15.

Burr DB, Hirano T, Turner CH, Hotchkiss C, Brommage R, Hock JM (2001) Intermittently administered human parathyroid hormone(1-34) treatment increases intracortical bone turnover and porosity without reducing bone strength in the humerus of ovariectomized cynomolgus monkeys. *J Bone Miner Res 16*, 157-65.

Carter DR, Hayes WC (1977) Compact bone fatigue damage II: a microscopic examination. *Clin Orthop* 1977, 265-74.

Cohen J, Harris WH (1958) The three-dimensional anatomy of haversian systems. *J Bone Joint Surg Am 40-A*, 419-34.

Cummings SR, Nevitt MC, Browner WS, et al. (1995) Risk factors for hip fracture in white women. Study of Osteoporotic Fractures Research Group. *N Engl J Med 332,* 767-73.

Currey J (1984) *The mechanical adaptations of bones,* Princeton University Press, Princeton.

Currey JD, Brear K, Zioupos P (1996) The effects of ageing and changes in mineral content in degrading the toughness of human femora. *J Biomech 29*, 257-60.

Dai RC, Liao EY, Yang C, Wu XP, Jiang Y (2004) Microcracks: an alternative index for evaluating bone biomechanical quality. *J Bone Miner Metab 22*, 215-23.

Forwood MR, Burr DB, Takano Y, Eastman DF, Smith PN, Schwardt JD (1995) Risedronate treatment does not increase microdamage in the canine femoral neck. *Bone 16*, 643-50.

Frost HM (1960) Presence of microscopic cracks in vivo in bone. *Bull Henry Ford Hospital 8*, 27-35.

Garnero P, Jamin C, Benhamou CL, Pelissier C, Roux C (2002) Effects of tibolone and combined 17beta-estradiol and norethisterone acetate on serum C-reactive protein in healthy post-menopausal women: a randomized trial. *Hum Reprod 17*, 2748-53.

Goulet RW, Goldstein SA, Ciarelli MJ, Kuhn JL, Brown MB, Feldkamp LA (1994) The relationship between the structural and orthogonal compressive properties of trabecular bone. *J Biomech 27*, 375-389.

Green JR (2002) Preclinical pharmacology of zoledronic acid. *Semin Oncol 29*, 3-11.

Guo XE, Kim CH (2002) Mechanical consequence of trabecular bone loss and its treatment: a three-dimensional model simulation. *Bone 30*, 404-11.

Hazenberg JG, Taylor D, Lee TC (2007) The role of osteocytes and bone microstructure in preventing osteoporotic fractures. *Osteoporos Int 18*, 1-8.

Hirano T, Burr DB, Turner CH, Sato M, Cain RL, Hock JM (1999) Anabolic effects of human biosynthetic parathyroid hormone fragment (1-34), LY333334, on remodeling and mechanical properties of cortical bone in rabbits. *J Bone Miner Res 14*, 536-45.

Hirano T, Turner CH, Forwood MR, Johnston CC, Burr DB (2000) Does suppression of bone turnover impair mechanical properties by allowing microdamage accumulation? *Bone 27*, 13-20.

Hui SL, Slemenda CW, Johnston CC, Jr. (1988) Age and bone mass as predictors of fracture in a prospective study. *J Clin Invest 81*, 1804-9.

Johnell O, Kanis JA (2006) An estimate of the worldwide prevalence and disability associated with osteoporotic fractures. *Osteoporos Int 17*, 1726-33.

Katz JL (1980) The structure and biomechanics of bone. *Symp Soc Exp Biol 34*, 137-68.

Kennedy OD, Brennan O, Rackard SM, Staines A, O'Brien FJ, Taylor D and Lee TC (2009) Effects of Ovariectomy on Bone Turnover, Porosity and Biomechanical Properties in Ovine Compact Bone 12-Months Post-Surgery. *J Orthop Res 27(3),* 303-9.

Kennedy OD, Brennan O, Rackard SM, Staines A, O'Brien FJ, Taylor D and Lee TC (2008) The Effects of Increased Intracortical Remodeling on Microcrack Behaviour in Compact Bone. *Bone 43(5)*, 889-93.

Klibanski A BT, Blair SN, Boden SD, Dickersin K, Gifford DR, Glasse L, Goldring SR, Hruska K, Johnson SR, McCauley LK, Russell WE (2001) Osteoporosis prevention, diagnosis, and therapy. *JAMA 285*, 785-95.

Latimer B (2005) The perils of being bipedal. *Ann Biomed Eng 33*, 3-6.

Lee TC, Myers ER, Hayes WC (1998) Fluorescence-aided detection of microdamage in compact bone. *J Anat 193* (Pt 2), 179-84.

Lee TC, Staines A, Taylor D (2002) Bone adaptation to load: microdamage as a stimulus for bone remodelling. *J Anat 201*, 437-46.

Martin RB (2000) Toward a unifying theory of bone remodeling. *Bone 26*, 1-6.

Martin RB, Burr DB (1982) A hypothetical mechanism for the stimulation of osteonal remodelling by fatigue damage. *J Biomech 15*, 137-9.

Mashiba T, Turner CH, Hirano T, Forwood MR, Johnston CC, Burr DB (2001) Effects of suppressed bone turnover by bisphosphonates on microdamage accumulation and biomechanical properties in clinically relevant skeletal sites in beagles. *Bone 28*, 524-31.

Melton LJ (1995) How many women have osteoporosis now? *J Bone Miner Res 10*, 175-177.

Meunier PJ, Boivin G (1997) Bone mineral density reflects bone mass but also the degree of mineralization of bone: therapeutic implications. *Bone 21*, 373-7.

Meurman KO, Elfving S (1980) Stress fracture in soldiers: a multifocal bone disorder. A comparative radiological and scintigraphic study. *Radiology 134*, 483-7.

Mosekilde L (1989) Sex differences in age-related loss of vertebral trabecular bone mass and structure--biomechanical consequences. *Bone 10*, 425-32.

Mosekilde L (1999). Bone Dynamics. www.lab.anhb.uwa.edu.au/mb140 /MoreAbout/bonedynamics.html

Noble BS, Stevens H, Loveridge N, Reeve J (1997) Identification of apoptotic changes in osteocytes in normal and pathological human bone. *Bone 20*, 273-82.

Norman TL, Wang Z (1997) Microdamage of human cortical bone: incidence and morphology in long bones. *Bone 20*, 375-9.

Nuzzo S, Peyrin F, Cloetens P, Baruchel J, Boivin G (2002) Quantification of the degree of mineralization of bone in three dimensions using synchrotron radiation microtomography. *Med Phys 29*, 2672-81.

O'Brien FJ, Taylor D, Clive Lee T (2005) The effect of bone microstructure on the initiation and growth of microcracks. *J Orthop Res 23*, 475-80.

O'Brien FJ, Taylor D, Lee TC (2003) Microcrack accumulation at different intervals during fatigue testing of compact bone. *J Biomech 36*, 973-80.

Parfitt AM (2002) High bone turnover is intrinsically harmful: two paths to a similar conclusion. The Parfitt view. *J Bone Miner Res 17*, 1558-9.

Prendergast PJ, Huiskes R (1996) Microdamage and osteocyte-lacuna strain in bone: a microstructural finite element analysis. *J Biomech Eng 118*, 240-6.

Reid IR, Brown JP, Burckhardt P, et al. (2002) Intravenous zoledronic acid in postmenopausal women with low bone mineral density. *N Engl J Med 346*, 653-61.

Reifenstein EC, Albright F (1947) The Metabolic Effects Of Steroid Hormones In Osteoporosis. *J Clin Invest 26*, 24-56.

Rice JC, Cowin SC, Bowman JA (1988) On the dependence of the elasticity and strength of cancellous bone on apparent density. *J Biomech 21*, 155-168.

Riggs BL, Melton LJ, 3rd (2002) Bone turnover matters: the raloxifene treatment paradox of dramatic decreases in vertebral fractures without commensurate increases in bone density. *J Bone Miner Res 17*, 11-4.

Riggs BL, Parfitt AM (2005) Drugs used to treat osteoporosis: the critical need for a uniform nomenclature based on their action on bone remodeling. *J Bone Miner Res 20,* 177-84.

Rosen CJ (2000) Pathogenesis of osteoporosis. *Baillieres Best Pract Res Clin Endocrinol Metab 14*, 181-93.

Salter R B (1970) *Textbook of Disorders and Injuries of the Musculoskeletal System,* Lippincott Williams and Wilkins.

Schaffler MB, Choi K, Milgrom C (1995) Aging and matrix microdamage accumulation in human compact bone. *Bone 17*, 521-525.

Seeman E, Delmas PD (2006) Bone quality--the material and structural basis of bone strength and fragility. *N Engl J Med 354*, 2250-61.

Soderman K, Bergstrom E, Lorentzon R, Alfredson H (2000) Bone mass and muscle strength in young female soccer players. *Calcif Tissue Int 67*, 297-303.

Sparidans RW, Twiss IM, Talbot S (1998) Bisphosphonates in bone diseases. *Pharm World Sci 20*, 206-13.

Turner CH (2002) Determinants of skeletal fragility and bone quality. *J Musculoskelet Neuronal Interact 2*, 527-8.

Turner RT, Evans GL, Wakley GK (1995) Spaceflight results in depressed cancellous bone formation in rat humeri. *Aviat Space Environ Med 66*, 770-4.

Verborgt O, Gibson GJ, Schaffler MB (2000) Loss of osteocyte integrity in association with microdamage and bone remodeling after fatigue in vivo. *J Bone Miner Res 15*, 60-7.

Waarsing JH, Day JS, van der Linden JC, et al. (2004) Detecting and tracking local changes in the tibiae of individual rats: a novel method to analyse longitudinal in vivo micro-CT data. *Bone 34*, 163-9.

Wolff J (1892) *Das Gesetz der Transformation der Knochen.,* Hirschwald, Berlin.

Zioupos P (2001) Ageing human bone: factors affecting its biomechanical properties and the role of collagen. *J Biomater Appl 15*, 187-229.

In: Osteoporosis: Etiology, Diagnosis and Treatment
Editors: Bilar E. Mattingly and Albert C. Pillare
ISBN 978-1-60692-397-9

Chapter 13

OSTEOPOROSIS AND FRACTURE RISK: NEW PERSPECTIVES FOR EARLY DIAGNOSIS AND TREATMENT ASSESSMENT

Annamaria Zaia
INRCA-Italian National Research Centers on Aging, Italy.

ABSTRACT

Osteoporosis is a major health concern for our growing elderly population. It represents one major health condition accounting for significant morbidity and mortality in postmenopausal women and an emerging health problem even in aging men.

Screening of the population at risk for bone demineralization and treatment of patients to prevent consequent fractures would be useful tools to increase quality of life in the elderly and to lighten the related socio-economic impact.

The most common approach to osteoporosis diagnosis in clinical practice is the estimate of bone mineral content (BMD) by means of dual-energy X-ray absorptiometry (DEXA). However, BMD alone is not a good predictor for fracture risk. From a clinical point of view, bone microarchitecture is an interesting aspect to study and to define patterns of bone alterations with aging and pathology. In fact, microarchitecture seems to be a determinant of bone fragility independent of bone density, and as a result is important to understand the mechanisms of bone fragility as well as the action of the drugs used to prevent osteoporotic fractures.

The rapid diffusion of medical imaging techniques in clinical practice as well as the surprising development of information technologies with an increased power calculation capacity has allowed proliferation of new methods to assess trabecular bone architecture changes with aging and osteoporosis. Recently, magnetic resonance imaging (MRI) has emerged as a means of measuring trabecular bone structure in vivo. Developments in high-resolution MRI techniques have opened up new perspectives for the characterization of trabecular bone architecture by non-invasive non-ionizing methods. However, texture analysis is not frequently used as the interpretation of the large number of calculated parameters is difficult.

A proper combination of medical imaging technique, texture analysis procedure, and mathematical approach to the study of trabecular bone architecture allows the development of computerized methods that, by providing a limited number of parameters sensitive to pathology onset and progression, would speed up their application into clinical practice.

The introduction in the biomedical field of paradigms, such as theory of complexity, chaos, and fractals, suggests new approaches and provides innovative tools to the study of aging phenomena. Taking into account the complexity of living beings and fractal properties of many anatomic and physiologic structures, it is possible to quantify morpho-functional changes with aging and pathology by means of fractal analysis. In this particular context, fractal lacunarity appears the most suitable tool to characterize trabecular bone texture as it is able to describe discontinuity of the bone network as well as sizes of bone marrow spaces, changes of which are an index of increased fracture risk.

INTRODUCTION

Osteoporosis is a major health concern for our growing elderly population (Lau, 2004). It represents one major health condition accounting for significant morbidity and mortality in postmenopausal women and an emerging health problem even in aging men (Gilbert & McKiernan, 2005; Wang et al., 2001). Perimenopausal women still represent the population with the highest risk of early osteoporosis onset. In fact, a physiologic progressive decline of bone mineral content occurs with aging in both women and men after 30 years of age. However, a faster kinetics of bone demineralization characterizes bone degenerative processes during the hormonal changing phase of perimenopausal women (Kiebzak, 1991; Mirza & Prestwood, 2004). The increased lifespan in the industrialized world accounts for the increasing incidence of osteoporosis and bone fractures with a perspective of additional years (at least 20) of disability osteoporotic women have to face in their later life.

For a long time, osteoporosis has been considered exclusively linked to the female gender. On the contrary, men have been believed to be holders of a more robust bone structure, therefore protected against osteoporosis. Nevertheless, despite a lack of well-known critical hormonal changes, responsible for a fast degenerative action on bone tissue, the male structure undergoes a slow progressive loss of bone mass and the risk of being affected by osteoporosis in late age is increasing even in men (Audran et al., 2001; Johnell et al., 2001; Seeman, 2001).

Osteoporosis is characterized by low bone mineral density (BMD), and microarchitectural deterioration of bone tissue with an increased fracture risk. Due to the silent progression of bone structure degeneration, osteoporosis diagnosis often follows a painful fracture event. Till now, only a small percentage of individuals have been known to be osteoporotic while the condition of most pathologic people had remained undiagnosed until a fracture occurs (Elliot-Gibson et al., 2004; Kanis et al., 2005; Solomon et al., 2003). It is worth noting that the first fracture event increases the risk and accelerates the onset of new ones (Lindsay et al., 2001).

Screening of the population at risk for bone demineralization and treatment of patients to prevent consequent fractures would be useful tools to increase quality of life in the elderly. In fact, early diagnosis of bone degenerative processes represents a suitable approach to prevent disability and reduce mortality in osteoporotic patients.

Osteoporosis and Medical Imaging

The most common approach to osteoporosis diagnosis in clinical practice is the estimate of bone mineral content by means of dual-energy X-ray absorptiometry (DEXA). However, BMD alone is not a good predictor for fracture risk (Hough, 1998). Recently, detection of BMD by means of ultrasound techniques has been obtaining more attention as a possible less invasive diagnostic tool for bone degenerative disorders. At present, echographic investigation in clinical practice remains the "alternative" way to assess bone mass only in those subjects who cannot undergo x-ray irradiations. However, quantitative ultrasound detection of bone degeneration is becoming ever more promising and potentially useful mainly in screening studies. This method, in fact, offers advantages over X-ray-based techniques, including low cost, portability, and no ionizing radiation exposure. In addition, it is known that ultrasound transmission depends not only on mineral content, but also on biomechanical properties of the bone, thus providing extremely useful information about bone structure properties. As a matter of fact, recent studies have highlighted that bone parameters measured by quantitative ultrasounds provide information about fracture risk independent of BMD (Bauer et al., 1997; Cheng et al., 1997; Hans et al., 1996; Pinheiro et al., 2003).

From a clinical point of view, microarchitecture is an interesting aspect to study and define patterns of bone alterations with aging and pathology. Microarchitecture seems to be a determinant of bone fragility independent of bone density: the incidence of fractures is not always correlated to diminished BMD (Helgason et al., 2008). In fact, too high of a mineral content could predispose to a higher risk of bone fractures, probably due to an increased rigidity of the structure. Moreover, pharmacological treatment with agents acting by preventing bone mineral content and/or reducing bone loss is not always able to reduce bone fracture risk (Seeman, 2007). Therefore, bone microarchitecture seems to be important to understand the mechanisms of bone fragility as well as the action of the drugs used to prevent osteoporotic fractures (Dalle Carbonare & Giannini, 2004).

For a long time, the unique font of information about bone microarchitecture in humans had been coming from studies on biopsies of bone tissue from autoptic samples. The rapid diffusion of medical imaging techniques in clinical practice as well as the surprising development of information technologies with an increased power calculation capacity has allowed proliferation of new methods to assess trabecular bone architecture changes with aging and osteoporosis. Several processing methods of axial radiographic images (Feltrin et al., 2001; Gregory et al., 2004) and computer tomography, CT, projections (Oka et al., 2002) have been reported as a suitable tool to quantify trabecular bone architecture not only in classical sites at high risk of fracture (spine and femur head) but even in mirror sites such as calcaneus and radius (Cortet et al., 1999; Gordon et al., 1996). Recently, magnetic resonance (MR) imaging has emerged as a means of measuring trabecular bone structure in vivo (Majumdar, 1998; Majumdar et al., 1997). In particular, MR-based diagnosis could be used to complement or even substitute standard BMD methods for assessing osteoporosis and evaluating longitudinal changes. Developments in high-resolution MR imaging techniques have opened up new perspectives for the characterization of trabecular bone architecture by non-invasive non-ionizing methods. However, texture analysis is not frequently used as the interpretation of the large number of calculated parameters is difficult (Boutry et al., 2003). Most methods, in fact, use classical histomorphometric techniques that provide a set of numerous parameters (up to 25) to be analyzed (Boutry et al., 2003; Cortet et al., 2000). A promising approach uses wavelet techniques (Daubechies, 1992). Wavelet analysis is successfully used in functional medical imaging and finds wide application with MR imaging (Bullmore et al., 2004). An always increasing application of wavelet-based texture analysis has been also reported for several biological structures (Faber et al., 2004; Lee et al., 2003). However, the time-cost is too high for a clinical routine application, in spite of attempts to reduce computational charge and speed the methods (Faber et al., 2004).

Recently, a method of MR image analysis has been proposed to provide a limited number of parameters sensitive to bone microarchitecture changes in aging and in pathology onset and progression (Zaia et al., 2005; 2006). It has been built taking into account the complexity of the living being and fractal properties of many anatomic and physiologic structures (Cross, 1997; Lipsitz & Goldberg, 1992; Losa & Nonnenmacher, 1997; Mandelbrot, 1982) and can be seen as a proper combination of medical imaging technique, texture analysis procedure, and mathematical approach to the study of trabecular bone architecture. In fact, it has been built by processing vertebral images obtained by MR imaging Spin-echo techniques. The mathematical solution proposed is one parameter calculated from the simple hyperbola formula that well describes the plot obtained from lacunarity analysis of trabecular network (Zaia et al., 2005).

Before introducing the original method of texture analysis on trabecular bone RM images, a glance at concepts dealing with complex systems and fractals would give insights into the innovative and fruitful approach to the study of aging and related pathologies, among them, osteoporosis.

Biocomplexity, Aging and Pathology

One most relevant aspect of aging populations is represented by the high degree of inter-individual variability. An ever increasing number of people are living longer, however, only a small percentage are aging well. In fact, more than 60% of elderly people experience a pathologic aging, often characterized by co-morbidity (Abate et al., 2007). Heterogeneity of the senescent phenotype has been for a long time considered as an obstacle to understanding "physiologic" aging, therefore making it hard to discriminate from pathological aging in subjects (Brenner & Arndt, 2004).

Sometimes, new ideas can emerge from difficulties and just those aspects considered as the problem(s) suggest more effective approaches. This is what is happening even in the gerontologic field: apparent contradictions, or phenomena apparently unexplainable become understandable in the light of new paradigms. As an example, the variability observed in the longevity phenotype, which creates serious problems of interpretation, can be explained in light of the theory of complexity by considering longevity as a "secondary product" of the evolution of a dynamic nonlinear system.

Due to its "complexity", the topic will be presented, in this context, mainly dealing with the link among several concepts useful to describe the behavior of a biologically complex system in particular, by recalling some basic characteristics and properties of complex systems.

Outline of Complex Systems

Nature is rich in complex shapes and functions, which represents the rule rather than the exception. The science of complexity has been emerging in biomedicine and offers powerful tools to study and analyze the global behavior of biologically complex systems. Complex systems are made up of a considerable number of sub-systems with various different mutual interactions; their global behavior results from all such interactions; they are characterized by a great number of freedom degrees in space and time; they are dissipative and nonlinear systems. Complex systems show a global emerging behavior: macro- cannot be inferred from micro-properties of single behaviors separately considered, rather they emerge from the interactions of local dynamics. Emerging global organization of a complex system occurs without a main controller, on the contrary, there is a self-organization, that is a spontaneous emerging of a global order (Flood & Carson, 1993).

One most remarkable feature of complex systems deals with nonlinearity and it is worth noting that most systems in nature are nonlinear (Kiriazis, 2003). In linear systems, little perturbations cause light reactions, great perturbations cause strong reactions. This is not the case of nonlinear systems where little perturbations induce no response, or a light or strong response, or oscillations, or chaotic behavior, that is a behavior characterized by apparently random dynamics that truly follow well-defined cause-effect laws. The kind of answer depends on the status of the system at the time the perturbation occurs. At certain stati, the so-called bifurcation points, the system can react in an unforeseeable manner, where the same little perturbation can cause completely different dynamics. Another consequence deals with the superposition principle (the whole is equal to the sum of the parts) peculiar to linear systems but not true for nonlinear ones: it follows that properties of nonlinear systems cannot be understood by analyzing single components separately. Therefore, the theory of complexity is completely in contrast with the reductionism approach (seeking the solution to a global behavior of a complex system by analyzing those of single subcomponents).

When a system is in a particular status, sudden changes (transitions of phase) can occur at different levels included among ordered and disordered dynamics. A special transition of phase is represented by the so-called point of criticity, or criticism, at which order and disorder coexist at any scale, at any spatio-temporal level of observation. It is worth noting that the apparent status of the matter can change by changing the scale of observation; as an example, micro-clusters of dishomogeneity can be found when changing the scale of observation from macro to micro. At the criticism point a very intriguing phenomenon can occur: all spatio-temporal properties become scale invariant (self-similarity). A possible basic principle of complexity is given from the concept of self-organized criticism: the system has the ability to evolve spontaneously, without control parameters, toward a critic status. When a complex system is in a status generating dynamic transitions of phase, it is said it enters the chaos bounder region, where there are not specific scales. Dealing with scale characteristics, there exist dynamic structures or processes showing systematic inter-scale correlations and a hierarchical order observable for a significant number of spatial and/or temporal scales (fractal properties) (Goldberger et al., 1990). Self-similarity, peculiar to fractal objects, reflects powerful constraints on the organization of complex systems - constraints which are consequences of a few basic physical, biological and mathematical principles. Structures and processes with self-similar properties over many orders of magnitude provide a means for extrapolating among scales: among large scales of the globe, region, ecosystem, or habitat where ecological relationships appear to be complex, and the small scales of the field or laboratory experiment where hypotheses can be tested and mechanisms can be studied. Most importantly, study of scaling is one powerful way of simplifying ecological complexity and understanding physical and biological principles that regulate biodiversity (Brown et al., 2002).

Aging of Biological Systems as the Temporal Evolution of Nonlinear Dynamic Systems

The high degree of inter-individual heterogeneity, a characteristic always present in any biological phenomenon, is often considered as inconvenient and troublesome. However, if not neglected, it can contribute to avoid interpretative errors of both theoretic and practical relevance. In addition, analysis of variability can become a powerful tool of deeper and wider understanding, or at least, an attempt of understanding biological aging. Therefore, heterogeneity from problem becomes a possible key of interpretation (Piantanelli et al., 2001).

Since few years interest to studies on very advanced ages has been growing. As an example, studies on centenarians, that represent subpopulations undergone selection all lifelong, can provide extremely precious information (Franceschi et al., 1991; 1992; 1995; Mari et al., 1996). Also in this case, we face the "problem" of inter-individual heterogeneity: genetic influence on the variance of the phenotype longevity within a given species appears lower than expected on the basis of the so clear genetic causes on different lifespan of several species (Finch & Tanzi, 1997; Herskind et al., 1996; Johnson, 1985). Environment, instead, with its intrinsic variability, seems to be the most useful aspect to be considered in the attempt to explain the variance observed even in homozygous twins. However, from the analysis of survival kinetics of experimental animals, it emerges that, also in this case, the curve tail shows a clear slowing-down (Carey et al., 1992; Economos, 1982; Piantanelli, 1986). It suggests a high degree of heterogeneity even for those populations made up of subjects with quite similar genetic background and bred under the same environmental conditions. Such a heterogeneity suggests that random fluctuations of genetics-environment interaction strongly affect longevity itself.

Heterogeneity as the Consequence of Complex System Variability

Biological systems, like complex systems, are made up of numerous sub-systems (nervous, cardiovascular, endocrine, ... systems), interacting with each other. Each sub-system is further subdivided into interacting lower components (organs, tissues, ...) and so on at lower levels of organization. They are highly dependent upon initial conditions; thus, in a cohort, even very small differences occurring at certain times can cause higher and higher differences at later ages in most characteristics of individual phenotype. In this view, considering living systems as complex systems (Pettersson, 1996), life trajectories of the various subjects in a population, whatever close at birth, will evolve fluctuating with time, progressively enlarging the variance of their phenotype characteristics, among which longevity. One major feature of complex systems is that of presenting 'emergent behavior', that is, a global behavior that cannot be understood on the basis of the knowledge of their micro-components behavior. Thus, even in the presence of genetically homogeneous backgrounds, inter-individual variability is always present independently of how large environmental changes are.

We have seen as biological systems, human beings in particular, can be considered complex systems and how the laws of chaos can be called in cause to explain their evolution, from development to maintenance of "homeostatic" dynamic equilibrium of all their integrated functions as an adaptive response to continuous noxae from both endogenous and exogenous environment. In the light of this holistic point of view, aging has been defined as the temporal evolution of a complex system, characterized by a nonlinear dynamic behavior governed by the laws of chaos (Figure 1).

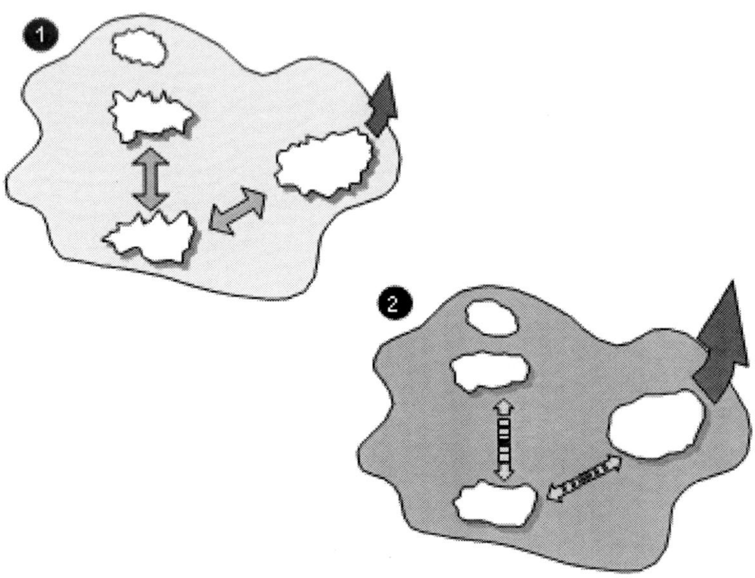

Figure 1. Schematic representation of a complex biosystem, made up of numerous sub-systems interacting with each other (1). The system evolves, under the influence of both endogenous and exogenous environments with loss of complexity during aging (2).

Changes in the very degree of complexity with advancing age could be a useful way to find some parameters describing global characteristics of the system as it is required in the search for determinants and/or biomarkers of aging (McClearn, 1997). A parallel, if not the same approach could be fruitful even in the search for diseases determinants and biomarkers. It is worth noting that attempts to measure the degree of complexity of biological systems have already been done at both structural and functional levels. In particular, experimental findings are available suggesting a decreasing trend of complexity with advancing age (Goldberger, 1996; Lipsitz et al., 1990; Nonnenmacher et al., 1990). The inadequacy of the Cartesian view that phenomena can be studied analyzing their components separately without losing any essential information, and the basic role played by the self-organization which overcomes the restricted view of genotype/phenotype dualism, have also been demonstrated during development; in particular, self-organizing processes give an essential contribute to increasing complexity just during development (Amzallag, 2000). This should sound very well to researchers figuring out parameters able to describe the global behavior of the evolving biological systems. We can hypothesize that complexity increases during development up to an individual maximum, then decreases again with advancing age.

Fractals in Biomedicine

The concept, previously introduced, that a complex system with a chaotic behavior often generates fractal structures, the so-called strange attractors (Grassberger & Procaccia, 1987), simply highlights the usefulness of fractal analysis as a suitable tool to measure biocomplexity and its changes with aging at both functional and structural levels and, potentially, to discriminate among "physiologic", pathologic, and successful aging (Figure 2). This approach could give insight into the search for biomarkers of aging and/or pathologies so important for the knowledge of primary aging processes.

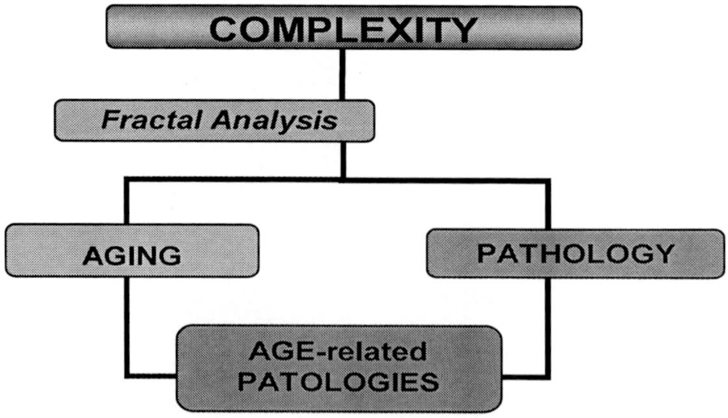

Figure 2. Hypothesis of work based on the new definition of aging as a temporal evolution of a complex system. Fractal analysis can measure variations of complexity in biosystems that evolve in the time by following different trajectories. Individual specific genetic-environment interactions define the senescent phenotype as normal aging, pathologic aging, or successful aging.

Many structures and processes in biology and medicine show fractal properties and fractal analysis has been becoming a common tool to measure biocomplexity. Among the numerous complex anatomic structures with fractal-like geometry are vessel trees (both arterial and venous), neural branching in the nervous system, tracheobronchial tree, kidney glomerula, biliary ducts, intestinal villi (Bassingthwaihte et al., 1994; Goldberger, 1997; Weibel, 1991). All these self-similar objects, as characterized by a sort of fractal-like branching or wrinkly structures, guarantee one of the fundamental physiologic functions: rapid and efficient transport by displaying a large interchange surface in a limited space. Fractal-like properties have been widely described also for different processes that generate irregular fluctuations with self-similarity characteristics observable at multiple time scale. Fractality has been observed at both space and time scales in the same system characterized by self-similarity or fractal-like properties at both morphologic and functional level. As an example, heartbeat with well established fractal properties is the result of cardiac muscle contraction under Purkinje neural control both described as fractal objects (Goldberger et al., 2002). Fractal properties have been also described for bronchial branching tree as well as for alveolar air flow or for vessel tree and blood flow at branching nodes.

Fractal Geometry

The term fractal (from Latin *fractus*, non-integer) applies to objects in space or fluctuations in time that possess a form of self-similarity and cannot be described within a single scale of measurement. Fractals are irregular in space or time, with details repeated at different levels of scales resembling the whole structure and fractal dimension was introduced to measure these forms with non-Euclidian geometry showing non–integer dimension (Figure 3). It measures the complexity of a fractal (Mandelbrot, 1982).

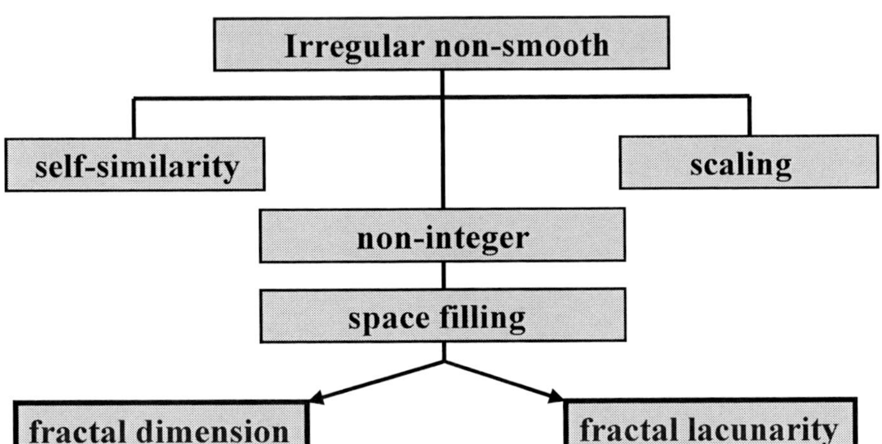

Figure 3. Schematic representation of fractals' properties. Fractal geometry provides mathematical tools, such as fractal dimension and fractal lacunarity, to measure fractal objects.

As briefly and effectively summarized by Waliszewski & Konarski (2002), fractal dimension can be defined as a real number equal to the limit of the quotient log n(ε)/log(1/ ε) at ε→0, where n(ε) is a minimum number of N-dimensional cubes of side ε necessary to cover the entire object, curve, or set of points. In particular, fractal dimension can be integer number if this is the limit of the quotient (Peano curve). Fractal dimension can also be defined by self-similarity of structure as described by the power law scaling of the algebraic form $y = ax^b$, in which y is a number of objects in the area covered by a single cube or circle of the linear grid, x stands for linear size of the cube or radius of the circle, a is scaling coefficient, and b is dimension of space occupied by the patterns analyzed (Brown et al., 2002). One can expect the co-existence of fractal dimension and self-similarity if coefficient of nonlinear regression R is greater than 0.95. This last definition underlies box counting method (Hastings & Sugihara, 1993), the most common computerized approach to measure fractal dimension. Fractal lacunarity further classifies fractals and measures space filling capacity. The term Lacunarity from Latin *Lacuna*, lack or hole, was coined by Mandelbrot referring to gap distribution in a fractal and lacunarity analysis was initially introduced to differentiate fractal objects displaying the same fractal dimension but a very different visual appears. In fact, fractal dimension gives an estimate of the complexity of the structure but doesn't provide any information on its shape (Mandelbrot, 82; 93).

While the concept of fractal geometry was introduced by Mandelbrot (1982) to describe natural objects irregularity of which cannot be fitted by Euclidian's regular shapes, fractals' mathematics was developed for ideal fractals. Thus, self-similarity and invariance of scale are properties belonging to ideal fractals. They show exact or approximate self-similarity at any scale of observation (comprised between 0 and ∞). When computerized methods of fractal analysis are considered, two limits are imposed by resolution capacity and calculus powerful. In particular, in a graphic representation of an ideal fractal (e.g. Cantor set or Kock snow flock) an upper limit is given by the finite size of the object as well as a lower limit is represented by pixel dimension.

When fractal structures are considered in biology and medicine we deal with statistical self-similarity in a limited range of scale. In addition, multifractal structures are more common.

Fractal Analysis in Aging and Pathology

Fractal analysis is a procedure already employed to the study of structural and physiological characteristics of very different biological objects: from neurons to vessels, from bacteria to fungi (Caserta et al., 1995; Cross et al., 1993; Landini et al., 1993; Losa and Nonnenmacher, 1996; Neale et al., 1993; Obert et al., 1990; Patankar et al., 1992). It can be applied to the study of many alterations occurring in different organs and tissues during disease and aging to measure changes in complexity at both structural and functional levels (Cross, 1997; Lipsitz & Goldberger, 1992; Piantanelli et al., 2002; Vaillancourt & Newell, 2002). As a matter of fact, loss of complexity in fractal structures has been observed as loss of neuron ramification with advancing age (Scheibel, 1985). It has also been shown that cardiac frequency signal presents a pattern with different degree of complexity in young and old people. On this basis, different mechanisms responsible for syncope in young and old individuals have been proposed from the study of chaotic phenomena (Lipsitz et al., 1990).

The advent of fractal mathematics to describe complex structures in biology and medicine has been accepted by most scientists and an always increasing number of fractal analysis techniques have been proposed and applied. However, the application of fractal techniques is often limited to fractal dimension. As a matter of fact, fractal dimension has been proposed and used as a suitable tool to measure complexity variation of most biomedical functions and structures during aging and disease (Link et al., 2004; Lipsitz, 2004; Losa & Nonnenmacher, 1996; Vaillancourt & Newell, 2002). This has been happening also in the case of bone structures and related pathologies among which is osteoporosis (Feltrin et al., 2001; Gilbert & McKirnan, 2005; Oka et al., 2002; Prouteau et al., 2004). While fractal dimension gives an estimate of the complexity of the structure, it alone is not sufficient to characterize a fractal object. Fractal's lacunarity, instead, describes the texture of a fractal and can measure fractal space filling capacity (Mandelbrot, 1993). Lacunarity analysis was initially introduced to differentiate fractal objects displaying the same fractal dimension but a very different appearance. More recently, lacunarity analysis has been presented as a more general technique able to describe random and fractal spatial patterns (Allain & Cloitre, 1991; Plotnick et al., 1996; Smith et al., 1996). Thus, it can be applied to complex objects with fractal, multifractal, and non-fractal properties.

Taking into account the limits of fractal analysis applied to natural objects (Mandelbrot, 1993; Plotnick et al., 1996) as well as the particular space pattern of trabecular bone, fractal lacunarity analysis has been used in the new method to determine relevant parameter(s) able to differentiate age-related physio-pathologic changes of trabecular bone structure from lumbar vertebra MR images. Fractal lacunarity analysis, in this particular context, appears the most suitable tool to characterize trabecular bone texture as it is able to describe discontinuity of the bone network as well as sizes of bone marrow spaces, changes of which are index of increased fracture risk.

OUTLINE OF THE METHOD

The method for bone microarchitecture texture characterization by lacunarity analysis is made up on three main steps: image acquisition by MR imaging Spin-Echo multislice technique; image processing of vertebral axial images to produce a binary representation of trabecular bone structure; quantitative lacunarity analysis of trabecular network by hyperbola function model approximation of the graph produced by gliding box technique.

The method has been developed on real images to avoid surprises during clinical application. In fact, often it happens that methods built up on simulation models fail when applied to real clinical images.

The procedure adopted to set up the method is described and discussed below and is schematically represented in Figure 4.

MR Imaging Acquisition

MR images of lumbar vertebrae were obtained by using a standard clinical 1.5-T whole-body imaging system (Gyroscan Intera; Philips Medical System, ACR-Nema 1.0). Once the fourth lumbar vertebra (L4) is spotted, a set of 9 axial images (512x512 pixels, pixel dimension equal to 0.469mm) of the vertebra was obtained by using Spin-Echo multislice technique (Figure 4A). Spin-Echo technique is not routinely used in clinical practice yet and images were obtained on purpose from patients underwent MR assessment for injuries of the column. The patients were classified as follows: healthy young (n. 4, mean age 33.7 years, age range 31-37); perimenopausal (n. 10, mean age 51.7 years, age range 43-65); osteoporotic, as defined by classical BMD method based diagnosis (n. 10, mean age 68.4 years, age range 64-74). Only one healthy old patient (80 years) occurred in the sample considered.

A B

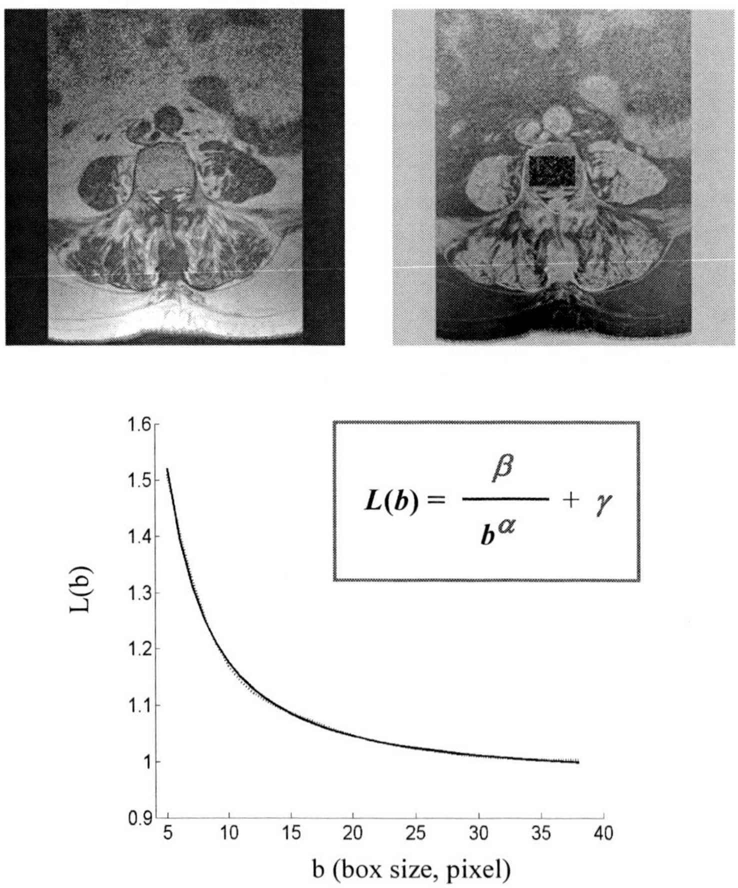

Figure 4. Schematic representation of the method. A-Fifth axial section image of the fourth lumbar vertebra. B- Rectangular ROI on reverse gray-scale image after an intermediate step of image processing to obtain binary representation of trabecular bone network. The plot represents the result of GBA application (dotted line) as fitted by hyperbola function used to calculate the triplet of parameters α, β, γ.

Image Processing and Analysis of MR Images

The data set was transferred from MR imaging system to a personal computer for image texture analysis and the fifth axial image was considered. The choice of the fifth axial section image stems from two main considerations: a certain degree of variability had to be expected among the nine axial images in each vertebra, thus, only one, namely the middle one was considered to build the method and compare results from different subjects. The limitation of the analysis to one image only would have the advantage to save time and increases the possibility of an easy transfer of the method in clinical practice. A pilot study supported the goodness of this choice as the method applied to all the nine axial images of different vertebrae produced sets of results with a certain degree of heterogeneity among the sections with the fifth one generally displaying intermediate values.

The algorithm developed for the characterization of trabecular bone was built on images processed as described in (Boutry et al., 2003) by the easy and available software ImageJ, version 1.26t. Briefly, reverse grey-scale display of the original image is used to ease visualization of the trabecular network, a rectangular ROI (region of interest) is chosen as large as possible to fit the inner perimeter of the trabecular network. The boundary between cortical bone and soft-tissue background is defined by using an automatic contour detection algorithm. Trabecular bone is then extracted from the bone marrow by using a Gaussian filter. This scheme generates a binary representation of the trabecular structure in which the dark regions represent bone marrow and the light regions represent bone. The Gaussian filter is applied first to the original ROI image and then to the thresholding one. The two resulting binary images are finally combined. This procedure allows either keeping or excluding the "false-positive finding" of trabeculae in the dark regions and also to remove the residual small artefacts.

Estimate of Lacunarity

Among the definitions and calculating procedures proposed to estimate lacunarity, the gliding box algorithm, GBA, based on the analysis of mass distribution in the set is the more popular (Allain & Cloitre, 1991). This method involves the variance of the box mass, M, at each step, wherein the box is moved one space unit at a time. The box mass is recounted till the whole region is traversed thus producing a frequency distribution of box masses, $n(M,b)$, where b is the size of the gliding box.

Assuming that, for each b, only a finite number of masses M_j, $j=1,2,\dots,\mu(b)$ are encountered in the various gliding boxes of size b, only a discrete frequency distribution $n(M_j,b)$, $j=1,2,\dots,\mu(b)$ has to be considered. Note that such an assumption holds for binary images, where the mass of a generic box on the image is given by the number of white pixels in the box, i.e. the pixels associated to the value one. From standard arguments the moments of order q of M, through the GBA, are given by:

$$Z_q(M,b) = \frac{1}{N(b)} \sum_{j=1}^{\mu(b)} M_j^q n(M_j,b), \qquad b > 0,$$

where the division by $N(b)$ needs to convert $n(M_j,b)$, $j=1, 2,\ldots,\mu(b)$ into a probability distribution. The definition of the lacunarity function Λ uses only the first and the second moments of M, that is

$$\Lambda(b) = \frac{Z_2(M,b)}{Z_1(M,b)^2}, \qquad b > 0.$$

The GBA method was implemented in software by using MATLAB version 6.1. The program begins to elaborate a binary image coming from the above mentioned processing of lumbar vertebra MR images. It calculates the values of lacunarity, for each integer value of b between b_{min} and b_{max}, where b_{min}, b_{max} are given integer multiples of the pixel size in the image under consideration. Once the lacunarity function $\Lambda(b)$, $b=b_{min}, b_{min}+1,\ldots, b_{max}$ is obtained, the program shows the results on a graph.

It was observed that, for all the images analyzed, the behavior of lacunarity function resembles the one of hyperbola (Figure 4, plot), therefore, the following model:

$$L(b) = \frac{\beta}{b^{\alpha}} + \gamma, \qquad b \in [b_{min}, b_{max}]$$

was chosen to approximate the lacunarity function where the three coefficients α, β, γ are suitable parameters.

Note that this observation is consistent with the theoretical behavior of lacunarity function Λ for self-similar fractals and for other different random sets. Moreover, for such fractals parameter α is related to the fractal dimension of the set and parameter β characterizes the lacunarity of the set, see (Allain & Cloitre, 1991) for details. In each particular example considered in this study, the best interpretation of lacunarity $\Lambda(b)$, $b=b_{min}$, $b_{min}+1,\ldots, b_{max}$, by the model function $L(b)$, $b \in [b_{min}, b_{max}]$, is computed as the solution of a least squares problem, where parameters α, β, γ are the independent variables. In particular, minimizer of this problem is a triplet of parameters (α^*, β^*, γ^*) of the model function that better represents the variation of mass density of pixels in that image.

Parameter β as an Estimate of Lacunarity

The method was applied to different types of bone trabecular structure. The subjects, representative for age and healthy status, were used to test the robustness of the method. In particular, thirty-year-old women were considered as bone starts loosing density approximately at that age. Pre- and post-menopause subjects were analyzed as representative of perimenopausal condition linked to a high risk of osteoporosis onset. Since the possibility exists, although rare, to physiologically grow old (in this context without clinical signs of osteoporosis), a healthy old woman was also included. The pathologic patients were classified as osteoporotic on the basis of classical BMD-diagnosis. Step by step application of the method to the same original image was repeated for six times. Results were obtained from the fifth axial section image by fixing b_{min} equal to 5 pixels and b_{max} equal to the nearest integer to 50% of ROIs' diagonal length, measured in pixels.

The three parameters α, β, γ define as univocal each function of lacunarity, *L(b)*. In particular, α represents the order of convergence of *L(b)*, β the concavity of the hyperbola, and γ the translation term. Parameters α and γ assume small values that slightly differ among the different bone structures analyzed while parameter β assumes values within a more wide numerical range. A low β value defines a hyperbola function with a wide concavity (high lacunarity), whereas a high β value defines a hyperbola function with a deeper concavity (low lacunarity) (Figure 5).

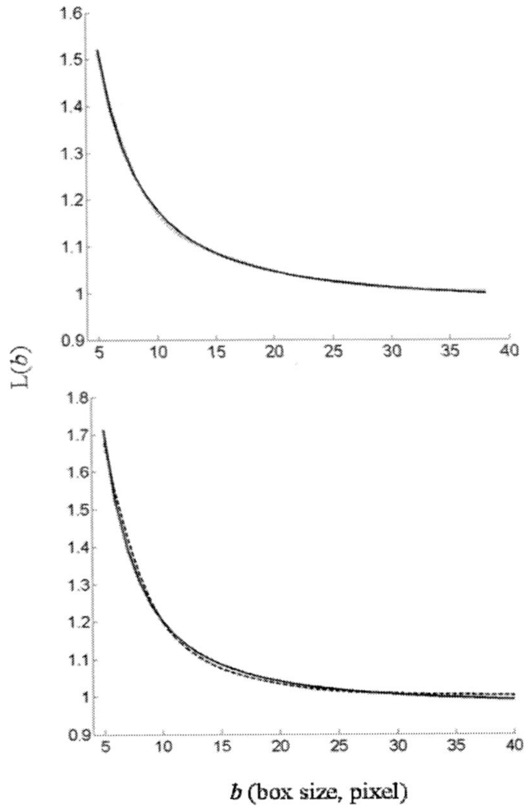

Figure 5. Comparison of two lacunarity GBA graph, as fitted by hyperbola function model, representative of two different trabecular bone structures: osteoporotic high lacunarity, β^* equal to 5.457 (top); healthy old lower lacunarity, β^* equal to 11,249 (bottom).

The Table summarizes the results of image processing from 24 women classified in three subgroups: healthy young, perimenopausal, and osteoporotic. Among the three coefficients, the parameter β undergoes the most significant variation. In particular, a correlation between parameter β and pathologic status exists with a decreasing trend of β values from healthy young to perimenopausal to osteoporotic patients.

Table. Parameters of lacunarity

Subjects (n, mean age)	α^*	β^*	γ^*
Healthy young (4, 33.7)	1.125±0.153	39.727±18.546	0.539±0.322
Perimenopause (10, 51.7)	0.949±0.356	16.158±3.142	0.643±0.179
Osteoporotic (10, 68.4)	1.848±0.269	4.636±1.350	0.748±0.168

Results are expressed as means ± SD of parameters values from each subgroup.

In spite of the small size of the sample, one-way Anova variance analysis followed by post hoc tests was performed. Results show that the three classes of trabecular bone structure considered (healthy young, perimenopausal, and osteoporotic) statistically differ from each other (probability significance value $p \leq 0.5$ for SNK multiple range test) as far as parameter β is concerned. A correlation also exists between parameter β and age with a decreasing trend from young to old subjects (Figure 6). It is worth noting that the healthy old subject shows a β value higher than the younger osteoporotic patients.

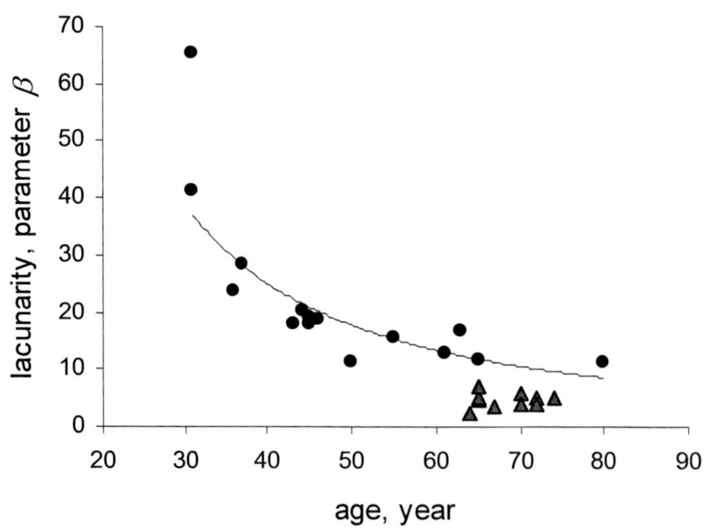

Figure 6. Representation of lacunarity changes with aging and osteoporosis as expressed by parameter β. Circles indicate healthy aging trabecular bone. Triangles represent osteoporotic bone. Decreasing β^* values correspond to increasing lacunarity. Osteoporotic trabecular structures show the highest lacunarity.

Improvements of the method need before to validate the goodness of parameter β as a marker of microarchitecture variation in aging and pathology on a conspicuous number of subjects. A more precise procedure of thresholding and segmentation are under consideration as well as ROI size and shape to improve robustness and reliability of the method.

CONCLUSION

Many advantages can be obtained from the clinical application of such a method to assess fracture risk in osteoporotic patients. First, it uses vertebral images. From comparative studies, where structural analysis was performed in different sites, among which are distal radius, calcaneus, and spine, spine remains the best site to predict osteoporotic fracture status (Prouteau et al., 2004). Second, the method uses MR images, in particular axial sections of the fourth vertebra (the best site to assess osteoporosis). MR imaging has been reported as to be ideally suited for analyzing texture of trabecular bone because bone marrow has uniform high signal intensity while bone appears with background intensity. These characteristics yield a binary tomographic system that makes easier thresholding of the spongy network (Wehrli et al., 2002). Using Spin-Echo technique, in addition, allows providing axial sections of trabecular bone by avoiding adulterate enlargement of the trabeculae as obtained by using gradient-echo MR imaging (Boutry et al., 2003; Majumdar et al., 1995).

The most intriguing advantage of the proposed method is given by the use of lacunarity analysis. Recently, fractal analysis has been becoming a common approach to assess complexity of trabecular bone structure. Only fractal dimension, however, is generally reported often expressed by the Hmean parameter (Boutry et al., 2003; Brown et al., 2005; Feltrin et al., 2001; Oka et al., 2002). As mentioned in this chapter, lacunarity represents the most suitable tool to characterize trabecular bone texture as it is able to describe discontinuity of the bone network as well as sizes of bone marrow spaces, changes of which are index of increased fracture risk. In addition, dealing with lacunarity analysis as a more general approach to analyze complex patterns with or without fractal properties (Allain & Cloitre, 1991; Plotnick et al., 1996; Smith & Lange, 1996), it allows overcoming biomedical limits of fractal analysis, responsible for misinterpretation if neglected. Human clinical application of lacunarity analysis of trabecular bone has been previously reported only for CT images and micro radiography images of bone biopsies (Chappard et al., 2001; Dougherty & Henebry, 2002). Application of lacunarity analysis to trabecular bone in the vertebra from MR images, therefore, provides a novel non-ionizing, non-invasive method to assess trabecular bone architecture (Zaia et al., 2005; 2006). Recently, a method for in vivo MR imaging assessment of osteoporosis in men has been proposed (Boutry et al., 2003). It uses the above-mentioned gradient-echo technique to obtain sagittal images of the calcaneus. As far as clinical application is concerned, choosing mirror sites, as it is the calcaneus, is justified when invasive and/or ionizing techniques are applied to assess osteoporosis. Once again, texture analysis of trabecular bone is performed by using histomorphometric methods that provide a set of numerous parameters to be analyzed. In particular, in the cited study (Boutry et al., 2003) 13 of 20 parameters are reported as significantly different in osteoporotic patients. Most studies performed in different sites with different image acquisition techniques propose histomorphometric-based methods and others (gray level histogram, runlength, gradient matrices, co-occurrence, anisotropy) for trabecular bone texture analysis (Chappard et al., 2005; Herlidou et al., 2004) that make their application hard in clinical routine because of the large number of parameters to be checked and analyzed. As a matter of fact, 8 parameters of 32 calculated in (Cortet et al., 1999) and 9 of 24 in (Cortet et al., 2000) have been reported as featuring bone trabecular architecture changes.

This observation highlights the last, but not least, advantage of the method, that is the result: a triplet of values corresponding to the three coefficients, α, β, γ, of the hyperbola model function which univocally characterize each single trabecular structure pattern considered. In particular, parameter β appears highly sensitive to bone microarchitecture variation, thus representing a suitable standard for an evaluation of trabecular bone architecture and a potential useful parametric index in early diagnosis of osteoporosis and therapeutic assessment to prevent bone fracture risk.

In this particular context, criteria for osteoporosis diagnosis, as recommended by World Health Organization (WHO), and related therapeutic treatments to care for the disease and prevent bone fracture deserve some discussion (for review see: Jordan & Cooper, 2002; Raisz, 2008). Just to give a taste, BMD-based diagnosis of osteoporosis expressed by a T score $\leq$ -2.5 as measured by means of DEXA presents at least three main limits. BMD alone is not a good predictor of fracture risk as other factors, such as bone geometry, microarchitecture, and size, also affect bone strength. Z scores vs. T score would be more informative, especially in young subjects, whereas both T and Z scores lose any significance when dealing with senescent people. In fact, taking into account the high degree of heterogeneity characterizing the senescent phenotype, chronological age does not correspond to the biological one. In addition, bone mineral content variations as absolute values are not predictive of increased bone fragility, rather they assume pathologic meaning when related to the individual maximal mineral content reached around thirty years of age; therefore, the rate of bone loss rather than bone density per se would be a better indicator of fracture risk. This aspect stresses another WHO recommendation needing revision: all people over 50 would undergo a bone mineral densitometry. The third but not last limit deals with DEXA technology: in spite of its wide clinical application, current DEXA utilization includes discrepancies among various manufacturers' devices and limitations of accuracy and reproducibility (Olson, 2007). It is worth noting that WHO recommended that diagnosis of osteoporosis be made a DEXA-based measurement of BMD when non-invasive technologies to assess in vivo bone architecture were not available yet.

The rapid development of medical imaging and information technologies have been opening up new perspectives to the study of etiopathogenesis of osteoporosis and bone fractures in the light of trabecular bone architecture degenerative processes with aging and pathology. It would also give insights into the search for therapeutical approaches, such as antiresorptive drugs or fracture healing agents, more effective in preventing and/or curing osteoporotic bone fractures (Bonnik, 2006; Fleurence et al., 2007; Schacht et al., 2007; Seeman, 2007; Silverman et al., 2008). Screening and follow-up studies enrolling a considerable number of subjects are obviously necessary.

The original and innovative method described in this chapter appears particularly promising. It provides only one parameter highly sensitive to trabecular bone architecture changes thus representing a suitable method for an easy and fast applicability into both research and clinical practice.

The intriguing and promising results obtained with this method further stresses the usefulness of interpreting aging phenomena in the light of new paradigms such as complexity, chaos, and fractals. The innovative hypothesis of work deals with the application of fractal analysis to gerontology studies. It is based on fractal analysis as a useful tool to measure complexity of biological structures and functions and its modification with aging and pathology. It could represent a suitable approach to discriminate between physiological and pathological aging as well as between age-related and age-associated diseases, two main tasks dealing with aging well.

References

Abate, M; Di Iorio, A; Di Renzo, D; Paganelli, R; Saggini, R; Abate, G. Frailty in the elderly: the physical dimension. *Eura Medicophys*, 2007, 43, 407-415.

Allain, C; Cloitre, M. Characterizing the lacunarity of random and deterministic fractal sets. *Phy Rev A*, 1991, 44, 3552-3558.

Amzallag, GN. Connectance in *Sorghum* development: beyond the genotype-phenotype duality. *BioSystem*, 2000, *56*, 1-11.

Audran, M; Chappard, D; Legrand, E; Libouban, H; Baslé, MF. Bone microarchitecture and bone fragility in men: DXA and histomorphometry in humans and in orchidectomized rat model. *Calcif Tissue Int*, 2001, 69, 214-217.

Bassingthwaihte, JB; Liebovitch, LS; West, BJ. *Fractal physiology*. New York: Oxford University Press; 1994.

Bauer, DC; Glüer, CC; Cauley, JA; Vogt, TM; Ensrud, KE; GenantHK; Black DM. Bone ultrasound predicts fractures strongly and independently of densitometry in older women: A prospective study. *Arch Intern Med*, 1997, 157, 629-634.

Bonnick, SL. Osteoporosis in men and women. *Clin Cornerstone*, 2006, 8, 28-39.

Boutry, N; Cortet, B; Dubois, P; Marchandise, X; Cotten, A. Trabecular Bone Structure of the calcaneus: Preliminary in Vivo MR Imaging Assessment in Men with Osteoporosis. *Radiology*, 2003, 227, 708-717.

Brenner, H; Arndt, V. Epidemiology in aging research. *Exp Gerontol*, 2004, 39, 679-86.

Brown, JH; Gupta, VK; Li, BL; Milne, BT; Restrepo, C; West, GB. The fractal nature of nature: power laws, ecological complexity and biodiversity. *Philos Trans R Soc London B Biol Sci*, 2002, 357, 619-626.

Brown, RA; Zhu, H; Mitchell, JR. Distributed vector processing of a new local multiscale Fourier transform for medical application. *IEEE Trans Med Imaging*, 2005, 24, 689-691.

Bullmore, E; Fadili, J; Maxim, V; Xendur, L; Mhitcher, B; Suckling, J; Brammer, MJ; Breakspear, MJ. Wavelets and functional magnetic resonance imaging of the human brain. *NeuroImage,* 2004, 23, 234-249.Cheng, S; Tylavsky, F; Carbone, L. Utility of ultrasound to assess risk of fracture. *J Am Geriatr Soc*, 1997, 45, 1382-1394.

Carey, JR; Liedo, P; Orozco, D; and Vaupel, JW. Slowing of mortality rates at older ages in large medfly cohorts. *Science*, 1992, 258, 457-461.

Caserta, F; Eldred, WD; Fernandez, E; Hausman RE; Stanford LR; Bulderev, SV; Schwarzer, S; Stanley, HE. Determination of fractal dimension of physiologically characterized neurons in two and three dimensions. *J Neurosci Methods*, 1995, 56, 133-144.

Chappard, C; Brunet-Imbault, B; Lemineur, G; Giraudeau, B, Basillais, A, Harba, R; Benhamou, CL. Anisotropy changes in post-menopausal osteoporosis: characterization by a new index applied to trabecular bone radiographic images. *Osteoporos Int*, 2005, 16, 1193-1202.

Chappard, D; Legrand, E; Haettich, B; Chales, G; Auvinet, B; Eschard, JP; Hamelin, JP; Basle, MF; Audran, M. Fractal dimension of trabecular bone: comparison of three histomorphometric computed techniques for measuring the architectural two-dimensional complexity. *J Pathol*, 2001, 195, 515-521.

Cortet, B; Dubois, P; Boutry, N; Bourel, P; Cotten, A; Marchandise, X. Image analysis of the distal radius trabecular network using computed tomography. *Osteoporos Int*, 1999, 9, 410-419.

Cortet, B; Dubois, P; Boutry, N; Varlet, E; Cotten, A; Marchandise, X. Does high-resolution computed tomography image analysis of the distal radius provide information independent of bone mass? *J Clin Densitom*, 2000, 3, 339-351.

Cross, SS. Fractals in pathology. *J Pathol*, 1997, 182, 1-8.

Cross, SS; Start, RD; Silcocks, PB; Bull, AD; Cotton, DW; Underwood, JC. Quantification of the renal arterial tree by fractal analysis. *J Pathol*, 1993, 170, 479-484.

Dalle Carbonare L; Giannini, S. Bone microarchitecture as an important determinant of bone strength. *Endocrinol Invest*, 2004, 27, 99-105.

Daubechies, I. Ten Lectures on Wavelets. *Society for Industrial and Applied Mathematics*, Philadelphia: 1992.

Dougherty, G; Henebry, GM. Lacunarity analysis of spatial pattern in CT images of vertebral trabecular bone for assessing osteoporosis. *Med Eng Phys*, 2002, 24, 129-138.

Economos, AC. Rate of aging, rate of dying and the mechanism of mortality. *Arch Gerontol Geriatr*, 1982 1, 3-27.

Elliot-Gibson, V; Bogoch, ER; Jamal, SA; Beaton, DE. Practice patterns in the diagnosis and treatment of osteoporosis after a fragility fracture: a systematic review. *Osteoporos Int*, 2004, 15, 767-778.

Faber, TD; Yoon, DC; Service, SK; White, SC. Fourier and wavelet analyses of dental radiographs detect trabecular changes in osteoporosis *Bone*, 2004, 35, 403-411.

Feltrin, GP; Macchi, V; Saccavini, C; Tosi, E; Dus, C; Fascina, A; Parenti, A; De Caro, R. Fractal analysis of lumbar cancellous bone architecture. *Clin Anat*, 2001, 14, 414-417.

Finch, CE; Tanzi, RE. Genetics of aging. *Science*, 1997, 278, 407-411.

Fleurence, RL; Iglesias, CP; Johnson; JM. The cost effectiveness of bisphosphonates for the prevention and treatment of osteoporosis: a structured review of the literature. *Pharmacoeconomics*, 2007, 25, 913-933.

Flood, RL; Carson, ER. *Dealing with complexity*. New York: Plenum Press; 1993.

Franceschi, C., Monti, D., Cossarizza, A., Fagnoni, F., Passeri, G., and Sansoni, P. Aging, longevity and cancer: studies in Down's syndrome and in centenarians. *Ann N Y Acad Sci*, 1991, 621, 428-440.

Franceschi, C; Monti, D; Sansoni, P; Cossarizza, A. The immunology of exceptional individuals: the lesson of centenarians. *Immunol Today*, 1995, 16, 12-16.

Franceschi, C; Monti, D; Scarfi, MR; Zeni, O; Temperani, P; Emilia, G; Sansoni, P; Lioi, MB; Troiano, L; Agnesini, C; et al. Genomics instability and aging. Studies in centenarians (successful aging) and in Down's syndrome patients (accelerated aging). *Ann N Y Acad Sci*, 1992, 663, 4-16.

Gilbert, SM; McKiernan, JM. Epidemiology of osteoporosis and prostate cancer. *Curr Opin Urol*, 2005, 15, 23-27.

Goldberger, AL. Non-linear dynamics for clinicians: chaos theory, fractals, and complexity at the bedside. *Lancet*, 1996, 347, 1312-1314.

Goldberger, AL. Fractal variability versus pathologic periodicity: complexity loss and stereotypy in disease. *Perspect Biol Med*, 1997, 40, 543-561.

Goldberger, AL; Peng, CK; Lipsitz, LA. What is physiologic complexity and how does it change with aging and disease? *Neurobiol Aging*, 2002, 23, 23-26.

Goldberger, AL; Rigney, DR; West, BJ. Chaos and fractals in human physiology. *Scintific American*, 1990, 262, 43-49.

Gordon, CL; Webber, CE; Adachi, JD; Christoforou, N. In vivo assessment of trabecular bone structure at the distal radius from high-resolution computed tomography images. *Phys Med Biol*, 1999, 41, 495-508.

Grassberger, A; Procaccia, I. Measuring the strangeness of strange attractors. *Physica D*, 1987, 9, 189-208.

Gregory, JS; Stewart, A; Undrill, PE; Reid, DM; Aspden, RM. Identification of hip fracture patients from radiograghs using Fourier analysis of the trabecular structure: a cross-sectional study. BMC Med Imaging, 2004, 4, 4. http://www.biomedcentral.com/1471-2342/4/4.

Hans, D; Dargent-Molina, P; Schott, AM; Sebert, JL; Cormier, C; Kotzki, PO; Delmas, PD; Pouilles, JM; Breart, G; Meunier, PJ. Ultrasonographic heel measurements to predict hip fracture in elderly women: the EPIDOS prospective study. *Lancet,* 1996, 348, 511-514.

Hastings HM; Sugihara G. *Fractals: A user's guide for the natural science*. Oxford: Oxford University Press; 1993.

Helgason, B; Perilli, E; Schileo, E; Taddei, F; Brynjolfsson, S; Viceconti, M. Mathematical relationships between bone density and mechanical properties: a literature review. *Clin Biomech*, 2008, 23, 135-146.

Herlidou, S; Grebe, R; Grados, F; Leuyer, N; Fardellone, P; Meyer, ME. Influence of age and osteoporosis on calcaneus trabecular bone structure: a preliminary in vivo MRI study by quantitative texture analysis. *Magn Reson Imaging*, 2004, 22, 237-243.

Herskind, AM; McGue, M; Iachine, IA; Holm, N; Sçrensen, TI.; Harvald, B; Vaupel, JW. Untangling genetic influences on smoking, body mass index and longevity: a multivariate study of 2464 Danish twins followed for 28 years. *Hum Genet*, 1996, 98, 467-475.

Hough, S. Fast and slow bone losers. Relevance to the management of osteoporosis. *Drugs Aging*, 1998, 12, Suppl. 1, 1-7.

Johnell, O; Kanis, J; Gullberg, G. Mortality, morbidity, and assessment of fracture risk in male osteoporosis. *Calcif Tissue Int*, 2001, 69, 182-184.

Johnson, HA. Is aging physiological or pathological ? In: Johnson HA editor. Relations between Normal Aging and Disease; *Aging Series, Vol 28*. New York: Raven Press; 1985; 239-247.

Jordan, KM; Cooper, C. Epidemiology of osteoporosis. *Best Pract Res Clin Rheumathol*, 2002, 16, 795-806.

Kanis, JA; Borgstrom, F; De Laet, C; Johansson, H; Johnell, O; Jonsson, B; Oden, A; Zethraeus, N; Pfleger, B; Khaltaev, N. Assessment of fracture risk. *Osteoporos Int*, 2005, 16, 581-589.

Kiebzak, GM. Age-related bone changes. *Exp Gerontol*, 1991, 26, 171-187.

Kyriazis, M. Practical applications of chaos theory to the modulation of human aging: nature prefers chaos to regularity. *Biogerontol*, 2003, 4, 75-90.

Landini, G; Misson, GP; Murray, PI. Fractal analysis of the normal human retinal fluorescein angiogram. *Curr Eye Res*, 1993, 12, 23-27.

Lau, EM. Preventing osteoporosis in everyday life. *Clin Calcium*, 2004, 14, 430-434.

Lee, WL; Chen, YC; Hsieh, KS. Ultrasonic liver tissues classification by fractal feature vector based on M-band wavelet transform. *IEEE Trans Med Imaging*, 2003, 22, 382-392.

Lindsay, R; Silverman, SL; Cooper, C; Hanley, DA; Barton, I; Broy, SB; Licata, A; Benhamou, L; Geusens, P; Flowers, K; Stracke, H; Seeman, E. Risk of new vertebral fracture in the year following a fracture. *JAMA*, 2001, 285, 320-323.

Link, TM; Bauer, J; Kollstedt, A; Stumpf, I; Hudelmaier, M; Settles, M; Majumdar, S; Lochmuller, EM; Eckstein, F. Trabecular bone structure of the distal radius, the calcaneus, and the spine: which site predicts fracture status of the spine best? *Invest Radiol*, 2004, 39, 487-489.

Lipsitz, LA. Physiological complexity, aging, and the path to frailty. Sci Aging Knowledge Environ, 2004, 16, pe16. http://sageke.sciencemag.org/cgi/content/full/2004/16/pe16.

Lipsitz, LA; Goldberger, AL. Loss of 'complexity' and aging: potential applications of fractals and chaos theory to senescence. *JAMA*, 1992, 267, 1806-1809.

Lipsitz, LA; Mietus, J; Moody, GB; Goldberger, AL. Spectral characteristics of heart rate variability before and during postural tilt. Relations to aging and risk of syncope. *Circulation*, 1990, 81, 1803-1810.

Losa, GA; Nonnenmacher, TF. Self-similarity and fractal irregularity in pathologic tissues. *Mod Pathol*, 1996, 9, 174-182.

Majumdar, S. A review of magnetic resonance (MR) imaging of trabecular bone micro-architecture: contribution to the prediction of biomechanical properties and fracture prevalence. *Technol Health Care*, 1998, 6, 321-327.

Majumdar, S; Genant, HK; Grampp, S; Newitt, DC; Truong, VH; Lin, JC; Mathur, A. Correlation of trabecular bone structure with age, bone mineral density, and osteoporotic status: in vivo studies in the distal radius using high resolution magnetic resonance imaging. *J Bone Miner Res*, 1997, 12, 111-118.

Majumdar, S; Newitt, D; Jergas, M; Gies, A; Osman, D; Keltner, J; Keyak, J; Genant, H. Evaluation of technical factors affecting the quantification of trabecular bone structure using magnetic resonance imaging. *Bone*, 1995, 17, 417-430.

Mandelbrot, BB. *The Fractal Geometry of Nature*, New York: W.H. Freeman, 1982.

Mandelbrot, BB. *A Fractal's Lacunarity, and how it can be Tuned and Measured. In Fractals in Biology and Medicine*. Nonnenmacher TF, Losa GA, Weibel ER editors. Basel: Birkhauser Press; 1993, 8-21.

Mari, D; Mannucci, PM; Duca, F; Bertolini, S; Franceschi, C. Mutant factor V (Arg506GIn) in healthy centenarians. *Lancet*, 1996, 347, 1044.

McClearn, GE. Biomarkers of age and aging. *Exp Gerontol*, 1997, 32, 87-94.

Mirza FS; Prestwood, KM. Bone health and aging: implications for menopause. *Endocrinol Metab Clin North Am*, 2004, 33, 741-759.

Neale, EA; Bowers, LM; Smith, Jr, TG., Early dendrite development in spinal cord cell cultures: a quantitative study. *J Neurosci Res*, 1993, 34, 54-66.

Nonnenmacher, TF, Baumann, G; Losa, GA. Self-organization and fractal scaling patterns in biological systems. In: Menon, J editor. *Trends in Biological Cybernetics. Trivandrum India: Publication Manager, Reserach Trends, Council of Scientific Research Integration*; 1990, 65-73.

Obert, M; Pfeifer, P; Sernez, M. Microbial growth patterns described by fractal geometry. *J Bacteriol*, 1990, 172, 1180-1185.

Oka, K; Kumasaka, S; Kashima, I. Assessment of bone feature parameters from lumbar trabecular skeletal patterns using mathematical morphology. *J Bone Miner Metab*, 2002, 20, 201-208.

Olson, AF. Osteoporosis. *Nurse Pract*, 2007, 32, 20-27.

Patankar, D; Oolman, T; Johnson, S; Berggren, M. Ultrasonic characterization of mycelial morphology as a fractal structure. *Ultrason Imaging*, 1992, 14, 86-95.

Pettersson, M. *Complexity and evolution*. Cambridge: Cambridge University Press; 1996.

Piantanelli, A; Serresi, S; Ricotti, G; Rossolini, G; Zaia, A; Basso, A; Piantanelli, L. Color-based method for fractal dimension estimation of pigmented skin lesion contour. In: Losa GA, Merlini D, Nonnenmacher TF, Weibel ER editors. *Fractals in biology and medicine; Mathematics and Biosciences in Interaction Series, vol. III*. Basel: Birkhauser Press; 2002, 127-136.

Piantanelli, L. A mathematical model of survival kinetics. I. Theoretical basis. *Arch Gerontol Geriatr*, 1986, 5, 107-118.

Piantanelli, L; Rossolini, G; Basso, A; Piantanelli, A; Malavolta, M; Zaia, A. Use of mathematical models of survivorship in the study of biomarkers of aging: the role of heterogeneity. *Mech Ageing Dev*, 2001, 122, 1461-1475.

Pinheiro, MM; Castro, CHM; Frisoli Jr, A; Szejnfeld, VL. Discriminatory ability of Quantitative ultrasound measurements is similar to Dual-energy x-ray absorptiometry in a Brazilian women population with osteoporotic fracture. *Calcif Tissue Int*, 2003, 73, 555-564.

Plotnick, RE; Gardner, RH; Hargrove, WW; Prestegard, K; Perlmutter, M. Lacunarity analysis: A general technique for the analysis of spatial patterns. *Phys Rev E*, 1996, 53, 5461-5468.

Prouteau, S; Ducher, G; Nanyan, P; Lemineur, G; Benhamou, L; Courteix, D. Fractal analysis of bone texture: a screening tool for stress fracture risk? *Eur J Clin Invest*, 2004, 34,137-142.

Raisz, LG. Screening for Osteoporosis. *N Engl J Med*, 2005, 353, 164-171.

Schacht, E. Dukas, L; Richy, F. Combined therapies in osteoporosis: bisphosphonates and vitamin D-hormone analogs. *J Musculoskelet Neuronal Interact*, 2007, 7, 174-184.

Scheibel, AB. Falls, motor dysfunction, and correlative neurohistologic changes in the elderly. *Clin Geriatr Med*, 1985, 1, 671-676.

Seeman, E. Unresolved issues in osteoporosis in men. *Rev Endocr Metab Disord*, 2001, 2, 45-64.

Seeman, E. Is a change in bone mineral density a sensitive and specific surrogate of anti-fracture efficacy? *Bone*, 2007, 41, 308-317.

Silverman, SL; Cummings, SR; Watts, NB; Consensus Panel of the ASBMR, ISCD, and NOF. Recommendations for the clinical evaluation of agents for treatment of osteoporosis: consensus of an expert panel representing the American Society for Bone and Mineral Research (ASBMR), the International Society for Clinical Densitometry (ISCD), and the National Osteoporosis Foundation (NOF). *J Bone Miner Res*, 2008, 23, 159-165.

Smith, Jr, TG; Lange, GD; Marks, WB. Fractal methods and results in cellular morphology-dimensions, lacunarity and multifractals. *J Neurosci Methods*, 1996, 69, 123-136.

Solomon, DH; Finkelstein, JS; Kats, JN; Mogun, H; Avorn, J. Underuse of osteoporosis medications in elderly patients with fractures. *Am J Med*, 2003, 115, 398-400.

Vaillancourt, DE; Newell, KM. Changing complexity in human behaviour and physiology through aging and disease. *Neurobiol Aging*, 2002, 23, 1-11.

Waliszewski, P; Konarski, J. Fractal structure of space and time is necessary for the emergence of self-organization, connectivity, and collectivity in cellular system. In: Losa GA, Merlini D, Nonnenmacher TF, Weibel ER editors. *Fractals in biology and medicine; Mathematics and Biosciences in Interaction Series, vol. III*; Basel: Birkhauser Press; 2002, 14-24.

Wang, CY; Bruder, JM; Rubin, D. Evaluation and treatment of postmenopausal osteoporosis. *Am J Manag Care*, 2001, 7, SP5-16.

Wehrli, FW; Saha, PK; Gomberg, BR, Song, HP; Snyder, PJ; Benito, M; A; Wright, Weening, R. Role of magnetic resonance for assessing structure and function of trabecular bone. *Top Magn Reson Imaging*, 2002, 13, 335-355.

Weibel, ER. Fractal geometry: a design principle for living organisms. *Am J Physiol*, 1991, 261, L361-L369.

Zaia, A; Eleonori, R; Maponi, P; Rossi, R; Murri, R. Medical Imaging and Osteoporosis: Fractal's Lacunarity Analysis of Trabecular Bone in MR Images. In: Tsymbal A, Cunningham P editors. *Proceedings - Eighteenth IEEE Symposium on Computer-Based Medical Systems–CBMS* 2005, Dublin, Ireland. Los Alamitos CA: IEEE Computer Society Press; 2005, 3-8.

Zaia, A; Eleonori, R; Maponi, P; Rossi, R; Murri, R. MR Imaging and Osteoporosis: Fractal Lacunarity Analysis of Trabecular Bone. *IEEE Trans Inf Tech Biom,* 2006, 10, 484-489.

In: Osteoporosis: Etiology, Diagnosis and Treatment
Editors: Bilar E. Mattingly and Albert C. Pillare
ISBN 978-1-60692-397-9

Chapter 14

TREATMENT OF OSTEOPOROTIC COMPRESSION FRACTURES WITH VERTEBROPLASTY

Bryan Tan Hsi Ming and Hee Hwan Tak*
National University Hospital, Singapore, Republic of Singapore.

ABSTRACT

Osteoporosis is a world wide problem and its incidence is rising as life expectancy increases. A common complication of osteoporosis is that of wedge compression fractures of the vertebrae. Traditionally, wedge compression fractures have been treated conservatively with analgesia, bed rest and subsequently back physiotherapy when the pain has subsided to an acceptable level.

Following its introduction in the 1980s, vertebroplasty has gained popularity in the management of osteoporotic compression fractures and is fast becoming the standard of care for painful compression fractures. Performance of the procedure is quick and simple yet affords rapid and efficacious pain relief, while maintaining an excellent safety profile. Despite its excellent safety profile, complications have been reported post vertebroplasty, some of which are potentially devastating. As such, one must practice careful patient selection in order to maximize benefits from the procedure while minimizing complications.

INTRODUCTION

The prevalence of osteoporosis around the world is rising. As bone mass peaks at age 35 and starts of decrease progressively after, increased life expectancy has also resulted in

* Correspondence concerning this article should be addressed to: A/P Hee HT, Senior Consultant and Deputy Head, Division of Spinal Surgery, Department of Orthopaedic Surgery, National University Hospital, Singapore. 5 Lower Kent Ridge Road, Singapore 119074, Republic of Singapore. Tel: +65-67724327; Fax: +65-67780720; Email: doshht@nus.edu.sg.

increased incidence of osteoporosis. It has been estimated that 90% of the population of women above the age of 75 are clinically osteoporotic. Complications which occur as a result of osteoporosis are also increasingly common. The lifetime risk of a symptomatic osteoporotic fracture has been reported as 15.6% for females and 5% for males. These figures do not reflect the true extent of the problem as asymptomatic fractures are often missed or only picked up incidentally. Complications resulting from osteoporotic compression fractures include chronic pain, spinal cord compression, ileus [1] and compromised pulmonary function [2]. These complications then result in often overlooked and neglected problems of reduced quality of life, insomnia and even depression. Studies have even shown a 30% increase in age-adjusted mortality [3]. The prevalence of this problem is expected to increase as medical science progresses and life expectancy increases.

The management of osteoporotic wedge compression fractures of the vertebrae has traditionally been non-interventional. Patients who present with painful compression fractures are treated symptomatically. For many, the pain associated with the fracture resolves slowly with time while bed rest, external support in the form of braces or corsets and mediations like analgesia and calcitonin are prescribed to make patients more comfortable while healing occurs. Gentle physiotherapy is also recommended when pain is more tolerable. In others, however, the fracture fails to heal and patients develop painful pseudarthrosis which results in persistent mechanical pain. In severe cases previously, intervention entailed major surgery which often involved fusion of the affected and adjacent levels with metallic implants. These surgeries, however, are associated with the attendant risks, morbidity and mortality of such extensive operations. As such, surgery is usually advocated only for severe cases where there is impending neurological compromise or gross spinal deformity. Hence, in order to avoid surgery, the group of patients who experience debilitating pain would almost certainly mean prolonged bed rest. Unfortunately, prolonged recumbence also has its own problems, including decubitus ulcers, impaired bowel function, urinary retention and urinary tract infections, deep vein thrombosis, pulmonary embolism, exacerbation of pre-existing osteoporosis etc.

Vertebroplasty refers to a procedure in which the integrity and structure of a damaged or destroyed vertebral body is augmented. This can be achieved either through bone grafts, insertion of metallic implants or with the use of bone cements. This procedure has gained widespread acceptance for many reasons including high efficacy, excellent safety profile, ability to be performed under local anaesthesia, rapidity of relief of symptoms, relative low cost and relatively low learning curve.

The technique of vertebroplasty through the injection of bone cement into the body of the affected vertebra was first developed and described by French surgeons Galibert and Deramond in 1984 [4]. It was first developed for the treatment of an aggressive cervical vertebral hemangioma. Subsequently, the same technique was used in the treatment of painful osteoporotic wedge compression fractures. Studies have shown up to 90% significant pain relief following the procedure [5] and since, vertebroplasty has grown to be the standard of care for painful wedge compression fractures [6], not only of osteoporotic aetiology, but also for painful pathological fractures resulting from tumor infiltration.

Patient Selection

Although vertebroplasty has been proven to be an extremely safe procedure, it is still an invasive procedure and is associated with potentially serious complications (which will be discussed in detail later in this chapter). The decision to perform vertebroplasty should not be taken lightly.

Careful patient selection is the key to achieving a high success rate. The first line of management of osteoporotic compression fractures is still conservative management. There are no definite guidelines as to how long one should persist with conservative management. Vertebroplasty can be considered if pain worsens or if the pain relief plateaus at an unacceptable level.

It is also of utmost importance to carefully assess the patient through a thorough history and physical examination. Pain resulting from compression fractures is often axial, mechanical, sharp and localized. Patients with radicular pain may not benefit from vertebroplasty. On examination, patients will complain of increased pain with movement. Getting on and off the examination couch will be laborious. Some will have localized pain in the spine on gentle percussion. A kyphotic posture from previous wedge compression fractures is also a common finding. Axial back pain in often exacerbated by forward flexion and partially relieved by extension. A careful neurological examination is also important as a more serious complication of osteoporosis is that of a senile burst fracture, which may be associated with retropulsion of bony fragments resulting in neurological impairment.

Chronicity of the fracture is another important factor to be considered. Again, no definite guidelines are available, but generally, results of vertebroplasty performed of fractures older than 3 months are poorer. This observation, however, does not apply to cases of re-fracture or pseudarthrosis.

Investigations

Standard radiographs of the spine taken in the antero-posterior and lateral views should be done. These should reveal the presence of a wedge compression fracture. It is important to differentiate a wedge compression fracture from a senile burst fracture as management of these 2 pathologies is very different. The severity of compression of the affected vertebral body should be assessed and noted. Severe loss of height is considered a relative contraindication to vertebroplasty [7] by some authors. Other factors to consider in assessing radiographs include age of the fracture, presence of compression fractures in other levels (which may make accurate identification of the painful compression fracture difficult), breaks in the pedicles and breaches in the posterior wall. Indications and contraindications to vertebroplasty will be discussed in detail later in this chapter.

In addition to standard radiographs, lateral views taken in flexion and extension may be taken if the patient is able to comply. These can help to identify fractures which are mobile.

In cases where multiple wedge compression fractures are present, a bone scan will often help to identify the problem level. An acute fracture will show up as a "hot spot", whereas a chronic, healed fracture will fail to "light up". Although helpful, a bone scan will not be able to furnish details about the integrity of the pedicles and posterior walls. Presence of retropulsed fragments with cord compression may also be missed. Hence, many surgeons now order magnetic resonance imaging (MRI) of the spine as part of the standard pre-operative workup prior to vertebroplasty. This excellent investigation not only accurately identifies acute fractures which will benefit from vertebroplasty, but also help to distinguish wedge compression fractures from burst fractures, picks up presence of other pathological processes like neoplastic disease and gives good information regarding the presence or absence of posterior wall breaches and pedicle fractures.

Technique of Vertebroplasty

Logistics

A radiolucent operating table will allow fluoroscopic images in both the AP as well as lateral views. A high quality, high resolution image intensifier is required for this procedure.

Positioning

The patient is placed prone with suitable padding of the bony prominences. Many operators advocate positioning of pillows/ cushions on either side of the level to be operated on to enhance postural reduction of the fracture and restoration of height.

Analgesia

This procedure is usually done under local anaesthesia with close monitoring of the patient's vital parameters in the presence of an anaesthetist. Intravenous sedation and analgesia in the form of 2 – 4 mg of midazolam and 50 to 100 mg of fentanyl titrated according to the needs of the patient (or similar pharmacological agents) is usually required. The patient should be given supplementary oxygen via either nasal prongs or a simple face mask during the procedure. Blood pressure, continuous electrocardiogram and pulse oxymetry monitoring should be ensured during the whole procedure. The procedure may also be performed under general anaesthesia in some patients but the patient would then be subjected to the attendant risks of general anaesthesia. It would also have the distinct disadvantage of inability to ask patients about whether or not they experience any lower limb symptoms, especially in cases of suspected or established cement leakage.

Antibiotics Prophylaxis

Skin organisms are covered, usually with the use of a first generation cephalosporin like intravenous cefazolin 1g. In patients who are allergic to penicillin, clindamycin 600mg or vancomycin 1g may be used instead.

Technique of Vertebroplasty

The most commonly used route to access the vertebral body is via a transpedicular route. There are multiple advantages to using this route. Spine surgeons would be thoroughly familiar with this route as this is the most commonly technique in the placement of pedicle screws in spinal instrumentation. It is also easy to ensure that an intra-pedicular position of the needle is maintained at all times checking intra-operative radiographs in 2 orthogonal planes during the insertion of the needle. By ensuring an intrapedicular position, risk of injury to surrounding structures like spinal nerves is greatly reduced. After injection of local anaesthetic agent (often 1:1 mixture of 1% lignocaine and 0.25% bupivacaine) taking extra care to ensure a generous subperiosteal infiltration to enhance patient comfort, a small stab incision is made on either side after localization using the image intensifier. An 11 gauge osteoplasty needle is inserted through the pedicle under fluoroscopic guidance. One should aim for the superolateral aspect of the pedicle as seen on the anteroposterior view (under fluoroscopy) as the insertion point of the osteoplasty needle. The needle is aimed in a slight supero-lateral to infero-medial direction and advanced. The objective is to position the needle tip at the junction of the anterior and middle third of the vertebral body. At this position, the vertebral body should be relatively devoid of venous plexuses. Care is taken to avoid breaching the walls of the pedicle as injury to adjacent nervous structures may result. This would also predispose to cement leakage. The needle should be inserted slowly, advancing several millimeters at a time and checking its position after every advancement. This would reduce the chances of pedicle wall breach and mal-position of the needle. The same procedure is repeated on the contralateral side.

Once optimal position is achieved, a vertebrogram (of venogram) is performed. In this on-table investigation, radio-opaque contrast media is injected into either needle slowly, while multiple fluoroscopic images are taken in both the antero-posterior and the lateral views, looking out for any signs of leakage. The contrast media routinely used are Omnipaque 300 or Isovue 300. The main objective of performing a vertebrogram is to detect the presence of leaks, through breaches in the pedicular walls, vertebral walls or even into the spinal canal via the plexus of vertebral veins. If a leak is detected, the needles are adjusted and the vertebrogram repeated till a leak is no longer present. Some authors do not routinely perform a vertebrogram prior to injection of the cement. The argument against performing a vertebrogram is that the viscosities of the contrast media and the final cement are so different that the vertebrogram does not accurately predict the possibility of a cement leak. Studies have even shown that performance of a vertebrogram does not add to the safety of the procedure [8]. We routinely perform a vertebrogram prior to injection of the cement despite other authors' claims to the contrary. In our experience, injection of the vertebrogram is indeed helpful in detecting the presence of a leak and necessary adjustments of the needle can then be made prior to cement injection. This technique has proven to be invaluable on multiple occasions and does not add to the morbidity, technical complexity or time required for the procedure.

After the needle is placed in a satisfactory position, a mixture of polymethylmethacrylate (PMMA) and barium sulphate can then prepared. Mixing of the polymer and monomer of the PMMA should only be done at this stage and not earlier as the surgeon must not feel pressured to attain optimal placement of the needle before the cement hardens. Many commercially available bone cements now have radio-opaque contrast media pre-mixed into the cement, making addition of barium sulphate unnecessary. One should wait till optimal consistency of the cement is achieved before injecting it. At optimal consistency, the cement should be of a honey-like consistency. Injecting the cement too early, while it is of low viscosity will result in possible leaking, while injecting the cement while it is too viscous will prove to be extremely difficult, if not impossible. Adequate filling is achieved when the cement fills to the posterior one quarter of the vertebral body. A total of 2 to 6 mls of cement should suffice. Studies have shown that there is no correlation between the volume of cement injected and pain reduction [9].

There is significant debate regarding whether to place a single transpedicular needle versus placing a transpedicular needle on either side. Studies have shown no significant differences in terms of clinical outcome using either technique [10]. The author of this chapter advocates using a bi-transpedicular technique for several reasons. Placement of 2 needles rather than just 1 does not significantly add to procedural time or complexity of the procedure. There are several advantages of having 2 accurately placed needles rather than 1. Also, with 2 needles in place, 1 may act as a "vent" while cement is injected through the other. In addition, should 1 needle be deemed unsuitable for use for injection of cement (should the needle become blocked or demonstrate signs of leakage), a second needle is readily available for use. Lastly, a more symmetrical injection of cement can be achieved by using a bi-transpedicular technique.

The patient should remain prone till the cement has hardened. There is no consensus regarding the immediate post-operative weight bearing status of the patient. Some authors do the procedure as a "Day Case" and patients are allowed to weight bear immediately post-operatively. Others prefer to keep the patient rested in bed and only allow weight bearing on the first post-operative day. In our practice, all patients are instructed to rest in bed for the rest of the day following the procedure, and only allowed weight bearing and discharge the next day.

Mode of Action

The most intuitive explanation for the proven efficacy of vertebroplasty in relieving pain from compression fractures is a mechanical one. Injection of bone cement imparts instantaneous stability to the fracture, not only providing structural stability, but also holding the fracture together and reducing micromovements between the fractured surfaces [11]. Assuming that this is the only mode of action, one might conclude that injecting the affected vertebral body with larger amounts of cement would yield better results. This, however appears to be an erroneous assumption. Studies have shown that there is a lack of correlation between the volume of cement injected [12] and the degree of pain relief achieved. Some postulate that in addition to the structural effect of cement injection, another possible effect includes ablation or alteration of the afferent nerve endings at the affected vertebral body by chemical toxicity and thermal injury [13] (during the exothermic reaction of cement curing).

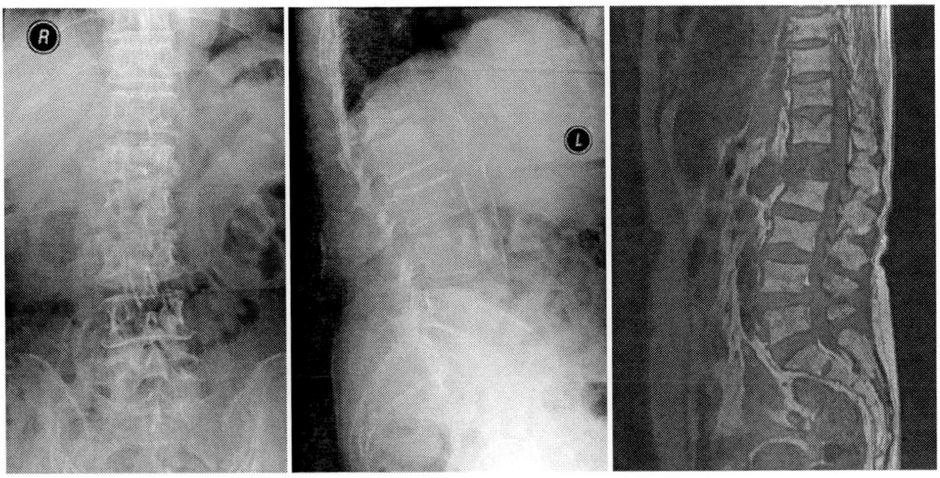

Pre vertebroplasty

The above x-rays show wedge compression fracture of the L1 vertebra.
The MRI confirms the fracture is new as evidenced by the reduced signal intensity on the T1 weighted image

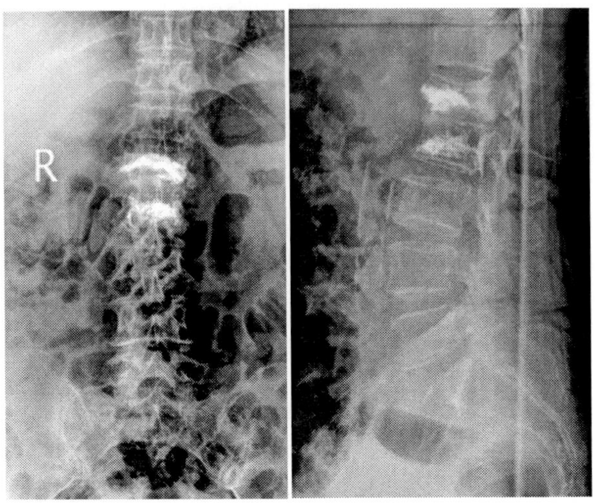

Post vertebroplasty

The x-rays show the appearance of vertebral bodies after treatment with vertebroplasty.

INDICATIONS AND CONTRAINDICATIONS

The main indication for vertebroplasty is persistent or debilitating pain from compression fractures of the vertebra, although some have extended the use of the procedure to treatment of continued collapse of an affected vertebral body and severe kyphosis especially at the thoracolumbar segment.

Contraindications to vertebroplasty can be broadly classified into patient factors and pathology. Young patients should not be treated with vertebroplasty for 2 main reasons. Firstly their potential for healing are superior to that of older patients and the fracture should be allowed to achieve stability by healing rather than by injection of bone cement which would permanently impede healing. The second reason is that younger patients presumably have a longer life expectancy and the long term effects of bone cement in vertebra is, as yet, unknown. Generally vertebroplasty should only be considered for patients under the age of 65. Pregnant patients are also not candidates for vertebroplasty as this subset of patients are invariably young. Also, they should not be subjected to repeated fluoroscopy, which is a requirement in vertebroplasty, as earlier described.

Allergy to either contrast media or bone cement will make some patients unsuitable for the procedure. Other patients may be unable to lie prone for the duration of the procedure which may take up to 45 minutes. Patients with any sources of infection should not undergo vertebroplasty till the source of infection is effectively eliminated. This applies to even somewhat simple lesions, for example, pimples, abrasions etc on the skin where the vertebroplasty needle would have to traverse. Introducing infection into the vertebral body would be troublesome, to say the least.

The pathology of the fracture is another factor to consider. Patients who have existing neurological deficit should not undergo vertebroplasty. This is because these patients already display signs of cord compression and as such, have lower "reserves". A minor cement leak which would have been asymptomatic in a more wisely chosen patient could potentially result in severe neurological compromise in these patients.

Patients presenting with burst fractures or Chance injuries should not undergo vertebroplasty. There is a real risk of cement leak with vertebroplasty in burst fractures and chance fractures often require surgical stabilization with instrumentation. Severe degrees of compression fractures (>70% reduction in height) used to be considered an absolute contraindication [14] but as experience and expertise in this procedure improves, cases of vertebral plana are increasingly treated with vertebroplasty [15]. Currently, even patients in whom the fracture line extends to the posterior wall can be considered candidates for the procedure, provided the surgeon has the requisite skill and experience to prevent development of a cement leak.

TIMING OF SURGERY

There are currently no strict guidelines as to when vertebroplasty should be offered or performed. Some authors have advocated waiting four to six weeks [16]. Others are offering the procedure as early as three weeks after the acute fracture. In view of the excellent safety profile of the procedure and the rapidity of the pain relief, it seems reasonable to offer the procedure early, especially to patients who experience such severe pain as to incapacitate them and confine them to bed with the attendant problems of prolonged recumbency. Clinical judgment must be exercised in these cases.

COMPLICATIONS

Although complications in vertebroplasty are not frequent, they can be potentially devastating. The main complications include anesthetic complications, misplacement of the vertebroplasty needle, cement extravasation, adjacent level fracture and infection. In addition, other authors have reported other serious complications including pulmonary embolism and myocardial infarction.

Cement leakage can occur via improperly placed needles, breaches in the vertebra (which can occur anywhere from its insertion point through the pedicles to the vertebral body) and through venous plexuses within the vertebral body. The reported incidence of cement leakage varies widely. This is likely due to the clarity and quality of the imaging modality used in performing the procedure. Procedures done under standard intra-operative fluoroscopic guidance or image intensifiers will be less sensitive for cement leakages as compared to CT guided vertebroplasty. Reports of cement leaks range from 6% to 25% for fluoroscopically done procedures [17,18]. Small leakages have been detected in CT guided procedures in up to 55.4% of cases [19]. The large majority of these small leaks is not significant clinically and is asymptomatic. The symptoms that patients suffer as a result of the leaks depend heavily on the site of extravasation. Leaks into the neural foramina or spinal canal could result in potentially devastating complications. Leaks into the epidural spaces have been associated with large volumes of cement injected [20,21].

Other serious complications occur only infrequently but deserve mention. Infections of the vertebral body are rare and till date, only several cases have been reported as case reports by different authors [22]. Needle biopsy for identification of the offending organism is indicated and may require surgical decompression. Pulmonary embolism has also been reported post vertebroplasty [5]. These are usually not symptomatic, but may rarely produce clinical symptoms accompanying pulmonary infarct.

There has also been concern regarding the possibility of increasing the risk of adjacent level fractures as a result of reduced local spinal flexibility especially in cases where cement leakage had occurred into the adjacent level discs. This could allow propagation of forces into the adjacent levels, predisposing them to fractures [23]. No studies have conclusively proven this hypothesis.

CONCLUSION

Percutaneous vertebroplasty is a safe and efficacious method of pain relief in the treatment of wedge compression fractures of the spine. Pain relief is often rapid and dramatic. This procedure has a definite role in the management of painful wedge compression fractures, which till the development of vertebroplasty, necessitated the often suboptimal management of analgesia, bed rest and gentle physiotherapy.

Although this technique has almost established itself as the standard of care for painful compression fractures in many tertiary centers, it must be recommended to patients only after careful consideration, as complications could potentially be devastating.

REFERENCES

[1] Bostrom MP, Lane JM. Future directions. Augmentation of osteoporotic vertebral bodies. *Spine* 1997;15:38–42.

[2] Leech JA, Dulberg C, Kellie S, Pattee L, Gay J. Relationship of lung function to severity of osteoporosis in women. *Am Rev Respir Dis* 1990;141:68–71.

[3] Kado DM, Browner WS, Palermo L. Vertebral fractures and mortality in older women: a prospective study. Study of osteoporotic fractures research group. *Arch Intern Med* 1999;159:1215–20.

[4] Galibert P, Deramond H, Rosat P, Le Gars D. Preliminary note on the treatment of vertebral angioma by percutaneous acrylic vertebroplasty. *Neurochir* 1987;33:166–8.

[5] Jensen ME, Evans AJ, Mathis JM, Kallmes DF, Cloft HJ, Dion JE. Percutaneous polymethylmethacrylate vertebroplasty in the treatment of osteoporotic vertebral body compression fractures: technical aspects. *AJNR Am J Neuroradiol* 1997;18:1897–904.

[6] Mathis JM, Barr JD, Belkoff SM. Percutaneous vertebroplasty: a developing standard of care for vertebral compression fractures. *AJNR Am J Neuroradiol* 2001;22:373–81.

[7] Cotten A, Boutry N, Cortet B. Percutaneous vertebroplasty: state of the art. *Radiographics* 1998;18:311–20.

[8] Gaughen JR, Jensen ME, Schweickert PA. Relevance of antecedent venography in percutaneous vertebroplasty for the treatment of osteoporotic compression fractures. *AJNR Am J Neuroradiol* 2002;23:594–600.

[9] Belkoff SM, Mathis JM, Jasper LE et al. The biomechanics of vertebroplasty. The effect of cement volume on mechanical behavior. *Spine* 2001;26(14):1537-41

[10]Kim AK, Jensen ME, Dion JE. Unilateral transpedicular percutaneous vertebroplasty: initial experience. *Radiology* 2002;222:737–41.

[11]Belkoff SM, Mathis JM, Fenton DC, Scribner RM, Reiley ME, Talmadge K. An ex vivo biomechanical evaluation of an inflatable bone tamp used in the treatment of compression fracture. *Spine* 2001;26:151–6.

[12]Dean JR, Ison KT, Gishen P. The strengthening effect of percutaneous vertebroplasty. *Clin Radiol* 2000;55:471–6.

[13]Mathis JM, Petri M, Naff N. Percutaneous vertebroplasty treatment of steroidinduced osteoporotic compression fracture. *Arthritis Rheum* 1998;41:171–5.

[14]Cotten A, Boutry N, Cortet B. Percutaneous vertebroplasty: state of the art. *Radiographics* 1998;18:311–20.

[15]Barr JD, Barr MS, Lemley TJ, McCann RM. Percutaneous vertebroplasty for pain relief and spinal stabilization. *Spine* 2000;25:923–8.

[16]Truumees E, Hilibrand A, Vaccaro AR. Percutaneous vertebral augmentation. *The Spine J* 2004;4:218–29.

[17]Grados F, Depriester C, Cayrolle G. Long-term observations of vertebral osteoporotic fractures treated by percutaneous vertebroplasty. *Rheumatology (Oxford)* 2000;39:1410–4.

[18]Layton KF, Thielen KR, Koch CA, Luetmer PH, Lane JI, Wald JT, Kallmes DF (2007) Vertebroplasty, first 1000 levels of a single center: evaluation of the outcomes and complications. *Am J Neuroradiol 28*:683–689.

[19]Pitton MB, Herber S, Koch U, Oberholzer K, Drees P, Düber C. CT-guided vertebroplasty: analysis of technical results, extraosseous cement leakages, and complications in 500 procedures. *Eur Radiol.* 2008 Jun 4.

[20]Baroud G, Crookshank M, Bohner M (2006) High-viscosity cement significantly enhances uniformity of cement filling in vertebroplasty: an experimental model and study on cement leakage. *Spine 31*:2562–2568.

[21]Ryu KS, Park CK, Kim MC, Kang JK (2002) Dose-dependent epidural leakage of polymethylmethacrylate after percutaneous vertebroplasty in patients with osteoporotic vertebral compression fractures. *J Neurosurg 96*(1 Suppl):56–61.

[22]Vats HS, McKiernan FE. Infected vertebroplasty: case report and review of literature. *Spine*. 2006 Oct 15;31(22):E859-62.

[23]Baroud G, Bohner M (2006) Biomechanical impact of vertebroplasty. Postoperative beiomechanics of vertebroplasty. *Joint Bone Spine 73*:144–150.

In: Osteoporosis: Etiology, Diagnosis and Treatment
Editors: Bilar E. Mattingly and Albert C. Pillare
ISBN 978-1-60692-397-9

Chapter 15

Drug Induced Osteoporosis Fracture Risk Associated with Drugs Other Than Corticosteroids

Peter Vestergaard* MD PhD DrMedSc, Lars Rejnmark MD PhD DrMedSc, Leif Mosekilde MD DrMedSc
Department of Endocrinology and Metabolism C, Aarhus Amtssygehus, Aarhus University Hospital

Abstract

Drugs may affect bone turnover and density in many ways. However, the disease for which the drugs are administered may also contribute to bone loss. Drugs against epilepsy may be associated with a limited increase in the risk of fractures. However, much of the increase may be linked to the underlying disease. Sedatives and anxiolytics may be associated with a limited increase in the risk of fractures, especially among the drugs with long half-lives. Among the antidepressants, especially those which inhibit serotonin reuptake (SSRI) are associated with an increase in the risk of fractures, possibly linked to the effect of serotonin on the bone cells, but also through an increased risk of falls. Neuroleptics may be associated with a limited increase in the risk of fractures. In contrast to mosh other psychotropic drugs, lithium seems associated with a decrease in the risk of fractures, possibly mediated through a bone anabolic effect via the Wnt signalling system. Type 1 diabetes is associated with a decrease in bone mineral, while type 2 diabetes is associated with an increase. The new class of thiazolidinediones (glitazones) has been associated with an increased loss of bone mineral. Most cardiovascular drugs (thiazide diuretics, nitrates, digoxin, antihypertensive drugs, and statins) are associated with a decrease in the risk of fractures, possibly though an amelioration of the negative effects of the underlying cardiovascular system on the

* Correspondence concerning this article should be addressed to: Peter Vestergaard MD PhD DrMedSc, The Osteoporosis Clinic, Aarhus Amtssygehus, Tage Hansens Gade 2, DK-8000 Aarhus C, Denmark. Telephone + 45 89 49 76 81; Fax + 45 89 49 76 84; E-mail p-vest@post4.tele.dk.

skeleton. A few exceptions are amiodarone, which is associated with an increased risk of fractures, and vitamin K antagonists, which do not seem to affect the risk of fractures much. Infection with human immunodeficiency virus leads to a loss of bone mineral, while treatment with highly active antiretroviral therapy does not seem to contribute to further bone loss. Proton pump inhibitors may lead to decreased calcium absorption and thus a decreased bone mineral and an increased risk of fractures. In breast cancer treatment tamoxifen is associated with an increased bone mineral, while the newer class of aromatase inhibitors through a decrease in serum estradiol are associated with an increased loss of bone mineral. Strong analgesics (opioids) may decrease bone mineral density through inhibition of gonadotrophins while weak analgesics such as the non-steroidal anti-inflammatory drugs may increase bone mineral through an effect on the prostaglandin system. However, possibly through an increased risk of falls, the weak analgesics are associated with an increased risk of fractures.

By analysing these differences much can be learned about signalling pathways in the skeleton much in the same way as through screening of the human genome.

1. Introduction

Drugs may affect calcium metabolism and thus bone mineral through a number of mechanisms. Several new classes of drugs have high lightened this by revealing negative effects on bone turnover and bone mineral density with an increased risk of fractures. Some of the older drugs classes have also been shown to have interesting effects on bone turnover, which have shown the significance of novel signal systems on bone physiology and turnover. Thus not all drugs may exert negative effects on the skeleton, and a systematic review of mechanisms of action of drugs may reveal new and interesting signalling mechanisms and may potentially lead to the discovery of new treatment principles against osteoporosis just in the same way as a screening of the genome may bring new potential targets for therapy against osteoporosis. Furthermore may new knowledge be achieved on drugs that may perhaps be preferred over other drugs in patients at risk of osteoporosis and fractures.

The aim of this review is to present the effects of some of the more widely used drugs on bone metabolism and the risk of fractures. This may also shed new light on some of the myths regarding fracture risk associated with some drugs. Table 1 presents an overview on the odds ratios (OR) for fracture associated with some of the more widely used drugs compared to non-users of the drug in question.

Table 1. Association between drugs and the risk of any fracture adjusted for fractures

Drug group	Drug	OR (95% CI)
Antiepileptics	Carbamazepine	1.18 (1.10-1.26)
	Phemobarbital	1.79 (1.64-1.95)
	Phenytoin	1.20 (1.00-1.43)
	Lamotrigine	1.04 (0.91-1.19)
	Oxcarbazepine	1.14 (1.03-1.26)
	Valproate	1.15 (1.05-1.26)

Table 1. (Continued)

Drug group	Drug	OR (95% CI)
	Topiramate	1.39 (0.99-1.96)
CNS active drugs	Anxiolytics and sedatives ≥0.33 DDD/dag	1.10 (1.07-1.13)
	Neuroleptics >0.1 DDD/dag	1.18 (1.12-1.25)
	Tricyclic antidepressants ≥0.75 DDD/dag	1.27 (1.13-1.42)
	Selective serotoin reuptake inhibitors ≥0.75 DDD/dag	1.40 (1.35-1.46)
	Lithium ≥850 DDD	0.72 (0.59-0.89)
Antidiabetics	Insulin ≥2.000 DDD	0.88 (0.76-1.02)
	Metformin ≥500 DDD	0.81 (0.70-0.93)
	Sulphonylureas ≥1.300 DDD	0.85 (0.76-0.95)
	Glitazones *	1.74 (1.31-2.31)
Cardiovascular drugs	Thiazide diuretics	0.90 (0.88-0.93)
	Loop diuretics	1.04 (1.01-1.07)
	Beta blockes	0.91 (0.88-0.93)
	Calcium antagonists	0.94 (0.91-0.96)
	Angiotensin converting enzym inhibitors (incl AT2-antagonists)	0.93 (0.90-0.96)
	Amiodarone	1.47 (1.21-1.78)
	Digoxin	0.75 (0.71-0.79)
	Oral anticoagulants	1.10 (1.03-1.18)
	Nitroglycerin	0.89 (0.86-0.92)
Drugs against ulcers	Proton pump inhibitors	1.18 (1.12-1.43)
	Histamine H2 receptor antagonists	0.88 (0.82-0.95)
Pain killers	Morphine	1.47 (1.37-1.58)
	Oxycodone	1.36 (1.08-1.59)
	Nicomorfin	1.57 (1.38-1.78)
	Pethidine	0.98 (0.89-1.08)
	Tramadol	1.54 (1.49-1.59)
	Codeine	1.16 (1.12-1.20)
	Acetaminophene	1.45 (1.41-1.49)
	Acetylsalicylic acid	0.92 (0.76-1.12)
	Ibuprofene	1.76 (1.72-1.81)
	Naproxene	1.37 (1.29-1.46)
	Celecoxib	0.94 (0.84-1.04)
	Rofecoxib	1.02 (0.96-1.07)
Drugs against cancer	Methotrexate	1.01 (0.91-1.12)
	Azathioprine	1.17 (1.03-1.33)
	Tamoxifen	N/A
	Aromatase inhibitors	1.21 (1.03-1.43)

OR: Odds ratio, CI: confidence interval.

2. Material and Methods

PubMed, EMBASE, and Web of Science were searched using the MESH terms: "fracture", and the disease/condition/syndrome that was relevant (say "epilepsy"). Furthermore, abstract books from J Bone Mineral Research, Bone, Osteoporosis Int og

Calcified Tissue Int were searched manually. Papers reporting on an association between the risk of fracture and any given drugs were retrieved.

3. CNS Active Drugs

3.1. Drugs Against Epilepsy

Patients with epilepsy have an increased risk of fractures mainly related to traumas sustained during seizures, i.e. spine fractures occurring from convulsions of the spine muscles or peripheral fractures from convulsions or traumas say a fall during a grand mal or petit mal seizure. The risk of fractures is thus associated with the severity of and the number of seizures.

Patients treated with antiepileptic drugs (AEDs) may have a limited reduction in bone mineral density (BMD), which may explain a minor part of the increased risk of fractures. The decrease in BMD is often limited (less than 0.5 T- or Z-scores). However, the decrease in BMD may also be linked to the underlying disease, and not just to the AEDs. This is in particular the case in children especially those with developmental disorders. Children with developmental disorders more often suffer from epilepsy, and children with developmental disturbances more often have growth disturbances, are malnourished, have vitamin D deficient due to their concomitant handicaps, and this in combination increase the risk of decreased BMD.

Epidemiological studies have shown a limited increase in the risk of fractures in subjects using AEDs. Carbamazepine, oxcarbazepine, clonazepam, og valproate were associated with a rather limited increase in the risk of fractures (OR in the range 1.1-1.2) while Phenobarbital was associated with a somewhat higher risk (OR 1.8) probably due to the sedative effect leading to an increased risk of sat falls, but also a liver inducing effect may play a role. Ethosuximide, lamotrigine, phenytoin, primidone, tiagabine, topiramate, and vigabatrin were not statistically significantly associated with risk of fractures. However, the confidence intervals were so wide that they overlapped the AEDs who were actually statistically significantly associated with the risk of fractures. Liver inducing AEDs (phenobarbital, phenytoin, mysoline) were associated with a somewhat higher risk of fractures than non liver inducing AEDs. This may be due to the increased vitamin D degradation inflicted by liver inducing AEDs. Also for these drugs the group at highest risk is institutionalized patients with severe co-morbidity and latent vitamin D deficiency.

It is not known if AEDs change the biomechanical competence of the skeleton, i.e. if the relationship between BMD and fracture risk changes. More research is thus needed as most studies are observational. In conclusion it is important to control the number and severity of seizures to prevent fractures. The decrease in BMD associated with AEDs is often limited. An adequate vitamin D status should be maintained.

3.2. Psychopharmacological Drugs

3.2.1. Antidepressants

Patients with depression may have a decreased BMD. However, not all studies have demonstrated a decreased BMD in patients with depression. The mechanisms behind the reduced BMD are not known, but a reduced nutrition with lack of vital nutrients such as calcium and vitamin D may also play a role.

No studies are available showing a direct effect of tricyclic antidepressants (TCAs) on bone metabolism, however recent studies have failed to show an effect on cross sectional BMD and rate of BMD loss, thus indicating that in terms of BMD TCAs may be safe.

Recent research has shown that osteoblasts have serotonin receptors, and inhibition of the serotonin system may lead to osteopenia in animal models. This may signal a reduction in BMD also in humans with the use of selective serotonin reuptake inhibitors (SSRIs) and thus perhaps an increased fracture risk. Recent human studies have added to this concern showing a reduction in BMD in a cross sectional study and an increased loss rate for BMD in a longitudinal study. Epidemiological studies have shown that the increase in risk of fractures in particular was associated with the serotonin effect of the antidepressants. SSRIs were thus associated with an increased risk of fractures, while TCA in general were not except for sedative TCAs. The group of other antidepressants (monoamine oxidase B inhibitors and drugs with effects on norepinephrine and other signalling systems) were not associated with an increased risk of fractures.

3.2.2. Anxiolytics, Sedatives, and Hypnotics

These drugs may increase the risk of falls through their sedative effect. One tablet may thus be sufficient to increase the risk of falls and thus fractures. An alternative possibility is that insomnia may be associated with an increased risk of falls and that hypnotics thus by confounding by indication may be associated with an increased risk of fractures. Epidemiological studies have shown an increase in the risk of fractures even at low doses. Longer half lives have been associated with a higher risk of fractures than shorter half lives. However, overall the clinical significance is low, but caution is advised in elderly fall prone individuals.

3.2.3. Neuroleptics

Due to their antodopaminergic effect, neuroleptics may increase serum prolactin, which possibly may lead to a decrease in BMD. Neuroleptics may potentially in combination with the underlying psychiatric disorder increase the risk of falls. Epidemiological studies have shown a limited increase in the risk of fractures in users of neuroleptics. The clinical significance is probably limited.

3.2.4. Lithium

In terms of bone turnover lithium is particularly interesting. Lithium may induce hyperparathyroidism by acting as a calcilytic on the calcium sensing receptor (CaSR). In early studies, lithium has been associated with a decreased bone mineral content (BMC) in the forearm and bone mineral density (BMD) of the lumbar spine possibly mediated through induction of hyperparathyroidism.

One prior study reported a decreased forearm BMC in bipolar patients, but not in unipolar patients. However, the daily lithium dose tended to be higher in bipolar (mean±SD 28.8±8.3 mmol/day) than in unipolar patients (26.0±5.0 mmol/day, $p=0.06$). The BMC in unipolar patients was a little higher than in normal controls (102%, non-significant), while the BMC of the bipolar patients was significantly reduced (88% of normal, $p<0.01$). Similarly, Cohen et al. reported normal BMD in the lumbar spine and femoral neck both in patients who had used lithium for less than 12 month (daily dose 22.3 mmol/day), and in patients treated for more than 3 years (daily dose 26.8 mmol/day). A negative correlation between duration of lithium treatment and femoral neck BMD has also been reported. However, no correlation between forearm BMC, and daily dose of lithium, duration of lithium treatment, total lithium dose, and serum lithium could be found in the study by Christiansen et al.. Eren et al. failed to show a correlation between serum lithium and spine or femoral neck BMD. The absence of a correlation with serum lithium may be due to the fact that in most patients, serum lithium was aimed at being in therapeutical levels, i.e. within a narrow interval.

On the cellular level lithium has been shown to affect Wnt signalling in a bimodal way – at low concentrations lithium increases the proliferation of human mesenchymal stem cells, whereas it inhibits the proliferation in high concentrations. At low concentrations lithium may thus possess bone anabolic properties. Lithium has been shown to inhibit bone resorption by inhibiting the effects of 1,25-dihydroxy-vitamin D. Lithium also interferes with the calcium sensing receptor (CaSR) by decreasing the sensitivity to calcium, i.e. the "set-point" is increased, and parathyroid hormone (PTH) secretion is increased. The increase in PTH secretion following administration of lithium may theoretically mimic the anabolic effects of PTH.

A large-scale case control study from Denmark (n=124,655 fracture cases and 373,962 controls, 1,403 [0.3%] users of lithium) reported a dose dependent decreased overall risk of fractures (OR decreasing from 0.96 with <250 DDD in the prior 5 years over 0.71 for 250-849 DDD to 0.72 with ≥850 DDD). At high doses ≥850 DDD there was a borderline significant decrease in the risk of forearm fractures, while a borderline insignificant decrease was present for spine fractures. No association was present for hip fractures.

A further epidemiological case-control study (n=231,778 fracture cases and n=231,778 controls, 1,027 [0.2%] users of lithium) from the UK also found a reduced risk of fractures among users of lithium (OR=0.85) in the same range as the prior study, but could not confirm a dose response effect and concluded that pharmacological effects of lithium could not explain the risk reduction.

However, given that lithium as the only drugs in the categories for treatment of manic depressive episodes was associated with a reduction in the risk of fractures even after adjustment for co-morbidity and use of other CNS active drugs makes lithium an attractive candidate for further research into the mechanisms, and if the difference is real perhaps a choice for patients with osteoporosis and manic depressive episodes in high risk for fractures. However, more research is needed.

3.2.5. Parkinson's Disease

Patients with Parkinsonism have an increased risk of fractures, and especially of femoral neck fractures. The risk of fractures is related to the increased risk of falls, related both to Parkinsonism per se and to concomitant dementia. However, the patients also have a decreased bone mineral density (BMD) linked to decreased vitamin D levels and secondary hyperparathyroidism, which may also contribute to the increased risk of fractures. Other factors such as vitamin K1 deficiency and high homocysteine levels may also contribute. An epidemiological study did not show any effect of drugs against Parkinsonism in alleviating the risk of fractures.

4. Drugs Against Diabetes

Diabetes mellitus per se is associated with disturbances in bone metabolism. The patophysiology is complex with many factors being active. One important factor is glucosuria, which through osmotic effects or prostaglandin mediated effects leads to an increased excretion of calcium in the urine. Vitamin D metabolism may be impaired both through the diabetes per se but also through impairment of renal function. Formation of advanced glycation end products (AGE) and their interaction with their receptor (RAGE) may interact with collagen formation and the cytokine system leading to osteoporosis. Body mass index modifies bone mineral density (BMD) as patients with type 1 diabetes (T1D) have a decreased BMD while patients with type 2 diabetes (T2D) have an increased BMD. In T1D an increased risk of fractures is seen, whereas in T2D a much smaller increase on the risk of fractures is seen.

Traditional drugs against diabetes such as insulin, sulphonylureas and metformin have been associated with a reversal of the negative effects of diabetes on bone metabolism and a decrease in the risk of fractures.

However, recent data for the new class of drugs against diabetes the thiazolidinediones (glitazones) have raised concern as an increased risk of fractures was seen in contrast to what should be expected from the effect on blood glucose control. The glitazones are ligands for perioxisome proliferators-activated receptor-gamma (PPARγ), and have effects on a number of organ systems leading to among others adipocyte differentiation. A prior study in mice with troglitazone has shown an increase in adipocyte volume in the bone marrow with a decrease in haematopoetic marrow, and a decrease in vascular sinusoid volume, while the bone volume and ash weight did not differ between troglitazone and placebo treated mice. The increased volume of adipocytes should theoretically decrease the number of osteoblasts in the bone marrow and thus bone formation as adipocytes and osteoblasts are derived from a common mesenchymal progenitor. Two studies in mice using rosiglitazone have reported a decreased bone mineral density (BMD) and a decrease in the number of osteoblasts and a decrease in bone formation expressed as wall width. The expression of key osteoblastogenic transcription factors such as Runx2 and Osterix was decreased leading to a diversion of progenitor cells away from osteoblastogesis to adipocytogenesis. The number of osteoclasts was unaffected. In humans use of glitazones (n=69 of 666 diabetic subjects, 22 users of troglitazone, 30 users of pioglitazone, and/or 31 users of rosiglitazone) has been associated with an increased loss of BMD in the spine, trochanter and whole body in women (n=32 users of glitazones), but not in men (n=37 users of glitazones) with diabetes. A randomised controlled trial using rosiglitazone, metformin, or glyburide (n=4360 in total followed for 4 years) reported an increased risk of limb fractures in women, but not in men. It has been concluded that this negative effect of the glitazones may be a class effect, as a similar increase in fracture risk has been seen with pioglitazone as with rosiglitazone. Caution must thus been taken with the use of glitazones and these should be avoided in individuals at risk of osteoporosis and fractures.

5. Cardiovascular Drugs

5.1. Diuretics

Thiazide diuretics (TD) and loop diuretics (LD) have opposing effects on calcium homeostasis. The renal calcium excretion is increased during treatment with LD, while it is reduced during treatment with TD. Randomised controlled trials (RCT) have shown that TD increases BMD, and case-control studies have shown a reduced risk of fractures in patients treated with TD. However, no RCT are available on the effect of TD on the risk of fractures in patients with osteoporosis. TD may thus not be used for preventing and treating osteoporosis. TD does not affect the plasma levels of parathyroid hormone (PTH), whereas LD increases PTH in a dose-dependent manner. Four to six hours after ingestion of LD PTH may be increased by up to 100% and 24 hours after ingestion, PTH is increased by 25% per 40 mg of furosemide (equivalent to 1 mg of bumetanide). As a consequence of the increased calcium loss in the urine and increased PTH several studies have reported a decreased BMD in subjects receiving LD, and a RCT showed a decrease of 2% in BMD in postmenopausal women without cardiovascular disease in comparison with placebo after one year of treatment with 2 mg of bumetanide per day. In accordance with this LD has been associated with a slight increase in the risk of fractures in case-control studies. If treatment with a diuretic is warranted a TD may perhaps be preferred over LD in patients at risk of osteoporosis and fractures if feasible.

5.2. Statins and other Lipid Lowering Drugs

Studies in animals have shown that statins may possess bone anabolic effect, and case-control studies have shown a significantly reduced risk of fractures in users of statins. However, studies in humans have not shown clear effects on BMD of statins or changes in biochemical markers of bone turnover that could explain a change in the risk of fractures. This has raised the question whether the reduced risk of fractures in users of statins was indeed the effect of the statins on bone tissue or rather a spurious effect not linked to the statins. As statins are recirculated in the enterohepatic circle it is possible that the concentration of statins in bone is too low to have bone anabolic effects in humans although such have been seen in animals. It has been suggested that the seemingly lower risk of fractures may be due to certain characteristics of the statin treated subjects (such as e.g. life style and body mass index) which may be associated with a decreased risk of fractures. However, some studies have shown that only lipophilic statins (such as simvastatin) and not hydrophilic statins (such as pravastatin) or non-statin lipid lowering drugs (e.g. the fibrates) are associated with a reduced risk of fractures, and this may point at a true pharmacological effect on bone.

5.3. Blood Pressure Lowering Drugs, Antiarrhythmics, and Nitroglycerin

Only few studies are available on the risk of fractures in relation to treatment with different blood pressure lowering drugs and antiarrhythmics. A limited reduction in the risk of fractures have been observed in patients using beta-blockers, calcium-antagonists, and angiotensin converting enzyme (ACE) inhibitors and angiotensin 2 receptor (AT2) blockers. Osteoblasts have receptors for these drugs, and a direct effect on bone turnover is thus possible. Patients treated with digoxin also have been reported to have a decreased risk of fractures, whereas amiodarone may be associated with an increased risk of fractures. The mechanisms for these observations are not known in detail. One possible explanation is that digoxin besides strengthening the heart muscle also exerts positive effects on peripheral skeletal muscles and thus decreases the risk of falls. Sensitizing of the skin to sun light is a known side effect of amiodarone, and amiodarone may thus through avoidance of direct sunlight be associated with vitamin D deficiency and an increased risk of fractures. Users of nitroglycerin have also been reported to have a decreased risk of fractures. The mechanism is not known in detail, but may be related to inhibition of pro-inflammatory cytokines decreasing bone resorption.

5.4. Anticoagulants

Anticoagulants act by inhibiting vitamin K (VKA – vitamin K antagonists). Vitamin K is an important co-factor in the post-translational carboxylation of several proteins that are a part of the bone matrix. Studies on the effects of VKA have not shown significant effects on BMD or fracture risk. A recent case-control study showed an increased risk of fractures in users of low accumulated doses of VKA (<100 defined daily doses), while no significant changes in the risk of fractures was seen at higher doses. Such an effect only at low doses is not a biological effect of VKA. One possible explanation is that the disease that necessitates initiation of VKA treatment (say atrial fibrillation or deep venous thromboembolism) may be associated with an increased risk of fractures, which subsequently returns to normal upon treatment of the underlying disease.

6. Drugs Against Ulcers

Drugs used to inhibit gastric acidity include proton pump inhibitors, histamine H2 receptor antagonists (H2 blockers), and other antacid medications including bicarbonate containing preparations, and preparations containing aluminium and magnesium along with agents with specific effects on prostaglandin synthesis.

These drugs may interfere with bone metabolism and thus affect the risk of fracture. Proton pump inhibitors (PPI) such as omeprazole, esomeprazole, pantoprazole etc. inhibit the proton pump in the gastric mucosa thus reducing acid output into the stomach and duodenum in contrast to H2 blockers, which decrease acid secretion by interfering with the H2 receptor. The osteoclasts also possess proton pumps, which are used during the excretion of H^+ ions for the resorption of bone. Osteoclast selective proton pump inhibitors may therefore in theory be interesting antiresorptive agents with a potential to prevent fractures. Omeprazole has been shown to inhibit gastric proton pumps at physiological concentrations, whereas the inhibition of osteoclast and other tissue H(+)-ATPase activity such as osteoclast proton pumps was much less pronounced. In humans administration of omeprazole has been shown to alter biochemical markers of bone turnover when patients with gastric ulcers on stable histamine H2 blocker therapy were switched to omeprazole (PPI) treatment. Among patients shifted from H2 blockers to omeprazole a decrease in urine hydroxyproline and calcium was observed in comparison to patients on continued H2 blocker therapy. However it should be noted that the study did not compare changes over time, and upon direct comparison, the changes over time in patients treated with proton pump inhibitors seemed similar to those in patients treated with H2 blockers. Serum intact PTH, alkaline phosphatase, osteocalcin, and tartrate resistant phosphatase (TRAP) all increased among patients shifted to omeprazole compared to patients on continued H2 blocker therapy suggesting combined antiresorptive and anabolic properties of PPIs. Again upon comparison of the changes over time in patients treated with proton pump inhibitors the results seemed similar to those in patients treated with H2 blockers. In the evaluation of this study, it should be remembered, that the effect was observed in patients already on H2 therapy, and may thus signal reactions to removal of the H2 blockers. In patients with cystic fibrosis on lanzoprazole, bone mineral content has been shown to increase. In rats no effect of omeprazole on bone mineral content has been observed. In clinical studies pump inhibitors were associated with an increase in fracture risk while H2 blockers were not. Theoretical considerations point at an antiresorptive potential, however the clinical effect on the osteoclast may be too low for a significant effect on bone mineral. The increased risk may be linked to a decrease in calcium absorption with secondary hyperparathyroidism leading to a negative calcium balance despite the decrease in urine calcium. The increase in PTH may induce bone loss and increased fracture risk. Further studies are thus needed.

In men, the use of cimetidine (a H2 blocker) has been linked to a 2.5 fold increase in hip fracture risk. However, H2 receptor blockers have been found to have no influence on BMD in humans. In rats, cimitidine has been shown to prevent osteopenia by preventing osteoclast differentiation induced by histamine. Furthermore, studies in rats on histamine H2 antagonists have demonstrated antiresorptive properties. In this context, H2 receptors seem to play a more central role for osteoclasts than H1 receptors, in accordance with our findings of no effects of H1 receptor blocking drugs (antihistamines). H2 blockers may thus increase BMD, and this could be one mechanism underlying the decrease in fracture risk. One epidemiological study showed a trend towards a decreased fracture risk with H2 blockers. At present the mechanism for this is not known in details.

Aluminum containing antacids may inhibit intestinal phosphate absorption inducing hypophosphataemia and impaired mineralisation. In patients with impaired renal function aluminium may per se impair mineralisation. Calcium containing antacids may increase calcium absorption and thus increase the bone mineral. One epidemiological study showed a trend towards an increased risk of fractures with the use of the group of other antacids.

7. Pain Medication

Pain medications are in widespread used both for acute and chronic pain. Any fracture risk associated with pain medication may thus have a significant impact on a population level. The pain killers may be subdivided into: 1) weak analgesics, which include acetaminophen, acetylsalicylic acid and the non-steroidal anti-inflammatory drugs (NSAIDs), and 2) strong analgesics, which include opiate like substances acting on the morphine receptors (morphine, opiate and derivatives, which may be agonists or partial agonists and antagonists on the morphine receptors).

In terms of BMD, the weak analgesics mainly act via the prostaglandin system, and the prostaglandin system may interact directly with bone cells and thus affect bone mineral density and bone fragility. Prostaglandins may stimulate bone resorption, and NSAIDs may in vitro inhibit bone resorption, which in theory should lead to an increased bone mineral density.

The effects of prostaglandins on bone turnover is complex, as say prostaglandin E2 (PGE2) may both have a stimulatory and an inhibitory effect on bone formation expressed as collagen formation in fetal fat calvariae. However, PGE2 may also stimulate osteoclastic bone resorption, although a transient reduction may also be seen.

However, it remains unclear if these effects are of significance in vivo. Increased inflammation lead to bone loss from increased production of prostaglandins, and this may be countered by NSAIDs, and similar conditions may be seen in postmenopausal women where an increased level of prostaglandins may be present and the increased bone resorption may be countered by NSAIDs. However, in the normal subject it is unclear if NSAIDs may increase BMD in the absence of inflammation. Several epidemiological studies have been performed. Carbone et al. in a cross sectional study of 2,853 subjects with a mean age of 73.6 years from the Health ABC cohort found that current use of relative COX-2 selective NSAIDs (defined as COX-1 IC_{50} to COX-2 IC_{50} ratio <1) with acetylsalicylic acid (ASA) was associated with a higher whole body (4.2%) and hip BMD (4.6%, n=47) than in non-users of NSAIDs or ASA (n=1,382). Current ASA use was associated with a higher whole body (1.1%) but not hip BMD. Use of COX-1 and COX-2 selective NSAIDS alone was not associated with changes in BMD after adjustment for confounders (age, gender, race, height, weight, smoking, rheumatoid arthritis, other forms of arthritis, calcium and vitamin D supplementation and Womac score). Bauer et al. in the SOF cohort of 7,786 white women aged 65 years or more observed an increased hip and spine BMD (1.0-5.8%) in current users of NSAIDs (n=1,413) or ASA (n=1,789) with a frequency of 5-7 times/week. Morton et al. in a study of 932 Caucasian community dwelling women aged 44-98 years found that users of propionic acid NSAIDs (n=84) had higher midshaft radius and lumbar spine BMD than non-users (n=818). There was no difference in ultradistal radius, femoral neck and total hip BMD. Users of acetic acid NSAIDs (n=30) did not differ from non-users at any site. Combined these cross-sectional studies adjusted for confounders indicate an increased BMD and thus a potentially lower fracture risk. However, epidemiological studies have pointed at an increased risk of fractures, possibly linked to an increased risk of falls.

No data are available on the direct effects of morphine and opiates on bone cells. Opioids have been shown to decrease sex steroid levels in both men and women. The effect may be medicated by suppression of gonadotropins by opioids, and the effect is reversible by opioid antagonists such as naloxone. However, other factors may also play a role. Among chronic i.v. abusers of opioids, malnutrition and hypogonadism secondary to this may also play a role. The underlying disease for which the opiates were administered may also contribute to the disturbances in BMD along with any concomitant treatment given for the disease in question (say chemotherapy). A large population based study has shown a decreased BMD among users of opioids with a decrease in BMD in the order of 0.3 Z or T-scores. However, dizziness leading to falls following the CNS effects of opiates may also contribute to the risk of fractures.

8. Drugs Against HIV

Most studies in patients with human immunodeficiency virus (HIV) infection have reported a decreased BMD. Only two studies did not report a decreased BMD. An increased risk of fractures has also been reported. The decrease in BMD may be linked to a number of factors such as lipodystrophy (loss of fat mass), malnutrition (wasting), use of corticosteroids, hypogonadism, central adiposity and decreased glucose tolerance. In relationship with hypogonadism, opiates may contribute to low BMD by suppressing LH and FSH. The precise mechanism behind the decreased BMD has not been completely elucidated. A histomorphometric study showed decreased parameters of formation and turnover with a correlation with disease severity. The findings regarding biochemical markers of bone turnover have been contradictory. Two studies reported low osteocalcin and thus decreased bone formation in children and adults, while one study reported high osteocalcin levels in children. Concern has been raised that treatment for HIV with highly active antiviral therapies (HAART) may lead to a decrease in BMD.

Vitamin D status is often impaired in patients with HIV, and HIV-protease inhibitors (ritonavir, indinavir, and nefinavir) have been shown to impair the 1-alpha-hydroxylase enzyme, and thus the formation of 1,25-dihydroxy-vitamin D in a cell model. They also seemed to impair formation of 25-hydroxy-vitamin D further contributing to vitamin D deficiency. However, the degradation of 1,25-dihydroxy-vitamin D was also affected but to a lesser degree than the formation of 1,25-dihydroxy-vitamin D leading to a net deficiency in the cell model. Further vitro evidence has pointed at a negative effect of HIV treatment on bone metabolism with an increased bone resorption (seen with nelfinavir, indinavir, saquinavir, and ritonavir, but not with lopinavir or amprinavir) and a decreased bone formation (seen with lopinavir and nelfinavir, but not with the other drugs) in users of HIV-protease inhibitors in vitro. However in vivo, evidence for a negative effect of HAART has been more scarce, and has so far been based on theoretical considerations. In fact BMD has been shown to be stable and not significantly reduced in patients treated with HAART in many studies. The use of HAART and duration of use has been similar in HIV patients with normal and decreased BMD. The decrease in weight and BMI in HIV patients may be more linked to the decreased BMD than the use of HAART. Bone mineral density (BMD) and content (BMC) has been shown to remain stable for two to six years in adults or even to increase in adult patients mainly treated with HAART. In children the increase in BMD was the same in the spine but lower in the total body in HIV infected children on HAART compared to normal controls. The drugs may thus not induce any major bone loss. However, more studies are needed on the differences between different types of HAART (HIV-protease inhibitors, nucleoside and non-nucleoside reverse transcriptase inhibitors, and fusion inhibitors), and differences within the individual classes of drugs (say HIV-protease inhibitors).

The mechanism by which the HAARTs maintain BMD is probably better general condition with increasing body weight and increasing fat mass. There are only case reports of fractures in HIV patients treated with HAART, and the underlying disease rather than the drugs may be responsible for this. No differences in fracture rates have been observed with different types of HAART. Treatment with bisphosphonates such as zoledronate and alendronate has been shown to increase BMD in patients on HAART.

9. Drugs Against Cancer

9.1. Breast Cancer

9.1.1. Aromatase Inhibitors

Aromatase inhibitors act by decreasing production of estradiol thereby inhibiting the growth of estrogen receptor positive tumours. However, by decreasing estradiol levels, they induce the same changes seen in menopause with an increased osteoclast activity with increased bone resorption mirrored in increasing biochemical markers of bone resorption and a negative calcium balance. This leads to a decreased bone mineral density and an increased risk of fractures. Similar effects have been seen for anastrozole, letrozole, and exemestane. Studies on aromatase inhibitors have shown an increased risk of fractures in users of aromatase inhibitors compared to users of tamoxifen. On the other hand are aromatase inhibitors significantly better tolerated with respect to endometrial cancer, hot flushes, cerebrovascular events and vaginal bleeding than tamoxifen. The balance between benefit and side effects must thus be carefully weighted.

Combining aromatase inhibitors with tamoxifen prevents much of the bone loss associated with aromatse inhibitors. However, the increase in BMD is much lower than with tamoxifen alone. When using aromatase inhibitors considerations should be given to preventive measures against bone loss and fractures in women who are at risk of osteoporosis and fractures.

9.2. Chemotherapy for Breast Cancer

Chemotherapy for breast cancer mainly consists of three principles: 1) Combination chemotherapy: CMF (cyclophosphamide, methotrexate, fluorouracil), CEF (cyclophosphamide, epirubicin, and fluorouracil) or other variations of these, 2) Taxanes (paclitaxel, docetaxel), and 3) Trastuzumab. The number of studies in the field is scarce, and few have specifically addressed women with breast cancer. The main detrimental effect on the skeleton by chemotherapy is mediated through loss of estrogen production induced by amenorrhoea in premenopausal women. The effects of chemotherapy in postmenopausal women are thus different from premneopausal women as postmenopausal women are already amenorrhoeic. Other detrimental mechanisms of chemotherapy are toxic effects of the drugs on the bone cells and decreased food intake and thus lack of vitamin D, calcium and other nutrients following nausea and vomiting. With the increasing survival among women with breast cancer, the prevention of bone loss and subsequent fractures is a priority.

9.2.1. Combination Chemotherapy

Most available studies have addressed the CMF regimen, and have demonstrated that induction of amenorrhoea was the key factor in subsequent bone loss in premenopausal women. One study on adjuvant chemotherapy for premenopausal breast cancer and axillary lymph node metastases showed that 71% of 44 women were postmenopausal at the time of the study compared to 16% of the 44 matched control women (risk difference 55%), and that most of the patients developed amenorrhoea following initiation of chemotherapy. The patients in this study had received six cycles of CMF (dose not stated). The mean lumbar spine BMD 3.5 years after treatment was 1.17 g/cm^2 in patients compared to 1.29 g/cm^2 in matched controls equalling a loss of around 1 Z-scores or an expected relative risk of any fracture around 1.5. In this study there was no difference in lumbar spine BMD in patients and controls (1.34 vs. 1.35 g/cm^2, n=11 in both groups) that were premenopausal at the time of the study, whereas patients who were postmenopausal at the time of the study had significantly lower lumbar spine BMD than controls who were premenopausal (1.17 vs. 1.29 g/cm^2, n=26 in both groups). In the small group where both patients and controls were postmenopausal (n=7 in both groups) the controls had a higher BMD than cases (1.30 vs. 1.2 g/cm^2), but significance was not stated.

All other studies have not used control groups but have reported longitudinal changes after initiation of CMF chemotherapy. A randomised controlled study in 96 patients with node positive early breast cancer compared two years with six cycles of CMF (n=43, cyclophosphamide 500 mg/m^2 i.v. on day 1 and 8 or 100 mg/m^2 orally on day 1-14, methotrexate 40 mg/m^2 i.v. on day 1 and 8, and fluorouracil 600 mg/m^2 i.v. on day 1 and 8 with an interval of 28 days between each cycle) with goserelin (a GnRH analogue, n=53, 3.6 mg s.c. with 28 days interval for two years, i.e. 26 injections). After two years this study showed a considerable decrease in bone mineral in both the spine and hip with goserelin (-

10.5% and –6.4%) and CMF (-6.5% and –4.5%). However, the bone loss with CMF seemed to be irreversible in contrast to goserelin where a partial recovery was observed after three years. At two years 100% of women on goserelin were amenorrhoeic compared to 69% of women on CMF, but after three years only 27% of women on goserelin were amenorrhoeic compared to 77% of women treated with CMF. After discontinuation the BMD levels with goserelin only increased to the same level as with CMF so that the loss of BMD at three years was the same with goserelin and CMF probably due to the recovery of menses among the goserelin treated women. The loss of BMD was closely related to amenorrhoea: women in the CMF group who had amenorrhoea had a loss of 6.4% in lumbar spine BMD and 5.2% in hip BMD after one year compared to losses of 1.6 and 3.1% in the spine and hip after one year in patients who had menstruations. It should be noted that although women maintained their menstruations a considerable loss was still seen in BMD.

Vehmanen et al. also reported a large loss in BMD after CMF (cyclophosphamide 600 mg/m^2 i.v. at day 1, methotrexate 40 mg/m^2 i.v. at day 1, fluorouracil 600 mg/m^2 i.v. on day 1 given in six cycles at an interval of three weeks) in amenorrhoeic patients (-10.4% in the lumbar spine and –5.8% in the femoral neck after 5 years) and a much smaller change in patients who maintained menstruations (-1.3% in the lumbar spine and –0.3% in the hip after 5 years). These findings are in contrast to the findings of Fogelman et al. of a large loss despite maintenance of menstruations. However, some of the patients in the study by Vehmanen et al. had received treatment with the bisphosphonate clodronate.

Saarto et al. conducted a comparable study on 148 premenopausal women with breast cancer without skeletal metastases treated with CMF. The patients were treated with six cycles of CMF (600 mg/m^2 of cyclophosphamide, 400 mg/m^2 of methotrexate, and 600 mg/m^2 of fluorouracil i.v. on day one with an interval of three weeks). This resulted in a loss of –9.5% in spine BMD and –3.9% in the femoral neck in patients with amenorrhoea vs. a loss of –0.3% in the spine and unchanged femoral neck BMD in patients with regular menstruations. Again these findings are in contrast to Fogelman et al..

For the CEF regimen one study exists using doxorubicin instead of epirubicin. Similar effects of menstrual and thus estrogen status were seen in this study with 6-10 cycles of cyclophosphamide (500 mg/m^2), doxorubicin (50 mg/m^2), and fluorouracil (500 mg/m^2). The study showed that women who became permanently amenorrheic had 14% lower BMD than women who maintained their menstrual cycles. In one study higher baseline BMD before CMF and larger decrease in serum estradiol were predictors of ovarian failure in breast cancer.

Given that the average loss of BMD after natural menopause is around 1-2% per year, the losses reported in these studies are large and gives rise to concern for fracture risk in long-term survivors. However, no fracture studies exist.

Even women who do not have amenorrhoea may lose bone, but more studies are needed. The effects on BMD of adjuvant chemotherapy in women already postmenopausal are not known in detail and needs further evaluation.

9.2.1.1. Individual drugs

9.2.1.1.1. Cyclophosphamide

In male Wistar rats cyclophosphamide (10-20 mg/kg/day) has been shown to cause disorders of bone remodelling, and decreases in bone mass and mineral content along with growth disturbances with decreases in length and diameter of the bones followed by decreases in bone. The synthesis of collagen has also been impaired with cyclophosphamide in rats, which may lead to increased bone fragility in the same way as seen with osteogenesis imperfects. Whether similar effects would occur in the adult skeleton is unknown. Cyclophosphamide also reduces fracture healing in rabbits. Human studies on cyclophosphamide in breast cancer are however lacking.

9.2.1.1.2. Methotrexate

Low dose oral methotrexate used in rheumatoid arthritis has not shown any effect on BMD. However, the doses in these studies were on average 7.5-11 mg methotrexate orally or i.v. per week, i.e. 23-44 mg per 3-4 weeks compared to around 65-70 mg i.v. in a standard adult female per 3-4 weeks with the CMF regimens. A study indicated that the effect of methotrexate on bone was dose dependent, as higher doses were associated with a lower forearm BMC. A rat study showed decreased cancellous bone volume with methotrexate. However, negative consequences of methotrexate in rat models, may be linked to folinic acid deficiency. In a cell culture study on human osteoblast like cells from children vincristine, etoposide, daunorubicin, and asparaginase all caused a decrease in the synthesis of collagen I, whereas methotrexate did not. An epidemiological study including mainly low dose oral methotrexate for rheumatoid arthritis and other non-malignant conditions did not find any increase in the overall risk of fractures, or in fractures of the hip, forearm or spine. In conclusion methotrexate per se may perhaps be less toxic to bone cells than other cytostatic agents, but more evidence is needed especially for higher doses before firm conclusions can be drawn.

9.2.1.1.3. Other Chemotherapeutics:

No studies specifically addressing fluorouracil alone exist. Existing studies on fluorouracil have all except one been performed with the fluorouracil as part of the CMF regimen (see above). One study was performed with the CEF regimen using doxorubicin instead of epirubicin. A study in dogs using doxorubicin, cisplatin and ifosfamide showed that the isolated effects of chemotherapy on the bone turnover may be limited and reversible (note that this study did not include hypogonadism). No data exist for epirubicin, taxanes, or trastuzumab. However, given that epirubicin and taxanes induce menopause in the same way as CMF, the risk of osteoporosis may also be high. The lack of data for trastuzumab is particularly troubling as this drug interacts with essential signalling pathways. Human data are thus needed.

9.3. Prostate Cancer

Prostate cancer is dependent on testosterone for its growth. Inhibition of testosterone is thus a cornerstone in the treatment of prostate cancer. This may be achieved through orchiectomy, through the use of LHRH agonists or antiandrogens. However, the lack of testosterone may lead to osteoporosis irrespective of the way it is induced.

In a few patients with hormone resistant prostate cancer chemotherapy may be indicated. In these patients the same considerations regarding hypogonadism as mentioned for breast cancer are present. As an experimental treatment, raloxifene has been used in patients with prostate cancer. No large-scale studies with hard end-points exist for raloxifene.

As prostate cancer is a frequent cancer in men the use of androgen deprivation therapy may thus be a major cause of bone loss and an increased risk of fractures.

10. Immunomodulator Drugs

These drugs may be used to suppress immune activity in rheumatoid arthritis and other rheumatological conditions, in inflammatory bowel disease, in kidney diseases, liver diseases, and in patients undergoing organ transplantation. Inflammatory diseases per se may be associated with an increased bone loss associated with the increased level of inflammatory cytokines and inflammation in general.

10.1. Prednisolone

Corticosteroids have a range of effects on the skeleton: They affect sex steroids, interfere with calcium turnover, affect collagen, and do perhaps alter bone biomechanical competence. Regarding the effects on sex steroids, corticosteroids inhibit sex steroid synthesis and secretion leading to relative sex steroid deficiency with increased osteoclastic bone resorption and a negative calcium balance. With respect to calcium balance corticosteroids antagonise the effects of vitamin D leading to decreased calcium absorption from the intestine and an increased calcium loss in the kidneys resulting in a negative calcium balance with secondary hyperparathyroidism. The corticosteroids have direct effects on the bone cells with decreased osteoblast activity leading to a decreased bone formation. Osteoclasts may also be affected with increased bone resorption. Corticosteroids also interfere with collagen synthesis leading to a decreased synthesis and a increased degradation resulting in bone fragility. The IGF system is also negatively affected by corticosteroids, which leads to a decreased osteoblast function and a decreased formation of bone matrix. Besides the mechanisms mentioned above, which affect bone mineral density (BMD), corticosteroids may also decrease bone biomechanical competence through effects on bone structure, i.e. corticosteroid treated patients may have a large risk of fractures at the same BMD than patients not treated with corticosteroids although not all studies have confirmed this.

Corticosteroids exist in several forms, prednisolone being the most commonly used, but variations such as budesonide, fluticasone etc. also being widely used for say inhaled preparations. To compare the effect of the different preparations an equipotency scale based on anti-inflammatory potential has been adopted in some studies. The different forms of administration also represent differences in absorption and first pass metabolism in the liver. After oral administration more than 80% of corticosteroids may undergo first pass metabolism limiting the systemic bioavailability. Topically administered corticosteroids do not undergo first pass metabolism, but the absorption may be very low. For rectally administered corticosteroids 3.1% are systemically available in healthy volunteers and 4.5% in patients probably due to the inflammation in the rectum in patients with inflammatory bowel disease. For nasal corticosteroids a bio-availability of 0.4% has been reported, and for dermal preparations <0.3% are absorbed into systemic circulation. For inhaled corticosteroids, systemic bioavailability is much higher (>15%). However, healthy controls may absorb inhaled corticosteroids better than patients with lung diseases. For inhaled corticosteroids, different methods of inhalation, different devices used for inhalation, and different operation of inhalation devices may all influence the amount of corticosteroid delivered in the lungs, and the amount going into the gastrointestinal tract. Furthermore, may the absorption from the gastrointestinal tract vary as well as the degree of first pass metabolism. These differences indicate that some of the topical preparations may have very limited systemic effects.

A rapid decrease in BMD has been observed upon initiation of corticosteroids (n=20) in comparison with patients randomised to placebo (n=20) in a randomised controlled trial in patients with rheumatoid arthritis. The decrease was more pronounced in trabecular (a loss of 9% compared to placebo after 20 weeks) than in cortical bone (a loss of 0.5% compared to placebo after 20 weeks). Upon discontinuation of oral corticosteroids a rapid increase was observed in trabecular BMD to pre-treatment levels. This indicates that bone is very susceptible to the effects of corticosteroids, but also seems able to repair the damages induced upon discontinuation of corticosteroids. This is in line with the results from other studies showing that it is daily rather than cumulated dose that is associated with fracture risk. A high cumulated dose may e.g. be seen if the corticosteroids are administered intermittently. In this case the bone may have time to restore normal BMD between the series of corticosteroids. This is illustrated by a study in children with nephrotic syndrome, which received high intermittent doses of prednisolone (23 grams cumulated). But despite the high accumulated dose many years later BMD was almost normal. In the context of nephrotic syndrome it should be pointed out that the underlying disease per se may be associated with a decreased BMD and that a decreased BMD may be seen during ongoing therapy. In accordance with the study showing that corticosteroids were more detrimental to trabecular than cortical bone, the impact of corticosteroids were more pronounced on vertebral than on hip fractures, with 72% of spine and 47% of hip fractures attributable to use of oral corticosteroids among users of oral corticosteroids. For oral corticosteroids even very small doses were associated with an increase in the risk of fractures, the increase already being seen at doses larger than 2.5 mg of prednisolone equivalents per day.

The underlying diseases e.g. lung disease may affect BMD in a number of ways. Patients with severe chronic obstructive pulmonary disease (COPD) and pulmonary emphysema may be less physically active due to their decreased lung function, which may lead to "disuse" osteoporosis. The patients may also be malnourished and underweight, which may lead to a deficiency in calcium and vitamin D. The retention of carbon dioxide with disturbances in acid balance in COPD and emphysema may lead to a decrease in bone mineral density (BMD). Some lung diseases may also be accompanied by an increased production of cytokines, which may increase bone resorption. A cross sectional study of inhaled corticosteroids in adults with asthma showed a weak but statistically significant decrease in lumbar spine BMD of 0.16 Z-scores with each doubling of inhaled corticosteroid dose after adjustment for confounders including indices of severity of the asthma such as lung function. A randomised controlled trial of inhaled corticosteroids vs. non-corticosteroid therapy in patients with mild asthma showed better symptom control and no additional bone loss with inhaled budesonide or beclomethasone vs. other therapy (beta-agonists, cromoglycate, theophylline or atropine like substances). A limited decrease in BMD and a very small increase in fracture risk may thus be seen at high doses, but the severity of the underlying lung disease may account for much of the increase in fracture risk.

10.2. Disease Modifying Antirheumatic Drugs (DMARD)

These drugs are primarily use to induce remission in rheumatoid arthritis, but may also be used in a number of other inflammatory diseases. They include methotrexate, azathioprine, cyclophosphamide, cyclosporine A, chloroquine, sulphasalazine, penicillamine, and gold salts. For methotrexate and cyclophosphamide see above for drugs against cancer.

In a rat model, cyclosporine was associated with an increased loss of bone. However, in a human study, addition of cyclosporine A in patients with methotrexate resistant rheumatoid arthritis led to a suppression of inflammation and an increase in BMD. Two studies indicated that cyclosporine A use in renal transplant recipients was associated with a trend towards an increase in BMD of the spine. However, another study has indicated that cyclosporine A may perhaps be responsible for the loss of bone in heart transplant recipients. Conversion of treatment with cyclosporine A to tacrolimus in liver transplant recipients was associated with an increase in spine BMD and a stable hip BMD. However, some of the detrimental effects associated with cyclosporine A may actually be linked to a higher need for prednisolone. Treatment with cyclosporine A in patients undergoing renal transplantation seemed associated with a higher bone turnover compared to sirolimus as evaluated by osteocalcin and urinary excretion of N-telopeptides. In a histomorphometric study cyslosporine A was associated with an increased bone resorption and a decreased bone formation when compared to azathiorpine and prednisolone.

In a rat model azathioprine was not associated with a decrease in bone mineral. In a multivariate analysis, neither azathioprine nor cyclosporine A were associated with hip or spine BMD in patients with juvenile systemic lupus erythematosus. In patients with Crohn's disease, one study indicated that azathioprine was associated with a decreased BMD in the spine and hip. However, this could not be confirmed by another study which indicated that azathiprine rather was corticoid sparing and thus not detrimental to bone per se. One study indicated that cyclosporine A monotherapy was less detrimental to bone than azathiorpine.

In patients receiving gold for rheumatoid arthritis little change in BMD has been observed. Patients treated with gold and penicillamine and other types of antirheumatic drugs for rheumatoid arthritis all had reduced forearm BMC compared to normal controls, while patients receiving corticosteroids had a further decrease in forearm BMC compared to gold, penicillamine, and other antirheumatic drugs. However, it remained unclear if the decrease was a result of the underlying rheumatoid arthritis or the drugs per se. Treatment with penicillamine for rheumatoid arthritis seemed to reverse the loss of BMD, a trend not seen with gold salts. In patients with systemic sclerosis, use of penicillamine did not seem to alter the changes in forearm bone mineral compared to other treatments (glutamine, hydralazine, phenytoin, chlorpromazine). In animal experiments large probably non-pharmacological doses of penicillamine induced a number of skeletal changes. Use of chloroquine treatment in patients with rheumatoid arthritis seems associated with a prednisolone sparing effect and possibly a positive effect on BMD.

Sulphasalazine did not seem to have a major negative effect on BMD in patients with rheumatoid arthritis. One study actually pointed at a high trochanteric BMD in patients receiving sulphasalazine.

In conclusion although differences seem to exist, the immunomodulators of this class may not have major detrimental effects on BMD per se, and some of the effect may be mediated through the underlying disease and the use of prednisolone. However, more research is needed.

10.3. TNF-alpha Inhibitors

A new class of immunomodulators have been introduced with the TNF-alpha inhibitors. These include adalimumab, etanercept, infliximab, and anakinra. They have been used for immunomodulation in a number of conditions including rheumatoid arthritis and inflammatory bowel disease.

An open label study of patients with rehumatoid arthritis treated with infliximab compared to controls showed a decrease in BMD of the spine and femoral neck in controls, whereas it had remained stable in infliximab treated patients. Two further uncontrolled study in patients with rheumatoid arthritis treated with infliximab showed no significant changes in spine and hip BMD. Treatment of patients with spondylarthropathy with infliximab led to an increase in spine and hip BMD at six month in a non-controlled study. The increase in BMD seemed to correlate with the decrease in erythrocyte sedimentation rate as a marker of inflammation control. In a study where patients with spondylarthropathy received etanercept an increase was seen in spine and hip BMD compared to a decrease in spine and hip BMD in patients treated conventionally. Maintenance therapy with infliximab in patients with Crohn's disease also seemed associated with an increase in spine and femoral neck BMD. Treatment with infliximab in patients with Crohn's disease also seemed to add to the benefit of bisphosphonates on spine BMD.

In conclusion it thus seems that the TNF-alpha inhibitors may halt or perhaps even reverse the bone loss associated with inflammatory diseases.

REFERENCES

[1] Vestergaard P. Epilepsy, osteoporosis and fracture risk - a meta-analysis. *Acta Neurol Scand* 2005;112:277-86.

[2] Souverein PC, Webb DJ, Weil JG, van Staa TP, Egberts AC. Use of antiepileptic drugs and risk of fractures: case-control study among patients with epilepsy. *Neurology*. 2006;66:1318-24.

[3] Vestergaard P, Tigaran S, Rejnmark L, et al. Fracture risk is increased in epilepsy. *Acta Neurol Scand* 1999;99:269-75.

[4] Wirrell EC, Camfield PR, Camfield CS, Dooley JM, Gordon KE. Accidental injury is a serious risk in children with typical absence epilepsy. *Arch Neuro*l 1996;53:929-32.

[5] Persson HBI, Alberts KA, Farahmand BY, Tomson T. Risk of extremity fractures in adult outpatients with epilepsy. *Epilepsia* 2002;43:768-72.

[6] Guo CY, Ronen GM, Atkinson SA. Long-term valproate and lamotrigine treatment may be a marker for reduced growth and bone mass in children with epilepsy. *Epilepsia* 2001;42:1141-7.

[7] Jekovec-Vrhovsek M, Kocijancic A, Prezelj J. Effect of vitamin D and calcium on bone mineral density in children with CP and epilepsy in full-time care. *Dev.Med Child Neurol* 2000;42:403-5.

[8] Pack AM, Morrell MJ, Marcus R, et al. Bone mass and turnover in women with epilepsy on antiepileptic drug monotherapy. *Ann Neurol* 2005;57:252-7.

[9] Gissel T, Poulsen CS, Vestergaard P. Adverse effects of antiepileptic drugs on bone mineral density in children. *Expert Opin Drug Saf* 2007;6:267-78.

[10] Vestergaard P, Rejnmark L, Mosekilde L. Fracture risk associated with use of anti-epileptic drugs. *Epilepsia* 2004;45:1330-7.

[11] Christiansen C, Kristensen M, Rodbro P. Latent osteomalacia in epileptic patients on anticonvulsants. *Br.Med J* 1972;3:738-9.

[12] Christiansen C, Rodbro P, Lund M. Effect of vitamin D on bone mineral mass in normal subjects and in epileptic patients on anticonvulsants: a controlled therapeutic trial. *Br.Med J* 1973;2:208-9.

[13] Christiansen C, Rodbro P. Initial and maintenance dose of vitamin D2 in the treatment of anticonvulsant osteomalacia. *Acta Neurol.Scand* 1974;50:631-41.

[14] Christiansen C, Rodbro P, Munck O. Actions of vitamins D2 and D3 and 25-OHD3 in anticonvulsant osteomalacia. *Br.Med J* 1975;2:363-5.

[15] Christiansen C, Rodbro P, Nielsen CT. Iatrogenic osteomalacia in epileptic children. A controlled therapeutic trial. *Acta Paediatr.Scand* 1975;64:219-24.

[16] Mussolino ME, Jonas BS, Looker AC. Depression and bone mineral density in young adults: results from NHANES III. *Psychosom Med* 2004;66:533-7.

[17] Wong SY, Lau EM, Lynn H, et al. Depression and bone mineral density: is there a relationship in elderly Asian men? Results from Mr. Os (Hong Kong). *Osteoporosis Int* 2005;16:610-5.

[18] Konstantynowicz J, Kadziela-Olech H, Kaczmarski M, et al. Depression in anorexia nervosa: a risk factor for osteoporosis. *J Clin Endocrinol Meta*b 2005;90:5382-5.

[19] Diem SJ, Blackwell TL, Stone KL, et al. Use of Antidepressants and Rates of Hip Bone Loss in Older Women: The Study of Osteoporotic Fractures. *Archives of Internal Medicine* 2007;167:1240-5.

[20] Haney EM, Chan BKS, Diem SJ, et al. Association of Low Bone Mineral Density With Selective Serotonin Reuptake Inhibitor Use by Older Men. *Archives of Internal Medicine* 2007;167:1246-51.

[21] Bliziotes M, Gunness M, Eshleman A, Wiren K. The role of dopamine and serotonin in regulating bone mass and strength: studies on dopamine and serotonin transporter null mice. *J Musculoskelet.Neuronal.Interact* 2002;2:291-5.

[22] Warden SJ, Robling AG, Sanders MS, Bliziotes MM, Turner CH. Inhibition of the serotonin (5-hydroxytryptamine) transporter reduces bone accrual during growth. *Endocrinology* 2005;146:685-93.

[23] Vestergaard P, Rejnmark L, Mosekilde L. Selective Serotonin Reuptake Inhibitors and Other Antidepressants and Risk of Fracture. *Calcif Tissue Int* 2008;82:92-101.

[24] Vestergaard P, Rejnmark L, Mosekilde L. Anxiolytics, sedatives, antidepressants, neuroleptics and the risk of fracture. *Osteoporosis Int* 2006;17:807-16.

[25] Vestergaard P, Rejnmark L, Mosekilde L. Anxiolytics and Sedatives and Risk of Fractures: Effects of Half-life. *Calcif Tissue Int* 2008;82:34-43.

[26] Higuchi T, Komoda T, Sugishita M, et al. Certain neuroleptics reduce bone mineralization in schizophrenic patients. *Neuropsychobiology* 1987;18:185-8.

[27] Ataya K, Mercado A, Kartaginer J, Abbasi A, Moghissi KS. Bone density and reproductive hormones in patients with neuroleptic-induced hyperprolactinemia. *Fertil Steril* 1988;50:876-81.

[28] Seely EW, Moore TJ, Leboff MS, Brown EM. A single dose of lithium carbonate acutely elevates intact parathyroid hormone levels in humans. *Acta Endocrinol* (Copenh) 1989;121:174-6.

[29] Baastrup PC, Christiansen C, Transbol I. Calcium metabolism in lithium-treated patients. Relation to uni-bipolar dichotomy. *Acta Psychiatr Scand* 1978;57:124-8.

[30] Christiansen C, Baastrup PC, Transbol I. Lithium-induced "primary" hyperparathyroidism. *Calcif Tissue Res* 1977;22 Suppl:341-3.

[31] Christiansen C, Baastrup PC, Transbol I. Osteopenia and dysregulation of divalent cations in lithium-treated patients. *Neuropsychobiology* 1975;1:344-54.

[32] Eren Y, Yyldyz M, Civi Y, Gundodar D, Ozcankaya R. The effects of lithium treatment on bone mineral density of bipolar patients. *European Neuropsychopharmacology* 2003;13:S249

[33] Christiansen C, Baastrup PC, Transbol I. Development of 'primary' hyperparathyroidism during lithium therapy: longitudinal study. *Neuropsychobiology* 1980;6:280-3.

[34] Cohen O, Rais T, Lepkifker E, Vered I. Lithium carbonate therapy is not a risk factor for osteoporosis. *Hormone and Metabolic Research* 1998;30:594-7.

[35] De Boer J, Wang HJ, Van Blitterswijk C. Effects of Wnt signaling on proliferation and differentiation of human mesenchymal stem cells. *Tissue Eng* 2004;10:393-401.

[36] Pepersack T, Corvilain J, Bergmann P. Effects of lithium on bone resorption in cultured foetal rat long-bones. *European Journal of Clinical Investigation* 1994;24:400-5.

[37] Pepersack T, Corazza F, Demulder A, et al. Lithium inhibits calcitriol-stimulated formation of multinucleated cells in human long-term marrow cultures. *J Bone Miner Res* 1994;9:645-50.

[38] Brown EM. Lithium induces abnormal calcium-regulated PTH release in dispersed bovine parathyroid cells. *J Clin Endocrinol Metab* 1981;52:1046-8.

[39] Neer RM, Arnaud CD, Zanchetta JR, et al. Effect of parathyroid hormone (1-34) on fractures and bone mineral density in postmenopausal women with osteoporosis. *N Engl J Med* 2001;344:1434-41.

[40] Vestergaard P, Rejnmark L, Mosekilde L. Reduced Relative Risk of Fractures Among Users of Lithium. *Calcif Tissue Int* 2005;77:1-8.

[41] Wilting I, de Vries F, Thio BM, et al. Lithium use and the risk of fractures. *Bone.* 2007;40:1252-8.

[42] Genever RW, Downes TW, Medcalf P. Fracture rates in Parkinson's disease compared with age- and gender-matched controls: a retrospective cohort study. *Age Ageing.* 2005;34:21-4.

[43] Johnell O, Melton LJ, III, Atkinson EJ, O'Fallon WM, Kurland LT. Fracture risk in patients with parkinsonism: a population-based study in Olmsted County, Minnesota. *Age Ageing.* 1992;21:32-8.

[44] Taylor BC, Schreiner PJ, Stone KL, et al. Long-term prediction of incident hip fracture risk in elderly white women: study of osteoporotic fractures. *J Am Geriatr.Soc.* 2004;52:1479-86.

[45] Johnell O, Melton LJ, III, Atkinson EJ, O'Fallon WM, Kurland LT. Fracture risk in patients with parkinsonism: a population-based study in Olmsted County, Minnesota. *Age Ageing.* 1992;21:32-8.

[46] Wielinski CL, Erickson-Davis C, Wichmann R, Walde-Douglas M, Parashos SA. Falls and injuries resulting from falls among patients with Parkinson's disease and other parkinsonian syndromes. *Mov Disord.* 2005;20:410-5.

[47] Williams DR, Watt HC, Lees AJ. Predictors of falls and fractures in bradykinetic rigid syndromes: a retrospective study. *J Neurol.Neurosurg.Psychiatry.* 2006;77:468-73.

[48] Melton LJ, III, Leibson CL, Achenbach SJ, et al. Fracture risk after the diagnosis of Parkinson's disease: Influence of concomitant dementia. *Mov Disord.* 2006;21:1361-7.

[49] Yamanashi A, Yamazaki K, Kanamori M, et al. Assessment of risk factors for second hip fractures in Japanese elderly. *Osteoporos Int.* 2005;16:1239-46.

[50] Di Monaco M, Vallero F, Di Monaco R, Tappero R, Cavanna A. Bone mineral density in hip-fracture patients with Parkinson's disease: a case-control study. *Arch Phys.Med Rehabil.* 2006;87:1459-62.

[51] Taggart H, Crawford V. Reduced bone density of the hip in elderly patients with Parkinson's disease. *Age Ageing.* 1995;24:326-8.

[52] Sato Y, Kikuyama M, Oizumi K. High prevalence of vitamin D deficiency and reduced bone mass in Parkinson's disease. *Neurology.* 1997;49:1273-8.

[53] Sato Y, Manabe S, Kuno H, Oizumi K. Amelioration of osteopenia and hypovitaminosis D by 1alpha-hydroxyvitamin D3 in elderly patients with Parkinson's disease. *J Neurol.Neurosurg.Psychiatry*. 1999;66:64-8.
[54] Sato Y, Honda Y, Kaji M, et al. Amelioration of osteoporosis by menatetrenone in elderly female Parkinson's disease patients with vitamin D deficiency. *Bone*. 2002;31:114-8.
[55] Sato Y, Kaji M, Tsuru T, Oizumi K. Risk factors for hip fracture among elderly patients with Parkinson's disease. *J Neurol.Sci*. 2001;182:89-93.
[56] Sato Y, Honda Y, Kaji M, et al. Amelioration of osteoporosis by menatetrenone in elderly female Parkinson's disease patients with vitamin D deficiency. *Bone*. 2002;31:114-8.
[57] Sato Y, Iwamoto J, Kanoko T, Satoh K. Homocysteine as a predictive factor for hip fracture in elderly women with Parkinson's disease. *Am J Med*. 2005;118:1250-5.
[58] Vestergaard P, Rejnmark L, Mosekilde L. Fracture risk associated with parkinsonism and anti-Parkinson drugs. *Calcif.Tissue Int*. 2007;81:153-61.
[59] Vestergaard P. Osteoporosis and fracture risk in patients with diabetes. SIIC 2006;11:1
[60] Raskin P, Stevenson MRM, Barilla DE, Pak CYC. The hypercalciuria of diabetes mellitus: its amelioration with insulin. *Clin Endocrinol* 1978;9:329-35.
[61] McNair P, Madsbad S, Christensen MS, et al. Bone mineral loss in insulin-treated diabetes mellitus: studies on pathogenesis. Acta Endocrinol 1979;90:463-72.
[62] Bouillon R. Diabetic bone disease [editorial]. *Calcif Tissue Int* 1991;49:155-60.
[63] Hein G, Weiss C, Lehmann G, et al. Advanced glycation end product modification of bone proteins and bone remodelling: hypothesis and preliminary immunohistochemical findings. *Ann Rheum Dis* 2006;65:101-4.
[64] Saito M, Fujii K, Soshi S, Tanaka T. Reductions in degree of mineralization and enzymatic collagen cross-links and increases in glycation-induced pentosidine in the femoral neck cortex in cases of femoral neck fracture. *Osteoporos Int* 2006;17:986-95.
[65] Yamagishi S, Nakamura K, Inoue H. Possible participation of advanced glycation end products in the pathogenesis of osteoporosis in diabetic patients. *Medical Hypotheses* 2005;65:1013-5.
[66] Vestergaard P. Discrepancies in bone mineral density and fracture risk in patients with type 1 and type 2 diabetes-a meta-analysis. *Osteoporos Int* 2007;18:427-44.
[67] Vestergaard P, Rejnmark L, Mosekilde L. Relative fracture risk in patients with diabetes mellitus, and the impact of insulin and oral antidiabetic medication on relative fracture risk. *Diabetologia* 2005;48:1292-9.
[68] Kahn SE, Haffner SM, Heise MA, et al. Glycemic durability of rosiglitazone, metformin, or glyburide monotherapy. *N Engl J Med* 2006;355:2427-43.
[69] Yki-Jarvinen H. Thiazolidinediones. *N Engl J Med* 2004;351:1106-18.
[70] Tornvig L, Mosekilde LI, Justesen J, Falk E, Kassem M. Troglitazone treatment increases bone marrow adipose tissue volume but does not affect trabecular bone volume in mice. *Calcif Tissue Int* 2001;69:46-50.
[71] Ali AA, Weinstein RS, Stewart SA, et al. Rosiglitazone causes bone loss in mice by suppressing osteoblast differentiation and bone formation. *Endocrinology* 2005;146:1226-35.

[72] Soroceanu MA, Miao D, Bai XY, et al. Rosiglitazone impacts negatively on bone by promoting osteoblast/osteocyte apoptosis. *J Endocrinol* 2004;183:203-16.

[73] Schwartz AV, Sellmeyer DE, Vittinghoff E, et al. Thiazolidinedione use and bone loss in older diabetic adults. *J Clin Endocrinol Metab* 2006;91:3349-54.

[74] Short R. Fracture risk is a class effect of glitazones. *BMJ* 2007;334:551

[75] Rejnmark L, Vestergaard P, Pedersen AR, et al. Dose-effect relations of loop- and thiazide diuretics on calcium homeostasis: a randomized, double blinded Latin-square multiple cross-over study in postmenopausal osteopenic women. *European Journal of Clinical Investigation* 2003;33:41-50.

[76] Jones G, Nguyen T, Sambrook PN, Eisman JA. Thiazide diuretics and fractures: can meta-analysis help? *J.Bone Miner.Res*. 1995;10:106-11.

[77] Rejnmark L, Vestergaard P, Mosekilde L. Reduced fracture risk in users of thiazide diuretics. *Calcif Tissue Int* 2005;76:167-75.

[78] LaCroix AZ, Ott SM, Ichikawa L, Scholes D, Barlow WE. Low-dose hydrochlorothiazide and preservation of bone mineral density in older adults. A randomized, double-blind, placebo-controlled trial. *Ann Intern Med*. 2000;133:516-26.

[79] Reid IR, Ames RW, Orr-Walker BJ, et al. Hydrochlorothiazide reduces loss of cortical bone in normal postmenopausal women: a randomized controlled trial. *Am J Med*. 2000;109:362-70.

[80] Rejnmark L, Vestergaard P, Heickendorff L, Andreasen F, Mosekilde L. Loop diuretics alter the diurnal rhytm of endogenous parathyroid hormone secretion. A randomized-controlled study on the effects of loop- and thiazide diuretics on the diurnal rhytms of calcitropic hormones and biochemical bone markers in postmenopausal women. *European Journal of Clinical Investigation* 2001;31:764-72.

[81] Rejnmark L, Vestergaard P, Heickendorff L, Andreasen F, Mosekilde L. Loop Diuretics Increase Bone Turnover and Decrease BMD in Osteopenic Postmenopausal Women: Results From a Randomized Controlled Study With Bumetanide. *J Bone Miner Res* 2006;21:163-70.

[82] Rejnmark L, Vestergaard P, Mosekilde L. Fracture risk in patients treated with loop diuretics. *Journal of Internal Medicine* 2006;259:117-24.

[83] Rejnmark L, Vestergaard P, Mosekilde L. Statin but not non-statin lipid-lowering drugs decrease fracture risk: a nation-wide case-control study. *Calcif Tissue Int* 2006;79:27-36.

[84] Mundy G, Garrett R, Harris S, et al. Stimulation of bone formation in vitro and in rodents by statins. *Science*. 1999;286:1946-9.

[85] Oxlund H, Andreassen TT. Simvastatin treatment partially prevents ovariectomy-induced bone loss while increasing cortical bone formation. *Bone*. 2004;34:609-18.

[86] Rejnmark L, Buus NH, Vestergaard P, et al. Effects of simvastatin on bone turnover and BMD: a 1-year randomized controlled trial in postmenopausal osteopenic women. *J Bone Miner Res* 2004;19:737-44.

[87] Ray WA, Daugherty JR, Griffin MR. Lipid-lowering agents and the risk of hip fracture in a Medicaid population. *Inj.Prev*. 2002;8:276-9.

[88] Rejnmark L, Vestergaard P, Mosekilde L. Treatment with beta-blockers, ACE inhibitors, and calcium-channel blockers is associated with a reduced fracture risk: a nationwide case-control study. *J Hypertens*. 2006;24:581-9.

[89] Rejnmark L, Vestergaard P, Mosekilde L. Fracture risk in patients treated with amiodarone or digoxin for cardiac arrhythmias: a nation-wide case-control study. *Osteoporos Int* 2006;18:409-17.

[90] Rejnmark L, Vestergaard P, Mosekilde L. Decreased fracture risk in users of organic nitrates: a nationwide case-control study. *J Bone Miner Res* 2006;21:1811-7.

[91] Szulc P, Meunier PJ. Is vitamin K deficiency a risk factor for osteoporosis in Crohn's disease? *Lancet* 2001;357:1995-6.

[92] Caraballo PJ, Gabriel SE, Castro MR, Atkinson EJ, Melton LJ. Changes in bone density after exposure to oral anticoagulants: a meta-analysis. *Osteoporosis Int* 1999;9:441-8.

[93] Jamal SA, Browner WS, Bauer DC, Cummings SR. Warfarin use and risk for osteoporosis in elderly women. Study of Osteoporotic Fractures Research Group. *Ann.Intern.Med.* 1998;128:829-32.

[94] Rejnmark L, Vestergaard P, Mosekilde L. Fracture risk in users of oral anticoagulants: A nationwide case-control study. *Int J Cardiol.* 2007;118:338-44.

[95] Farina C, Gagliardi S. Selective inhibition of osteoclast vacuolar H(+)-ATPase. *Curr Pharm Des* 2002;8:2033-48.

[96] Sahara T, Itoh K, Debari K, Sasaki T. Specific biological functions of vacuolar-type H(+)-ATPase and lysosomal cysteine proteinase, cathepsin K, in osteoclasts. *Anat Rec A Discov. Mol Cell Evol.Biol* 2003;270:152-61.

[97] Sasaki T. Recent advances in the ultrastructural assessment of osteoclastic resorptive functions. *Microsc. Res Tech.* 1996;33:182-91.

[98] Shibata T, Amano H, Yamada S, Ohya K. Mechanisms of proton transport in isolated rat osteoclasts attached to bone. *J Med Dent.Sc*i 2000;47:177-85.

[99] Gagliardi S, Nadler G, Consolandi E, et al. 5-(5,6-Dichloro-2-indolyl)-2-methoxy-2,4-pentadienamides: novel and selective inhibitors of the vacuolar H+-ATPase of osteoclasts with bone antiresorptive activity. *J Med Chem* 1998;41:1568-73.

[100] Rzeszutek K, Sarraf F, Davies JE. Proton pump inhibitors control osteoclastic resorption of calcium phosphate implants and stimulate increased local reparative bone growth. *J Craniofac.Surg* 2003;14:301-7.

[101] Sundquist K, Lakkakorpi P, Wallmark B, Vaananen K. Inhibition of osteoclast proton transport by bafilomycin A1 abolishes bone resorption. *Biochem Biophys. Res Commun.* 1990;168:309-13.

[102] Visentin L, Dodds RA, Valente M, et al. A selective inhibitor of the osteoclastic V-H(+)-ATPase prevents bone loss in both thyroparathyroidectomized and ovariectomized rats. *J Clin Invest* 2000;106:309-18.

[103] Xu J, Feng HT, Wang C, et al. Effects of Bafilomycin A1: an inhibitor of vacuolar H (+)-ATPases on endocytosis and apoptosis in RAW cells and RAW cell-derived osteoclasts. *J Cell Biochem* 2003;88:1256-64.

[104] Mattsson JP, Vaananen K, Wallmark B, Lorentzon P. Omeprazole and bafilomycin, two proton pump inhibitors: differentiation of their effects on gastric, kidney and bone H(+)-translocating ATPases. *Biochim.Biophys.Acta* 1991;1065:261-8.

[105] Mizunashi K, Furukawa Y, Katano K, Abe K. Effect of omeprazole, an inhibitor of H+,K(+)-ATPase, on bone resorption in humans. *Calcif Tissue Int* 1993;53:21-5.

[106] Tran TM, Van den NA, Hendriks JJ, Forget P, Forget PP. Effects of a proton-pump inhibitor in cystic fibrosis. *Acta Paediatr*. 1998;87:553-8.

[107] Persson P, Gagnemo-Persson R, Chen D, et al. Gastrectomy causes bone loss in the rat: is lack of gastric acid responsible? *Scand J Gastroenterol* 1993;28:301-6.

[108] Vestergaard P, Rejnmark L, Mosekilde L. Proton pump inhibitors, histamine h(2) receptor antagonists, and other antacid medications and the risk of fracture. *Calcif Tissue Int* 2006;79:76-83.

[109] Yang Y-X, Lewis JD, Epstein S, Metz DC. Long-term Proton Pump Inhibitor Therapy and Risk of Hip Fracture. *JAMA* 2006;296:2947-53.

[110] Vestergaard P, Mollerup CL, Frøkjær VG, et al. Cohort study of risk of fracture before and after surgery for primary hyperparathyroidism. *BMJ* 2000;321:598-602.

[111] Grisso JA, Kelsey JL, O'Brien LA, et al. Risk factors for hip fracture in men. Hip Fracture Study Group. *Am J Epidemiol*. 1997;145:786-93.

[112] Adachi Y, Shiota E, Matsumata T, et al. Bone mineral density in patients taking H2-receptor antagonist. *Calcif Tissue Int* 1998;62:283-5.

[113] Yamaura K, Yonekawa T, Nakamura T, Yano S, Ueno K. The histamine H2-receptor antagonist, cimetidine, inhibits the articular osteopenia in rats with adjuvant-induced arthritis by suppressing the osteoclast differentiation induced by histamine. *J Pharmacol Sci* 2003;92:43-9.

[114] Lesclous P, Guez D, Saffar JL. Short-term prevention of osteoclastic resorption and osteopenia in ovariectomized rats treated with the H(2) receptor antagonist cimetidine. *Bone* 2002;30:131-6.

[115] Lesclous P, Guez D, Baroukh B, Vignery A, Saffar JL. Histamine participates in the early phase of trabecular bone loss in ovariectomized rats. *Bone* 2004;34:91-9.

[116] Dobigny C, Saffar JL. H1 and H2 histamine receptors modulate osteoclastic resorption by different pathways: evidence obtained by using receptor antagonists in a rat synchronized resorption model. *J Cell Physiol* 1997;173:10-8.

[117] Shearn MA. 1987 Nonsteroidal Anti-inflammatory Agents; Nonopiate Analgesics; Drugs used in gout. In: Katzung BG (ed) *Basic and Clinical Pharmacology.3. ed.* Appleton & Lange,Norwalk, pp 396-413.

[118] Way WL, Way EL. 1987 Opioid Analgesics & Antagonists. In: Katzung BG (ed) B*asic and Clinical Pharmacology.3. ed.* Appleton & Lange, Norwalk, pp 336-349.

[119] Raisz LG. Physiologic and pathologic roles of prostaglandins and other eicosanoids in bone metabolism. *J Nutr* 1995;125:2024S-7S.

[120] Raisz LG. Prostaglandins and bone: physiology and pathophysiology. Osteoarthritis. *Cartilage*. 1999;7:419-21.

[121] Raisz LG. Potential impact of selective cyclooxygenase-2 inhibitors on bone metabolism in health and disease. *Am J Med* 2001;110 Suppl 3A:43S-5S.

[122] Kawaguchi H, Pilbeam CC, Harrison JR, Raisz LG. The role of prostaglandins in the regulation of bone metabolism. *Clin Orthop Relat Res* 1995;36-46.

[123] Kawaguchi H, Pilbeam CC, Gronowicz G, et al. Transcriptional induction of prostaglandin G/H synthase-2 by basic fibroblast growth factor. *J Clin Invest* 1995;96:923-30.

[124] Hurley MM, Lee SK, Raisz LG, Bernecker P, Lorenzo J. Basic fibroblast growth factor induces osteoclast formation in murine bone marrow cultures. *Bone* 1998;22:309-16.

[125] Raisz LG, Fall PM. Biphasic effects of prostaglandin E2 on bone formation in cultured fetal rat calvariae: interaction with cortisol. *Endocrinology* 1990;126:1654-9.

[126] Bell NH, Hollis BW, Shary JR, et al. Diclofenac sodium inhibits bone resorption in postmenopausal women. *Am J Med* 1994;96:349-53.

[127] Carbone LD, Tylavsky FA, Cauley JA, et al. Association between bone mineral density and the use of nonsteroidal anti-inflammatory drugs and aspirin: impact of cyclooxygenase selectivity. *J Bone Miner Res* 2003;18:1795-802.

[128] Bauer DC, Orwoll ES, Fox KM, et al. Aspirin and NSAID use in older women: effect on bone mineral density and fracture risk. Study of Osteoporotic Fractures Research Group. *J Bone Miner Res* 1996;11:29-35.

[129] Morton DJ, Barrett-Connor EL, Schneider DL. Nonsteroidal anti-inflammatory drugs and bone mineral density in older women: the Rancho Bernardo study. *J Bone Miner Res* 1998;13:1924-31.

[130] Vestergaard P, Rejnmark L, Mosekilde L. Fracture risk associated with use of nonsteroidal anti-inflammatory drugs, acetylsalicylic Acid, and acetaminophen and the effects of rheumatoid arthritis and osteoarthritis. *Calcif Tissue Int* 2006;79:84-94.

[131] Azizi F, Vagenakis AG, Longcope C, Ingbar SH, Braverman LE. Decreased serum testosterone concentration in male heroin and methadone addicts. *Steroids* 1973;22:467-72.

[132] Giri M, Kaufman JM. Opioidergic modulation of in vitro pulsatile gonadotropin-releasing hormone release from the isolated medial basal hypothalamus of the male guinea pig. *Endocrinology* 1994;135:2137-43.

[133] Abs R, Verhelst J, Maeyaert J, et al. Endocrine consequences of long-term intrathecal administration of opioids. *J Clin Endocrinol Metab* 2000;85:2215-22.

[134] Finch PM, Roberts LJ, Price L, Hadlow NC, Pullan PT. Hypogonadism in patients treated with intrathecal morphine. *Clin J Pain* 2000;16:251-4.

[135] Roberts LJ, Finch PM, Pullan PT, Bhagat CI, Price LM. Sex hormone suppression by intrathecal opioids: a prospective study. *Clin J Pain* 2002;18:144-8.

[136] Daniell HW. Hypogonadism in men consuming sustained-action oral opioids. *J Pain* 2002;3:377-84.

[137] Sikharulidze ZD, Kopaliani MG, Kilasoniia LO. [Comparative evaluation of clinical symptoms and status of bone metabolism in patients with heroin and buprenorphine addiction in the period of withdrawal]. *Georgian.Med News*. 2006;72-6.

[138] Pedrazzoni M, Vescovi PP, Maninetti L, et al. Effects of chronic heroin abuse on bone and mineral metabolism. *Acta Endocrinol* (Copenh). 1993;129:42-5.

[139] Kinjo M, Setoguchi S, Schneeweiss S, Solomon DH. Bone mineral density in subjects using central nervous system-active medications. *Am J Med* 2005;118:1414

[140] Lovell SJ, Taira T, Rodriguez E, et al. Comparison of valdecoxib and an oxycodone-acetaminophen combination for acute musculoskeletal pain in the emergency department: a randomized controlled trial. *Acad Emerg.Med* 2004;11:1278-82.

[141] Arnsten JH, Freeman R, Howard AA, et al. HIV infection and bone mineral density in middle-aged women. *Clin Infect.Dis* 2006;42:1014-20.

[142] Loiseau-Peres S, Delaunay C, Poupon S, et al. Osteopenia in patients infected by the human immunodeficiency virus. A case control study. *Joint Bone Spine* 2002;69:482-5.

[143] Bonnet E, Delpierre C, Sommet A, et al. Total body composition by DXA of 241 HIV-negative men and 162 HIV-infected men: proposal of reference values for defining lipodystrophy. *J Clin Densitom* 2005;8:287-92.

[144] Brown TT, Ruppe MD, Kassner R, et al. Reduced bone mineral density in human immunodeficiency virus-infected patients and its association with increased central adiposity and postload hyperglycemia. *J Clin Endocrinol Metab* 2004;89:1200-6.

[145] Dolan SE, Kanter JR, Grinspoon S. Longitudinal analysis of bone density in human immunodeficiency virus-infected women. *J Clin Endocrinol Metab* 2006;91:2938-45.

[146] Ellis KJ, Shypailo RJ, Hardin DS, et al. Z score prediction model for assessment of bone mineral content in pediatric diseases. *J Bone Miner Res* 2001;16:1658-64.

[147] Fairfield WP, Finkelstein JS, Klibanski A, Grinspoon SK. Osteopenia in eugonadal men with acquired immune deficiency syndrome wasting syndrome. *J Clin Endocrinol Metab* 2001;86:2020-6.

[148] Jacobson DL, Spiegelman D, Duggan C, et al. Predictors of bone mineral density in human immunodeficiency virus-1 infected children. *J Pediatr Gastroenterol Nutr* 2005;41:339-46.

[149] Ozcakar L, Guven GS, Unal S, Akinci A. Osteoporosis In Turkish HIV/AIDS patients: comparative analysis by dual energy X-ray absorptiometry and digital X-ray radiogrammetry. *Osteoporos Int* 2005;16:1363-7.

[150] Pitukcheewanont P, Safani D, Church J, Gilsanz V. Bone measures in HIV-1 infected children and adolescents: disparity between quantitative computed tomography and dual-energy X-ray absorptiometry measurements. *Osteoporos Int* 2005;16:1393-6.

[151] Rosenthall L, Falutz J. Bone mineral and soft-tissue changes in AIDS-associated lipoatrophy. *J Bone Miner Metab* 2005;23:53-7.

[152] Teichmann J, Stephan E, Discher T, et al. Changes in calciotropic hormones and biochemical markers of bone metabolism in patients with human immunodeficiency virus infection. Metabolism 2000;49:1134-9.

[153] Paton NI, Macallan DC, Griffin GE, Pazianas M. Bone mineral density in patients with human immunodeficiency virus infection. *Calcif Tissue Int* 1997;61:30-2.

[154] Serrano S, Marinoso ML, Soriano JC, et al. Bone remodelling in human immunodeficiency virus-1-infected patients. A histomorphometric study. *Bone* 1995;16:185-91.

[155] Arnsten JH, Freeman R, Howard AA, et al. Decreased bone mineral density and increased fracture risk in aging men with or at risk for HIV infection. *AI*DS 2007;21:617-23.

[156] Bongiovanni M, Tincati C. Bone diseases associated with human immunodeficiency virus infection: pathogenesis, risk factors and clinical management. *Curr Mol Med* 2006;6:395-400.

[157] Brown TT, McComsey GA. Osteopenia and osteoporosis in patients with HIV: a review of current concepts. *Curr Infect.Dis Rep* 2006;8:162-70.

[158] Glesby MJ. Bone disorders in human immunodeficiency virus infection. *Clin Infect.Dis* 2003;37 Suppl 2:S91-S95

[159] Panayotakopoulos GD, Day S, Peters BS, Kulasegaram R. Severe osteoporosis and multiple fractures in an AIDS patient treated with short-term steroids for lymphoma: a need for guidelines. *Int J STD AID*S 2006;17:567-8.

[160] Dobs A. Role of testosterone in maintaining lean body mass and bone density in HIV-infected patients. *Int J Impot.Res* 2003;15 Suppl 4:S21-S25

[161] Brown TT, Ruppe MD, Kassner R, et al. Reduced bone mineral density in human immunodeficiency virus-infected patients and its association with increased central adiposity and postload hyperglycemia. *J Clin Endocrinol Metab* 2004;89:1200-6.

[162] Cooper OB, Brown TT, Dobs AS. Opiate drug use: a potential contributor to the endocrine and metabolic complications in human immunodeficiency virus disease. *Clin Infect.Dis* 2003;37 Suppl 2:S132-S136

[163] Serrano S, Marinoso ML, Soriano JC, et al. Bone remodelling in human immunodeficiency virus-1-infected patients. A histomorphometric study. *Bone* 1995;16:185-91.

[164] Zamboni G, Antoniazzi F, Bertoldo F, et al. Altered bone metabolism in children infected with human immunodeficiency virus. *Acta Paediatr* 2003;92:12-6.

[165] Serrano S, Marinoso ML, Soriano JC, et al. Bone remodelling in human immunodeficiency virus-1-infected patients. A histomorphometric study. *Bone* 1995;16:185-91.

[166] Tan BM, Nelson RP, Jr., James-Yarish M, Emmanuel PJ, Schurman SJ. Bone metabolism in children with human immunodeficiency virus infection receiving highly active anti-retroviral therapy including a protease inhibitor. *J Pediatr* 2001;139:447-51.

[167] Pan G, Yang Z, Ballinger SW, McDonald JM. Pathogenesis of osteopenia/osteoporosis induced by highly active anti-retroviral therapy for AIDS. *Ann N Y Acad Sci* 2006;1068:297-308.

[168] Garcia Aparicio AM, Munoz FS, Gonzalez J, et al. Abnormalities in the bone mineral metabolism in HIV-infected patients. *Clin Rheumatol* 2006;25:537-9.

[169] Cozzolino M, Vidal M, Arcidiacono MV, et al. HIV-protease inhibitors impair vitamin D bioactivation to 1,25-dihydroxyvitamin D. *AIDS* 2003;17:513-20.

[170] Cozzolino M, Vidal M, Arcidiacono MV, et al. HIV-protease inhibitors impair vitamin D bioactivation to 1,25-dihydroxyvitamin D. *AIDS* 2003;17:513-20.

[171] Cozzolino M, Vidal M, Arcidiacono MV, et al. HIV-protease inhibitors impair vitamin D bioactivation to 1,25-dihydroxyvitamin D. *AIDS* 2003;17:513-20.

[172] Jain RG, Lenhard JM. Select HIV protease inhibitors alter bone and fat metabolism ex vivo. *J Biol Chem* 2002;277:19247-50.

[173] Pan G, Yang Z, Ballinger SW, McDonald JM. Pathogenesis of osteopenia/osteoporosis induced by highly active anti-retroviral therapy for AIDS. *Ann N Y Acad Sci* 2006;1068:297-308.
[174] Bolland MJ, Grey AB, Horne AM, et al. Bone mineral density is not reduced in HIV-infected Caucasian men treated with highly active antiretroviral therapy. *Clin Endocrinol (Oxf)* 2006;65:191-7.
[175] Bolland MJ, Grey AB, Horne AM, et al. Bone mineral density remains stable in HAART-treated HIV-infected men over 2 years. *Clin Endocrinol (Oxf)* 2007;67:270-5.
[176] Brown TT, Ruppe MD, Kassner R, et al. Reduced bone mineral density in human immunodeficiency virus-infected patients and its association with increased central adiposity and postload hyperglycemia. *J Clin Endocrinol Metab* 2004;89:1200-6.
[177] Cassetti I, Madruga JV, Suleiman JM, et al. The Safety and Efficacy of Tenofovir DF in Combination with Lamivudine and Efavirenz Through 6 Years in Antiretroviral-Naive HIV-1-Infected Patients. *HIV Clin Trials* 2007;8:164-72.
[178] Cirelli A, Cirelli G, Balsamo G, et al. Body habitus changes, metabolic abnormalities, osteopenia and cardiovascular risk in patients treated for human immunodeficiency virus infection. *Ann Ital.Med Int* 2003;18:238-45.
[179] Dube MP, Qian D, Edmondson-Melancon H, et al. Prospective, intensive study of metabolic changes associated with 48 weeks of amprenavir-based antiretroviral therapy. *Clin Infect.Dis* 2002;35:475-81.
[180] Fausto A, Bongiovanni M, Cicconi P, et al. Potential predictive factors of osteoporosis in HIV-positive subjects. *Bone* 2006;38:893-7.
[181] Mondy K, Yarasheski K, Powderly WG, et al. Longitudinal evolution of bone mineral density and bone markers in human immunodeficiency virus-infected individuals. *Clin Infect.Dis* 2003;36:482-90.
[182] Mora S, Zamproni I, Beccio S, et al. Longitudinal changes of bone mineral density and metabolism in antiretroviral-treated human immunodeficiency virus-infected children. *J Clin Endocrinol Metab* 2004;89:24-8.
[183] Tebas P, Yarasheski K, Henry K, et al. Evaluation of the virological and metabolic effects of switching protease inhibitor combination antiretroviral therapy to nevirapine-based therapy for the treatment of HIV infection. *AIDS Res Hum Retroviruses* 2004;20:589-94.
[184] Brown TT, Ruppe MD, Kassner R, et al. Reduced bone mineral density in human immunodeficiency virus-infected patients and its association with increased central adiposity and postload hyperglycemia. *J Clin Endocrinol Metab* 2004;89:1200-6.
[185] Bolland MJ, Grey AB, Horne AM, et al. Bone mineral density is not reduced in HIV-infected Caucasian men treated with highly active antiretroviral therapy. *Clin Endocrinol (Oxf)* 2006;65:191-7.
[186] Fausto A, Bongiovanni M, Cicconi P, et al. Potential predictive factors of osteoporosis in HIV-positive subjects. *Bone* 2006;38:893-7.
[187] Mondy K, Yarasheski K, Powderly WG, et al. Longitudinal evolution of bone mineral density and bone markers in human immunodeficiency virus-infected individuals. *Clin Infect.Dis* 2003;36:482-90.

[188] Bolland MJ, Grey AB, Horne AM, et al. Bone mineral density remains stable in HAART-treated HIV-infected men over 2 years. *Clin Endocrinol (Oxf)* 2007;67:270-5.

[189] Cassetti I, Madruga JV, Suleiman JM, et al. The Safety and Efficacy of Tenofovir DF in Combination with Lamivudine and Efavirenz Through 6 Years in Antiretroviral-Naive HIV-1-Infected Patients. *HIV Clin Trials* 2007;8:164-72.

[190] Cirelli A, Cirelli G, Balsamo G, et al. Body habitus changes, metabolic abnormalities, osteopenia and cardiovascular risk in patients treated for human immunodeficiency virus infection. *Ann Ital.Med Int* 2003;18:238-45.

[191] Dube MP, Qian D, Edmondson-Melancon H, et al. Prospective, intensive study of metabolic changes associated with 48 weeks of amprenavir-based antiretroviral therapy. *Clin Infect.Dis* 2002;35:475-81.

[192] Mora S, Zamproni I, Beccio S, et al. Longitudinal changes of bone mineral density and metabolism in antiretroviral-treated human immunodeficiency virus-infected children. *J Clin Endocrinol Metab* 2004;89:24-8.

[193] Guaraldi G, Ventura P, Albuzza M, et al. Pathological fractures in AIDS patients with osteopenia and osteoporosis induced by antiretroviral therapy. *AIDS* 2001;15:137-8.

[194] Gallant JE, Staszewski S, Pozniak AL, et al. Efficacy and safety of tenofovir DF vs stavudine in combination therapy in antiretroviral-naive patients: a 3-year randomized trial. *JAMA* 2004;292:191-201.

[195] Tebas P, Yarasheski K, Henry K, et al. Evaluation of the virological and metabolic effects of switching protease inhibitor combination antiretroviral therapy to nevirapine-based therapy for the treatment of HIV infection. *AIDS Res Hum Retroviruses* 2004;20:589-94.

[196] Bolland MJ, Grey AB, Horne AM, et al. Annual zoledronate increases bone density in highly active antiretroviral therapy-treated human immunodeficiency virus-infected men: a randomized controlled trial. *J Clin Endocrinol Metab* 2007;92:1283-8.

[197] Negredo E, Martinez-Lopez E, Paredes R, et al. Reversal of HIV-1-associated osteoporosis with once-weekly alendronate. *AIDS* 2005;19:343-5.

[198] Eastell R, Hannon RA, Cuzick J, et al. Effect of an aromatase inhibitor on bmd and bone turnover markers: 2-year results of the Anastrozole, Tamoxifen, Alone or in Combination (ATAC) trial (18233230). *J Bone Miner Res* 2006;21:1215-23.

[199] Baum M, Budzar AU, Cuzick J, et al. Anastrozole alone or in combination with tamoxifen versus tamoxifen alone for adjuvant treatment of postmenopausal women with early breast cancer: first results of the ATAC randomised trial. *Lancet.* 2002;359:2131-9.

[200] Perez EA, Josse RG, Pritchard KI, et al. Effect of letrozole versus placebo on bone mineral density in women with primary breast cancer completing 5 or more years of adjuvant tamoxifen: a companion study to NCIC CTG MA.17. *J Clin Oncol.* 2006;24:3629-35.

[201] Coleman RE, Banks LM, Girgis SI, et al. Skeletal effects of exemestane on bone-mineral density, bone biomarkers, and fracture incidence in postmenopausal women with early breast cancer participating in the Intergroup Exemestane Study (IES): a randomised controlled study. *Lancet Oncol.* 2007;8:119-27.

[202] Shapiro CL, Recht A. Side effects of adjuvant treatment of breast cancer. *N Engl J Med* 2001;344:1997-2008.

[203] Bruning PF, Pit MJ, Jong-Bakker M, et al. Bone mineral density after adjuvant chemotherapy for premenopausal breast cancer. *Br J Cancer* 1990;61:308-10.

[204] Bruning PF, Pit MJ, Jong-Bakker M, et al. Bone mineral density after adjuvant chemotherapy for premenopausal breast cancer. *Br J Cancer* 1990;61:308-10.

[205] Bruning PF, Pit MJ, Jong-Bakker M, et al. Bone mineral density after adjuvant chemotherapy for premenopausal breast cancer. *Br J Cancer* 1990;61:308-10.

[206] Marshall D, Johnell O, Wedel H. Meta-analysis of how well measures of bone mineral density predict occurrence of osteoporotic fractures. *BMJ* 1996;312:1254-9.

[207] Bruning PF, Pit MJ, Jong-Bakker M, et al. Bone mineral density after adjuvant chemotherapy for premenopausal breast cancer. *Br J Cancer* 1990;61:308-10.

[208] Bruning PF, Pit MJ, Jong-Bakker M, et al. Bone mineral density after adjuvant chemotherapy for premenopausal breast cancer. *Br J Cancer* 1990;61:308-10.

[209] Fogelman I, Blake GM, Blamey R, et al. Bone mineral density in premenopausal women treated for node-positive early breast cancer with 2 years of goserelin or 6 months of cyclophosphamide, methotrexate and 5-fluorouracil (CMF). *Osteoporos Int* 2003;14:1001-6.

[210] Fogelman I, Blake GM, Blamey R, et al. Bone mineral density in premenopausal women treated for node-positive early breast cancer with 2 years of goserelin or 6 months of cyclophosphamide, methotrexate and 5-fluorouracil (CMF). *Osteoporos Int* 2003;14:1001-6.

[211] Fogelman I, Blake GM, Blamey R, et al. Bone mineral density in premenopausal women treated for node-positive early breast cancer with 2 years of goserelin or 6 months of cyclophosphamide, methotrexate and 5-fluorouracil (CMF). *Osteoporos Int* 2003;14:1001-6.

[212] Fogelman I, Blake GM, Blamey R, et al. Bone mineral density in premenopausal women treated for node-positive early breast cancer with 2 years of goserelin or 6 months of cyclophosphamide, methotrexate and 5-fluorouracil (CMF). *Osteoporos Int* 2003;14:1001-6.

[213] Fogelman I, Blake GM, Blamey R, et al. Bone mineral density in premenopausal women treated for node-positive early breast cancer with 2 years of goserelin or 6 months of cyclophosphamide, methotrexate and 5-fluorouracil (CMF). *Osteoporos Int* 2003;14:1001-6.

[214] Fogelman I, Blake GM, Blamey R, et al. Bone mineral density in premenopausal women treated for node-positive early breast cancer with 2 years of goserelin or 6 months of cyclophosphamide, methotrexate and 5-fluorouracil (CMF). *Osteoporos Int* 2003;14:1001-6.

[215] Vehmanen L, Saarto T, Elomaa I, et al. Long-term impact of chemotherapy-induced ovarian failure on bone mineral density (BMD) in premenopausal breast cancer patients. The effect of adjuvant clodronate treatment. *Eur J Cancer* 2001;37:2373-8.

[216] Fogelman I, Blake GM, Blamey R, et al. Bone mineral density in premenopausal women treated for node-positive early breast cancer with 2 years of goserelin or 6

months of cyclophosphamide, methotrexate and 5-fluorouracil (CMF). *Osteoporos Int* 2003;14:1001-6.

[217] Vehmanen L, Saarto T, Elomaa I, et al. Long-term impact of chemotherapy-induced ovarian failure on bone mineral density (BMD) in premenopausal breast cancer patients. The effect of adjuvant clodronate treatment. *Eur J Cancer* 2001;37:2373-8.

[218] Saarto T, Blomqvist C, Valimaki M, et al. Chemical castration induced by adjuvant cyclophosphamide, methotrexate, and fluorouracil chemotherapy causes rapid bone loss that is reduced by clodronate: a randomized study in premenopausal breast cancer patients. *J Clin Onco*l 1997;15:1341-7.

[219] Saarto T, Blomqvist C, Valimaki M, et al. Chemical castration induced by adjuvant cyclophosphamide, methotrexate, and fluorouracil chemotherapy causes rapid bone loss that is reduced by clodronate: a randomized study in premenopausal breast cancer patients. *J Clin Oncol* 1997;15:1341-7.

[220] Saarto T, Blomqvist C, Valimaki M, et al. Chemical castration induced by adjuvant cyclophosphamide, methotrexate, and fluorouracil chemotherapy causes rapid bone loss that is reduced by clodronate: a randomized study in premenopausal breast cancer patients. *J Clin Oncol* 1997;15:1341-7.

[221] Fogelman I, Blake GM, Blamey R, et al. Bone mineral density in premenopausal women treated for node-positive early breast cancer with 2 years of goserelin or 6 months of cyclophosphamide, methotrexate and 5-fluorouracil (CMF). *Osteoporos Int* 2003;14:1001-6.

[222] Headley JA, Theriault RL, LeBlanc AD, Vassilopoulou-Sellin R, Hortobagyi GN. Pilot study of bone mineral density in breast cancer patients treated with adjuvant chemotherapy. *Cancer Invest* 1998;16:6-11.

[223] Shapiro CL, Phillips G, Van Poznak CH, et al. Baseline bone mineral density of the total lumbar spine may predict for chemotherapy-induced ovarian failure. *Breast Cancer Res Trea*t. 2005;90:41-6.

[224] Alexeeva L, Burkhardt P, Christiansen C, et al. 1994. *Assessment of fracture risk and its application to screening for postmenopausal osteoporosis: report of a WHO Study Group. 1.* ed. WHO Technical Report Series 843, Geneva.

[225] Cegiela U, Piatek A, Janiec W, et al. [Effect of cyclophosphamide on bone remodeling in rats]. *Przegl.Lek.* 2003;60:329-33.

[226] Wie H, Beck EI. Synthesis and solubility of collagen in rats during recovery after high-dose cyclophosphamide administration. *Acta Pharmacol Toxicol* (Copenh) 1981;48:294-9.

[227] Glorieux F, Bishop NJ, Plotkin H, et al. Cyclic asministration of pamidronate in children with severe osteogenesis imperfecta. *N Engl J Med* 1998;339:947-52.

[228] Langendorff HU, Sauer HD, Schottle H, Ringe JD, Jungbluth KH. [The influence of cyclophosphamide upon the healing of fractures in the rabbit (author's transl)]. *Unfallchirurgie* 1981;7:231-5.

[229] Buckley LM, Leib ES, Cartularo KS, Vacek PM, Cooper SM. Effects of low dose methotrexate on the bone mineral density of patients with rheumatoid arthritis. *J Rheumatol* 1997;24:1489-94.

[230] Carbone LD, Kaeley G, McKown KM, et al. Effects of long-term administration of methotrexate on bone mineral density in rheumatoid arthritis. *Calcif Tissue Int* 1999;64:100-1.

[231] Cranney AB, McKendry RJ, Wells GA, et al. The effect of low dose methotrexate on bone density. *J Rheumatol* 2001;28:2395-9.

[232] di Munno O, Mazzantini M, Sinigaglia L, et al. Effect of low dose methotrexate on bone density in women with rheumatoid arthritis: results from a multicenter cross-sectional study. *J Rheumatol 2004*;31:1305-9.

[233] Mazzantini M, di Munno O, Incerti-Vecchi L, Pasero G. Vertebral bone mineral density changes in female rheumatoid arthritis patients treated with low-dose methotrexate. *Clin Exp Rheumatol* 2000;18:327-31.

[234] Tascioglu F, Oner C, Armagan O. The effect of low-dose methotrexate on bone mineral density in patients with early rheumatoid arthritis. *Rheumatol Int* 2003;23:231-5.

[235] Buckley LM, Leib ES, Cartularo KS, Vacek PM, Cooper SM. Effects of low dose methotrexate on the bone mineral density of patients with rheumatoid arthritis. *J Rheumatol* 1997;24:1489-94.

[236] Gnudi S, Butturini L, Ripamonti C, Avella M, Bacci G. The effects of methotrexate (MTX) on bone. A densitometric study conducted on 59 patients with MTX administered at different doses. *Ital.J Orthop Traumatol.* 1988;14:227-31.

[237] Wheeler DL, Vander Griend RA, Wronski TJ, et al. The short- and long-term effects of methotrexate on the rat skeleton. *Bone* 1995;16:215-21.

[238] Laurindo IM, Mendes FL, Novaes GS, et al. Methotrexate inhibition of bone mineral density increase in growing rabbits: prevention by folinic acid. *Clin Exp Rheumatol* 2003;21:581-6.

[239] Davies JH, Evans BA, Jenney ME, Gregory JW. Effects of chemotherapeutic agents on the function of primary human osteoblast-like cells derived from children. *J Clin Endocrinol Metab* 2003;88:6088-97.

[240] Vestergaard P, Rejnmark L, Mosekilde L. Methotrexate, azathioprine, cyclosporine, and risk of fracture. *Calcif Tissue Int* 2006;79:69-75.

[241] Virolainen P, Inoue N, Nagao M, Frassica FJ, Chao EY. The effect of a doxorubicin, cisplatin and ifosfamide combination chemotherapy on bone turnover. *Anticancer Res* 2002;22:1971-5.

[242] Goodwin PJ, Ennis M, Pritchard KI, Trudeau M, Hood N. Risk of menopause during the first year after breast cancer diagnosis. *J Clin Oncol* 1999;17:2365-70.

[243] Virolainen P, Inoue N, Nagao M, Frassica FJ, Chao EY. The effect of a doxorubicin, cisplatin and ifosfamide combination chemotherapy on bone turnover. *Anticancer Res* 2002;22:1971-5.

[244] Cross SS. The molecular pathology of new anti-cancer agents. *Current Diagnostic Pathology* 2005;11:329-39.

[245] Alibhai SM, Gogov S, Allibhai Z. Long-term side effects of androgen deprivation therapy in men with non-metastatic prostate cancer: a systematic literature review. *Crit Rev Oncol.Hematol.* 2006;60:201-15.

[246] Berruti A, Dogliotti L, Terrone C, et al. Changes in bone mineral density, lean body mass and fat content as measured by dual energy x-ray absorptiometry in patients with prostate cancer without apparent bone metastases given androgen deprivation therapy. *J Urol.* 2002;167:2361-7.

[247] Daniell HW. Osteoporosis after orchiectomy for prostate cancer. *J Urol.* 1997;157:439-44.

[248] Diamond TH, Bucci J, Kersley JH, et al. Osteoporosis and spinal fractures in men with prostate cancer: risk factors and effects of androgen deprivation therapy. *J Uro*l. 2004;172:529-32.

[249] Greenspan SL, Coates P, Sereika SM, et al. Bone loss after initiation of androgen deprivation therapy in patients with prostate cancer. *J Clin Endocrinol Metab.* 2005;90:6410-7.

[250] Lopez AM, Pena MA, Hernandez R, et al. Fracture risk in patients with prostate cancer on androgen deprivation therapy. *Osteoporos Int* 2005;16:707-11.

[251] Melton LJ, III, Alothman KI, Khosla S, et al. Fracture risk following bilateral orchiectomy. J Urol. 2003;169:1747-50.

[252] Morote J, Orsola A, Abascal JM, et al. Bone mineral density changes in patients with prostate cancer during the first 2 years of androgen suppression. *J Urol.* 2006;175:1679-83.

[253] Morote J, Morin JP, Orsola A, et al. Prevalence of osteoporosis during long-term androgen deprivation therapy in patients with prostate cancer. *Urology*. 2007;69:500-4.

[254] Smith MR, Lee WC, Brandman J, et al. Gonadotropin-releasing hormone agonists and fracture risk: a claims-based cohort study of men with nonmetastatic prostate cancer. *J Clin Oncol.* 2005;23:7897-903.

[255] Smith MR, Boyce SP, Moyneur E, et al. Risk of clinical fractures after gonadotropin-releasing hormone agonist therapy for prostate cancer. *J Urol.* 2006;175:136-9.

[256] Stoch SA, Parker RA, Chen L, et al. Bone loss in men with prostate cancer treated with gonadotropin-releasing hormone agonists. *J Clin Endocrinol Metab*. 2001;86:2787-91.

[257] Vordos D, Paule B, Vacherot F, et al. Docetaxel and zoledronic acid in patients with metastatic hormone-refractory prostate cancer. *BJU.Int*. 2004;94:524-7.

[258] Smith MR, Fallon MA, Lee H, Finkelstein JS. Raloxifene to prevent gonadotropin-releasing hormone agonist-induced bone loss in men with prostate cancer: a randomized controlled trial. *J Clin Endocrinol Metab*. 2004;89:3841-6.

[259] Vestergaard P. Bone loss associated with gastrointestinal disease: prevalence and pathogenesis. *Eur J Gastroenterol Hepatol* 2003;15:856

[260] Vestergaard P. Prevalence and pathogenesis of osteoporosis in patients with inflammatory bowel disease. *Minerva Me*d 2004;95:469-80.

[261] Hyams JS, Fitzgerald JE, Wyzga N, et al. Relationship of interleukin-1 receptor antagonist to mu*cosal inflammation in inflammatory bowel disease.* J Pediatr Gastroenterol Nutr 1995;21:419-25.

[262] Hyams JS, Wyzga N, Kreutzer DL, Justinich CJ, Gronowicz GA. Alterations in bone metabolism in children with inflammatory bowel disease: an in vitro study [see comments]. *J Pediatr Gastroenterol Nutr* 1997;24:289-95.

[263] Sylvester FA, Wyzga N, Hyams JS, Gronowicz GA. Effect of Crohn's disease on bone metabolism in vitro: a role for interleukin-6. *J Bone Miner Res* 2002;17:695-702.

[264] Canalis E. Mechanisms of glucocorticoid action in bone: implications to glucocorticoid-induced osteoporosis. *J Clin Endocrinol Metab* 1996;81:3441-6.

[265] Patschan D, Loddenkemper K, Buttgereit F. Molecular mechanisms of glucocorticoid-induced osteoporosis. *Bone* 2001;29:498-505.

[266] van Staa TP, Laan RF, Barton IP, et al. Bone density threshold and other predictors of vertebral fracture in patients receiving oral glucocorticoid therapy. *Arthritis Rheum* 2003;48:3224-9.

[267] Selby PL, Halsey JP, Adams KRH, et al. Cortocosteroids do not alter the threshold for vertebral fracture. *J Bone Miner Res* 2000;15:952-6.

[268] Vestergaard P, Rejnmark L, Mosekilde L. Fracture risk associated with systemic and topical corticosteroids. *J Intern Med* 2005;257:374-84.

[269] Edsbacker S, Andersson T. Pharmacokinetics of budesonide (Entocort EC) capsules for Crohn's disease. *Clin Pharmacokinet.* 2004;43:803-21.

[270] Tromm A, Mollmann H, Barth J, et al. Pharmacokinetics and rectal bioavailability of hydrocortisone acetate after single and multiple administration in healthy subjects and patients. *J Clin Pharmacol* 2001;41:536-41.

[271] Daley-Yates PT, Kunka RL, Yin Y, et al. Bioavailability of fluticasone propionate and mometasone furoate aqueous nasal sprays. *Eur J Clin Pharmacol* 2004;60:265-8.

[272] Mizuchi A, Miyachi Y, Tamaki K, Kukita A. Percutaneous absorption of betamethasone 17-benzoate measured by radioimmunoassay. *J Invest Dermatol* 1976;67:279-82.

[273] Dahlstrom K, Thorsson L, Larsson P, Nikander K. Systemic availability and lung deposition of budesonide via three different nebulizers in adults. *Ann Allergy Asthma Immunol* 2003;90:226-32.

[274] Pedersen S. Do Inhaled Corticosteroids Inhibit Growth in Children? *Am.J.Respir.Crit.Care Med.* 2001;164:521-35.

[275] Singh SD, Whale C, Houghton N, et al. Pharmacokinetics and systemic effects of inhaled fluticasone propionate in chronic obstructive pulmonary disease. *Br J Clin Pharmacol* 2003;55:375-81.

[276] Laan RF, van Riel PL, van de Putte.L.B., et al. Low-dose prednisone induces rapid reversible axial bone loss in patients with rheumatoid arthritis. A randomised controlled study. *Ann Intern Med* 1993;119:963-8.

[277] van Staa TP, Leufkens HGM, Abenhaim L, Zhang B, Cooper C. Fractures and oral corticosteroids: relationship to daily and cumulative dose. *Rheumatol* 2000;39:1383-9.

[278] Leonard MB, Feldman HI, Shults J, et al. Long-term, high-dose glucocorticoids and bone mineral content in childhood glucocorticoid-sensitive nephrotic syndrome. *N Engl J Med* 2004;351:868-75.

[279] Leonard MB, Feldman HI, Shults J, et al. Long-term, high-dose glucocorticoids and bone mineral content in childhood glucocorticoid-sensitive nephrotic syndrome. *N Engl J Med* 2004;351:868-75.

[280] Leonard MB. Glucocorticoid-induced osteoporosis in children: impact of the underlying disease. *Pediatrics* 2007;119 Suppl 2:S166-S174

[281] Lettgen B, Jeken C, Reiners C. Influence of steroid medication on bone mineral density in children with nephrotic syndrome. *Pediatr Nephrol* 1994;8:667-70.

[282] van Staa TP, Abenhaim L, Cooper C, Zhang B, Leufkens HGM. Public health impact of adverse bone effects of oral corticosteroids. *Br J Clin Pharmacol* 2001;51:601-7.

[283] van Staa TP, Leufkens HGM, Abenhaim L, Zhang B, Cooper C. Use of oral corticosteroids and risk of fractures. *J Bone Mineral Res* 2000;15:993-1000.

[284] Abramson AS, Delagi EF. Influence of weight-bearing and muscle contraction on disuse osteoporosis. *Arch Phys Med Rehab* 1961;42:147-51.

[285] Dimal HP, Domej W, Leb G, Lau K-HW. Bone loss in patients with untreated chronic obstructive pulmonary disease is mediated by an increase in bone resorption associated with hypercapnia. *J Bone Miner Res* 2001;16:2132-41.

[286] Doucet C, Brouty-Boye D, Pottin-Clemenceau C, et al. Interleukin (IL) 4 and IL-13 act on human lung fibroblasts. Implication in asthma. *J.Clin.Invest.* 1998;101:2129-39.

[287] Wong CA, Walsh LJ, Smith CJ, et al. Inhaled corticosteroid use and bone-mineral density in patients with asthma. *Lancet* 2000;355:1399-403.

[288] Tattersfield AE, Town GI, Johnell O, et al. Bone mineral density in subjects with mild asthma randomised to treatment with inhaled corticosteroids or non-corticosteroid treatment for two years. *Thorax* 2001;56:272-8.

[289] Bryer HP, Isserow JA, Armstrong EC, et al. Azathioprine alone is bone sparing and does not alter cyclosporin A-induced osteopenia in the rat. J Bone Miner Res 1995;10:132-8.

[290] Ferraccioli G, Casatta L, Bartoli E. Increase of bone mineral density and anabolic variables in patients with rheumatoid arthritis resistant to methotrexate after cyclosporin A therapy. *J Rheumatol 1996*;23:1539-42.

[291] Ezaitouni F, Westeel PF, Fardellone P, et al. [Long-term stability of bone mineral density in patients with renal transplant treated with cyclosporine and low doses of corticoids. Protective role of cyclosporine?]. *Presse Med.* 1998;27:705-12.

[292] Aroldi A, Tarantino A, Montagnino G, et al. Effects of three immunosuppressive regimens on vertebral bone density in renal transplant recipients: a prospective study. *Transplantation* 1997;63:380-6.

[293] Thiebaud D, Krieg MA, Gillard-Berguer D, et al. Cyclosporine induces high bone turnover and may contribute to bone loss after heart transplantation. *European Journal of Clinical Investigation* 1996;26:549-55.

[294] Ott R, Bussenius-Kammerer M, Koch CA, et al. Does conversion of immunosuppressive monotherapy from cyclosporine A to tacrolimus improve bone mineral density in long-term stable liver transplant recipients? *Transplant Proc* 2003;35:3032-4.

[295] Monegal A, Navasa M, Guanabens N, et al. Bone mass and mineral metabolism in liver transplant patients treated with FK506 or cyclosporine *A. Calcif Tissue Int* 2001;68:83-6.

[296] Campistol JM, Holt DW, Epstein S, et al. Bone metabolism in renal transplant patients treated with cyclosporine or sirolimus. *Transpl.Int* 2005;18:1028-35.

[297] Cueto-Manzano AM, Konel S, Crowley V, et al. Bone histopathology and densitometry comparison between cyclosporine a monotherapy and prednisolone plus

azathioprine dual immunosuppression in renal transplant patients. *Transplantation* 2003;75:2053-8.

[298] Cueto-Manzano AM, Konel S, Hutchison AJ, et al. Bone loss in long-term renal transplantation: histopathology and densitometry analysis. *Kidney Int* 1999;55:2021-9.

[299] Bryer HP, Isserow JA, Armstrong EC, et al. Azathioprine alone is bone sparing and does not alter cyclosporin A-induced osteopenia in the rat. *J Bone Miner Res 1995*;10:132-8.

[300] Compeyrot-Lacassagne S, Tyrrell PN, Atenafu E, et al. Prevalence and etiology of low bone mineral density in juvenile systemic lupus erythematosus. *Arthritis Rheum* 2007;56:1966-73.

[301] Frei P, Fried M, Hungerbuhler V, et al. Analysis of risk factors for low bone mineral density in inflammatory bowel disease. *Digestion* 2006;73:40-6.

[302] Floren CH, Ahren B, Bengtsson M, Bartosik J, Obrant K. Bone mineral density in patients with Crohn's disease during long-term treatment with azathioprine. *J Intern Med* 1998;243:123-6.

[303] McIntyre HD, Menzies B, Rigby R, et al. Long-term bone loss after renal transplantation: comparison of immunosuppressive regimens. *Clin Transplant* 1995;9:20-4.

[304] Als OS, Christiansen C, Hellesen C. Prevalence of decreased bone mass in rheumatoid arthritis. Relation to anti-inflammatory treatment. Clin Rheumatol 1984;3:201-8.

[305] Schorn D. Osteoporosis in the rheumatoid hand--the effects of treatment with D-penicillamine and oral gold salts. *S Afr Med J* 1983;63:121-3.

[306] Hagdrup H, Serup J, Tvedegaard E. Does long-term treatment with D-penicillamine alter calcium and phosphorus metabolism in patients with systemic sclerosis? *Acta Derm.Venereol.* 1983;63:447-9.

[307] Merker HJ, Franke L, Gunther T. The effect of D-penicillamine of the skeletal development of rat foetuses. *Naunyn Schmiedebergs Arch Pharmacol* 1975;287:359-76.

[308] Riede UN. [Cells and matrix of epiphyseal plate after administration of D-penicillamine]. *Virchows Arch B Cell Patho*l 1971;9:322-32.

[309] Trzenschik K, Hahnel H, Muhlbach R, et al. [Animal experiments on the action of D-penicillamine with reference to its effects on the skeletal system]. *Dtsch Gesundheitsw.* 1972;27:289-91.

[310] Lakshminarayanan S, Walsh S, Mohanraj M, Rothfield N. Factors associated with low bone mineral density in female patients with systemic lupus erythematosus. *J Rheumatol* 2001;28:102-8.

[311] van Schaardenburg D, Valkema R, Dijkmans BA, et al. Prednisone treatment of elderly-onset rheumatoid arthritis. Disease activity and bone mass in comparison with chloroquine treatment. *Arthritis Rheum* 1995;38:334-42.

[312] van Schaardenburg D, Valkema R, Dijkmans BA, et al. Prednisone treatment of elderly-onset rheumatoid arthritis. Disease a*ctivity and bone mass in comparison with chloroquine treatment.* Arthritis Rheum 1995;38:334-42.

[313] Tascioglu F, Oner C, Armagan O. The effect of low-dose methotrexate on bone mineral density in patients with early rheumatoid arthritis. *Rheumatol Int* 2003;23:231-5.

[314] Tengstrand B, Hafstrom I. Bone mineral density in men with rheumatoid arthritis is associated with erosive disease and sulfasalazine treatment but not with sex hormones. *J Rheumatol* 2002;29:2299-305.

[315] Marotte H, Pallot-Prades B, Grange L, et al. A 1-year case-control study in patients with rheumatoid arthritis indicates prevention of loss of bone mineral density in both responders and nonresponders to infliximab. *Arthritis Res Ther* 2007;9:R61

[316] Vis M, Voskuyl AE, Wolbink GJ, Dijkmans BA, Lems WF. Bone mineral density in patients with rheumatoid arthritis treated with infliximab. *Ann Rheum Dis* 2005;64:336-7.

[317] Vis M, Havaardsholm EA, Haugeberg G, et al. Evaluation of bone mineral density, bone metabolism, osteoprotegerin and receptor activator of the NFkappaB ligand serum levels during treatment with infliximab in patients with rheumatoid arthritis. *Ann Rheum Dis* 2006;65:1495-9.

[318] Vis M, Havaardsholm EA, Haugeberg G, et al. Evaluation of bone mineral density, bone metabolism, osteoprotegerin and receptor activator of the NFkappaB ligand serum levels during treatment with infliximab in patients with rheumatoid arthritis. *Ann Rheum Dis* 2006;65:1495-9.

[319] Allali F, Breban M, Porcher R, et al. Increase in bone mineral density of patients with spondyloarthropathy treated with anti-tumour necrosis factor alpha. *Ann Rheum Dis* 2003;62:347-9.

[320] Allali F, Breban M, Porcher R, et al. Increase in bone mineral density of patients with spondyloarthropathy treated with anti-tumour necrosis factor alpha. *Ann Rheum Dis* 2003;62:347-9.

[321] Marzo-Ortega H, McGonagle D, Haugeberg G, et al. Bone mineral density improvement in spondyloarthropathy after treatment with etanercept. *Ann Rheum Dis* 2003;62:1020-1.

[322] Bernstein M, Irwin S, Greenberg GR. Maintenance infliximab treatment is associated with improved bone mineral density in Crohn's disease. *Am J Gastroenterol* 2005;100:2031-5.

[323] Pazianas M, Rhim AD, Weinberg AM, Su C, Lichtenstein GR. The effect of anti-TNF-alpha therapy on spinal bone mineral density in patients with Crohn's disease. *Ann N Y Acad Sci* 2006;1068:543-56.

[324] Vestergaard P, Rejnmark L, Mosekilde L. Fracture risk associated with use of morphine and opiates. *J Intern Med* 2006;260:76-87.

[325] Mincey BA, Duh MS, Thomas SK, et al. Risk of cancer treatment-associated bone loss and fractures among women with breast cancer receiving aromatase inhibitors. *Clin Breast Cancer*. 2006;7:127-32.

In: Osteoporosis: Etiology, Diagnosis and Treatment
Editors: Bilar E. Mattingly and Albert C. Pillare
ISBN 978-1-60692-397-9

Chapter 16

SECONDARY OSTEOPOROSIS: THE ROLE OF THYROID HORMONES AND THYROID STIMULATING HORMONE IN BONE LOSS. A NEW APPROACH TO AN OLD CONCEPT

Z. E. Belaya, L. Y. Rozhinskaya and G. A. Melnichenko
The National Research Centre for Endocrinology, Moscow, Russia.

ABSTRACT

In recent years, it has been suggested that not only thyroid hormone excess but also thyroid stimulating hormone (TSH) deficiency may be the cause of bone loss in patients with hyperthyroidism.

The excess of thyroid hormone (T3) leads to increased bone remodeling, characterized by an imbalance between bone resorption and formation which results in net bone loss and an increased risk of fragile fractures. A brief overview of the molecular actions of thyroid hormone in adult bone is provided as well as a review of the clinical effects of excess levels of thyroid hormones and the long-term effects of the treated manifest hyperthyroidism on the skeleton.

Since thyrotropin receptors have been demonstrated in several extrathyroidal tissues and cells, including human and rat osteosarcoma cell lines and primary cultures of human osteoblast-like (hOB) cells, its role in bone metabolism has been discussed. In this article, we will evaluate the results of different research concerning molecular actions of TSH on bone and estimate its input in comparison to thyroid hormones.

With the development of sensitive thyrotropin assays, subclinical hyperthyroidism has become a commonly diagnosed endocrine disorder especially in the elderly population in iodine deficient areas. Whereas manifest thyrotoxicosis is usually diagnosed and treated at a very early stage, subclinical thyroid dysfunction has often remained undiagnosed and even artificially maintained with suppressive thyroid hormone therapy in patients after surgical treatment for differentiated thyroid cancer. The clinical significance of subclinical hyperthyroidism on bone mineral density and fracture risk and the first experience in the antiosteoporotic treatment of these patients will be discussed.

INTRODUCTION

An association between thyroid gland disorder and bone disease was first suggested in 1891 when German pathologist Friedrich Daniel von Recklinghausen reported a patient with untreated hyperthyroidism and multiple fractures [73]. While the clinical consequences of overt hyperthyroidism on the skeleton have been known for many years and the term "secondary osteoporosis" has been used to represent the effects of thyroid hormone excess on bone, an understanding of the molecular mechanism of bone loss due to thyroid disorders has remained incomplete.

Earlier recognition of thyroid disease and effective treatment for clinical symptoms has meant that severe bone loss is now rarely seen [63]. Recently, with the development of more sensitive TSH assays and the recognition that even subclinical thyroid disease, associated with suppressed thyrotropine (TSH) but normal fT3 and fT4 levels, may have effects on fracture risk, there has been a renewed interest in the role of thyroid disorders in bone. The major issue is that subclinical hyperthyroidism, without elevated thyroid hormones, is associated with substantial bone loss [92]. It has, therefore, been suggested that there could be a relationship between low TSH levels and bone disease, although this has traditionally been attributed to an elevation in thyroid hormones [52]. Consistent with this, the high bone mass and increased cortical width noted in hypothyroid patients has been thought to result from low thyroid hormone levels, rather than from accompanying elevations in serum TSH. However, recently TSH deficiency or excess has been suggested as the important cause of bone disorders.

This paper reviews the recent developments in molecular action of thyroid hormones and TSH in bone tissue and the clinical consequences of overt and subclinical hyperthyroidism in the adult skeleton.

The Molecular Action of Thyroid Hormones in Bone

The actions of thyroid hormones play a key role in the normal development of endochondral and intramembranous bone, linear growth in children as well as in the maintenance of bone mass in the adult skeleton [14]. The pro-hormone thyroxine (T4) is synthesized in the thyroid gland together with a small amount of the active hormone 3,5,3-L-triiodothyronine (T3) [12]. At the same time, the majority of circulating T3 is generated by pre-receptor ligand metabolism resulting from activity of the iodothyronine deiodinase enzymes D1 and D2 which convert T4 to T3 by 5' monodeiodination. In contrast, the D3 enzyme inactivates T4 and T3. Thus, the intracellular level of T3 is dependent on the relative activities of these three deiodinases [18]. The thyroid hormone receptors (TRs) are members of the nuclear receptor superfamily and act as hormone-inducible transcription factors. The THRA and THRB genes are transcribed as multiple mRNA isoforms. TRα1, TRα2, TRβ1 and TRβ3 are widely synthesized, whereas TRβ2 is restricted predominantly to the hypothalamic-pituitary axis, where it negatively regulates TSH α- and β-subunit synthesis. TRα1, TRα2 and TRβ1 are synthesized in osteoblasts and in reserve and proliferative chondrocytes [75,91]. The thyroid hormone receptors compete with the retinoic acid receptor, vitamin D receptor, and peroxisome proliferator-activated receptor (PPAR) for heterodimeric partnership with RXR [14]. Studies on animals have shown that in bones TRα1 is expressed at a 12-fold higher concentration than TRβ1, indicating that TRα1 is the functionally predominant thyroid receptor in bones [64]. Detailed analysis of TR knockouts has not only highlighted the functional differences between the TRα and TRβ with respect to their effects on bone cells, but has also yielded unexpected bone phenotypes in adult mice. For example, biochemically euthyroid $TR\alpha^{0/0}$ mice with no α isoforms, display delayed chondrocyte maturation including growth and ossification defects in young mice, but show osteosclerosis in adults [13]. By contrast, $TR\beta^{-/-}$ mice, which have elevated thyroid hormone and TSH levels, exhibit accelerated chondrocyte maturation, but induce osteoporosis in adults [13].

Thus, osteoblasts synthesize TRα1 and TRα2, whereas the synthesis of TRβ varies with differentiation [104]. In studies of osteoblastic bone marrow stromal cells and osteoblast cell lines, T3 induced interleukin 6 (IL-6), IL-8, prostaglandin E2 (PGE2) and other cytokines involved in osteoclastogenesis, and augmented IL-1 stimulation of IL-6 [48,86]. It also stimulated the synthesis of insulin-like growth factor (IGF-1) and its regulatory binding proteins (IGF1BP-2 and -4) [57]. The effects of T3 in osteoblastic cells has been associated with the increased synthesis of osteocalcin (OC), type 1 collagen and alkaline phosphatase (ALP) as well as induction of the proangiogenic factor collagenase 3/matrix metalloproteinase 13 (MMP13), gelatinase B (MMP9) and the tissue inhibitor of MMP [70,80]. It also modulates parathyroid hormone-related peptide receptor (PTHrPR) synthesis and, therefore, regulates the osteoblastic parathyroid hormone response [35], increases osteoblast differentiation and apoptosis and induces receptor activator of nuclear factor-κB ligand (RANKL) synthesis [58]. The gene encoding fibroblast growth factor receptor 1 (FGFR1) was identified as a T3 target gene in osteoblasts that might have a role in the pro-proliferative and pro-apoptotic actions of T3 [90].

These studies indicate osteoblasts as the primary T3 target cells. T3 stimulates osteoblast activity both directly and indirectly via numerous growth factors and cytokines. By contrast, osteoclasts only resorb bone in response to T3 in the presence of cocultured osteoblasts, and osteoclastic bone resorptive actions of T3 are probably mediated indirectly in part by IL-6, PGs and RANKL [14]. The molecular actions of thyroid hormone and TSH in bone are summarized in Figure 1.

During bone remodeling, the bone structural unit, or osteon, is characterized by a certain structural thickness. In hyperthyroidism, the activation frequency is increased. The resorptive and formative phases are shortened in length. Resorption depth is normal, but completed wall thickness at the end of each cycle is reduced, leading to a loss of thickness with each cycle [60]. Reconstruction of the bone remodeling sequence in uncontrolled hyperthyroid patients indicates that the duration of remodeling is significantly reduced with a negative balance between resorption and formation, resulting in a net loss of about 10-15% of mineralized bone per cycle, with an ultimate reduction in BMD.

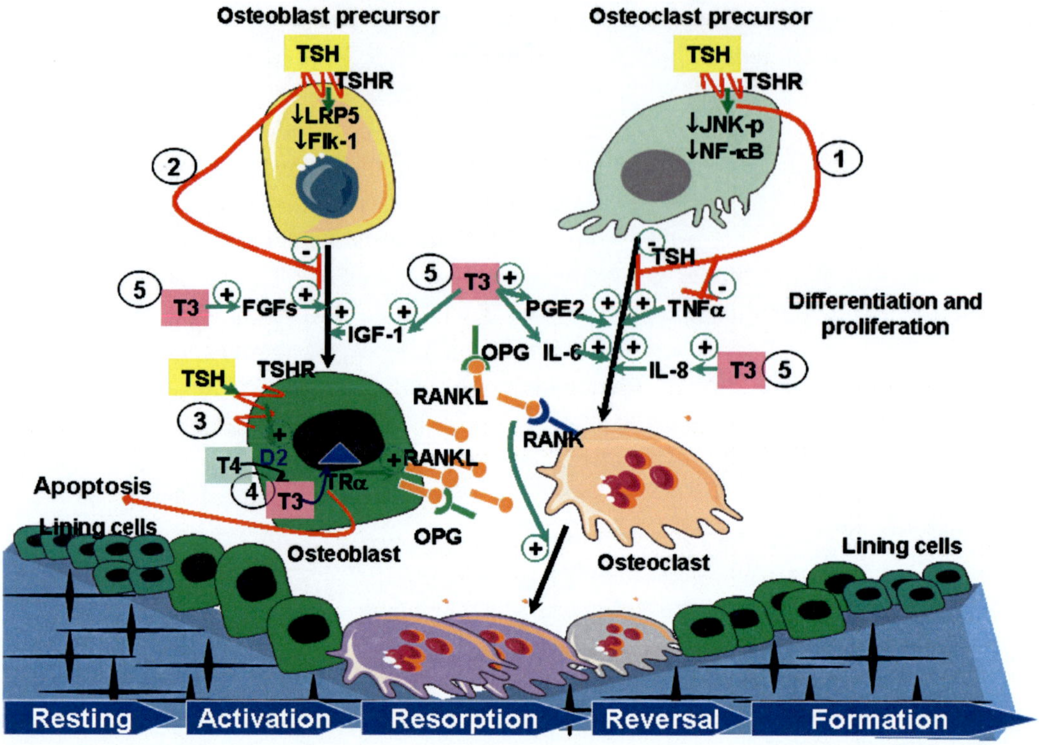

Figure 1. The current understanding of molecular actions of thyroid hormone and TSH in bone. The bone remodeling cycle is characterized by osteoclastic bone resorption followed by osteoblast invasion and bone formation. Direct osteoblast-osteoclast communication is required for osteoclast differentiation, and is mediated by the receptor activator of nuclear factor-κB (RANK) and its ligand (RANKL). This interaction is antagonized by osteoprotegerin (OPG), a soluble decoy receptor for RANKL, secreted by osteoblasts. Compelling evidence has been provided for the following molecular targets through which thyroid hormones and TSH influence bone tissue. 1. Tumor necrosis factor α (TNFα) as an osteoclastogenic signal is suppressed by TSH. The interaction of TNFα with its receptors results in the activation of Akt, MAP (Mitogen-Activated protein kinase) kinases (JNK, ERK, and p38) and nuclear factor kappa B (NFκB) which increase osteoclast differentiation. Consequently TSH decreases the nuclear translocation of the NFκB heterodimers, potently inhibits basal and RANKL-stimulated JNK and IκBα phosphorylation. Likewise TSH attenuates both basal and RANKL-induced c-jun translocation, and inhibits RANKL-induced nuclear translocation of p65. Therefore, TSH suppresses osteoclastogenesis [1]. 2. TSH inhibits osteoblast differentiation through the downregulation of the prodifferentiation factors, LRP5 and Flk-1 [1]. 3. TSH increases D2 mRNA and D2 activity in human osteoblasts and therefore influences on the intracellular level of T3 [59]. 4. T3 promotes osteoblastic proliferation, differentiation and apoptosis directly rough TRα and by inducing RANKL expression in osteoblasts indirectly stimulates osteoclastic differentiation and activity [58]. 5. T3 stimulates osteoblastogenesis indirectly by induction of insulin-like growth factor I (IGF-I) and modulation of fibroblast growth factor (FGF) signaling. Osteoclastogenesis is also indirectly stimulated by T3 through the induction of interleukin 6 (IL-6) and prostaglandin E2 (PGE2) [48,86,90].

Clinical Consequences of Overt Hyperthyroidism on the Adult Bone

The actions of thyroid hormones on bone and their effects on calcium homeostasis result in an increased urinary calcium excretion, increased urinary phosphate reabsorbtion, increased fecal calcium loss, and reduced intestinal calcium and phosphate absorbtion [37,60]. Serum albumin concentrations are reduced, resulting in elevated mean ionized calcium and phosphate concentrations. Marked hypercalcemia is uncommon but may occur in up to 5% of subjects; but even mild hypercalcemia, which occurs in up to 20% of patients, suppresses parathyroid hormone (PTH) secretion and serum PTH concentrations. Consequently, there is reduced renal conversion of 25(OH)-vitamin D3 to 1α25(OH)2-vitamin D3 and their levels are further decreased by increased metabolic clearance in thyrotoxicosis. In combination with the calcium-mobilizing effects of thyroid hormones on bone, these changes all contribute to a significant negative calcium balance [37] (Figure 2).

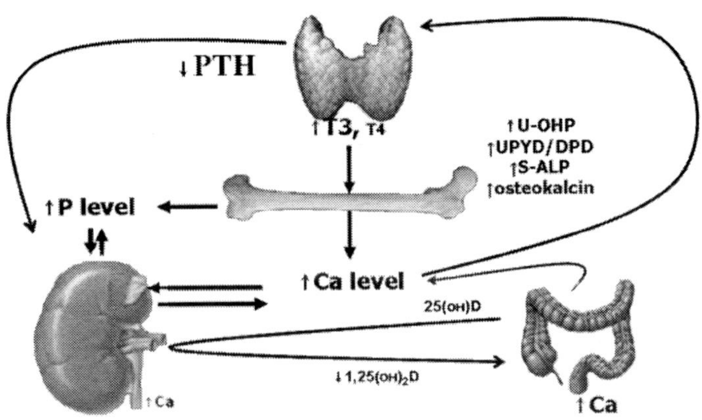

Figure 2. Clinical effects of thyroid hormones in bone. In thyrotoxicosis bone resorption and formation are increased, as is the frequency of remodeling this is reflected by high levels of the markers of bone metabolism. The duration of resorption is maintained, but that of bone formation is reduced by two-thirds which leads to excessive calcium release from bone tissue. Hypercalciemia is observed in 20% of patients. High calcium levels suppress parathyroid hormones and decrease vitamin D conversion into active D-hormone in kidneys which causes reduced intestinal absorption of calcium and increased renal and faecal losses. Consequently, active thyrotoxicosis is associated with a negative calcium balance and BMD loss.

Biochemical markers of bone turnover are elevated in hyperthyroidism and reflect increased activities of both osteoblasts and osteoclasts [6,37]. Statistically significant positive correlations have been found between urinary pyridinoline (Pyr) [65], deoxypyridinaline (Dpyr) [5,65], urinary type I collagen degradation products (CTx) [65], serum osteocalcin (OC) [11,65] and free T3, T4 levels in patients with overt hyperthyroidism. Hence, the severity of thyrotoxicosis influences the activity of bone metabolism and, therefore, the degree of bone loss. Changes in bone density occur differently in sites that contain metabolically active trabecular bone compared with cortical bone sites such as the femoral neck and radius. Histomorphometric studies indicate that thyrotoxic bone loss is greater in cortical bone [37,60]. The degree of reduction in bone mineral density in patients with thyrotoxicosis varies widely between reports but is approximately 12-15% in the lumbar spine, 13-17% at the hip, 15-20% in the forearm, and up to 25% in the calcaneus [37]. Thus, untreated hyperthyroidism causes severe osteoporosis and pathologic fractures. The long-term risk of fracture in patients previously treated for hyperthyroidism is less understood [103]. A mortality study of 7209 previously hyperthyroid patients treated with radioiodine over 30 years, revealed an increased risk of death due to fracture, with the majority of the higher death risk attributable to fractures of the femur [34]. This finding supported a prospective study which followed 9516 white women over 65 for an average of 4 years for incidents of fractures of the femur and found a 1,8 –fold increased relative risk amongst those with previous hyperthyroidism (95%Cl 1,2-2,6) [23]. In accordance with these findings, a retrospective study of 864 previously hyperthyroid patients treated with radioiodine showed an increased risk of self-reported fractures [101]. These findings are in contrast to another large prospective study of over 9000 post-menopausal women, which failed to show an association of thyrotoxicosis with fractures of the ankle and foot [83]. Nevertheless, a case control study of 11776 hyperthyroid subjects demonstrated an increased risk of fractures around the time of diagnosis (RR 1,26-2,29), but no increased risk after the diagnosis was made. Those patients treated with thyroidectomy had a significantly lower risk of fracture after diagnosis [99]. In more recent (2005) study 124655 consecutive patients who had had fractures were evaluated. An increased risk of fracture was found within 5 years of the diagnosis of hyperthyroidism and within 10 years of the diagnosis of hypothyroidism. Levothyroxine therapy was not associated with fractures and the use of antithyroid medications was associated with a significantly reduced risk of fracture [100]. This data was confirmed by the meta-analysis of 5 studies (62830 people including the control group) which showed a significant increase in risk of hip fracture for patients with previous hyperthyroidism when compared with the control group [98]. In addition, the risk of hip fracture increased with the age when hyperthyroidism was diagnosed [23,98].

TSH – an Independent Regulator of Bone Metabolism

The glycoprotein hormone, TSH, interacts with a seven transmembrane, glycosylated G protein-coupled TSH receptor (TSHR) on thyroid follicular cells to regulate the synthesis and secretion of thyroid hormones [24]. The TSHR, long known to signal via cAMP [105], can induce both the phospholipase C (PLC) and the protein kinase A signal transduction systems. Intracellular Ca^{2+} and PLC regulate iodine efflux, H_2O_2 production, and thyroglobulin iodination, while adenylate cyclase and cAMP regulate iodine uptake and transcription of thyroglobulin (Tg), and the sodium-iodine symporter in thyroid follicular cells [32,74]. In addition to thyroid glands, TSHR have been documented in the thymus [62,88], lymphocytes [8], pituitary [21], testis [25], kidney [84], brain [22], adipose/fibroblast cells [9,29], heart [28] and bone [1,44,59] as well as in some other organs. Though the extrathyroidal functions of TSH have been speculated on in recent years, few of these conjectures have been proven. Tsai et al., identified TSHRs in cultures of primary bone marrow-derived osteoblasts (hOB). In hOB cells, the basal intracellular cAMP levels increased 282% after stimulation with 10 U/L TSH, free cytoplasmic calcium did not change in response to TSH in hOB cells. The authors concluded that there is only weak evidence for the presence of functionally active hTSHR in hOB cells [96]. At the same time a Rotterdam study showed that elderly people (1600 Caucasian men and women age 68,5±7,4) with the TSHR-Glu727 variant, which results in an increased cAMP response of the receptor to TSH in vitro, have significantly higher BMD and BMC (bone mineral content) at the femoral neck [26]. In addition, the marker of bone resorption – C-terminal telopeptide of type I collagen (CTx) was found to be significantly lower in patients with high TSH level (10 patients with TSH secreting pituitary adenoma, 40 patients with thyroid hormone resistance, 31 patients with primary hypothyroidism before treatment) and higher in patients with low TSH [71].

Abe, et al. has found an abundant expression of TSHRs on both osteoclast and osteoblast precursors and reported direct effects of TSH on bone remodeling by demonstrating that TSHR haploinsufficient mice with normal circulating thyroid hormone levels have osteoporosis and focal osteosclerosis. To explore the role of TSH in bone remodeling, Abe, et al. deleted exon 1 of the TSHR gene and replaced it with a green fluorescent protein (GFP) cassette [1,2,92]. Heterozygote mice, haploinsufficient in the TSHR, were euthyroid, had a normal growth pattern, and unchanged circulating thyroid hormone and TSH levels. Homozygotic TSHR null mice, in contrast, had runted growth, low thyroid hormone levels, a high circulating TSH, and required thyroid extracts for growth and survival. The thyroid follicular pattern in the homozygotes was disorganized. In contrast, thyroid follicles in the heterozygotes were normal, as expected from a biochemically euthyroid state. Consequently, a 50% reduction in TSHR levels in heterozygote mice affected neither thyroid follicular growth or development, nor the secretion of thyroid hormones. With normal thyroid function established, the heterozygotes showed evidence of reduced bone mineral density (BMD) at all sites. Therefore, it was suggested that TSH is a single necessary molecular switch that negatively regulates both components of skeletal remodeling. In addition to the generalized osteopenia, there was also surprising evidence for focal osteosclerosis. This dual phenotype consisting of high-turnover osteoporosis and focal sclerosis is unusual and to some extent comprised areas reminiscent of human Paget's bone disease. Thus, it has been suggested that oseoblastic activity is pronounced, autonomous, and dissociated spatially from resorption. There was "ectopic" bone formation at sites that had not been resorbed previously [1,2]. It is unknown whether focal osteosclerosis also occurs in human hyperthyroidism because of the lack of histological information in these patients.

Ex vivo studies also indicated that TSH affects osteoclast and osteoblast function and formation. TSH decreased osteoblast differentiation and collagen synthesis [1,7]. RANKL-induced osteoclastogenesis was inhibited by recombinant TSH at two signal transduction steps involving inhibitor IκBα and JNK. This in turn, caused depressed nuclear levels of the proosteoclastogenic transcription factors c-jun and p65. The depressed c-jun levels impaired tartrate-resistant acidic phosphotase (TRAP) and cathepsin K gene transcription, which are critical to osteoclastic bone resorption [43,46,85,89].

Further experiments defined TNF-α as the critical cytokine mediating the downstream effects of TSH [38,87]. Specifically TSH inhibited cytokine-induced TNF-α production in the bone marrow microenvironment. Crossing the TSHR-/- animals to TNF-α -/- animals showed that the effect of TSHR inactivation on bone could be reversed, thus providing in vivo evidence for the role of TNF-α in the osteopenia associated with TSH receptor deficiency [38]. The effects of TSH and T3 on osteoblast and osteoclast precursors and bone remodeling cycle are summarized in Figure 1.

Sampath et al. have demonstrated that TSH suppresses bone remodeling in rats and consequently restores the bone loss in ovariectomised female rats [81]. Similarly, a single injection of human TSH given to postmenopausal women reduced markers of bone turnover to premenopausal levels within 2 days [56]. It is notable that, where measured, serum thyroid hormone levels did not change, again confirming a direct effect of TSH on bone remodeling in vivo. Ideas about TSH's influence in bone come from other studies as well. Thus, functional roles of the bone morphogenic protein (BMP) system in thyrotropin signaling was investigated [94]. BMP ligands belong to the TGF-β superfamily and were originally identified as the active components in bone extracts capable of inducing bone formation at ectopic sites [10]. A novel function of BMP-2, -4, -6, -7 in suppressing TSH-R expression by porcine thyroid cells was uncovered. Furthermore, TSH, in turn, inhibits BMP actions by suppressing ALK-6 receptor expression [94]. Hofbauer et al, investigating the role of receptor activator of NF-κB (RANK) ligand (RANKL) and osteoprotegerin (OPG), which are essential for bone metabolism, in the human thyroid gland, found that OPG mRNA levels and protein secretion were upregulated by TSH (threefold), whereas RANKL mRNA was inhibited by TSH [41].

The authors suggested that negative regulation between TSH and BMP ligands could be involved in the tumorigenesis of thyroid follicular adenomas [94] and RANKL/OPG system could represent local immunoregulatory factors in the thyroid gland [41]. However, whether these regulatory findings reflect the interactions between TSH and BMPs, OPG/RANKL system in bone tissue requires further investigation.

Furthermore, studies have revealed, previously unrecognized roles of TSHR and local T3 production by type 2 iodothyronine deiodinase (D2) in the pathophysiology of human osteoblasts [59]. To exert its biological activity, T4 needs to be converted to T3 by iodothyronine deiodinase. In human thyroid gland D2 expression is regulated by a TSH receptor-cAMP-mediated mechanism [18]. In the present study TSHR mRNA as well as D2 mRNA expression and D2 activity were demonstrated in normal human osteoblast (NHOst) cells. D2 activity was stimulated by TSH in NHOst cells. Based on the present observation, TSH positively regulates and thyroid hormones negatively regulate intracellular T3 production by contolling D2 in human osteoblasts, suggesting that intracellular T3 concentration provided by D2 may modulate the function of osteoblasts regulated by TSH via TSH receptors expressed in osteoblasts [59].

Clinical Relevance of TSH for Human Bones

Subclinical hyperthyroidism, defined as free triiodothyronine (fT3) and free thyroxine (fT4) concentrations within the reference range but serum TSH level below the reference range [20,69,93], seems to be an appropriate model to examine the direct effects of TSH on bone in clinical practice. The primary causes of subclinical hyperthyroidism include excessive doses of L-thyroxine, Graves disease, multinodular goiter, and solitary thyroid nodule. The prevalence of subclinical hyperthyroidism varies depending on age, sex and the level of iodine deficiency in the area [93]. Thus, on some date, the prevalence of subclinical hyperthyroidism is about 1% (95% Cl, 0,4%-1,7%) in men over 60 years of age and 1,5% (95% Cl, 0,8%-2,5%) in women over 60 years of age [39]. According to other data, 3,2% of the population (among people older than 12) in the United States are defined as having subclinical hyperthyroidism [42]. Subclinical hyperthyroid disease is more common in women than men, in blacks than whites, in the elderly [67] and in patients with low iodine intake [53]. For example, the spectrum of thyroid disorders was investigated in an iodine-deficient community of Southern Italy. Endogenous subclinical hyperthyroidism (thyroid functional autonomy due to multinodular goiter) was found in 67 of 1411 (4,7%) of subjects, with no difference between females (5,2%) and males (4,1%). Its frequency progressively increased with age from 0,7% in children to 15,4% in elderly subjects (>75 years old); the overall prevalence in the adult population was 6,4% [4]. Exogenous subclinical hyperthyroidism is common in individuals treated with levothyroxine, being present in 14% to 21% of such patients [68,77].

Several studies designed with the aim of finding new risk factors for osteoporosis, have shown that postmenopausal women with low TSH level (the etiology of subclinical hyperthyroidism was not specified) have lower bone mineral density (BMD) and higher fracture risk compared to women with normal TSH [45,47,54]. Thus, a secondary analysis of data collected as part of the Fracture Intervention Trial (FIT), which included 15316 postmenopausal women, concluded that women with TSH<0,1 mlU/l as well as TSH<0,5 mlU/l had significantly lower BMD at the femoral neck and in total body as compared to women with normal TSH [45]. Additionally, a cross-sectional study in Seoul, Korea, which enrolled 413 postmenopausal women, found that femoral neck BMD was significantly reduced both in the subclinical hyperthyroid group and in the subclinical hypothyroid patients as compared with euthyroid control [54]. Furthermore, a cross-sectional survey, in which 959 healthy postmenopausal women were enrolled, showed that even women with low normal TSH levels (0,5-1,1mU/l) had significantly lower BMD at the lumbar spine and femoral neck than those with high normal TSH levels (2,8-5,0) [47]. However, a prospective cohort study of 458 women over age 65 participating in the multicenter Study of Osteoporotic Fractures, found no consistent evidence that low TSH was associated with low BMD or accelerated bone loss in older ambulatory women [16]. Nevertheless prospective observation of 686 women over 65 (mean follow-up 3,5 years) showed that women with a low TSH level (≤0,1 mU/l) had a threefold increased risk for hip fracture (relative hazard 3.6 (95% Cl 1,0-12,9)) and a fourfold increased risk for vertebral fracture (odds ratio, 4,5 Cl 1,3-15,6) compared with women who had normal TSH levels (0,5-5,5 mU/l) [15]. Use of thyroid hormones in itself does not increase risk for fracture if TSH levels are normal [15]. At the same time, according to a summary of the evidence for the US Preventive Services Task Force and several other reviews the issue of whether subclinical hyperthyroidism has a clinically significant effect on BMD and fracture risk remains controversial [20,40,66].

Indeed, when looking at studies on the effects of subclinical hyperthyroidism with certain etiologies, some questions still remain. Thus, studies examining the effects of exogenous subclinical hyperthyroidism (for years TSH suppression with exogenous L-T4 therapy was recommended in most guidelines for the postoperative management of papillary or folliculare thyroid cancer) [19,36] on bone density have been inconsistent. Although most authors have come to the conclusion that there is no significant change in bone mineral density for premenopausal women or men receiving L-T4 suppressive therapy, the situation with postmenopausal women is still debated. The results of two meta-analyses (1994 and 1996) showed significant bone loss in postmenopausal women on LT4 suppressive therapy versus the control group [30,97]. However, two systematic reviews (2002 and 2003) of the literature showed that BMD changes in postmenopausal women on LT4 suppresive therapy remain unclear and require further evaluation [72,82].

Results of bone density studies in subjects with endogenous subclinical hyperthyroidism are scarce. One case-control study showed a significant increase in bone turnover markers and a decrease in bone mass in postmenopausal women with endogenous subclinical hyperthyroidism due to toxic multinodular goiter [95], whereas such an outcome was only suggestive in another paper which included both postmenopausal and premenopausal women [33].

In order to compare bone metabolism and BMD in postmenopausal women in relation to the etiology of subclinical hyperthyroidism, data of 88 postmenopausal women with different cause of the thyroid disease was analyzed [17]. The first group (1) consisted of 20 women with toxic multinodular goiter without history of clinical hyperthyroidism; the second group (2) included 25 patients on levothyroxine suppressive therapy after thyroidectomy due to differentiated thyroid cancer; the third group (3), which included 21 women with Graves' disease, (GD) received antithyroid drugs and the fourth group (4), the control group, included 22 healthy women matched for age and duration of menopause. Patients in the four groups did not differ on age, menopause status (all subjects were at least 5 years post menopause), body mass index as well as other osteoporotic fracture risk factors. Biochemical markers of bone turnover were significantly higher in all three groups of patients with subclinical hyperthyroidism compared to the control group. OC level was more than 50% higher in groups 1 and 3 ($p<0.001$for both groups), and 28% higher in group 2 ($p=0.005$) when compared to group 4. CTx level was more than 80% higher in groups 1 and 3 ($p<0.001$for both groups), and 36% higher in patients with exogenous subclinical hyperthyroidism. For all patients enrolled in this study TSH exhibited a significant negative correlation with both markers of bone metabolism. The significant decrease in BMD was observed only in patients with endogenous subclinical hyperthyroidism (groups 1 and 3) predominantly in distal and proximal cortical bones, whereas subjects receiving suppressive LT4 therapy did not differ from the control group (Figure 3).

This finding can be explained by the following. The study, mentioned above, proved the expression of D2 in human osteoblasts, which is regulated by TSH. Hence, this study presumed that TSH receptors in bone cells are responsible for the local T3 production by D2. Most of the plasma pool of T3 is derived from the peripheral metabolism of T4 [18]. Thus, the low TSH level may cause the decrease of intracellular T3 production in all patients with subclinical hyperthyroidism, but relatively higher T3 production might be expected in patients with endogenous subclinical hyperthyroidism, which is not observed in patients after total thyroidectomy.

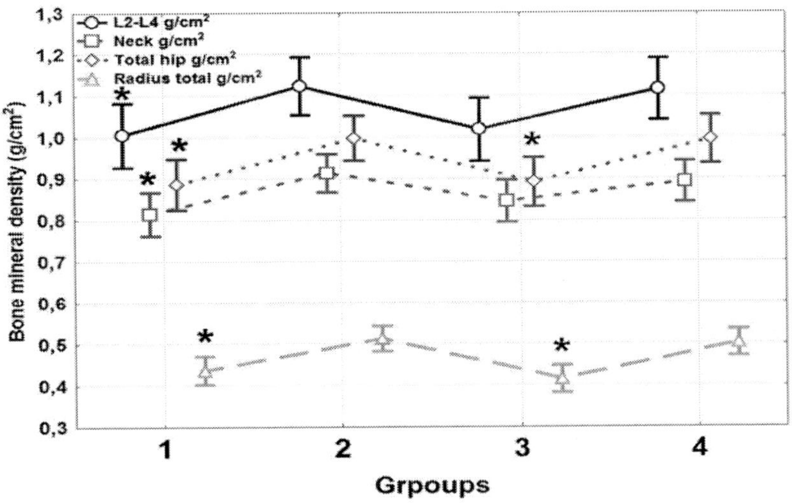

Figure 3. Comparative analysis of BMD in patients with different cause of subclinical hyperthyroidism. BMD at Total Hip and Total Radius was significantly lower in patients with endogenous subclinical hyperthyroidism (groups 1 and 3) than in the control group and in patients receiving suppressive doses of thyroxine ($p<0.05$). Patients from group 1 had significantly greater BMD loss in L1-L4 and the femoral neck when compared with the control group and patients with exogenous subclinical hyperthyroidism ($p<0.05$). No significant differences were found between groups 1 and 3 or between groups 2 and 4.

Antiosteoporosic Treatment in Patients with Hyperthyroidism

A number of studies have shown that the achievement of euthyroidism itself in patients with manifest and subclinical hyperthyroidism leads to decreased bone loss and even some improvement in BMD [3,7,31,61,98]. However, BMD loss in postmenopausal women due to thyrotoxicosis and other risk factors might be so profound that normalization of serum thyrotrophin level only is not sufficient to prevent low traumatic fracture. Although bone histomorphometry studies were not performed in humans with low TSH level, even a 50% reduction of TSHR in mice lead to high-turnover osteoporosis with focal osteosclerosis, which is typically associated with uncoupling between bone formation and resorption. Therefore, subclinical hyperthyroidism might alter bone quality even more than bone mass. Indeed, not all studies have shown BMD loss in postmenopausal women with low TSH versus a control group, but several studies have revealed a significant increase in risk for fragile fractures in women with subclinical hyperthyroidism and in those who had thyrotoxicosis in anamnesis when compared with postmenopausal women with normal thyroid function [15,23,45,98]. It has been suggested that the treatment tactic for hyperthyroidism influences fracture risk in future. Surgical treatment of Graves' disease appeared to be better for fracture risk reduction than radioactive iodine or antithyroid drugs [99,101]. This result may be explained by the fact that younger patients usually receive surgical treatment. Surgical treatment is the only thing that can lead to a prompt and stable decrease in TSHR autoantibody on bone, though research on the effects of TSHR autoantibody is minimal. Significant negative correlation has been found between BMD and the level of TSHR autoantibody in women [102] and men [55] with Graves' disease and a positive correlation has been shown between the markers of bone metabolism and TSHR autoantibody levels in postmenopausal women receiving antithyroid drugs [49].

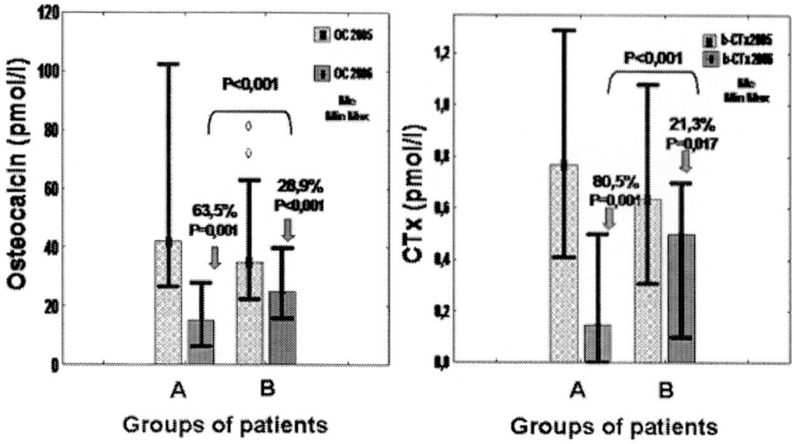

Figure 4. Markers of bone metabolism after one year of euthyroidism and bisphosphonate treatment in postmenopausal women with subclinical hyperthyroidism. The achievement of euthyroidism in postmenopausal women with endogenous subclinical hyperthyroidism led to a decrease in bone metabolism markers. At the same time, even half of the therapeutic dose of alendronate a week led to a significantly larger decrease when compared to calcium and vitamin D supplementation only.

Thus, pathogenesis of bone loss in patients with sublicincal and manifest hyperthyroidism has not been fully understood. At the same time, there is no doubt that these conditions cause a dramatic increase in bone turnover. Hence, antiresorptive treatment seems the most appropriate option among antiosteoporotic medicine. However only a few studies have been done to investigate its effectiveness. A prospective study on 46 postmenopausal Chinese women, receiving L-thyroxine suppressive therapy after surgical treatment on thyroid cancer, showed that both Miacalcic 200 IU five times a week and a 1000 mg calcium supplement are equally effective for preserving BMD [51]. In experimental study on a rat model of thyroid hormone-induced bone loss, natrium etidronate but not calcitonin, preserve bone loss [50]. Fifty-five middle-aged men and women taking suppressive doses of levothyroxine were randomized to treatment with pamidronate 30mg iv every 3 month for 2 years or placebo. There was no significant bone loss at any site of the skeleton in the placebo/T4 group, at the same time BMD even significantly increased in pamidronate/T4 group [76]. The effectiveness of oral bisphosphonate was investigated in postmenopausal women with subclinical hyperthyroidism and osteoporosis. Thirty postmenopausal women with subclinical hyperthyroidism (77% with endogenous subclinical hyperthyroidism and 23% on L-thyroxine suppressive therapy) were randomly assigned into two groups: group A – (14 women) received alendronate 35 mg a week with Calcium (500 mg) and Vitamin D (400UI) supplementation daily and group B – (16 women) received Calcium (1000 mg) and Vitamin D (800 UI) daily [79]. At the baseline visit, no differences were found between two groups. After 12 month of treatment, the markers of bone metabolism decreased in both groups, though the decreases were significantly greater ($p<0.001$ for both OC and CTx) in group A than in group B (Figure 4). BMD increased by 7,6% at L1-L4 (p=0,003), 2,6% at FN (p=0,013), 3,6% at TH (p=0,012) and 3,0 % at RT (p=0,047) in group A. BMD did not significantly change in group B after one year of observation. The improvement in BMD in group A compared to group B was significant at L1-L4 (p=0,001) (Figure 5). Therefore, even 35 mg of alendronate a week can be effective for the treatment of osteoporosis in postmenopausal women with subclinical hyperthyroidism provided compensation of endogenous subclinical hyperthyroidism [79].

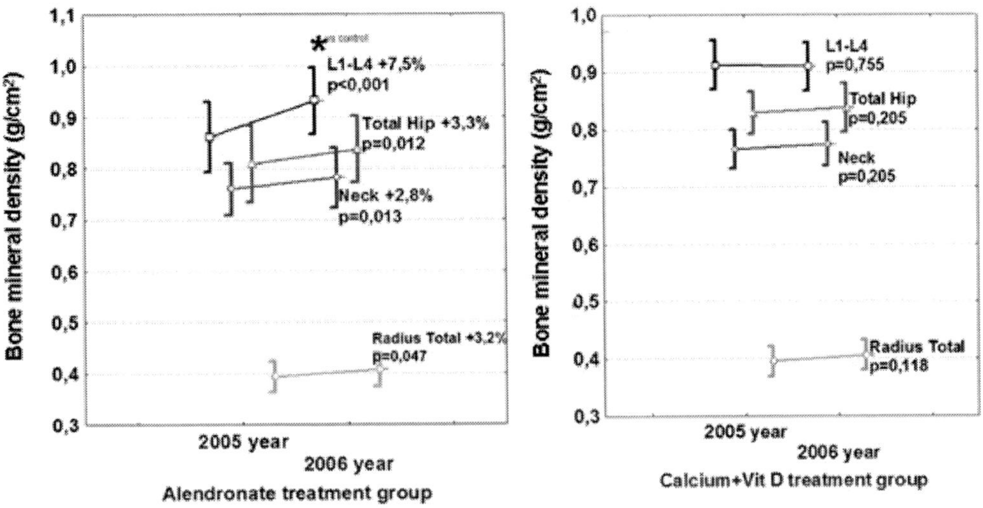

Figure 5. Bone mineral density after 12 months of euthyroidism and bisphosphonate treatment in postmenopausal women with subclinical hyperthyroidism. Normalization of TSH level prevented further bone lose in postmenopausal women with osteoporosis and subclinical hyperthyroidism. However, alendronate at 35 mg per week was associated with significant increase in BMD after one year of treatment (at L1-L4 p=0.001 versus control group) in these patients.

Conclusion

In summary, T3 and TSH independently affect bone condition in the adult skeleton. T3 effects seem to be mediated primarily by TR α. TSH has its own receptor on osteoblasts and osteoclasts precursors as well as on mature bone cells. There is convincing evidence that TSH inhibits both bone resorption and formation and also mediates intracellular T3 level in mature osteoblasts through the expression of D2.

Clinically, manifest thyrotoxicosis is associated with a negative calcium balance, high bone turnover that results in the loss of at least 10% of mineralized bone per cycle with the consequent development of secondary osteoporosis and increased risk for low traumatic fractures. Treatment of hyperthyroidism improves BMD but does not necessarily bring it to a normal level. Moreover, previously treated hyperthyroidism is likely a long-term risk factor for fractures, particularly of the hip. Thyroidectomy seems to be more beneficial for fracture risk reduction than radioactive iodine.

No studies reported any effects of subclinical thyrooxicosis on calcium or phosphorous balance. However, significantly higher levels of markers of bone metabolism are observed in patients with low TSH and normal thyroid hormone. The effects of subclinical hyperthyroidism on BMD are more controversial. Most likely, postmenopausal women with endogenous subclinical hyperthyroidism are at high risk of BMD loss predominantly in proximal and distal cortical bone, whereas suppressive levothyroxine therapy exerts less influence on BMD. At the same time, low TSH level seems to be an important risk factor for low traumatic vertebral and hip fractures in postmenopausal women. This may be additional proof that a high level of bone metabolism is an independent risk factor for future fractures. Taking into account the high-turnover bone metabolism in these patients, bisphosphonate seems to be the most appropriate antiosteoporotic drugs. Indeed, the achievement of euthyroidism and alendronate, even 35 mg a week, increased BMD in all regions of the skeleton in postmenopausal women with osteoporosis and subclinical hyperthyroidism and reduced bone resorption significantly better than only normalization of TSH level and calcium and vitamin D supplementation.

Fracture risk does not seem to be related to levothyroxine replacement in hypothyroid patients.

Further studies are needed to gain for better understanding of TSH effects in human bone and to develop the best therapeutic approach for preventing fragile fractures in patients with subclinical hyperthyroidism.

REFERENCES

[1] Abe E, Marians RC, Yu W, Wu X, Ando T, Li Y, Iqbal J, Eldeiry L, Rajendren G, Blair HC, Davies TF, Zaidi M.: TSH is a negative regulator of skeletal remodeling. // *J. Cell*, 2003, Vol. 115, pp. 151-162

[2] Abe E, Sun L, Mechanick J, Iqbal J, Yamoah K, Baliram R, Arabi A, Moonga BS, Davies TF, Zaidi M.: Bone loss in thyroid disease Role of low TSH and high thyroid hormone.// *J. Ann. N.Y. Acad. Sci*, 2007, Vol. 1116, pp. 383-391

[3] Acotto CG, Niepomniszcze H, Vega E, Mautalen CA.: Ultrasound parametrs and markers of bone turnover in hyperthyroidism: a longitudinal study. // *J. Clinical Densitometry*, 2004, Vol. 7, pp. 201-208

[4] Aghini-Lombardi F, Antonanceli L, Martino E, Vitti P, Maccherini D, Leoli F, Rago T, Grasso L, Valeriano R, Balestrieri A, Pinchera A.: The spectrum of thyroid disorders in an iodine-deficient community: the Pescopagano survey. // *J. Clinical Endocrinology Metabolism*, 1999, Vol. 84, pp. 561-566

[5] Akalin A, Colakt O, Alatast O, Efe B.: Bone remodeling markers and serum cytokines in patients with hyperthyroidism. // *J. Clinical Endocrinology*, 2002, Vol. 57, pp. 125-129

[6] Allain TJ, McCregor AM.: Thyroid hormones and bone. // *J. Endocrinology*, 1993, Vol. 139, pp. 9-18

[7] Arata N, Momotani N, Maruyama H, Saruta T, Tsukatani K, Kubo A, Ikemoto K, Ito K.: Bone mineral density after surgical treatment for Graves' disease. // *J. Thyroid*, 1997, Vol. 7, pp. 547-554

[8] Bagriacik EU, Klein JR.: The thyrotropin (thyroid stimulating hormone) receptor is expressed on murine dendritic cells and on a subset of CD45RBhigh lymph node T cells: functional role for thyroid-stimulating hormone during immune activation. // *J. Immunology*, 2000, Vol. 164, pp. 6158-6165

[9] Bahn RS, Dutton CM, Natt N, Joba W, Spitzweg C, Heufelder AE.: Thyrotropin receptor expression in Graves' orbital adipose/ connective tissues: potential autoantigen in Graves' ophthalmopathy. // *J. Clinical Endocrinology and Metabolism*, 1998, Vol. 83, pp. 998-1002

[10] Baker JC, Harland RM: From receptor to nucleus: the Smad pathway. // *J. Current Opinion in Genetics and Development*, 1997, Vol. 7, pp. 467-473

[11] Barsal G, Taneli F, Atay A, Hekimsoy Z, Erciyas F.: Serum osteocalcin levels in hyperthyroidism before and after antithyroid therapy. // *Tohoku J. Experimental Medicine*, 2004, Vol. 203, pp. 183-188

[12] Bassett JHD, Harvey CB, Williams GR.: Mechanisms of thyroid hormone receptor-specific nuclear and extra nuclear actions.// *Molecular and Clinical Endocrinology*, 2003, Vol. 213, pp. 1-11

[13] Bassett JHD, O'Shea PJO, Sriskantharajah S, Rabier B, Boyde A, Howell PGT, Weiss RE, Roux J-P, Malaval L, Clement-Lacroix P, Samarut J, Chasande O, Williams GR.: Thyroid hormone excess rather than TSH deficiency induces osteoporosis in hyperthyroidism.// *J. Molecular Endocrinology*, 2007, Vol.21, pp. 1095-1107

[14] Bassett JHD, Williams GR.: The molecular actions of thyroid hormone in bone.// *TRENDS in Endocrinology and Metabolism*, 2003, Vol.14, pp 356-364

[15] Bauer DC, Ettinger B, Nevitt MC, Stone KL.: Risk for fracture in women with low serum levels of thyroid-stimulating hormone.// *J. Annual Internal Medicine*, 2001, Vol. 134, pp. 561-568

[16] Bauer DC, Nevitt MC, Ettinger B, Stone K.: Low thyrotropin levels are not associated with bone loss in older women: a prospective study. // *J. Clinical Endocrinology and Metabolism*, 1997, Vol. 82, pp. 2931-2936

[17] Belaya ZE, Melnichenko GA, Rozhinskaya LY, Fadeev VV, Alekseeva TM, Dorofeeva OK, Sasonova NI, Kolesnikova GI.: Subclinical hyperthyroidism of variable etiology and its influence on bone in postmenopausal women.// *J. Hormones*, 2007, Vol. 6, pp. 62-70

[18] Bianco AC, Salvatore D, Gereben B, Berry MJ, Larsen PR.: Biochemistry, cellular and molecular biology, and physiological roles of the iodothyronin selenodeiodinases. // *J. Endocrine Review,* 2002, Vol. 23 pp. 38-89

[19] Biondi B, Filetti S, Schlumberger M.: Thyroid-hormone therapy and thyroid cancer: a reassessment.// *J. Nature clinical practice endocrinology and metabolism*, 2005, Vol. 1, pp. 32-40

[20] Biondi B, Palmeri EA, Klain M, Schlumberger M, Filetti S, Lombardi G.: Subclinical hyperthyroidism: clinical features and treatment options. // *European J. Endocrinology*, 2005, Vol.152, pp. 1-9

[21] Brokken LJ, Scheenhart JW, Wiersinga WM, Prummel MF.: Suppression of serum TSH by Graves'Ig: evidence for a functional pituitary TSH receptor. // *J. Clinical Endocrinology and Metabolism*, 2001, Vol. 86, pp. 4814-4817

[22] Crisanti P, Omri B, Hughes E, Meduri G, Hery C, Clauser E, Jacquemin C, Saunier B.: The expression of thyrotropin receptor in the brain. // *J. Endocrinology*, 2001, Vol. 142, pp. 812-822

[23] Cummings SR, Nevitt MC, Browner WS, Stone K, Fox KM, Ensrud KE, Cauley J, Black D, Vogt TM.: Risk factors for hip fracture in white women. Study of Osteoporotic Fractures Research Group. // *New England J. Medicine*, 1995, Vol. 332, pp. 767-773

[24] Davies T, Marians R, Latif R.: The TSH receptor reveals itself.// *J. Clin. Invest*, 2002, Vol. 110, pp. 161-164

[25] Davies TF, Smith BR, Hall R.: Binding of thyroid stimulators to guinea pig testis and thyroid. // *J. Endocrinology*, 1978, Vol. 103, pp. 6-10

[26] Deure VWM. Uitterlinden AG. Pols HAP. Peeters RP. Visser TJ.: The TSH receptor ASP727GLU polymorphism is associated with higher bone mineral density and bone mineral content.// *J Thyroid*, 2005, Vol. 15. s20-s21

[27] Diamond T, Vine J, Smart R, Butler P.: Thyrotoxic bone diesease in women: a potentially reversible disorder. // *J. Annual Internal Medicine*, 1994, Vol. 120, pp. 8-11

[28] Drvota V, Janson A, Norman C, Sylven C, Haggblad J, Bronnegard M, Marcus C.: Evidence for the presence of functional thyrotropin receptor in cardiac muscle. // *J. Biochemical Biophysical Research Communications*, 1995, Vol. 211, pp. 426-431

[29] Endo T, Ohta K, Haraguchi K, Onaya T.: Cloning and functional expression of a thyrotropin receptor cDNA from rat fat calls. // *J. Biological Chemistry*, 1995, Vol. 270, pp. 10833-10837

[30] Faber J, Galloe AM.: Changes in bone mass during prolonged subclinical hyperthyroidism due to L-thyroxine treatment: a meta-anaysis. // *European J. Endocrinology*, 1994, Vol. 130, pp. 350-356

[31] Faber J, Jensen IW, Petersen L, Nygaard B, Hegedus L, Siersbaek-Nielsen K.: Normalization of serum thyrotrophin by means of radioiodine treatment in subclinical hyperthyroidism: effect on bone loss in postmenopausal women. // *J. Clinical Endocrinology (Oxford)*, 1998, Vol. 48, pp. 285-290

[32] Field JB, Ealey PA, Marshall NJ, Cockcroft S.: Thyroid-stimulating hormone stimulates increases in inositol phosphates as well as cyclic AMP in the FRTL-5 rat thyroid cell line.// *Biochem. J*, 1987, Vol. 247, pp. 519-524

[33] Foldes J, Tarjan G, Szathmari M, Varga F, Krasznai I, Horvath C.: Bone mineral density in patients with endogenous subclinical hyperthyroidism: is this thyroid status a risk factor for osteoporosis? // *J. Clinical Endocrinology (Oxford)*, 1993, Vol. 39, pp. 521-527

[34] Franklyn J, Maisonneuve P, Sheppard M, Betteridge J, Boyle P.: Mortality after the treatment of hyperthyroidism with radioactive iodine.// *New England J. Medicine*, 1998, Vol. 338, pp. 712-718

[35] Gu WX, Stern PH, Madison LD, Du GG.: Mutual up-regulation of thyroid hormone and parathyroid hormone receptors in rat osteoblastic osteosarcoma 17/2.8 cells. // *J. Endocrinology*, 2001, Vol. 142, pp. 157-164

[36] Guidelines for the management of thyroid cancer in adult. // *British Thyroid Association and Royal College of Physicians*, 2002, www.british-thyroid-association.org

[37] Harvey CB, O'Shea PJ, Scott AJ, Robson H, Siebler T, Shalet SM, Samarut J, Chassande O, Williams GR.: Molecular mechanisms of thyroid hormone effects on bone growth and function.// *Molecular Genetics and Metabolism*, 2002, Vol. 75, pp. 17-30

[38] Hase H, Ando T, Eldeiry L, Brebene A, Peng Y, Liu L, Amano H, Davies TF, Sun L, Zaidi M, Abe E..: TNFalpha mediates the skeletal effects of thyroid-stimulating hormone.// *Proc. Natl. Acad. Sci. USA*, 2006, Vol. 103, pp. 12849-12854

[39] Helfand M, Redfern CC.: Clinical guideline, part 2. Screening for thyroid disease: an update. American College of Physicians.// *Ann Intern Med.*, 1998, Vol. 129, pp. 144-158

[40] Helfand M.: Screening for subclinical thyroid dysfunction in nonpregnant adults: a summary of the evidence for the US Preventive Services Task Force. // *J. Annual Internal Medicine*, 2004, Vol. 140, pp. 128-141

[41] Hofbauer LC, Kluger S, Kuhne CA, Dunstan CR, Burchert A, Schoppet M, Zielke A, Heufelder AE.: Detection and characterization of RANK ligand and osteoprotegerin in the thyroid gland.// *J. Cellular Biochemestry*, 2002, Vol. 86, pp. 642-650

[42] Hollowell JC, Staehling NW, Flanders WD, Hannon WH, Gunter EW, Spencer CA, Braverman LE.: Serum TSH, T(4), and thyroid antibodies in the United States population (1988 to 1994): National Health and Nutrition Examination Survey (NHANES III).// *J. Clinical Endocrinology Metabolism*, 2002, Vol. 87, pp. 489-499

[43] Ikeda F, Nishimura R, Matsubara T, Tanaka S, Inoue J, Reddy SV, Hata K, Yamashita K, Hiraga T, Watanabe T, Kukita T, Yoshioka K, Rao A, Yoneda T.: Critical roles of c-Jun signaling in regulation of NFAT family and RANKL-regulated osteoclast differentiation.// *J. Clinical Investigation*, 2004, Vol. 114, pp. 475-484

[44] Inoue M, Tawata M, Yokomori N, Endo T, Onaya T.: Expression of thyrotropin receptor on clonal osteoblast-like rat osteosarcoma cells.// *Thyroid*, 1998, Vol. 8, pp. 1059-1064

[45] Jamal SA, Leiter RE, Bayoumi AM, Bauer DC, Cummings SR.: Clinical utility of laboratory testing in women with osteoporosis. // *J. Osteoporosis International*, 2005, Vol. 16, pp. 534-540

[46] Kawaida R, et.al.: Jun dimerization protein 2 (JDP2), a member of the AP-1 family of transcription factor, mediates osteoclast differentiation induced by RANKL.// *J. Exp. Med.*, 2003, Vol. 197, pp. 1029-1035

[47] Kim DJ, Khang YH, Koh JM, Shong YK, Kim CS: Low normal TSH levels are associated with low bone mineral density in healthy postmenopausal women.// *J. Clinical Endocrinology (Oxford)*, 2006, Vol. 64, pp. 86-90

[48] Kim IS, Otto F, Zabel B, Mundlos S: Regulation of chondrocyte differentiation by Cbfa1.// *Mechanism of Development*, 1999, Vol.80, pp. 159-170

[49] Kumeda Y, Inaba M, Tahara H, Kurioka Y, Ishikawa T, Morii H, Nishizawa Y.: Persistent increase in bone turnover in Graves' patients with subclinical hyperthyroidism. // *J. Clinical Endocrinology and Metabolism*, 2000, Vol. 85, pp. 4157-4161

[50] Kung AW, Ng F.: A rat model of thyroid hormone-induced bone loss: effect of antiresorptive agents on regional bone density and osteocalcin gene expression. // *J. Thyroid*, 1994, Vol. 4, pp. 93-98

[51] Kung AWC, Yeung SSC.: Prevention of bone loss induced by thyroxine suppressive therapy in postmenopausal women: the effect of calcium and calcitonin. // *J. Clinical Endocrinology and Metabolism*, 1996, Vol. 81, pp. 1232-1236

[52] Lakatos P.: Thyroid hormones: beneficial or deleterious for bone?// *Calcif. Tissue Int*, 2003, Vol. 73, pp. 205-209

[53] Lauberg P, Pedersen KM, Vestergaard H, et al.: High incidence of multinodular toxic goiter in the elderly population in a low iodine intake area vs high incidence of Graves' disease in the young in a high iodine intake area: comparative surveys of thyrotoxicosis epidemiology in East-Jutland Denmark and Iceland.// *J. Internal Medicine*, 1991, Vol. 229, pp. 415-420

[54] Lee WY, Oh KW, Rhee EJ, Jung CH, Kim SW, Yun EJ, Tae HJ, Baek KH, Kang MI, Choi MG, Yoo HJ, Park SW.: Relationship between subclinical thyroid dysfunction and femoral neck bone mineral density in women.// *J. Archives of Medical Research*, 2006, Vol. 37, pp. 511-516

[55] Majima T, Komatsu Y, Doi K, Takagi C, Shigemoto M, Fukao A, Morimoto T, Corners J, Nakao K.: Negative correlation between bone mineral density and TSH receptor antibodies in male patients with untreated Graves' disease.// *J. Osteoporosis International*, 2006, Vol. 17, pp. 1103-1110

[56] Mazziotti G, Sorvillo F, Piscopo M, Cioffi M, Pilla P, Biondi B, Iorio S, Giustina A, Amato G, Carella C.: Recombinant human TSH modulates in vivo C-telopeptides of type-1 collagen and bone alkaline phosphatase, but not osteoprotegerin production in postmenopausal women monitored for differentiated thyroid carcinoma.// *J. Bone Mineral Research*, 2005, Vol. 20, pp. 480-486

[57] Milne M, Quail JM, Rosen CJ, Baran DT.: Insulin-like growth factor binding proteins in femoral and vertebral and vertebral bone marrow stromal cells: expression and regulation by thyroid hormone and dexamethasone.// *J. Cellular Biochemistry*, 2001, Vol. 81, pp. 229-240

[58] Miura M, Tanaka K, Komatsu Y, Suda M, Yasoda A, Sakuma Y, Ozasa A, Nakao K.: A novel interaction between thyroid hormones and 1,25(OH)2D3 in osteoclast formation.// *Biochem. Biophys. Res. Commun.*, 2002, Vol. 291, pp. 987-994

[59] Morimura T, Tsunekawa K, Kasahara T, Seki K, Ogiwara T, Mori M, Murakami M.: Expression of type 2 iodothyronine deiodinase in human osteoblast is stimulated by thyrotropin. // *J. Endocrinology*, 2005, Vol. 146 pp. 2077-2084

[60] Mosekilde L, Eriksen EF, Charles P.: Effects of thyroid hormones on bone and mineral metabolism. // *J. Endocrinology and Metabolism Clinical North America*, 1990, Vol. 19, pp. 35-63

[61] Mudde AH, Houben AJ, Nieuwenhuijzen KAC.: Bone metabolism during anti-thyroid drug treatment of endogenous subclinical hyperthyroidism. // *J. Clinical Endocrinology (Oxford)*, 1994, Vol. 41, pp. 421-424

[62] Murakami M, Hosoi Y, Negishi T, Kamiya Y, Miyashita K, Yamada M, Iriuchijima T, Yokoo H, Yoshida I, Tsushima Y, Mori M.: Thymic hyperplasia in patients with Graves disease. Identification of thyrotropin receptors in human thymus. // *J. Clinical Investigation*, 1996, Vol. 98, pp. 2228-2234

[63] Murphy E, Williams GR.: The thyroid and the skeleton // *J. Clinical Endocrinology*, 2004, Vol. 61, pp. 285-298

[64] O'Shea PJ, Harvey CB, Suzuki H, Kaneshige M, Kaneshige K, Cheng S-Y, Williams GR.: A thyrotoxic skeletal phenotype of advanced bone formation in mice with resistance to thyroid hormone.// *J. Molecular Endocrinology*, 2003, Vol. 17, pp. 1410-1424

[65] Oikawa M, Kushida K, Takahashi M, Ohishi T, Hoshino H, Suzuki M, Ogihara H, Ishigakit J, Inoue T.: Bone turnover and cortical bone mineral density in the distal radius in patients with hyperthyroidism being treated with antithyroid drugs for various periods of time. // *J. Clinical Endocrinology*, 1999, Vol. 50, pp. 171-176

[66] Papi G, Pearce EN, Braverman LE, Betterle C, Roti E.: A clinical and theraupeutic approach to thyrotoxicosis with thyroid-stimulating hormone suppression only.// *American J Medicine*, 2005, Vol. 118, pp. 349-361

[67] Parle JV, Franklyn JA, Cross KW, Jones SC, Shepard MC.: Prevalence and follow-up of abnormal thyrotropin (TSH) concentrations in the elderly in the United Kingdom.// *Clin Endocrinol (Oxf)*, 1991, Vol. 34, pp. 77-83

[68] Parle JV, Franklyn JA, Cross KW, Jones SR, Sheppard MC.: Thyroxine prescription in the community: serum thyroid stimulating hormone level assays as an indicator of undertreatment or overtreatment.// *Br J. Gen Pract*, 1993, Vol. 43, pp. 107-109

[69] Pearce EN, Braverman LE.: Subclinical hypertheroidism. // J. Thyroid International, 2001, Vol. 5, pp. 1-12; Ross DS.: Serum thyroid-stimulating hormone measurement for assessment of thyroid function and disease. // *J. Endocrinology Metabolism Clinics North America*, 2001, Vol. 30, pp. 245-264

[70] Pereira RC, Jorgetti V, Canalis E.: Triiodothyronine induces collagenase-3 and gelatinase B expression in murine osteoblasts.// *Am. J. Physiol*, 1999, Vol. 277, E496-E504

[71] Persani L, Preziati D, Matthews CH, Sartorio A, Chatterjee VK, Beck-Peccoz P.: Serum levels of carboxyterminal cross-linked telopeptide of type I collagen (ICTP) in the differential diagnosis of the syndromes of inappropriate secretion of TSH.// *J. Clinical Endocrinology (Oxford)*, 1997, Vol. 47, pp. 207-214

[72] Quan ML, Pasieka J, Rorstad O.: Bone mineral density in well-differentiated thyroid cancer patients treated with suppressive thyroxine: a systematic overview of the literature.// *J. Surgical Oncology*, 2002, Vol. 79, pp. 62-70

[73] Recklinghausen FD.: Die fibrose oder deformierende ositis, die osteomalazie und die osteoplastische carzinose in ihren gegenseitigen beziehungen.// *Festchrift Rudolf Virchow. George Reimer*, Berlin, 1891, p.1

[74] Riedel C, Levy O, Carrasco N.: Post-transcriptional regulation of the sodium/iodine symporter by thyrotropin.// *J. Biol. Chem.*, 2001, Vol. 276, pp. 21458-21463

[75] Robson H, Siebler T, Stevens DA, Shalet SM, Williams GR.: Thyroid hormone acts directly on growth plate chondrocytes to promote hypertrophic differentiation and inhibit clonal expansion and cell proliferation.// *J. Endocrinology*, 2000, Vol. 141, pp. 3887-3897

[76] Rosen HN, Moses AC, Garber J, Ross DS, Lee SL, Ferguson L, Chen V, Lee K, Greenspan SL.: Randomized trial of pamidronate in patients with thyroid cancer: bone density is not reduced by suppressive doses of thyroxine, but is increased by cyclic intravenous pamidronate. // *J. Clinical Endocrinology and Metabolism*, 1998, Vol. 83, pp. 2324-2330

[77] Ross DS, Daniels GH, Gouveia D.: The use and limitations of a chemiluminescent thyrotropin assay as a single thyroid function test in an outpatient endocrine clinic.// *J. Clin Endocrinol Metab*, 1990, Vol. 71, pp. 764-769

[78] Ross DS.: Hyperthyroidism, thyroid hormone therapy, and bone.// *Thyroid*, 1994, Vol. 4, pp. 319-326

[79] Rozhinskaya LY, Melnichenko GA, Belaya ZE, Kolesnikova GS, Ilyin AV, Sasonova NI.: The efficacy of Fosamax 35 mg a week for the treatment of osteoporosis in postmenopausal women with subclinical hyperthyroidism.// J. *Osteoporosis International*, 2008, Vol. 19, suppl. 1, s45-s46

[80] Salto C, Kindblom JM, Johansson C, Wang Z, Gullberg H, Nordström K, Mansén A, Ohlsson C, Thorén P, Forrest D, Vennström B.: Ablation of TRα2 and a concomitant over-expression of α1 yields a mixed hypo- and hyperthyroid phenotype in mice.// *J. Mol. Endocrinol.*, 2001, Vol. 15, pp. 2115-2128

[81] Sampath TK, Simic P, Sendak R, Draca N, Bowe AE, O'Brien S, Schiavi SC, McPherson JM and Vukicevic S.: Thyroid-stimulating hormone restores bone volume, microarchitecture, and strength in aged ovariectomised rats.// *J. Bone Mineral Research*, 2007, Vol. 22, pp. 849-859

[82] Schneider R, Reiners C.: The effect of Levothyroxine therapy on bone mineral density: a systematic review of the literature. // *J. Experimental Clinical Endocrinology and Diabetes*, 2003, Vol. 111, pp. 455-470

[83] Seeley DG, Kelsey J, Jergas M, Nevitt MC.: Predictors of ankle and foot fractures in older women. The study of Osteoporotic Fractures Research Group//*J. Bone and Mineral Research*, 1996, Vol.11, pp. 1347-1355

[84] Sellitti DF, Hill R, Doi SQ, Akamizu T, Czaja J, Tao S, Koshiyama H.: Differential expression of thyrotropin receptor mRNA in the porcine heart. // *J. Thyroid*, 1997, Vol. 7, pp. 641-646

[85] Shevde NK, Bendixen AC, Dienger KM, Pike JW..: Estrogens suppress RANK ligand-induced osteoclast differentiation via a stromal cell independent mechanism involving c-Jun repression.// *Proc. Natl. Acad. Sci. USA*, 2000, Vol. 97, pp. 7829-7834

[86] Siddiqi A, Burrin JM, Wood DF, Monson JP.: Tri-iodothyronine regulates the production of interleukin-6 and interleukin-8 in human bone marrow stromal and osteoblat-like cells.// *J. Endocrinology*, 1998, Vol. 157, pp. 453-461

[87] Simsek G, Karter Y, Aydin S, Uzun H..: Osteoporotic cytokines and bone metabolism on rats with induced hyperthyroidism; changes as a result of reversal to euthyroidism.// *Chinese. J. Physiology*, 2003, Vol. 46, pp. 181-186

[88] Spitzweg C, Joba W, Heufelder AE.: Expression of thyroid-related genes in human thymus. // *J. Thyroid*, 1999, Vol. 9, pp. 133-141

[89] Srivastava S, Toraldo G, Weitzmann M N, Cenci S, Ross FP, Pacifici R: Estrogen decreases osteoclast formation by downregulating receptor activator of NF-kappa B ligand (RANKL)-induced JNK activation.// *J. Biol Chem.*, 2001, Vol. 276, pp. 8836-8840

[90] Stevens DA, Harvey CB, Scott AJ, O'Shea PJ, Barnard JC, Williams AJ, Brady G, Samarut J, Chassande O, Williams GR.: Thyroid hormone activates fibroblast growth factor receptor-1 in bone.// *Mol. Endocrinology*, 2003, Vol. 17, pp. 1751-1756

[91] Stevens DA, Hasserjian RP, Robson H, Siebler T, Shalet SM, Williams GR.: Thyroid hormones regulate hypertrophic chondrocyte differentiation and expression of parathyroid hormone-related peptide and its receptor during endochondral bone formation.// *J. Bone Mineral Research*, 2000, Vol.15, pp. 2431-2442

[92] Sun L, Davies TF, Blair HC, Abe E, Zaidi M.: TSH and bone loss.// *Annals New York Academy of Science*, 2006, Vol. 1068, pp. 309-318

[93] Surks MI, Ortiz E, Daniels GH, Sawin CT, Col NF, Cobin RH, Franklin JA, Hershman JM, Burman KD, Denke MA, Gorman C, Cooper RS, Weissman NJ.: Subclinical thyroid disease. Scientific review and guidelines for diagnosis and management. // *J. American Medical Association*, 2004, Vol. 291, pp. 228-238

[94] Suzuki J, Otsuka F, Takeda M, Inagaki K, Miyoshi T, Mimura Y, Ogura T, Doihara H, Makino H.: Functional roles of the bone morphogenetic protein system in thyrotropin signaling in porcine thyroid cells. // *J. Biochemical and Biophysical Research Communications*, 2005, Vol. 327, pp. 1124-1130

[95] Tauchmanova L, Nuzzo V, Puente AD, Fonderico F, Puente AE, Padulla S, Rossi A, Bifulco G, Lupoli G, Lombardi G.: Reduced bone mass detected by bone quantitative ultrasonometry and DEXA in pre- and postmenopausal women with endogenous subclinical hyperthyroidism. // *J. Maturitas*, 2004, Vol. 48, pp. 299-306

[96] Tsai JA, Janson A, Bucht E, Kindmark H, Marcus C, Stark A, Rawet Zemack H, Torring O.: Weak evidence of thyrotropin receptors in primary cultures of human osteoblast-like cells. // *J. Calcified Tissue International*, 2004, Vol. 74, pp. 486-491

[97] Uzzan B, Campos J, Cucherat M, Nony P, Boissel JP, Perret GY.: Effects on bone mass of long term treatment with thyroid hormones: a meta-analysis. // *J. Clinical Endocrinology and Metabolism*, 1996, Vol. 81, pp. 4278-4289

[98] Vestegaard P, Mosekilde L.: Hyperthyroidism, bone mineral and fracture risk – a meta-analysis. // *J. Thyroid*, 2003, Vol. 13, pp. 585-593

[99] Vestergaard P, Mosekilde L.: Fractures in patients with hyperthyroidism and hypothyroidism: a nationwide follow-up study in 16249 patients. // *J. Thyroid*, 2002, Vol. 12, pp. 411-419

[100] Vestergaard P, Rejnmark L, Mosekilde L.: Influence of hyper- and hypothyrodism, and the effects of treatment with antithyroid drugs and levothyroxine on fracture risk.// *J. Calcif. Tissue International*, 2005, Vol. 77, pp. 139-144

[101] Vestergaard P, Rejnmark L, Weeke J, Mosekilde L.: Fracture risk in patients treated for hyperthyroidism. // *J. Thyroid*, 2000, Vol. 10, pp. 341-348

[102] Wakasugi M, Wakao R, Tawata M, Can N, Koizumi K, Onaya T.: Bone mineral density in patients with hyperthyroidism measured by dual energy X-ray absorptiometry. // *J. Clinical Endocrinology (Oxford)*, 1994, Vol. 38, pp. 283-286

[103] Wexler JA, Sharrets J.: Thyroid and bone.// *Endocrinol Metab Clin N Am*, 2007, Vol. 36, pp. 673-705

[104] Williams GR, Bland R, Sheppard MC.: Characterization of thyroid hormone (T3) receptors in three osteosarcoma cell lines of distinct osteoblast phenotype: interactions among T3, vitamin D3 and retinoid signaling.// *Endocrinology*, 1994, Vol. 135, pp. 2375-2385

[105] Wilson B, Raghupathy E, Tonoue T, Tong W.: TSH-like actions of dibutyryl-cAMP on isolated bovine thyroid cells.// *Endocrinology*, 1968, Vol. 83, pp. 877-884

In: Osteoporosis: Etiology, Diagnosis and Treatment
Editors: Bilar E. Mattingly and Albert C. Pillare
ISBN 978-1-60692-397-9

Chapter 17

NEW PERSPECTIVES IN OSTEOPOROSIS DIAGNOSIS: THE ROLE OF MRI IMAGING

E. Fanucci, N. Fusco, T. Volpi, E. Gaspari and G. Simonetti
University of Rome "Tor Vergata", Rome, Italy.

ABSTRACT

Osteoporosis is the most frequent metabolic bone disorder. Defined as a reduction of bone tissue compared to the anatomic volume of the bone with a preserved ratio between the mineral content and the organic matrix, this pathology leads to an enhanced bone fragility and a consequent increased susceptibility to spontaneous fractures even in the case of low energy traumas; the most frequent sites of these fractures are skeletal portions with a high trabecular content such as the spine, hip and wrist.

Up till now, the quantitative evaluation of osteoporosis and the assessment of fracture risk have been essentially based on the measurement of bone mineral density (BMD) that can be obtained with radiological techniques such as Dual X-Ray Absorpiometry (DEXA) and Quantitative Computed Tomography (QCT). The main limit of this kind of evaluation is that it exclusively considers the amount of mineral content without assessing the structure of the bone. The structure of the trabecular bone is in fact an important parameter to determine bone strength. For this reason the use of Magnetic Resonance imaging has been proposed since, by means of different techniques, it provides important morfological and structural information on the bone as well as on the presence and evolution of contingent fractures.

Besides 3 Tesla high field MR, which is a direct imaging method of the bone structure that can provide a quantitative evaluation, the trabecular bone network may be assessed with Diffusion Tensor Imaging (DTI) and spectroscopic analysis. These techniques identify early changes in the microarchitecture of cancellate bone before such phenomenon can be detected with DEXA.

It has been demonstrated that an increased marrow fat content with a decreased unsaturated lipidic component and a reduced Apparent Diffusion Coefficient (ADC) correlate to a reduction of trabecular bone, typical of this disease. The aforementioned MR techniques, by evaluating these biological characteristics through which important structural information is provided, may therefore be useful not only in fracture risk assessment, but in pre- and post- operative diagnostics for joint prosthesis placement as well. In pre-collapse osteoporotic vertebrae there is a narrowing and a rarefaction of the bone trabeculae, with a growth of inter-trabeculary spaces that are then filled by fat and liquids. Anisotropy calculation and colorimetric vectorial evaluation provide a new intuitive non-invasive instrument for the evaluation of osteoporotic levels to be treated with vertebroplasty before any difference is grossly assessable with conventional imaging.

1. Introduction

Bone mineral density (BMD) is perhaps the best index available for assessing the risk of osteoporotic fracture. Lindsay et al. reported that each reduction of one standard deviation of BMD corresponds to a 60% increase in the risk of vertebral fractures [1]. Dual X-ray absorptiometry (DXA) measures areal bone density and does not capture all factors contributing to bone strength. In addition to bone mass, density, and content, the trabecular and cortical bone architecture, mineralization, micro-fracture, and damage repair also contribute to bone strength. Site-specific bone structure information would significantly contribute to further understanding the determinants of fracture risk, and influence optimization of therapy. Considerable effort is being expended in developing techniques to assess trabecular bone micro-architecture non-invasively.

Many studies have shown that changes in bone quality and structure independent of BMD influence both bone strength and propensity to fracture. Furthermore, bone strength has been shown to depend not only on bone mineral density (BMD) but also marrow quality [2]. Both of these factors have implications in osteoporosis, although it is still unclear why some people are susceptible to osteoporosis and what role the marrow plays.

The influence of these other factors may partially explain the observed overlap in bone mineral measurements between patients with and patients without osteoporotic fractures. Thus, several emerging techniques have been aimed at quantifying trabecular bone structure in addition to BMD. Magnetic resonance (MR) imaging is a non-ionizing modality that utilizes a strong magnetic field and a sequence of radiofrequency pulses to produce three-dimensional images. The interactions between protons, gradient fields, and radiofrequency pulses allow an image to be created based on spatial frequency encoding. Hydrogen, present in musculoskeletal tissue water, is the most frequently studied component in biological MR imaging. Bone tissue has very low water content. Additionally, protons within bone tissue matrix have very short T2 relaxation time, a MR measure reflecting the chemical environment of the protons. As a result, bone gives no signal in standard MR. Osteoporotic fractures after minor trauma occur in the distal radius, proximal femur, humeral neck and spine. Radiological diagnosis by plain radiographs is usually straight forward. Hip fractures may be occult on plain radiographs and, by applying a single T1-w pulse sequence, MR imaging is helpful. Quite often in the elderly patients, osteoporotic and pathologic fractures secondary to malignant infiltration may coexist. MR imaging has been accurate in the correct differential diagnosis either by using morphologic criteria such as the "fluid" sign or by applying diffusion weighted imaging [2,3]. MR imaging is also capable of demonstrating the age of a vertebral fracture by depicting bonemarrow edema which is present in the acute and subacute phase. In osteoporosis the diagnostic goal is not to identify a present fracture, but trying to prevent the future fractures; this challenge ask for new imaging modalities. Over the two last decades, clinical and experimental studies have shown that magnetic resonance (MR) has the potential to be a useful tool for the assessment of skeletal status by means of measurements addressed for the study of trabecular bone. The techniques can be summarized in four categories namely: high resolution MR imaging (HR-MRI), MR relaxometry, in vivo MR spectroscopy, diffusion MR imaging and perfusion MR imaging.

A number of studies have been performed that applied magnetic resonance imaging (MRI) to the study of trabecular bone and bone quality. Bone quality is dependent on macroarchitecture, microarchitecture, modelling and remodelling (i.e. bone turnover), microfracture accumulation, mineralization and matrix. Currently, MRI can be used to examine two of these parameters, i.e. macroarchitecture and microarchitecture [5].

Macroarchitectural features refer to bone geometry; for instance, in the proximal femur they refer to hip axis length, femoral neck cross sectional area, femoral neck width and femoral neck shaft angle. These parameters could be measured by oblique coronal and sagittal magnetic resonance (MR) imaging. Although bone geometry is more frequently evaluated by dual-energy absorpiometry (DXA), computed tomography (CT) or radiogrammetry.

Magnetic resonance imaging, in addition to assessing bone macroarchitecture and microarchitecture as described above, can investigate three other aspects of bone physiology not measurable by other techniques, namely MR spectroscopy, perfusion and diffusion [5-11]. Magnetic resonance spectroscopy allows one to measure the relative ratio of fat vs water in bone marrow. Magnetic resonance perfusion provides a measure of perfusion indices in bone marrow and it is an indirect measure of blood flow in bone marrow. Marrow diffusion allows one to measure the rate of diffusion of water molecules within bone marrow.

2. High Resolution MRI

High-resolution MR imaging (HR-MRI) is referred to as a direct two-dimensional or three-dimensional imaging method of trabecular bone network, i.e. the microarchitecture [12-14]. Trabecula measure from 100 to 400 mm in width. Any imaging technique must have a resolution of 100 mm or less to be able to accurately resolve individual trabeculae. This resolution can now be achieved with high-field strength (1.5 or more), high-gradient (30mTlm or more) clinical MR units or micro-MRI units [15,16]. With the advent of 3 T MRI imaging of trabecular bone is getting more feasible. The higher field strength increases signal-to-noise-ratios two-fold compared to standard 1.5-T MRI, thus imaging time may be reduced and/or spatial resolution may be increased for high resolution imaging of trabecular bone.

In high-resolution T2-weighted MR images, bone tissue appears black while marrow — by virtue of containing sufficient amounts of water and fat — produces a high intensity signal within the trabecular spaces (Figure 1) Clinical MRI units using high-resolution gradient-echo sequences can achieve an isotropic resolution of 150μm. The advantage of gradient echo sequences is a faster acquisition time but more artifacts, while spin-echo sequences require longer acquisition time and have lower signal-to-noise-ratio yet less artifacts [17,18].

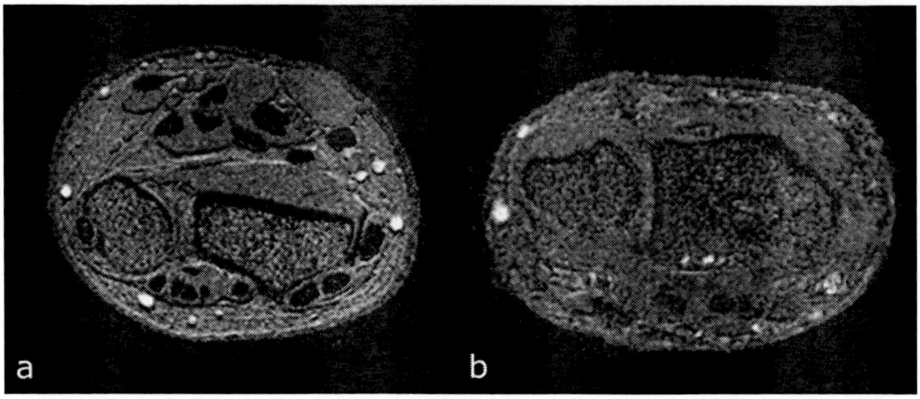

Figure 1. Axial image (obtained at 3 T, using a Philips scanner) of the distal radio at a resolution of 200×200×200 μm. Trabecular bone is depicted as dark striations amidst bright bone marrow. Images such as these may be quantified to characterize the complex trabecular bone network (a) Healthy volunteer and (b) trabecular bone structure of a patient with an osteoporotic fracture of the radio. The marrow spaces between the trabeculae, the number of the trabeculae and their thickness appear disomogeneus and wider in the image of the fracture.

To acquire this high resolution, a small local coil yielding a small field of view needs to be used; therefore, MRI is used currently to study the trabecular pattern in peripheral bones such as the radius and calcaneum. [19,20] Krug et al. reported the use of high-field MR imaging (3T) in the study of the proximal femur with excellent results. [21] Phan et al. concluded that MR imaging at 3T provided a better measure of trabecular bone structure than did MR imaging at 1.5 T [16]. However, in addition to a better depiction of the bone structure it should also be noted that trabeculae appear more amplified at 3 T, meaning that trabeculae are 2-fold thicker at 3T while they are only 1.6-fold thicker at 1.5 T as compared to the dimensions obtained with MicroCT. This amplification is due to increased susceptibility effects at the higher field strength.

At resolutions to the order of the trabecular dimension, partial volume effects arise, due to voxels consisting partially of bone and bone marrow spins. Therefore, MR-derived structural measures are similar but not identical to true histological dimensions [22,23]. Additionally, the susceptibility difference between bone and fatty marrow is approximately 3 ppm and thus leads to off-resonance effects, resulting in a signal attenuation near the transitions between bone and bone marrow [24]. These differences have to be taken into account and the MR pulse sequence best suited for trabecular bone imaging is still a topic of ongoing research since they differ in their ability to depict the trabecular network accurately [25,26]. However, the trabecular parameters can still be reproducibly measured and correlate well with μCT data [27]. This is because the trabecular spacing (~800–1,000 μm) is usually much larger than the size of the image voxel.

The first 7-T whole body MR scanners are now also available and researchers are starting to explore the potential of these machines. Future research will be dedicated to pushing the limits of trabecular bone imaging using this equipment. Trabecular structural measures analysed on MRI examination have been shown to be better than bone mineral density in differentiating patients with and without osteoporotic fractures in transplant patients [19].

A disadvantage of HR-MRI in vivo are relatively long acquisition times of up to 6–15 min. In addition, fast gradients are required together with dedicated coils with a small field of view and a high signal-to noise ratio (SNR). These conditions limit the clinical use of HR-MRI. Structure analysis of high resolution MR images can give additional information to BMD in differentiating patients with and without osteoporotic fractures [17,18,20]. HR-MR images may be used to characterize fracture incidence in patients with renal failure and renal transplantation; and the structural implications of metabolic bone disease, potentially providing a noninvasive tool for the evaluation of therapies for renal osteodystrophy. Quantitative estimations can be directly applied to a HR-MRI image; following image acquisition several computerized image processing steps are undertaken. These may include region-of-interest extraction, registration with baseline images for longitudinal studies, segmentation of the image in to trabecular bone and marrow and ultimately quantification of the trabecular bone structure. Several parameters have evolved over the last 10 years for characterizing trabecular bone. Measures such as apparent Bone Volume Fraction (app BV/TV), trabecular Number (App TbN), trabecular spacing (TbSp) are synonymous to histomorphometric measures.

An inherent problem assigned to this method is the comparable size of the bone trabeculae (70–200 μm) with the best reported spatial resolution (80 μm) of the HR-MRI technique [14]. Due to this fact, partial volume effects significantly affect MR image segmentation and therefore quantitative estimations.

Studies have shown that MR-derived trabecular bone structure measures correlate with age, menopausal status (in women), osteoporotic or fracture status, show moderate to poor correlation with DXA-derived bone mineral density, and when combined with DXA measures provide improved discrimination between individuals with and without fractures [28-32]. Imaging trabecular bone micro-architecture holds considerable promise for characterizing the features of trabecular bone for monitoring osteoporosis, and assessing fracture risk and post-therapeutic response. Trabecular bone comprises 20% of the skeleton, but is highly responsive to metabolic stimuli; thus, the assessment of trabecular bone alone, rather than a composite of trabecular and cortical bone as in DXA, is important

3. MR- Relaxometry

Magnetic resonance relaxometry is another MR-based method whereby trabecular structure can be indirectly assessed from studying the relaxation time T2* of the bone marrow [15]. This method uses standard MRI techniques and can be used in the wrist, calcaneus, spine, and femur. The technical principles of this technique may be explained by differences in magnetic susceptibility at the interface of bone trabeculae and marrow, which result in spatial inhomogeneities in the magnetic field. These inhomogeneities result in dephasing of the transverse magnetization, which leads to a decrease in the marrow T2* values. The decrease in T2* and its decay characteristics provide information about the density and structure of the surrounding trabecular network. Since spatial resolution is not a prerequisite for this technique, it can be performed on clinical MR unit and more quickly than high-resolution MRI.

Several studies showed that T2* increases with age [33,34,35]. In the proximal femur Link et al. (1998b) showed that correlations between T2* and age were stronger than correlations between BMD and age. These finding are supported by results in the distal radius; T2* compared to BMD determined by dual-energy X-ray absorptiometry (DXA) and peripheral quantitative CT was the most sensitive parameter by which to predict age related changes in this study [35]. While the authors did not find significant differences in the distal radius between T2* in healthy subjects and that in osteoporotic postmenopausal patients with spine fractures, the results of Link et al. showed that healthy subjects and osteoporotic postmenopausal patients with hip fractures could be distinguished using T2* measurements of the proximal femur However it is not clear whether the T2* characteristics provide additional informations to that supplied by BMD in the prediction of fracture risk and so future applications of this technique to clinical practice appears unlikely.

4. Proton (1H) MR Spectroscopy

In vivo 1H MR spectroscopy is a non-invasive technique suitable for the study of metabolic changes in disease processes; as applied to osteoporosis reflects measurable changes in the direct content of water and lipid molecules within bone tissues. Lipid and water are, for different aspects, both of great importance in determining the bone quality. There is substantial evidence that osteoporotic and "normal" bone, for example, differ significantly in their chemical make-up [36]. Next to osteoid and mineral, water occupies the largest volume fraction in bone. Bone water occurs at various locations and in different binding states. It is associated with the mineral phase, bound to the organic phase (collagen and cement substance), and a large fraction occurs in more or less free form (bulk water). The most tightly bound water is the one occupying the calcium ion coordination sites in the apatite-like crystals (about 35 mg of water/g mineral) [37]. A significant, less tightly bound fraction, is water associated with collagen fibrils. In the unmineralized state as the bone matrix is laid down by obsteoblasts, the collagen fibers produced contain a large volume fraction of water (up to 60%). During calcification, however, apatite crystals are deposited in the organic matrix, gradually displacing the osteoid water and reducing it down to a 20% volume fraction. Eventually, this fraction drops to 10% in senile bone suggesting the reduced impact strength in old age. It is thus plausible that the volume occupied by mineral cannot vary in a manner independent of that of collagen-bound water since the total volume has to be preserved. Any change in the mineral fraction will result in a compensatory change in the water fraction. Thus, a measurement of the water fraction can provide information— albeit in an inferential manner—on mineralization density [37,38,39]. Lipid are contained in marrow; Hematopoietically active red marrow is composed of two components: cells with myeloid, erythroid, and lymphoid elements produce a water signal, and fat cells are the origin of a lipid signal. The relative proportion of fat cells in red marrow is low at birth and increases with age. There is a well-established age-related conversion of red to yellow bone marrow, a process that occurs first in peripheral and later in the axial skeleton [40]. At any age a sustained increase in demand can lead to the reappearance of hematopoiesis in the extremities. Clearly, a complete characterization of all normal patterns and distributions of marrow is essential before pathologic conditions can be identified. Thus, as a unique feature, in adults red marrow yields signals from water and fat of about the same intensity.

Red and yellow marrow is readily distinguishable and marrow composition may be qualitatively assessed from signal intensity variations on MRI. Previous work has demonstrated the age-related conversion in cranium, femur, vertebral bodies, epiphyses, and pelvis. In particular, Ricci et al. described three distinct signal intensity patterns in the lumbar spine that changed with age [41-45].

The idea of gender differences in marrow content is less well established. Although Schellinger et al. and Kugel et al. demonstrated an increase in fat content in men using MRS, these results remain at odds with the many more imaging studies that have not observed any variation [6,43,46,47,48].

Spectroscopy allows a separate analysis of water and fat signals; thus, in addition to assessment of relative quantities, determinations of line widths and relaxation times become possible. Previous studies have shown that diseases of the hematopoietic system are indicated in the spectrum as an increased ratio of the water resonance to the fat signal, due to the displacement of fat by tumor cells and reactive stimulation. Investigations have been performed at 1.5 T in the iliac and vertebral bone marrow with stimulated echo acquisition mode (STEAM) and point-resolved spectroscopy (PRESS) sequences [49,50,51,52,53,54,55].

Quantitative histological studies performed on bone biopsies with regard to the changes in bone with age have shown the progressive, gradual and constant increase in the content of fats in bone marrow, with greater evidence found in osteoporotic subjects [56,57]. Bone marrow is known to consist primarily of saturated, monounsaturated and polyunsaturated fatty acids, but it is unknown if (and how) that composition varies in osteoporosis [58]. A very recent study carried out by Yeung et al. with a 1.5-T MR scanner compared the results of spectroscopy performed at the level of L3 on a population of postmenopausal osteoporotic women, with the spectrum obtained from a phantom of maize oil [9]. The findings demonstrated that the content of unsaturated fatty acids in bone marrow, calculated as a portion of the total FF, was clearly lower in osteoporotic subjects than in healthy subjects of the same age and gender, whereas the level of saturated fats was higher in the first group. The data obtained in several spectroscopic studies enable improved separation of the various molecular components of the spectrum and increased accuracy of assessing the individual fat peaks [9,11]. In a study performed using very high magnetic fields (3Tesla) water peak in healthy subjects was significantly higher than the fat peak, with an inverse progression as patient age increased and T-score decreased (inversion of the water/fat ratio). The spectral resolution of the sequence also revealed a notably higher increase in saturated fatty acids (especially methylene: 1.3 ppm) than unsaturated fatty acids (olefinic protons: 5.25 ppm) in osteoporotic patients compared with healthy patients (Figure 2) [59]. Healthy subjects in the premenopausal age range also had a mean fat content in the bone marrow significantly lower than healthy subjects older than 50 years ($p<0.001$). No statistically significant differences were found between osteoporotic patients without vertebral fractures and patients with vertebral fractures ($p<0.827$) A highly significant difference, however, was found between the FF value in healthy patients and osteoporotic patients ($p<0.001$), with a significant increase in FF in the latter group. Postmenopausal patients with a T score ≤ -2.5 reveal a consistent increase in FF when compared with healthy postmenopausal subjects Fat fraction values, however, were not significantly different from those of patients with a normal T score of the same gender and age [11]. Spectroscopic analysis of vertebral bodies with a clearly hyperintense signal in the T2-weighted sequences in osteoporotic patients, however, revealed an apparently retained water/fat ratio. This finding is likely due to the presence of bone marrow oedema within the vertebral body under study. The relationship between the fraction of bone marrow fats and bone weakening can be explained by a variety of factors. Firstly, trabecular thinning, which causes an increase in the intertrabecular spaces, is often given as the main cause of bone weakening in osteoporosis. A number of authors have suggested the presence of a compensatory mechanism that fills those spaces with yellow marrow [56,60,61]. In particular, Dunnill et al. suggested that with increasing age, the increase in bone marrow fats is even more marked than the reduction in red marrow, probably because the yellow marrow tends not only to replace the loss of bone but also the loss of red marrow [56]. A greater quantity of fat cells is therefore required to replace the loss of cancellous bone and the spaces formerly occupied by red marrow. Secondly, increased adipogenesis competes with osteogenesis, thus reducing the population of osteoblasts. Indeed, there is a reciprocal relationship between fat cells and osteoblasts, with the result of a loss of bone mass. This theory has found support in animal studies [62]. Thirdly, bone marrow fats can directly influence the quality of bone trabeculae. In fact, it is thought that the quality of bone marrow quality itself is an important determinant of mechanical vertebral strength and increased bone marrow fat negatively may affect the biomechanical strength of bone plays. Bone marrow that fills the intratrabecular spaces functions as a shock absorber and acts as a biomechanical support structure for the cancellous bone. Yellow marrow, due to its high fat content, is a weaker means of biomechanical support than is red marrow [63]. Red marrow contributes to hydrostatic strengthening, and fatty marrow causes greater compressibility of vertebrae. The combination of hematopoietic marrow (red), collagen, and hydroxyapatite forms a comparatively tough material.

The increase in marrow fat in osteoporotic and osteopenic subjects, as compared to normal subjects, was also observed in a study published by Griffith et al. [5] Yeung et al. reported that osteoporosis is associated with increased marrow fat content and decreased marrow fat unsaturation [9]. These Authors concluded that the increase in marrow fat seen in either osteoporotic or osteopenic subjects appears to be the result of a preferential increase in saturated lipids as compared to unsaturated lipids of fatty marrow.

Although best performances in MR spectroscopy can be achieved using very high field strength, today, 1H MR spectroscopy allows noninvasive quantitative bone marrow fat evaluation on all standard clinical MRI units with no magnet strength restrictions. The advantages of higher magnetic field are an increase in both signal-to-noise ratio and chemical shift dispersion. The former may be translated into improved spatial resolution, which is crucial in the examination of small vertebral bodies and those that are anatomically more difficult to prescribe (e.g., L5), or reduced scan times, enabling the examination of multiple

VBs. An increase in chemical shift dispersion is of benefit as it increases the separation of metabolite peaks and improves the potential for assessing the role of other fat resonances.

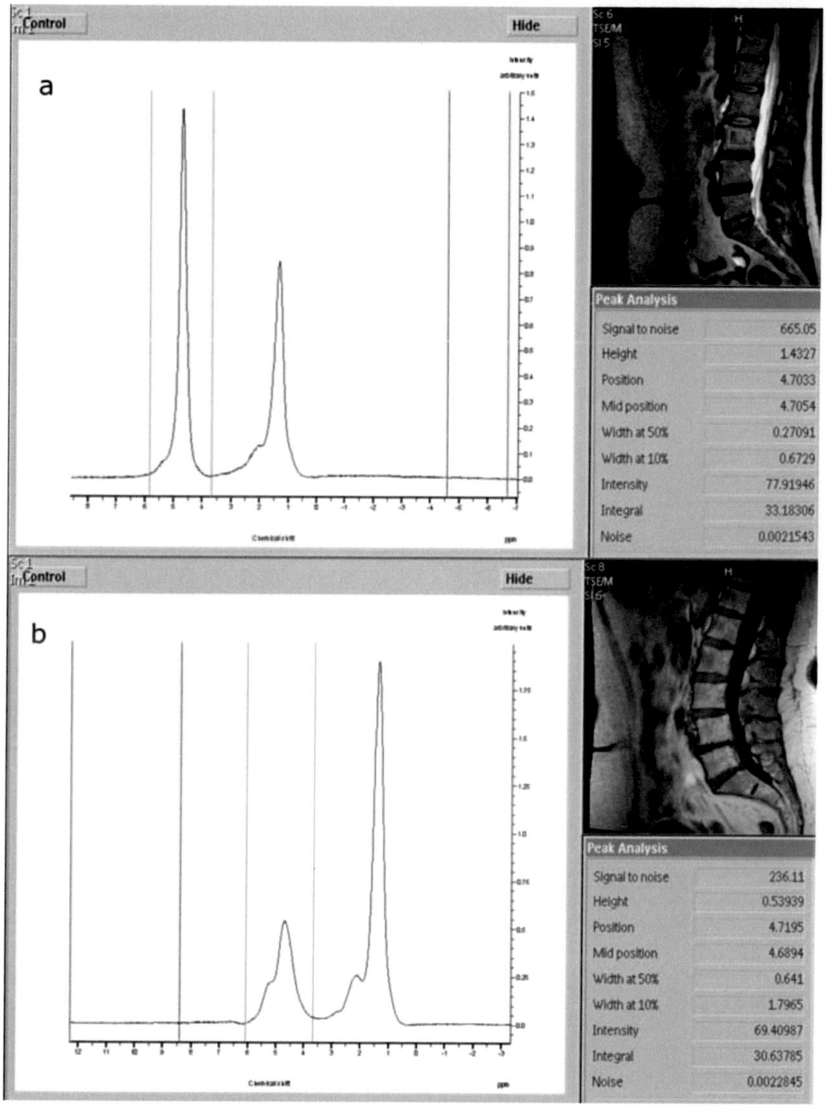

Figure 2. Spectroscopic analysis showing (a) a normal water/lipids ratio (FF 40.5%) in a healthy 39 year old woman and (b) an inverted water/lipids ratio (FF 72.5%) in a 79 year old osteoporotic woman.

Multiple vertebrae spectra can be acquired within a few minutes. Proton MR spectroscopy easily can be added to routine lumbar MRI with little time penalty. Patients undergoing diagnostic MRI evaluation of the spine can be screened simultaneously for bone marrow fat. The entire skeleton is accessible, and no ionizing radiation is involved. In a recent research Schellinger proposed a a new measuring unit of bone weakness: this interesting diagnostic opportunity that combines the diagnostic potential of bone marrow fat and that of BMD in a single expression: the bone marrow fat/BMD ratio. This ratio proved to be a valid indicator of bone weakening ($p = 0.02$), showing significant diagnostic value even at a small sample size [64]. As for the vertebrae, a correlation between fat fraction and bone mineral density have been found in the femoral neck (Fanucci et al. unpublished data) (Figure 3). Proximal femur fracture are more strongly associated with decreased BMD and cause more disability than any other type of osteoporotic fracture. Joining morphological and spectroscopic study is another diagnostic goal of MR imaging in osteoporosis.

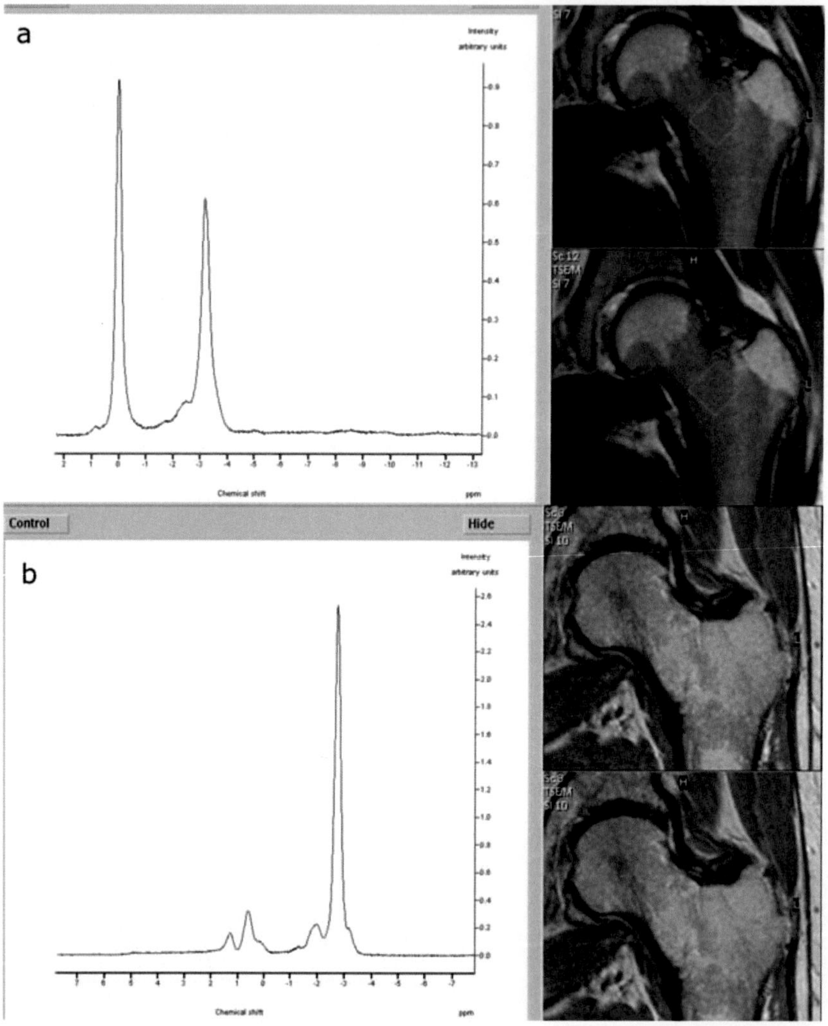

Figure 3. Spectroscopic analysis showing (a) a normal water/lipids ratio in a healthy 37 year old woman and (b) an inverted water/lipids ratio in a 76 year old osteoporotic woman (T-score $\geq$ -2.5).

5. MR Diffusion-Weighted Imaging

Diffusion-weighted imaging (DWI) is a technique that is sensitive to the mobility or diffusion of water in biological tissues; when applied to osteoporosis, measuring the random motion of Water molecules within the marrow may indirectly assess changes in the cellular composition of bone marrow .

To quantitate the effect of diffusion, strong external gradient fields have to be applied. The presence of strong magnetic field gradients helps in differentiating pure random motion from the combined T2 shortening effect observed in moving nuclei. MR voxel signal loss in the presence of such gradients is due to the combined effects of water diffusion within intra-cellular and extra-cellular spaces and perfusion associated with blood flowing within capillaries.

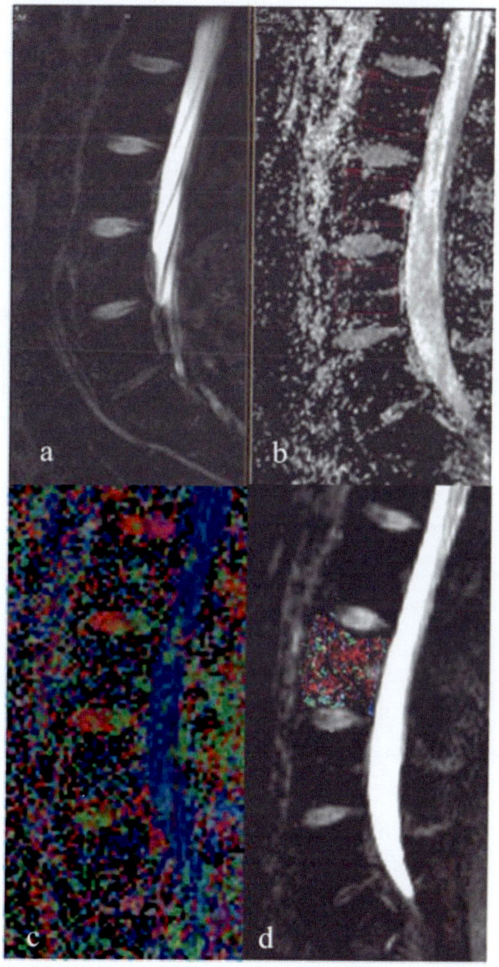

Figure 4. Images of a healthy 39 year old volunteer: a) a diffusion-weighted image; b) a grey-scale map of MD (Mean Diffusivity), which expressed as a value of ADC (apparent diffusion coefficient); c) Colorimetric map: anisotropy was also visualised by the generation of a 24-bit RGB colour map, which depicted the relative size of each vector value; d) Tractographic map which describes the directions of water molecules diffusion.

Images obtained with a DWI sequence were can generate 4 maps (Figure 4):

- A grey-scale map of MD (Mean Diffusivity), which expressed as a value of ADC (apparent diffusion coefficient)

- A grey-scale map of FA (Fractional Anisotropy) which is a parameter that describes the degree of variation of diffusion in space
- A Colour map : where anisotropy is visualised by the generation of a 24-bit RGB colour map, which depicted the relative size of each vector value
- A Tractographic map: which describes the directions of water molecules diffusion.

Results of diffusion measurements, expressed as apparent diffusion coefficient (ADC) values, serve as an indirect index for measuring the true random motion of water molecules within tissues. Initially applied in differentiating between benign and pathologic compression fractures, the method has been used by Yeung et al. to correlate ADC with osteoporosis; they found that ADC values were significantly reduced in post-menopausal osteoporotic subjects as compared to premenopausal normal control subjects [65,66]. This reduction of the ADC is due to the increased fat packing of bone marrow taking place in the dilated inter-trabecular space as a consequence of osteoporosis. A significant reduction of extracellular diffusion has been demonstrated in osteoporosis [11,67]. The decrease in the ADC and diffusion signal-intensity values might be explained by the reduction of extracellular diffusion as a result of increase in the fatty marrow [10,72]. The empty spaces are filled with fatty bone marrow after the architectural deterioration secondary to bone attenuation loss in osteoporosis. Nonomura et al. further indicated that there was a positive correlation between ADC values and the cellularity of bone marrow [68]. One possible explanation of this phenomenon is the perfusion effect. More blood supply and microcirculation are likely when active hemapoietic cells are abundant in the marrow. Therefore, hematopoietically active marrow (cellular marrow) has more intracellular water and adjacent free water than less-active marrow. The conversion of hematopoietic to fatty marrow is known to correlate with a physiologic decrease in intramedullary blood flow [69]. The Diffusion Tensor Imaging (DTI) is another attractive prospective in the study on bone marrow. By means of suitable MR sequences it is possible to measure an apparent diffusion coefficient value (ADC); this coefficient is not a true measure of the intrinsic diffusion because it depends on the diffusing time during which the molecular motion is observed and it depends on the interaction of diffusing molecules with the various type of obstacles and constraints to their free motion [70]. Because diffusion is a three dimensional process, a diffusion tensor is needed to describe the mobility of Brownian particles along the different directions. Estimating diffusion tensor imaging from MR images enables us to create parametric images where pixel intensity is proportional either to mean diffusivity (MD map) or to the degree of anisotropy (fractional anisotropy map) of the sample. The set of MRI techniques that allow to determine the elements of such a tensor and to display the informations contained in each voxel, is known as diffusion tensor imaging [11]. During the last decade DTI methods have been used to investigate cerebral morphology and white matter diseases; because of the trabecular bone emphasizes all the peculiar features of porous media, DTI allow to obtain bone network structural informations in normal and pathological issues. Fanucci et al. evidenced in normal bone marrow of a lumbar vertebra the absence of a preferential pathway of diffusion, visually shown by the lack of a dominant colour, while in the collapsed vertebral body and the underlying vertebra, a preferential craniocaudal diffusion direction visually demonstrated by the presence of blue-coloured fibres was shown (Figure 5) [11]. This findings correlate with values of ADC and FA and it means the presence of an intermediate anisotrophy. Authors supposed that the preferential craniocaudal directions could be explained by the reduction in vertical axis of bone trabeculae, as it happens in osteoporosis. DTI is a very promising tool in the study of bone architecture and in the assessment of the geometrical organization of anisotropic systems.

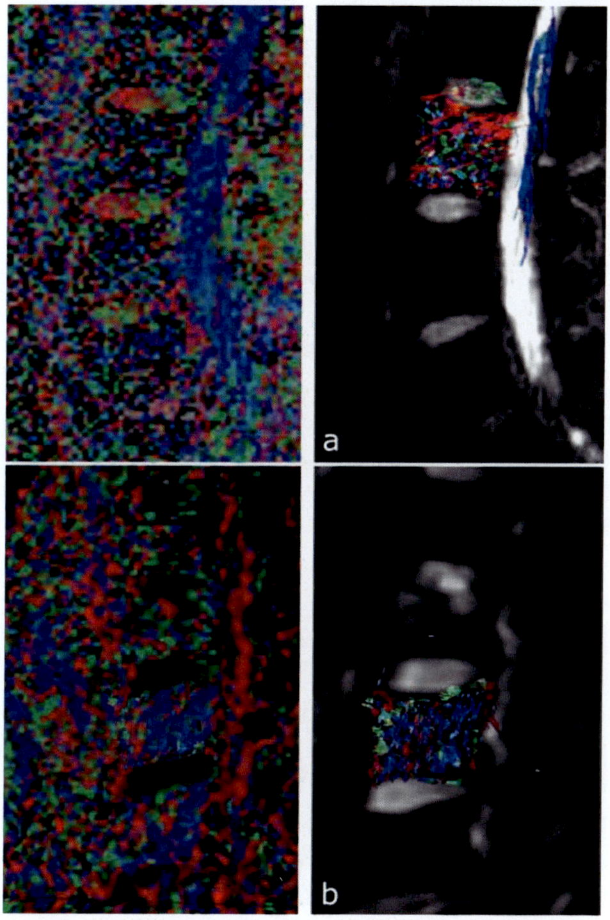

Figure 5. Diffusion Tensor Image showing (a) a healthy vertebra presenting a reduced diffusivity, absence of a preferential diffusion direction and absence of a dominant color and (b) an osteoporotic vertebra evidenced by the prevalence of the blue color and a preferential cranio-caudal diffusion direction

6. MR Perfusion Imaging

Dynamic contrast-enhanced MR imaging, applied clinically to measure perfusion in the brain, myocardial ischemia, breast tumors, prostate tumors, and liver disorders is another technique that may be useful in the study of perfusion changes associated with osteoporosis and of the relationship between BMD and perfusion [71-76]. An association of decreased vascular blood flow with osteoporosis has been described many times in the literature; patients with peripheral vascular disease of the lower extremities, reported mean bone mineral density (BMD) significantly lower in the more severely affected limb than in the less severely affected limb; an epidemiologic study of elderly women with osteoporosis, found diminished BMD associated with increased risk of death from stroke [77-80]. Low BMD independently predicts coronary artery disease in women undergoing coronary angiography with a higher predictive value than traditional risk factors such as age, hypertension, diabetes, high fasting glucose level, smoking, family history, or dyslipidemia [81].

MR perfusion imaging involves intravenous injection of a bolus of gadolinium contrast agent followed by rapid sequential MR scanning of the same region of interest over a specified time period (60–120 s). The first pass of gadolinium bolus, considered to represent arrival of the contrast material into the arteries and capillaries of the vertebral marrow and its diffusion into the extracellular space, is monitored. The amount and rate of contrast arrival into the tissues influences the maximum peak and slope of the time intensity perfusion curve [82]. Reports in the literature show a close correlation between osteoporosis and perfusion. Firstly, osteoporosis and osteopenia in vertebral body and proximal femur is associated with reduced bone perfusion compared with normal BMD subjects [5,8,10]. Secondly , the reduced perfusion observed in osteoporosis of the spine and hip region is an intraosseous occurrence rather than a reflection of a more generalized circulatory impairment. Whereas bone perfusion decreased with reduced BMD both in the proximal femur, acetabulum and lumbar vertebrae, no corresponding changes was observed in the adductor thigh and paravertebral muscles with the same blood supply [83]. This change between intraosseous and extraosseous perfusion in normal and osteoporotic patients may explain some of the different patterns of bone deposition and apposition seen in osteoporosis. Bone resorption, with aging, occurs preferentially on the trabecular and endocortical surfaces, whereas bone apposition occurs preferentially on the periosteal surface [84,85].

The third finding is that, as bone marrow perfusion decreased, there was a reciprocal rise in marrow fat content. Marrow fat content, quantifiable by proton MR spectroscopy through assessment of the relative signal contribution from fat in the spectrum, increases with age and osteoporosis. The latter may simply reflect increased size or number of fat cells replacing lost bone [86,87]. An effect of perfusion on differentiation of marrow mesenchymal stem cells may explain this observation. The mesenchymal stem cell acts as a common precursor for osteoblasts and adipocytes in the bone marrow; differentiation along osteoblast or adipocyte lines is influenced by oxygen tension and oxidative stress [88-92]. Decreased oxygen tension or increased oxidative stress favors adiopocyte over osteoblast precursor development [89-92]. Reduced marrow perfusion, as shown in the study of Griffith et al., is likely to decrease oxygen tension and increase oxidative stress within the marrow [83]. This change in microenvironment may effect mesenchymal stem cell maturation inducing adipocyte formation (increasing marrow fat) over osteoblast formation (decreasing BMD) [93].

Magnetic resonance imaging has the potential to investigate many aspects of bone physiology, namely bone fat content, perfusion and molecular diffusion. Investigation of these parameters may unlock new ways of studying and evaluating bone physiology and bone health.

REFERENCES

[1] Lindsay, R; Silverman, Sl; Cooper, C et al. (2001) Risk of new vertebral fracture in the year following a fracture. *Jama*, *285*, 320–323.

[2] Eriksson, SA; Isberg, BO; Lindgren, JU. (1989) Prediction of vertebral strength by dual photon absorptiometry and qualitative computed tomography. *Calcif Tissue Int*, *44*, 243–250.

[3] Baur, A; Stabler, A; Arbogast, S; Duerr, HR; Barti, R; Reiser, M. (2002) Acute osteoporotic and neoplastic vertebral compression fractures: fluid sign at MR imaging. *Radiology*, *25*, 730–735 .

[4] Baur, A; Dietrcich, O; Reiser, M. (2003) Diffusion-weighted imaging of bone marrow: current status. *Eur Radiol*, *13*, 1699–1708.

[5] Griffith, JF; Yeung, DK; Antonio, GE; Lee, FK; Hong, AW; Wong, SY; Lau, EM; Leung, PC. (2005) Vertebral bone mineral density, marrow perfusion, and fat content in healthy men and men with osteoporosis: dynamic contrast-enhanced MR imaging and MR spectroscopy. *Radiology*, *236*, 945-951.

[6] Kugel, H; Jung, C; Schulte, O; Heindel, W. (2001) Age- and sex-specific differences in the 1H-spectrum of vertebral bone marrow. *J Magn Reson Imaging*, *13*, 263-268.

[7] Schellinger, D; Lin, CS; Hatipoglu, HG; Fertikh, D. (2001) Potential value of vertebral proton. MR Spectroscopy in determining bone weakness. *Am J Neuroradiol*, *22*, 1620-1627.

[8] Shih, TT; Liu, HW; Chang, CJ; Wei, SY; Shen, LC; Yang, PC. (2004) Correlation of MR lumbar bone marrow perfusion with bonemineral density in female subjects. *Radiology*, *233*, 121-128.

[9] Yeung, DK; Griffith, JF; Antonio, GE; Lee, FK; Woo, J; Leung, PC. (2005) Osteoporosis is associated with increased marrow fat content and decreased marrow fat unsaturation: a proton MR spectroscopy study. *J Magn Reson Imaging*, *22*, 279-285.

[10] Griffith, JF; Yeung, DK; Antonio, GE; Wong, SYS; Kwok, T; Woo, J; Leung, PC. (2006) Marrow perfusion, diffusion and fat content in post-menopausal women of varying bone density. *Radiology*, *241*(3), 831-8.

[11] Fanucci et al. (2007) Multiparameter characterisation of vertebral osteoporosis with 3-T MR. *La Radiologia medica*, *112*(2), 208-223.

[12] Link, TM; Majumdar, S; Grampp, S; Guglielmi, G; van Kuijk, C; Imhof, H; Gluer, C; Adams, JE. (1999) Imaging of trabecular bone structure in osteoporosis. *Eur Radiol*, *9*, 1781–1788.

[13] Link, TM; Vieth, V; Matheis, J; Newitt, D; Lu Ying; Rummeny, EJ; Majumdar, S. (2002) Bone structure of the distal radius and the calcaneus vs. BMD of the spine and proximal femur in the prediction of osteoporotic spine fractures. *Eur Radiol*, *12*, 401–408.

[14] Jara, H; Wehrli, F; Chung, H; Ford, J. (1993) High resolution variable flip angle 3D MR imaging of trabecular microstructure in vivo. *Magn Reson Med*, *29*, 528–539.

[15] Link, TM; Majumdar, S. (2004) Current diagnostic techniques in the evaluation of bone architecture. *Curr Osteoporos Rep*, *2*(2), 47-52.

[16]Wehrli, F; Gomberg, B; Saha, P; Song, H; Hwang, S; Snyder, P. (2001a) Digital topological analysis of in vivo magnetic resonance microimages of trabecular bone reveals structural implications of osteoporosis. *J Bone Miner Res*, *16*, 1520–1531.

[17]Link, TM; Vieth, V; Matheis, J; Newitt, D; Lu, Y; Rummeny, E; Majumdar, S. (2002b) Bone structure of the distal radius and the calcaneus versus BMD of the spine and proximal femur in the prediction of osteoporotic spine fractures. *Eur Radiol*, *12*, 401–408.

[18]Link, TM; Lotter, A; Beyer, F et al. (2000) Changes in calcaneal trabecular bone structure after heart transplantation: an MR imaging study. *Radiology*, *217*, 855-862.

[19]Wehrli, FW; Ilwang, SN; Ma, J et al. (1998) Cancellous bone volume and structure in the forearm: noninvasive assessment with MR microimaging and image processing. *Radiology*, *206*, 347-357.

[20]Krug, R; Banerjee, S; Han, ET; Newitt, DC; Link, TM; Majumdar, S. (2005) Feasibility of in vivo structural analysis of high-resolution magnetic resonance images of the proximal femur. *Osteoporos Int*, *16*, 1307–1314.

[21]Phan, CM; Matsuura, M; Bauer, JS; Dunn, TC; Newitt, D; Lochmueller, EM; Eckstein, F; Majumdar, S; Link, TM. (2006) Trabecular bone structure of the calcaneus: comparison of MR imaging at 3.0 and 1.5T with micro-CT as the standard of reference. *Radiology*, *239* (2):488–496.

[22]Majumdar, S. (2002) Magnetic resonance imaging of trabecular bone structure. *Top Magn Reson Imaging*, *13*, 323–334.

[23]Hipp, JA; Jansujwicz, A; Simmons, CA; Snyder, BD. (1996) Trabecular bone morphology from micro-magnetic resonance imaging. *J Bone Miner Res*, *11*, 286–297.

[24]Jara, H; Wehrli, FW; Chung, H; Ford, JC. (1993) High-resolution variable flip angle 3D MR imaging of trabecular microstructure in vivo. *Magn Reson Med*, *29*, 528–539.

[25]Krug, R; Han, ET; Banerjee, S; Majumdar, S. (2006) Fully balanced steady-state 3D-spin-echo (bSSSE) imaging at 3 Tesla. *Magn Reson Med*, *56*, 1033–1040.

[26]Techawiboonwong, A; Song, H; Wehrli, FW; Saha, PK. (2004) Relative performance of FLASE, TrueFISP and gradient echo in micro-MRI of trabecular bone. *International Society for Magnetic Resonance in Medicine, Kyoto*

[27]Laib, A; Beuf, O; Issever, A; Newitt, DC; Majumdar, S. (2001) Direct measures of trabecular bone architecture from MR images. *Adv Exp Med Biol*, *496*, 37–46.

[28]Majumdar, S; Genant, H; Grampp, S et al. (1997) Correlation of trabecular bone structure with age, bone mineral density and osteoporotic status: in vivo studies in the distal radius using high resolution magnetic resonance imaging. *J Bone Miner Res 12*, 111–118.

[29]Link, TM; Majumdar, S; Augat, P et al. (1998) In vivo high resolution MRI of the calcaneus: differences in trabecular structure in osteoporosis patients. *J Bone Miner Res 13*(7), 1175–1182.

[30]Majumdar; S; Link, T; Augat, P et al. (1999) Trabecular bone architecture in the distal radius using MR imaging in subjects with fractures of the proximal femur. *Osteoporos Int*, *10*, 231–239.

[31]Laib, A; Newitt, DC; Lu, Y; Majumdar, S. (2002) New model-independent measures of trabecular bone structure applied to in vivo high-resolution MR images. *Osteoporos Int*, *13*(2), 130–136.

[32]Boutry, N; Cortet, B; Dubois, P; Marchandise, X; Cotten, A. (2003) Trabecular bone structure of the calcaneus: preliminary in vivo MR imaging assessment in men with osteoporosis. *Radiology*, *227*(3), 708–717.

[33]Wehrli, F; Ford, J; Attie, M; Kressel, H; Kaplan, F. (1991) Trabecular structure: preliminary application of MR interferometry. *Radiology*, *179*,615–621.

[34]Funke, M; Bruhn, H; Vosshenrich, R; Rudolph, O; Grabbe, E. (1994) Bestimmung der T2*-Relaxationszeit zur Charakterisierung des trabekulären Knochens. *Fortschr Roentgenstr*, *161*, 58–63.

[35]Grampp, S; Majumdar, S; Jergas, M; Newitt, D; Lang, P; Genant, H. (1996) Distal radius: in vivo assessment with quantitative MR imaging, peripheral quantitative CT and dual X-ray absorptiometry. *Radiology*, *198*, 213–218.

[36]Paschalis, EP;Boskey, AL; Kassem, M; Eriksen, EF. (2003) Effect of hormone replacement therapy on bone quality in early postmenopausal women. *J. Bone Miner. Res*, *18*(6), 955–959.

[37]Neuman, W. F. and Neuman M.W. *Skeletal Dynamics the Chemical Dynamics of Bone Mineral*. Chicago: Univ. Of Chicago Press; 1958, pp. 101.

[38]Robinson, R.A. and Elliot S.R. (1957) The water content of bone. *J.Bone Joint Surg*, *39*, 167–188.

[39]Timmins P.A. and Wall J.C. (1977)vBone water. *Calcif. Tissue Res*, *23*(1), 1–5.

[40]Piney, A. (1922) The anatomy of bone marrow. *Br Med J*, *2*, 792–795.

[41]Okada, Y; Aoki, S; Barkovich, AJ et al. (1989) Cranial bone marrow in children: Assessment of normal development with MR imaging. *Radiology*, *171*, 161–164.

[42]Moore, SG; Dawson, KL. (1990) Red and yellow marrow in the femur: agerelated changes in appearance at MR imaging. *Radiology*, *175*,219–223.

[43]Ricci, C; Cova, M; Kang YS et al. (1990) Normal age-related patterns of cellular and fatty bone marrow distribution in the axial skeleton: MR imaging study. *Radiology*, *177*, 83–88.

[44]Jaramillo, D; Laor, T; Hoffer, FA et al. (1991) Epiphyseal marrow in infancy: MR imaging. *Radiology*, *180*, 809–812.

[45]Dawson, KL; Moore, SG; Rowland, JM. (1992) Age-related marrow changes in the pelvis: MR and anatomic findings. *Radiology*, *183*, 47–51.

[46]Schellinger, D; Lin, CS; Fertikh, D et al. (2000) Normal lumbar vertebrae: anatomic, age and sex variance in subjects at proton MR spectroscopy— initial experience. *Radiology*, *215*, 910–916.

[47]Vande; Berg, BC; Lecouvert, FE; Malghem, J. (1998) Sex-related difference in marrow conversion in the proximal femur: does it exist? *Radiology*, *209*, 587–588.

[48]Jenkins, JPR; Stehling, M; Sivewright, G; Hickey, DS; Hillier, VF; Ishwerwood, I. (1989) Quantitative magnetic resonance imaging of vertebral bodies: a T1 and T2 study. *Magn Reson Imaging*, *7*, 17–23.

[49]Jensen, KE; Jensen, M; Grundtvig, P; Thomsen, C; Karle, H; Henriksen, O. (1990) Localized in vivo spectroscopy of the bone marrow in patients with leukemia. *Magn Reson Imaging*, *8*, 779–789.

[50]Ballon, D; Jakubowski, A; Gabrilove, J et al. (1991) In vivo measurements of bone marrow cellularity using volume-localized proton NMR spectroscopy. *Magn Reson Med*, *19*, 85–95.

[51]Schick, F; Bongers, H; Jung, WI et al. (1992) Volume-selective proton MRS in vertebral bodies. *Magn Reson Med*, *26*, 207–217.

[52]Schick, F; Einsele, H; Kost, R et al. (1994) Hematopoietic reconstitution after bone marrow transplantation: assessment with MR imaging and H-1 localized spectroscopy. *J Magn Reson Imaging*, *4*, 71–78.

[53]Bongers, H; Schick, F; Skalej, M; Jung WI; Einsele, H. (1992) Localized in vivo 1H spectroscopy and chemical shift imaging of the bone marrow in leukemic patients. *Eur Radiol*, *2*, 350–356.

[54]De Bisschop, E; Luypaert, R; Louis, O; Osteaux, M. (1993) Fat fraction of lumbar bone marrow using in vivo proton nuclear magnetic resonance spectroscopy. *Bone*, *14*, 133–136.

[55]LeBlanc, A; Lin, C; Evans, H et al. (1999) T2 vertebral bone marrow changes after space flight. *Magn Reson Med*, *41*, 495–498.

[56]Dunnill, MS; Anderson, JA; Whitehead, R. (1967) Quantitative histological studies on age changes in bone. *J Pathol Bacteriol*, *94*, 275–291.

[57]Verna, S; Rajaratnam, JH; Denton J et al. (2002) Adipocytic proportion of bone marrow is inversely related to bone formation in osteoporosis. *J Clin Pathol*, *55*, 693–698.

[58]Gunstone, FD; Harwood, JL; Padley, FB. *The lipid handbook*. 2nd ed. London: Chapman and Hall; 1994.

[59]Guillen, MD; Ruiz, A. (2003) Rapid simultaneous determination by proton NMR of unsaturation and composition of acryl groups in vegetable oils. *Eur J Lipid Sci Technol*, *105*, 688–696.

[60]Lang, P; Steiger, P; Faulkner, K et al. (1991) Osteoporosis: current techniques and recent developments in quantitative bone densitometry. *Radiol Clin North Am*, *29*, 49–76.

[61]Dooms, GC; Fisher, MR; Hricak, H et al. (1985) Bone marrow imaging: magnetic resonance studies related to age and sex. *Radiology*, *155*, 429–432.

[62]Beresford, JN; Bennett, JH; Delvin, C et al. (1992) Evidence for an inverse relationship between the differentiation of adipocytic and osteogenic cells in rat marrow stromal cell cultures. *J Cell Sci*, *102*, 341–351.

[63]Kazarian, L; Graves, GA. (1977) Compressive strength characteristics of the human vertebral column. *Spine*, *2*, 1–13.

[64]Schellinger et al. (2004) Bone marrow fat and bone mineral density on proton MR spectroscopy and dual-energy X-ray absorptiometry: their ratio as a new indicator of bone weakening. *AJR American journal of roentgenology*, *183*(6), 1761-5.

[65]Baur, A; Stabler, A; Bruning, R; Bartl, R; Krodel, A; Reiser, M; Deimling, M. (1998) Diffusion-weighted MR imaging of bone marrow: differentiation of benign versus pathologic compression fractures. *Radiology*, *207*, 349–356.

[66]Yeung, KWD; Wong, YSS; Griffith, FJ; Lau, MCE. (2004) Bone marrow diffusion in osteoporosis: evaluation with quantitative MR diffusion imaging. *J Magn Reson Imaging*, *19*, 222–228.

[67]Hatipoglu et al. (2007) Quantitative and diffusion MR imaging as a new method to assess osteoporosis. *AJNR American journal of neuroradiology*, *28*(10), 1934-7.

[68]Nonomura, Y; Yasumoto, M; Yoshimura, R, et al. (2001) Relationship between bone marrow cellularity and apparent diffusion coefficient. *J Magn Reson Imaging*, *13*, 757–60.

[69]Trabowitz, S; Davis, S. The bone marrow matrix. In: The Human Bone Marrow: Anatomy, Physiology, and Pathophysiology. Boca Raton, Fla: CRC; *182*, 43–76.

[70]Beaulieu, C. (2002) The basis of anisotropic water diffusion in the nervous system — a technical review. *NMR Biomed*, *15*, 435 – 55.

[71]Law, M; Oh, S; Babb, JS; Wang, E; Inglese, M; Zagzag, D; Knopp, EA; Johnson, G. (2006) Low-grade gliomas: dynamic susceptibility-weighted contrast-enhanced perfusion MR imaging--prediction of patient clinical response. *Radiology*, *238*(2),658-67.

[72]Wolff, SD; Schwitter, J; Coulden, R; Friedrich, MG; Bluemke, DA; Biederman, RW, Martin, ET; Lansky, AJ; Kashanian, F; Foo, TK; Licato, PE; Comeau, CR. (2004) Myocardial first-pass perfusion magnetic resonance imaging: a multicenter dose-ranging study. *Circulation*, *110*(6), 732-7.

[73]Kvistad, KA; Rydland, J; Vainio, J; Smethurst, HB; Lundgren, S; Fj¯sne, HE; Haraldseth, O. (2000) Breast lesions: evaluation with dynamic contrast-enhanced T1-weighted MR imaging and with T2*-weighted first-pass perfusion MR imaging. *Radiology*, *216*(2), 545-53.

[74]Engelbrecht, MR; Huisman, HJ; Laheij, RJ; Jager, GJ; van Leenders, GJ; Hulsbergen-Van De Kaa, CA; de la Rosette, JJ; Blickman, JG; Barentsz, JO. (2003) Discrimination of prostate cancer from normal peripheral zone and central gland tissue by using dynamic contrast-enhanced MR imaging. *Radiology*, *229*(1), 248-54.

[75]Guan, S; Zhao, WD; Zhou, KR; Peng, WJ; Tang, F; Mao, J. (2007) Assessment of hemodynamics in precancerous lesion of hepatocellular carcinoma: evaluation with MR perfusion. *World J Gastroenterol*, *13*(8), 1182-6.

[76]Chen, WT; Shih, TT; Chen, RC; Lo, SY; Chou, CT; Lee, JM; Tu, HY. (2001) Vertebral bone marrow perfusion evaluated with dynamic contrast-enhanced MR imaging: significance of aging and sex. *Radiology*, *220*(1), 213-8.

[77]Laroche, M. (1996) Arteriosclerosis and osteoporosis (editorial). *Presse Med*, *25*, 52–54. [French]

[78]Laroche, M; Pouilles, JM; Ribot, C et al. (1994) Comparison of the bone mineral content of the lower limbs in men with ischaemic atherosclerotic disease. *Clin Rheumatol*, *13*, 611– 614.

[79]Browner, WS; Seeley, DG; Vogt, TM; Cummings, SR. (1991) Non-trauma mortality in elderly women with low bone mineral density. *Lancet*, *338*, 355–358.

[80]Browner, WS; Pressman, AR; Nevitt, MC; Cauley, JA; Cummings, SR. (1993) Association between low bone density and stroke in elderly women: the study of osteoporotic fractures. *Stroke*, *24*, 940 –946.

[81]Marcovitz, PA; Tran, HH; Franklin, BA; O'Neill, WW; Yerkey, M; Boura, J; Kleerekoper, M; Dickinson, CZ. (2005) Usefulness of bone mineral density to predict significant coronary artery disease. *Am J Cardiol*, *96*(8), 1059-63.

[82]Luypaert, R; Boujraf, S; Sourbron, S; Osteaux, M. (2001) Diffusion and perfusion MRI: basic physics. *Eur J Radiol*, *38*(1), 19-27.

[83]Griffith, JF; Yeung, DK; Tsang, PH; Choi, KC; Kwok, TC; Ahuja, AT; Leung, KS; Leung, PC. (2008) Compromised bone marrow perfusion in osteoporosis. *J Bone Miner Res*, *23*(7), 1068-75.

[84]Seeman, E. (2002) Pathogenesis of bone fragility in women and men. *Lancet*, *359*(9320), 1841-50.

[85]Seeman, E. (2007) The periosteum--a surface for all seasons. *Osteoporos Int.*,*18*(2), 123-8.

[86]Rozman, C; Feliu, E; Berga, L; Reverter, JC; Climent, C; Ferrán, MJ. (1989) Age-related variations of fat tissue fraction in normal human bone marrow depend both on size and number of adipocytes: a stereological study. *Exp Hematol. 17*(1),34-7.

[87]Justesen, J; Stenderup, K; Ebbesen, EN; Mosekilde, L; Steiniche, T; Kassem, M. (2001) Adipocyte tissue volume in bone marrow is increased with aging and in patients with osteoporosis. *Biogerontology 2*(3),165-71.

[88]Gimble, JM; Nuttall, ME. Bone and fat: old questions, new insights. *Endocrine 23*(2-3),183-8

[89]D'Ippolito, G; Diabira, S; Howard, GA; Roos, BA; Schiller, PC. (2006) Low oxygen tension inhibits osteogenic differentiation and enhances stemness of human MIAMI cells. *Bone*, *39*(3), 513-22

[90]Fatokun, AA; Stone, TW; Smith, RA. (2006) Hydrogen peroxide-induced oxidative stress in MC3T3-E1 cells: The effects of glutamate and protection by purines. *Bone*, *39*(3), 542-51.

[91]Shouhed, D; Kha, HT; Richardson, JA; Amantea, CM; Hahn, TJ; Parhami, F. (2005) Osteogenic oxysterols inhibit the adverse effects of oxidative stress on osteogenic differentiation of marrow stromal cells. *J Cell Biochem*, *95*(6), 1276-83.

[92]Kha, HT; Basseri, B; Shouhed, D; Richardson, J; Tetradis, S; Hahn, TJ; Parhami F. (2004) Oxysterols regulate differentiation of mesenchymal stem cells: pro-bone and anti-fat. *J Bone Miner Res*, *19*(5),830-40.

[93]Duque, G. (2007) As a matter of fat: New perspectives on the understanding of age-related bone loss. *BoneKEy-Osteovision*, *4*,129-140.

In: Osteoporosis: Etiology, Diagnosis and Treatment
Editors: Bilar E. Mattingly and Albert C. Pillare
ISBN 978-1-60692-397-9

Chapter 18

Bone Mineral Density in Young Females – The Impact of Menstrual Dysfunction

William W. K. To[1] *and Margaret W. N. Wong*[2]
[1]United Christian Hospital, Hong Kong;
[2]The Chinese University of Hong Kong, Hong Kong.

Abstract

Young females have a high incidence of menstrual irregularities, and one of the most common forms of menstrual dysfunction is oligomenorrhea and amenorrhea as a result of prolonged anovulation. The common underlying causes include idiopathic hypothalamic amenorrhea, polycystic ovarian syndrome, exercise induced hypothalamic dysfunction, eating disorders, and other rarer congenital anomalies such as gonadal dysgenesis. Each of these conditions would have specific implications on bone mineral density (BMD) changes in affected women. While those with idiopathic hypothalamic amenorrhea are at risk of osteoporosis because of prolonged hypo-oestrogenism, the high androgen states in those with polycystic ovarian syndrome would compensate for the estrogen deficiency, so that BMD is preserved or better than eumenorrhoeic women. In exercise-induced amenorrhea, the positive stimulating effects of weight-bearing exercises would stimulate bone accrual and again off-set the negative effects of anovulation on BMD. Those with eating disorders suffer not only from the effects of amenorrhea, but also from the associated low energy intake and malnutrition. Women affected with gonadal dysgenesis, such as Turner's syndrome, would require long term hormonal therapy to maintain bone accretion and BMD, as well for induction of pubertal development. While genuine osteoporosis and its sequalae would only be expected in later life in these young women, the implications of menstrual dysfunction at this early reproductive age would need to be explored.

Introduction

Adolescence is a critical period for bone accretion as over half of peak bone mass is achieved during the teenage years. In an adolescent girl, it has been estimated that up to 90 % of total body mineral content would have accrued by age 16.9 $\pm$ 1.3 years [1], and the rates of calcium absorption and bone formation then decrease significantly with post-menarcheal age following onset of menses. Genetic predisposition is a very crucial factor determining bone mineral density, and can account for up to 80% of the variance in bone mass [2]. For instance, it has also been reported that black teenage girls had higher calcium absorption compared to whites, which may account in part for the higher bone density generally seen in black adolescents compared with other ethnic groups [3]. Other important modifiable factors are also at work during the adolescent period. Factors that would optimize bone accretion during this period include calcium intake, vitamin D, nutrition, and exercise [4]. With the onset of puberty and menarche, the effects of reproductive hormones such as oestrogen play an important role in determining further bone accrual and peak bone density in females.

Regular monthly menstruation in females has only been observed as the norm in modern society after the introduction of effective contraception to control the number and the timing of pregnancies. The length, regularity and frequency of normal menstrual cycles have been studied in large scale population studies [5]. The mean menstrual cycle length between the young reproductive age of 20 and 34 years varies from 28 to 30.7 days (range 19.7 to 43.5 days, 5th to 95th centiles). Regular monthly cycles represent cyclical ovarian activity, which in turn is dependent on the normal physiological hypothalamic pituitary axis, the uterus and endometrium as end organs, and a patent lower genital tract. Oligomenorrhea and amenorrhea are thus usually symptoms of ovarian and reproductive dysfunction.

Menstrual Dysfunction in the Form of Oligomenorrhoea and Amenorrhoea and Bone Mineral Density

Amenorrhea is defined as the complete absence or cessation of menstrual periods for greater than 6 months that is not due to pregnancy. Primary amenorrhoea is defined as the absence of menses by the age of 14 in the absence of secondary sexual characteristics, or in the presence of normal development, by the age of 16 [6]. Secondary amenorrhoea has been defined as the absence of menses for 6 months if the patient has previously experienced regular menses or for 12 months or more if the patient has oligomenorrhoea [7]. Oligomenorrhea is the reduction in frequency of menstruation where menstrual intervals may vary between 6 weeks and 6 months. However, regular but long cycles of up to 6 weeks are often physiologically indistinguishable from normal shorter 28 day cycles in terms of follicular formation, ovulation and hormonal profile. On the other hand, long irregular cycles often signify chronic anovulation, absence of mid cycle gonadotrophin surges and prolonged hypo-oestrogenism. Thus, the definition of oligomenorrhea as such includes a wide spectrum of conditions ranging from virtual normality to true amenorrhea and all its implications. In a clinical gynaecological setting, it is normal practice to initiate investigations for any woman with no menses for 3 months or more.

In adolescents, menstrual irregularity is common particularly in the first 2-3 years after menarche as the hypothalamic-pituitary axis continues to develop and mature [8]. Historically, it was reported that the 95th centile for cycle length was 90 days in the first menarcheal year [9]. Based on these definitions, it can be seen that the incidence of menstrual dysfunction in young females in their late adolescent period would be expected to be very high.

The World Health Organization has defined three categories of BMD values, namely osteopenia, osteoporosis and severe (established) osteoporosis, recognizing that low bone mineral density and a history of previous fractures both contribute to increased risk of future fractures [10]. Nevertheless, the WHO criteria are intended to be applied to postmenopausal women and not to premenopausal females, so that in this age group, Z scores should be preferable to T scores. In addition, a low BMD in premenopausal women may represent a low peak bone mass rather than bone loss. Healthy pre-menopausal women with low bone mass may not have any higher fracture risk than their counterparts with normal bone mass, though their fracture risk could be expected to be higher as they entered their menopause with a lower BMD value [11].

Using the WHO criterion, only 0.6% of all pre-menopausal females would be classified as having osteoporosis. However, approximately 15% of young women would be classified as osteopenic (between 1.0 and 2.5 SD below the mean for 30-40 years of age). The typical menopause-related bone loss would cause many of these women to sink into the high-risk osteoporotic category if their bone loss proceeded at the expected trend and rate [12]. It is in the context of this background that young females with menstrual dysfunction are considered to be at risk of osteoporosis in later life.

PREMATURE OVARIAN FAILURE AND RELATIONSHIP TO BONE MINERAL DENSITY

Clinically, primary amenorrhoea associated specific anatomical abnormalities, such as the Mayer-von Rokitansky-Kuster-Hauser syndrome, or those with obstruction to the outflow tract [13], are not associated with ovarian endocrine function, and should thus have no impact on BMD. On the other hand, amenorrhoea that is associated with chronic anovulatory cycles, as in the case of gonadal dysgenesis or premature ovarian failure, would be related to hypo-oestrogenism and its implications on BMD (Table 1).

A common clinical presentation of gonadal dysgenesis in adolescents reaching the age of puberty would be primary amenorrhoea, with or without incidental findings of associated morphological abnormalities and short stature. The underlying chromosomal abnormalities are usually Turner syndrome and its mosaic forms. Turner syndrome is a genetic condition which results from a total or partial absence of one of the X chromosomes. It has an incidence of around 1 in 2500 to 3000 live female births [14]. The most prominent clinical features of Turner syndrome are short stature and gonadal dysgenesis which leads to primary or premature ovarian failure, absence of, or delayed or incomplete pubertal development, and infertility. A myriad of dysmorphic features and congenital abnormalities can also be observed amongst patients with Turner syndrome. They are at risk of congenital heart defects such as coartation of the aorta, bicuspid aortic valves, and may have progressive aortic root dilatation or dissection. They are also at risk of congenital lymphoedema, renal malformations, sensorineural hearing loss, osteoporosis, obesity, diabetes mellitus, and artherogenic lipid profile. Patients usually have normal intelligence but may have problems with nonverbal, social and psychomotor skills. Turner syndrome should be suspected in girls presenting with primary amenorrhea and short stature [15].

Table 1. Causes of and amenorrhoea and oligomenorrhoea and relationship to BMD

Group	Aetiology	Impact on BMD
Delayed Puberty	Familial or Constitutional	Unlikely
	Nutritional	Possible
Anatomical congenital abnormalities	Imperforate hymen (crytomenorrhea) Mullerian agenesis (absent uterus/ absent vagina)	No
Karyotype abnormalities	Turner syndrome (45 XO) / mosaics XO/ XY mosaics	Yes
	Testicular feminization syndrome (46 XY)	Unknown
Hypothalamic pituitary axis	Kallman's syndrome Intense physical exercises Anorexia nervosa and weight loss Hyperprolactinemia Ablation by irradiation, surgery, compression by tumors or vascular infarction (Sheehan's syndrome)	Yes
Ovarian causes	Ablation by surgery, irradiation or chemotherapy Premature ovarian failure (including autoimmune causes) Polycystic ovarian syndrome Resistant ovary syndrome	No
Uterine causes	Ablation by surgery (hysterectomy or endometrial ablation) or pelvic irradiation (destroying functional endometrium) Ashermann syndrome and cervical stenosis Infections (such as tuberculosis endometritis)	No

A recent study of 50 women who had been previously diagnosed to have spontaneous premature ovarian failure, a semi-structured interview survey showed a significant delay in arriving at a definitive diagnosis (some for as long as 5 years) despite repeated clinical consultations. The need for earlier and more aggressive evaluation and management of the amenorrhoea was raised [16], and the potential aggravation of bone loss due to the delay to institute oestrogen replacement therapy was forewarned. Treatment for girls with Turner syndrome mainly aims at increasing their height and promoting sexual maturation. They would thus be treated with growth hormone therapy for short stature from early childhood, and supplementary oestrogen is initiated by adolescence for pubertal development and for prevention of osteoporosis. Life-long follow-up for Turner syndrome patients are generally recommended for management of commonly occurring conditions such as thyroid diseases, hypertension and diabetes mellitus [17]. However, the data on the incidence of osteoporosis or fracture risks in later life this group of individuals has been scanty in the literature, largely because of the difficulty in establishing long term study cohorts for follow up of Turner patients into their fifties or beyond. The effectiveness of long term oestrogen replacement therapy in these women with gonadal dysgenesis remains to be evaluated.

DRUG INDUCED AMENORRHOEA, HYPERPROLACTINAEMIA AND RELATIONSHIP TO BONE MINERAL DENSITY

Causes of amenorrhoea and oligomenorrhoea that are associated with chronic anovulatory cycles, including medications, hyperprolactinaemia, polycystic ovary syndrome, or hypothalamic dysfunction, can all be related to hypo-oestrogenism and its implications on bone mineral density (BMD).

Iatrogenic amenorrhoea from drugs such as gonadotrophin-releasing hormones (GnRH) analogue and depot medroxy-progesterone acetate has been associated with deleterious effects on BMD. Findings have shown that adolescents who are prescribed these drugs had significant losses in BMD compared to controls that are not exposed to these agents. In particular, a mean BMD loss of -1.5% to -1.8% was found after 1 year of treatment by depoprovera in these adolescents and up to -4.8% after 2 years of therapy, while untreated controls in contrast still showed gains of +1.20% to 2.85 % over 1 year or up to +9.49% over 2 years [18, 19]. Thus, the long term usage of such medication to inhibit endogenous ovulation does have a negative impact on bone mineral density in reproductive age women. Further studies are on-going to evaluate the degree of recovery in pre-menopausal women after the medications are withdrawn to allow resumption of spontaneous ovulation.

Hyperprolactinaemia is another frequent cause of secondary amenorrhoea in young women. The cause of hyperprolactinaemia is often idiopathic, or is related to a microadenoma of the pituitary gland demonstrable on computerized tomography or magnetic resonance imaging, and only rarely would it be related to a pituitary macroadenoma. Hyperprolactinaemia induces chronic anovulation, and thus have the same implications of hypo-oestrogenism and bone mineral density loss if left untreated. A study that utilized quantitative ultrasound measurements of the os calcis compared a group of premenopausal women with hyperprolactinaemia and amenorrhoea with healthy controls, and confirmed lower BMD in these women after controlling for age differences and body mass index [20]. However, hyperprolactinaemia is readily treatable with dopamine agonists such as bromocriptine, which should allow return of normal ovulatory cycles and menstruation, and thus alleviating the possible negative effects on BMD.

Hypothalamic Dysfunction, Polycystic Ovary Syndrome and Relationship to Bone Mineral Density

Similar patterns of menstrual dysfunction can result from anovulation related to hypothalamic or pituitary dysfunction or in those with polycystic ovaries. Polycystic ovarian syndrome (PCOS) is probably one of the most common causes for such menstrual dysfunction in reproductive age group women. Using ultrasound criteria, polycystic ovaries has been shown to account for 57% of women with anovulation, and definite associations have been shown between ultrasound appearance of polycystic ovaries, cycle irregularities and hormonal derangements [21].

Table 2. Polycystic Ovarian Syndrome and its manifestations

Possible clinical manifestations	Obesity Oligomenorrhea and secondary amenorrhea Infertility Hirsutism Asymptomatic
Possible hormonal disturbances	Hyperandrogenism (raised testosterone and androstenedione levels) Raised luteinizing hormone levels Raised fasting insulin levels Mild hyperprolactinemia Low sex hormone-binding globulin Raised estradiol levels
Possible medical complications	Diabetes mellitus Hyperlipidaemia Hypertension and cardiovascular disorders Carcinoma of the breast Carcinoma of the endometrium
Possible Impact on BMD	*Positive impact –* Hyperandrogenism Hyperinsulinaemia Increased peripheral conversion of oestrogens Persistent low levels of circulating oestrogens *Negative impact –* Lack of ovulatory cycles and chronic anovulation Absence of mid-cycle oestrogen surge Low mean circulating oestrogen levels Mild hyperprolactinaemia

It is apparent from the literature that the impact of hypothalamic menstrual dysfunction and PCOS on BMD was significantly different. Typically, women with PCOS have acyclical production of oestradial at levels similar to those seen in follicular phase, but considerably lower than the mean concentration across the normal menstrual cycle of normal menstruating women [22]. This static level of oestradiol, with the absence of the oestradiol surge associated with ovulation, would be expected to negatively affect bone density. Testosterone and androstenedione, however, are produced in excess by the PCOS ovary and the adrenals, and the chronic elevation in androgens may exert a positive influence on bone in PCOS women [23]. Moreover, elevated circulating insulin levels associated with PCOS may also offer some positive influence on bone through direct stimulation of osteoblastic activity, or indirectly via its effect on sex hormone-binding globulin or insulin-like growth factor binding proteins. A direct relationship between BMD and insulin levels and insulin resistance has been shown in a small series [24], and in some women with severe insulin resistance, over-growth of bone and features of acromegaly have been reported. Moreover, those with polycystic ovaries were found to be more oestrogenized at peripheral sites as compared to non-PCOS women, indicating that PCOS patients with menstrual dysfunction might not suffer the same degree of hypo-oestrogenism as in those with hypothalamic amenorrhoea. As these factors of hyperandrogenaemia, hyperinsulinaemia and peripheral oestrogenization will not be at work in those with hypothalamic pituitary anovulation, it becomes apparent that polycystic ovarian syndrome in post-adolescent women with secondary amenorrhea may have a protective effect on bone mineral loss compared to those with no polycystic ovaries [25] (Table 2).

In a cross-sectional observational study comparing girls between 16 to 19 years of age with oligomenorrhoea or amenorrhea due to either polycystic ovaries or normal ovaries (the hypothalamic dysfunction group), it was found that those with normal ovaries had lower BMD than eumenorrhoeic ones, but those with polycystic ovaries had BMD values comparable to eumenorrhoeic controls despite their menstrual dysfunction [26]. Thus, the group with menstrual dysfunction and normal ovaries should more typically represent the effects of hypo-oestrogenism as a result of chronic anovulation, while those with polycystic ovaries apparently did not suffer the negative impact on their BMD.

Menstrual Dysfunction Induced by Eating Disorders, Intensive Exercises and the Relationship to BMD

Another common underlying aetiology for oligomenorrhoea and secondary amenorrhoea is hypothalamic dysfunction related to the sequalae of eating disorders and low body fat composition. A variety of risk factors have been found to be conducive to low bone mass in young females with anorexia nervosa [27], which can result from a simultaneous increase in bone resorption as well as decrease in bone formation in these women. In particular, levels of anabolic hormones such as insulin-like growth factors (IGF-1) are low, and a close correlation between IGF-1 levels and biochemical bone formation markers have been found

[28]. The abnormal bone formation could be explained in part by abnormal osteoblast function found in these women with anorexia nervosa. Moreover, classical studies have shown that serum levels of dehydroepiandrosterone was subnormal in patients with anorexia nervosa [29], and could correlate inversely with urinary levels of N-telopeptides, a bone resorption marker, indicating that the hormone may modulate the increased bone resorption in these women. Contrarily, serum levels of interleukin-6, tumour necrosis factor-alpha and other pro-resorptive cytokines, markers shown to contribute to increased bone resorption in postmenopausal women, were at very low or undetectable levels in adolescents with anorexia nervosa [27]. Thus, the mechanisms that are at work to produce bone loss in these young women may be somewhat different from the older postmenopausal woman. The role of other mechanisms, such as disturbances in neurotransmitter and neuropeptides which may also be directly related to bone loss in these young women would also need to be explored (Table 3).

Table 3. Eating Disorders and relationship to BMD

Pathophysiology	Probable mechanisms
Insufficient caloric intake	Poor nutritional status, low body fat composition and catabolic metabolism
Insufficient calcium intake	Insufficient biochemical stimuli for osteogenic activity
Amenorrhoea and chronic anovulation	Hypothalamic pituitary axis suppression Hypo-oestrogenism and postmenopausal type of bone loss
Psychological Stress and depression	Immobility and lack of adequate physical exercises to stimulate proper osteogenic activity
Low metabolic rate	Retardation of proper age-appropriate bone accrual

Epidemiologically, adolescents who develop anorexia nervosa prior to menarche were found to have lower BMD than those who develop the disorder later in adolescence. In a cross-sectional sample of adolescent girls with anorexia nervosa with a mean age of 14.7 years, low total body BMD was found in 23.7% of them and low spinal BMD was found in 36.6%. The age of menarche has been found to be the most important factor predicting BMD in these young anorexic women [30]. In a detailed study of a cohort of adolescents with anorexia nervosa, when these are classified according to their stage of illness, it was found that osteopenia was more prevalent when patients presented at younger ages and when the duration of amenorrhoea was longer [31]. Amenorrhoea for 20 months was identified as a threshold above which the most severe osteopenia was seen. Serum IGF-1 levels were also directly correlated with bone formation markers, and levels of oestradiol negatively correlated with bone resorption markers. A further study that examined predictors of low bone density in young women with anorexia nervosa found a direct correlation between BMD and serum oestradiol, weight, body mass index and lean body mass [32]. As the duration of amenorrhoea and dieting were associated with a low BMD, it was concluded that essentially it was the timing of onset of dieting that is most relevant to bone density.

Adolescents who both reported dieting at degrees not qualified to be anorexia nervosa and who also had amenorrhoea were at similar risks for low bone density as those with true anorexia nervosa as judged by the standard diagnostic criteria. This implies that adolescents with eating disorders that do not qualify as anorexia nervosa still run similar risks of low bone density once they exhibit menstrual dysfunction. Given the widespread problem of eating disorders among teenage females, such information could have important implications on the general health of this young population.

While hypo-oestrogenism and disordered eating with poor nutrition are all associated with increased risks of bone loss in young women with anorexia nervosa, the appropriate management for preventing the development of osteoporosis is still controversial. When a group of young women with anorexia nervosa were given oral contraceptives for 23 months and compared with a similar group who received standard therapy with no hormones, no significant increases in BMD was seen in either groups. Such findings question the common practice of prescribing hormonal replacement therapy to increase bone mass in young women with anorexia nervosa [32], and the role for standard hormonal replacement regimes has been debated. In a randomized control trial, when postmenopausal doses of oestrogen replacement together with progestogens (Premarin 0.625 mg, days 1-25, Provera 5 mg days 16-25) were administered, bone mass was found to increase in a small subgroup of young women with the lowest initial body weight. [33]. On the other hand, in an open study that utilized contraceptive doses of ethinyl oestradiol (50 ug) that are substantially more potent than the postmenopausal hormonal replacement regimes, there was still no demonstrable increase in BMD after treatment after 12 months of treatment and partial weight recovery [34]. In a prospective observational study that compared a lower dosage of 20-35 ug ethinyl oestradiol oral contraceptives with no hormones, it was again found that despite weight gain in both groups, there was no BMD increase seen in either group. Bone density was nevertheless maintained over the 2 year treatment period at both the spine and hip regions in those taking oral contraceptives [35]. When a 20 ug ethinyl oestradiol oral contraceptive was compared with 50 mg of oral micronized dehydroepiandrosterone in a double-blinded randomized control trial, the investigators again found no significant increase in BMD over a period of 1 year, though maintenance of hip and spinal BMD was seen in both groups. [36]. When the anabolic effects of IGF-1 combined with oestrogen and progestin was examined as an anti-resorptive agent and compared with standard oestrogen/progestin HRT, a significant increase in spinal BMD was seen after 9 months of combined therapy, but no significant changes in BMD was seen in the group on oestrogen/progestin HRT alone [28]. While the above quoted studies have shown quite consistently that oestrogen replacement alone is not effective in preventing bone loss in anorexia nervosa patients, bone density was at least maintained in the women during the time they were taking the oestrogen. It appears likely that other hormonal mechanisms are responsible for the low BMD in these women. Proper nutrition, restoration of weight, introduction of exercises, are probably all essential to increase BMD in these women.

Menstrual Dysfunction Induced by Physical Exercises and Relationship to BMD

Two important modifiable factors that can influence menstrual function and produce oligo/amenorrhoea are low energy intake and intensive physical training [37]. The well known female athlete triad is a syndrome consisting of disordered eating, amenorrhoea and osteoporosis, which in turn is well known for its association with osteoporosis [38] and an increased risk of stress fractures. Athletes with voluntary dieting and restricted calorie intake mimic the picture of young women with anorexia nervosa. In addition, they have high energy expenditures as a result of their physical exercises and thus can develop an imbalance of energy intake and output. Menstrual dysfunction in the form of amenorrhoea or oligomenorrhoea results as hypothalamic-pituitary-ovarian axis dysfunction occurs similar to patients with anorexia nervosa, and hypo-oestrogenism ensues with increased bone resorption and reductions on peak bone mass as in those with anorexia nervosa (Table 4). Similar to athletes, dancers also fit into the high risk category for the development of the athlete triad, with a relatively high incidence of eating disorders due to the need for aesthetic body shapes, regular physical training that by its nature involves intensive weight bearing exercises and the resulting high rates of menstrual dysfunction [39].

Table 4. Exercise Related Menstrual Dysfunction and relation to BMD changes

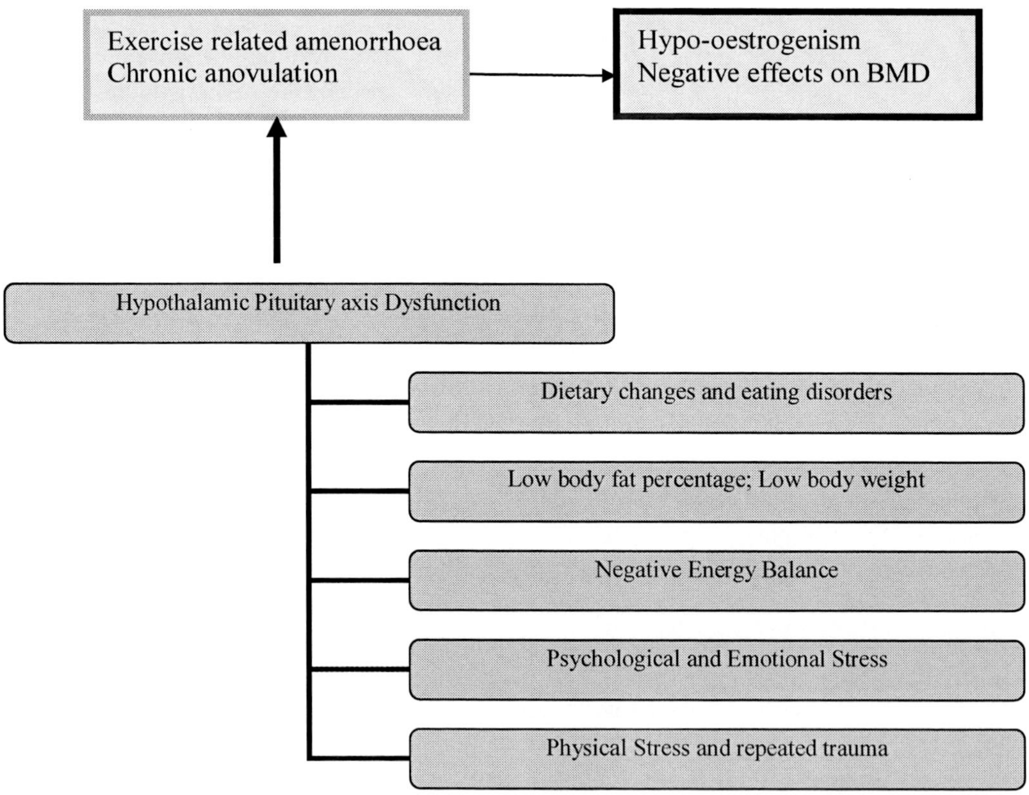

On the other hand, positive effects of mechanical loading via exercise on bone mineral density (BMD) have been well documented in humans. Weight bearing exercise is known to be an important contributor to the establishment of peak bone mass and to maintenance of bone mass after this peak is attained. It is commonly accepted that weight-bearing exercise provides an osteogenic stimulus to bones. The osteogenic stimulation of such activities could be seen in a variety of sports, such as athletics, weight lifting, high impact sports such as basketball or volley ball, medium impact sports such as soccer or track. On the contrary, this effect was not observed in sports activities that involved extensive energy expenditure and muscle strength but no true weight bearing, such as in swimming [40]. Studies have also shown that the benefits of exercise in promoting bone accrual and a higher peak bone mass are greatest before the completion of puberty. Participation in exercise and training before the onset of menses appears to increase BMD significantly more than when started after initiation of menses. A study of Canadian children showed that physically active girls had a 17 % higher total body BMD as compared to sedentary peers [40], while a retrospective study of young adult women showed that those who participated in high-school sports exhibited only a 7% increase in femoral neck BMD as compared to controls [41]. However, when hypo-oestrogenism occurs together with menstrual dysfunction resulting from excessive exercises, the benefits of the physical activity may be lost and the net effects of these opposing forces may be difficult to predict.

Healthy athletes have been shown to have better than average BMD, but amenorrhoeic athletes have been shown to have vertebral BMD some 9-31% lower than eumenorrhoeic ones. Stress fractures were significantly associated with a long duration of amenorrhoea in athletes [42]. In dancers, delayed menarche and prolonged amenorrhea was shown to be associated not only with increased risks of fractures, but also of scoliosis in these young women [43]. While it is still controversial whether low bone mineral density associated with prolonged hypo-estrogenic states are accountable for the increased incidence of scoliosis, the role of exercise in such amenorrhoeic states and the resulting impact on bone mineral density appears complex. A comparative study between young Chinese dancers and age matched non-athletic women that did not take into account menstrual status showed no difference in bone mineral density. The authors concluded that the dancers were significantly thinner than the controls and the negative effect of a lower bodyweight may neutralize the positive effects of the physical training, particularly in the femoral neck [44]. In contrast, a study on ballet dancers [38] has demonstrated significantly lower areal bone mass in young ballet dancers with exercise-associated amenorrhea and delayed menarche despite their intensive exercises, pointing to the importance of normal hormonal function on bone mineral density in these young individuals, and the inability for exercises to compensate for the detrimental effects of menstrual dysfunction on bone mineral density. On the other hand, when comparing bone mineral density in ballet dancers with aged-matched amenorrhoeic young women with anorexia nervosa, it has been found that weight-bearing exercise may off-set the effects of hypogonadism at predominantly cortical weight-bearing sites, while both non-weight bearing sites and weight bearing sites containing substantial amounts of trabecular bone, such as the lumbar spine, may still be adversely affected by the hypo-oestrogenism [45]. It appears therefore, that while exercise might have been able to offset some of the negative effects of hypo-oestrogenism on BMD, such protective effects could be incomplete.

In terms of therapy, weight gain and gradual resumption of menses with associated rises in endogenous oestrogen production are apparently the best approaches to increasing bone density in these underweight exercising females. However, the effect of oestrogen replacement in exercise-induced hypothalamic amenorrhoea still remains controversial. When oral contraceptives were given to a group of physically active women aged between 18-31 years, bone loss was still observed at the spine and hip [46]. Other studies, however, showed that cortical bone BMD responded favourably to oestrogen replacement, while supplementation with dietary calcium at a dose of 1200 mg per day appeared to be effective in minimizing bone loss in these women [1]. Thus, the available data on the effects of oral contraceptives in adolescents with exercise induced hypothalamic amenorrhoea appears to be conflicting, as is the effect of oral contraceptives on the BMD of healthy non-exercising women. It was speculated that endogenous gonadal oestrogen secretion was suppressed by the oral contraceptive, but the replacement dose administered was inadequate for achievement of peak bone mass [47]. In a prospective series, BMD increased by 2.33% over 1 year in healthy young women with a 35 ug ethinyl oestradiol norethindrone pill compared to a non-significant +0.33% increase in those on a 30 ug ethinyl oestradiol desogestrol pill, while the untreated group had a -0.37% BMD loss [48]. Further studies on the impact and dosage of oral contraceptive pills on the BMD in both exercising adolescents and non-exercising young women are indicated.

Comparison of BMD Density Differences in Exercising and Non-exercising Young Women

The responsiveness to either an increase or decrease in mechanical strain is probably greater in growing bones in adolescents than in adults, so that weight bearing exercises should still have an important impact on stimulating bone accrual in strategic weight bearing sites [40, 49] in young females as compared to older women. While most cross-sectional data support the benefits of exercise in children and adolescents, these findings were not consistent in all longitudinal studies relating bone mass to physical activity [50,51]. There is also doubt as to the extent the greater areal BMD gains in response to exercise could be translated into a commensurate increase in volumetric BMD increase or an increase in bone strength. In a cross sectional study comparing young eumenorrhoeic and oligo/amenorrhoeic dancers with non-dancing eumenorrhoeic controls (mean age 18 years), it was found that the lumbar spine and hip BMD values, and the tibial trabecular volumetric BMD values were significantly higher in the eumenorrhoeic dancers as compared to non-exercising controls. However, when oligo/amenorrhoeic dancers were compared to controls, such differences were no longer observed. It was concluded that young women undergoing regular intensive weight-bearing exercises have higher BMD in the axial and appendicular skeleton as compared to non-exercising females of similar age. The positive effects of exercise on BMD are apparently diminished if oligo/amenorrhoea occurred [39]. Similarly, a longitudinal study of a small group of adolescent gymnasts have also shown that despite lower body fat composition and weight, they were able to have enhanced BMD values over a period of three years as compared to controls [52]. Thus, it can be seen from such data that the majority of these young exercising women have been able to benefit from the physical training to enhance their bone mineral density accrual as compared to sedentary controls of the same age.

Data from other longitudinal studies have shown that during pubertal maturation, the accumulation rate of areal bone mineral density (BMD) as measured by dual energy X-ray absorptiometry at major sites of the axial skeleton such as the lumbar spine or the hip, increases by four to six fold over a 3 year period from 11 to 14 years in females [53]. The increase in BMD in the appendicular skeleton tend to be less marked, with only a twofold increase measured in the forearm [54] or midshaft of the femur [55]. From menarche onwards, the increase in BMD declines rapidly as peak bone mass is achieved any time before the end of the second decade to the early third decade, so that a large biological variability in the BMD values in both the axial and appendicular skeleton will exist by that time [56]. When the interval BMD changes of the axial and appendicular skeleton in a group of collegiate dance students undergoing intensive physical training over an 18 months interval were compared to non-exercising young females, it was found that the exercising group showed larger interval increments in lumbar spine BMD as well hip BMD values as compared to the controls, which had minimal increments. When the exercising group was subdivided into those that were eumenorrhoeic within the 18 month interval and those that were oligo/amenorrhoeic, the latter group showed significantly lower core (trabecular) BMD increments in the appendicular skeleton than those that remained eumenorrhoeic. It was apparent that these young women undergoing regular intensive weight-bearing exercises have higher BMD increments as compared to non-exercising females of the same age group, indicating that the stimulus of intensive weight bearing exercises could result in further bone accrual even in this age period of 17 -22 years when bone accrual would have decelerated to a very slow rate. However, the lower bone accrual at trabecular sites in the appendicular skeleton in oligo/amenorrhoeic dancers could be manifestations of chronic hypo-oestrogenism in these intensely exercising young females, attenuating the positive effects of physical exercises [57]. Similarly, sub-elite female adolescent runners have been shown not to suffer from any detrimental effect on bone accrual despite delayed pubertal development [52]. In addition, a longitudinal study of adolescent gymnasts have also shown that despite lower body fat composition and weight, they were able to have enhanced BMD values over a period of three years as compared to controls [58]. Again, it can be seen that despite the potential association of osteoporosis to oligo/amenorrhoea in young women undergoing intensive physical training, the majority of these young women have been able to benefit from such activity to enhance their bone mineral density accrual as compared to sedentary controls of the same age. Moreover, while the theoretical threat of the athlete triad and associated BMD loss has been repeatedly emphasized in earlier studies, recent data showed that true osteoporosis appears to be rare in these women, to the extent that it has been proposed that the criteria for athlete triad syndrome should be amended to use osteopenia rather than osteoporosis [59].

The long-term implications of lower BMD in these exercising females remains speculative. A review of available literature showed that some dancers continue to have an advantage of higher BMD in later life [60], particularly when they remained eumenorrhoeic during their training, while other studies showed no difference with non-exercising females [61]. While the general belief is that regular exercises should enhance bone health, the benefits of such physical training in the presence of menstrual dysfunction in later reproductive life or postmenopausal age remains to be evaluated.

Conclusion

The evidence from the literature confirmed the negative effects of menstrual dysfunction in certain forms of amenorrhoea and oligomenorrhoea on bone mineral density in young women, such as gonadal dysgenesis, anorexia nervosa, drug induced or idiopathic hypothalamic dysfunction. Polycystic ovary syndrome appears to have a protective effect on BMD despite the presence of menstrual dysfunction. The positive effects of physical exercises on BMD have been shown, particularly in major weight bearing sites as the hip or lumbar spine. The athletic triad syndrome and its association with osteopenia or osteoporosis has been implied in various forms of intensive physical training, but the positive benefits of exercise on bone density and peak bone mass apparently offset the detrimental effects of menstrual dysfunction to a large extent in many individuals. However, the available data cannot be linked directly to prediction of fracture risks for these young females, nor could be extrapolated to predict the incidence of postmenopausal osteoporosis or osteopenia in these women in later life.

References

[1] Weaver CM. Adolescence: the period of dramatic bone growth. *Endocrine* 2002; 17: 43-8.

[2] Recker RR, Deng HW. Role of genetics in osteoporosis. *Endocrine* 2002; 17: 55-66.

[3] Bryant RJ, Wastney ME, Martin BR *et al.* Racial differences in bone turnover and calcium metabolism in adolescent females. *J Clin Endocrinol Metab* 2003; 88: 1043-7.

[4] Gordon CM, Nelson LM. Amenorrhoea and bone health in adolescents and young women. *Curr Opin Obstet Gynecol* 2003; 15: 377-84.

[5] Harlow SD, Ephross SA. Epidemiology of menstruation and its relevance to women's health. *Epidemiologic Rev* 1995; 17: 256-286

[6] Gordon CM, Neinstein LS. Amenorrhoea. In: Neinstein LS, Editor. *Adolescent health care: a practical guide.* Fourth edition. Philadelphia: Lippincott, Williams and Wilkins; 2002; p973-93.

[7] Critchley HOD. In: Shaw RW, Soutter WP, Stanton SL, Editors. *Gynaecology* 3rd Edition. London: Churchill Livingstone; 2003; p 229-244.

[8] Hillard PA. Menstruation in young girls: a clinical perspective. *Obstet Gynecol* 2002; 99: 655-662.

[9] Treloar AE, Boynton RE, Behn BG, Brown BW. Variation of the human menstrual cycle through reproductive life. *Int J Fertil* 1967; 12: 77-126.

[10]Cumings SR, Nevitt MC, Browner WS, Stone K, Fox KM, Ensrud KE, Cauley J, Black D, Vogt TM. Risk factors for hip fracture in white women. *N Engl J Med* 1995; 332; 767-73.

[11]Arlot ME, Sornay-Rendu E, Garnero P Vey-Marty B, Delmas PD. Apparent pre- and post-menopausal bone loss evaluated by DXA at different skeletal sites in women: the OLEFY cohort. *J Bone Miner Res* 1997; 12: 683-90.

[12]Adams JE. Single and dual energy X ray absorptiometry. In: Genant HK, Gulielmi M, Jergas M (eds). *Bone densitometry and osteoporosis*. Berlin: Springer; 1998; p305-334.

[13]Laufer MR. Congenital absence of the vagina: in search of the perfect solution. When, and by what technique should a vagina be created? *Curr Opin Obstet Gynecol* 2002; 14:441-4.

[14]Sybert VP, McCauley E. Turner's syndrome. *N Engl J Med* 2004; 351: 1227-38.

[15]Morgan T. Turner syndrome: diagnosis and management. *Am Fam Physician* 2007; 76: 405-410

[16]Alzubaidi NH, Chapin HL, Vanderhoof VH, Calis KA, Nelson LM. Meeting the needs of young women with secondary amenorrhoea and spontaneous premature ovarian failure. *Obstet Gynecol* 2002; 99: 720-5.

[17]Conway GS. The impact and management of Turner's syndrome in adult life. *Baillieres Best Pract Res Clin Endocrinol Metab* 2002; 16: 243-261

[18]Cromer BA. Bone mineral density in adolescent and young adult women using injectable or oral contraception. *Curr Opin Obstet Gynecol* 2003; 15: 353-7.

[19]Cromer B, Blair J, Mahan J. A prospective comparison of bone density in adolescent girls receiving depot medroxyprogesterone acetate (Depoprovera), levonorgestrel (Norplant) or oral contraceptives. *J Pediatr* 1996; 129: 671-6.

[20]Vartej P, Poiana C, Vartej I. Effects of hyperprolactinemia on osteoporotic fracture risk in premenopausal women. *Gynecol Endocrinol* 2001; 15: 43-7.

[21]Van Hooff MH, Voorhorst FJ, Kaptein MB, Hirasing RA, Koppenaal C, Schoemaker J. Polycystic ovaries in adolescents and the relationship with menstrual cycle patterns, luteinizing hormone, androgens and insulin. *Fertility Steril* 2000; 74: 49-58.

[22]Gulekli B, Turhan NO, Senöz S, Kükner S, Oral H, Gökmen O. Endocrinological, ultrasonographic and clinical findings in adolescent and adult polycystic ovary patients; a comparative study. *Gynecol Endocrinol* 1993; 7: 273-7

[23]Zborowski JV, Cauley JA, Talbott EO, Guzick DS, Winters SJ. Bone mineral density, androgens and the polycystic ovary; the complex and controversial issue of androgenic influence in female bone. *J Clinical Endocrin Metab* 2000; 85: 3496-3506.

[24]Cresswell J, Fraser RB, Bruce C, Egger P, Phillips D, Barker DJ.Relationship between polycystic ovaries, body mass index and insulin resistance. *Acta Obstet Gynecol Scand* 2003; 82: 61-4.

[25]DiCarlo C, Shoham Z, MacDougall J, Patel A, Hall ML, Jacobs HS. Polycystic ovaries as a relative protective factor for bone mineral density loss in young women with amenorrhea. *Fertil Steril* 1992; 57: 314-9.

[26]To WWK, Wong MWN. A comparison of bone mineral density in oligomenorrhoeic adolescents with polycystic ovaries and normal ovaries. Gynecol Endocrin 2005; 20: 237-42.

[27]Gordon CM, Goodman E, Emans SJ, Grace E, Becker KA, Rosen CJ, Gundberg CM, LeBoff MS. Physiologic regulators of bone turnover in young women with anorexia nervosa. *J Pediatr* 2002; 141: 64-70.

[28]Grinspoon SK, Thomas L, Miller K, Herzog D, Klibanski A. Effects of recombinant human IGF-I and oral contraceptive administration on bone density in anorexia nervosa. *J Clin Endocrinol Metab* 2002; 87: 2883-91.

[29]Zumoff B, Walsh BT, Katz JL, Levin J, Rosenfeld RS, Kream J, Weiner H. Subnormal plasma dehydroepiandrosterone to cortisol ratio in anorexia nervosa: a second hormonal parameter of ontogenic regression. *J Clin Endocrinol Metab* 1983; 56: 668-71.

[30]Jagielska G, Wolanczyk T, Komender J, Tomaszewicz-Libudzic C, Przedlacki J, Ostrowski K. Bone mineral density in adolescent girls with anorexia nervosa: a cross sectional study. *Eur Child Adolesc Psychiatry* 2002; 11: 57-62.

[31]Audi L, Vargas DM, Gussinye M, Yesye D, Marti G, Carrascosa A. Clinical and biochemical determinants of bone metabolism and bone mass in adolescent female patients with anorexia nervosa. *Pediatr Res* 2002; 51: 497-504.

[32]Turner JM, Bulsara MK, McDermott BM, Byrne GC, Prince RL, Forbes DA. Predictors of low bone density in young adolescent females with anorexia nervosa and other dieting disorders. *Int J Eat Disord* 2001; 30: 245-51.

[33]Klibanski A, Biller BM, Schoenfield DA, Herzog DB, Saxe VC. The effects of oestrogen administration on trabecular bone loss in young women with anorexia nervosa. *J Clin Endocrinol Metab* 1995; 80: 898-904

[34]Munoz MT, Morande G, Garcia-Centenera JA, Hervas F, Pozo J, Argente J. The effects of estrogen administration on bone mineral density in adolescents with anorexia nervosa. *Eur J Endocrinol* 2002; 146: 45-50

[35]Golden NH, Lanzkowsky L, Schebendach J, Palestro CJ, Jacobson MS, Shenker IR. The effect of estrogen-progestin treatment on bone mineral density in anorexia nervosa. *J Adolesc Gynecol* 2002; 15: 135-143

[36]Gordon CM, Grace E, Emans SJ *et al.* Effects of oral dehydroepiandrosterone on bone density in young women with anorexia nervosa: a randomized trial. *J Clin Endocrinol Metab* 2002; 87: 4935-4941.

[37]Weimann E. Gender-related differences in elite gymnasts: the female athlete triad. *J Applied Physio* 2002; 92: 2146-52.

[38]Warren MP, Brooks-Gunn J, Fox RP, Holderness CC, Hyle EP, Hamilton WG. Osteopenia in exercise-associated amenorrhea using ballet dancers as a model: a longitudinal study. *J Clin Endocrin Metab* 2002: 3162-8.

[39]To WWK, Wong MWN, Lam IYL. Bone mineral density differences between adolescent dancers and non-exercising adolescent females. *J Pediatr Adolesc* Gynecol 2005; 18: 337-342.

[40]Emslander HC, Sinaki M, Muhs JM *et al.* Bone mass and muscle strength in female college athletes (runners and swimmers). *Mayo Clin Proc* 1998; 73: 1151-60.

[41]Bailey DA, McKay HA, Mirwald RL, Crocker PR, Faulkner RA. A six-year longitudinal study of the relationship of physical activity to bone mineral accrual in growing children: the University of Saskatchewan Bone Mineral Accrual study. *J Bone Miner Res* 1999; 14: 1672-9.

[42]Myburgh KH, Hutchins J, Fataar AB, Hough SF, Noakes TD. Low bone density is an etiologic factor for stress fractures in athletes. *Ann Intern Med* 1990; 113: 754-9.

[43]Warren MP, Brooks-Gunn J, Hamilton LH, Warren LF, Hamilton WG. Scoliosis and fractures in young ballet dancers; relation to delayed menarche and secondary amenorrhoea. *New Engl J Med* 1986; 314: 1348-50.

[44]Tsai SC, Hsu HC, Fong YC, Chiu CC, Kao A, Lee CC. Bone mineral density in young female Chinese dancers. *International Ortho* 2001; 25: 283-5.

[45]Young N, Formica C, Szmukler G, Seeman E. Bone density at weight-bearing and non-weight-bearing sites in ballet dancers: the effect of exercise, hypogonadism and body weight. *J Clin Endocrinol Metab* 1994; 78: 449-454.

[46]Burr DB, Yoshikawa T, Teegarden D, Lyle R, McCabe G, Weaver CM. Exercise and oral contraceptive use suppress the normal age-related increase in bone mass and strength of the femoral neck in women 18-31 years of age. *Bone* 2000; 20: 855-63.

[47]Polatti F, Perotti F, Filippa N, Gallina D, Nappi RE. Bone mass and long-term monophasic oral contraceptive treatment in young women. *Contraception* 1995; 51: 221-4.

[48]Berenson AB, Radecki CM, Grady JJ, Rickert VI, Thomas A. A prospective controlled study of the effects of hormonal contraception on bone mineral density. *Obstet Gynecol* 2001; 98: 576-82.

[49]Bass S, Pearce G, Bradney M, Hendrich E, Delmas PD, Harding A, Seeman E. Exercise before puberty may confer residual benefits in bone density in adulthood: studies in active prepubertal and retired female gymnasts. *J Bone Miner Res* 1998; 13: 500-7.

[50]Kroger H, Kotaniemi A, Kroger L, Alhava E. Development of bone mass and bone density of the spine and femoral neck: a prospective study of 65 children and adolescents. *Bone Miner* 1993; 23: 171-82.

[51]Bradney M, Pearce G, Naughton G, Sullivan C, Bass S, Beck T, Carlson J, Seeman E. Moderate exercise during growth in prepubertal boys: changes in bone mass, size, volumetric density and bone strength; a controlled prospective study. *J Bone Miner Res* 1998; 13:1814-21.

[52]Laing EM, Massoni JA, Nickols-Richardson SM, Modlesky CM, O'Connor JP, Lewis RD. A prospective study of bone mass and body composition in female adolescent gymnasts. *J Pediatr* 2002; 141: 211-6.

[53]Theintz G, Buchs B, Rizzoli R, Slosman D, Clavien H, Sizonenko PC, Bonjour JP. Longitudinal monitoring of bone mass accumulation in healthy adolescents: evidence for a marked reduction after 16 years of age at the levels of lumbar spine and femoral neck in female subjects. *J Clin Endocrinol Metab* 1992; 75: 1060-5.

[54]Glastre C, Braillon L, David P, Cochat P, Meunier PJ, Delmas PD. Measurement of bone mineral content of the lumbar spine by dual energy X-ray absorptiometry in normal children: correlation with growth parameters. *J Clin Endocrinol Metab* 1990; 70: 1330-3

[55]Bonjour JP, Theintz G, Buchs B, Solsman D, Rizzolo R. Critical years and stages of puberty for spinal and femoral bone mass accumulation during adolescence. *J Clin Endocrinol Metab* 1991; 73: 555-63.

[56]Hopper JL, Green RM, Nowson CA, Young D, Sherwin AJ, Kaymakci B, Larkins RG, Wark JD. Genetic, common environment, and individual specific components of variance for bone mineral density in 10-26 year-old females: a twin study. *Am J Epidemiol* 1998; 147: 17-29.

[57]MWN Wong, To WWK. Interval changes in bone mineral density in exercising young women with or without menstrual dysfunction – an 18-month longitudinal study. *HK J Gynecol Obstet Midwifery* 2006; 6: 16-23.

[58]Dyson K, Blimkie CJ, Davison KS, Webber CE, Adachi JD. Gymnastic training and bone density in pre-adolescent females. *Med Sci Sports Exerc* 1997; 29: 443-50.

[59]Khan KM, Liu-Ambrose T, Sran MM, Ashe MC, Donaldson MG, Wark JD. New criteria for female athlete triad syndrome? As osteoporosis is rare, should osteopenia be among the criteria for defining the female athlete triad syndrome? *Br J Sports Med* 2002; 36: 10-3.

[60]Keay N, Fogelman I, Blake G. Bone mineral density in professional female dancers. *Br J Sports Medicine* 1997; 31: 143-7.

[61]Khan KM, Green RM, Saul A, Bennell KL, Crichton KJ, Hopper JL, Wark JD. Retired elite female ballet dancers and non-athletic controls have similar bone mineral density at weight-bearing sites. *J Bone Miner Res* 1996; 11: 1566-74.

In: Osteoporosis: Etiology, Diagnosis and Treatment
Editors: Bilar E. Mattingly and Albert C. Pillare

ISBN 978-1-60692-397-9

Chapter 19

EXCESSIVE IRON ACCUMULATION: A NEW THERAPEUTIC TARGET OF POSTMENOPAUSAL OSTEOPOROSIS BY CHELATION

Gang Liu and Ping Men*

University of Utah, Salt Lake City, UT 84108, USA.

ABSTRACT

Postmenopausal osteoporosis is one of the most common diseases to confront elderly women. The disease is characterized by low bone mass and micro-architectural deterioration, hence resulting in increased fracture risk. In fact, this risk is greater than breast, cervical and endometrial cancer combined. Unfortunately, the exact causes of osteoporosis are not very clear although multifactorial pathology is recognized as contributors to development of the disease. Iron is ubiquitous in the human body and its homeostasis strictly relates to human health and wellbeing. What is observable in postmenopausal women, however, is the moderate, but significant, increase in stored body iron. This increase has been suggested as a risk factor of several chronic diseases such as atherosclerosis albeit with controversy. While the relationship between the moderate elevations of stored body iron and postmenopausal osteoporosis has been rarely explored, in this chapter we have provided evidence that iron concentrations increase in osteoporotic and osteopenic bones of postmenopausal women and estrogen-deficient animals, respectively. Importantly, we have also shown that iron reduction in bone through chelation therapy mitigates the osteopenic development in estrogen-deficient rats. These strongly suggest that iron buildup plays a causal role in the development of postmenopausal osteoporosis, thus providing novel preventive and therapeutic strategies.

---

* Correspondence concerning this article should be addressed to: Gang Liu and Ping Men, Department of Radiology, School of Medicine, University of Utah, 729 Arapeen Dr. Suite 2334, Salt Lake City, UT 84108, USA. Tel: 801-581-3429. Fax: 801-581-7008.

Moreover, the evidence may further help raise awareness about iron nutrition, iron supplements and Western diets that may be associated with excessive iron accumulation, and thereby increase the risks of postmenopausal and senile osteoporosis.

Introduction

Postmenopausal osteoporosis is a more dangerous disease than previously thought and is one of the most common diseases in older women. Osteoporosis means porous bone, reflecting the loss of bone density and strength, which increase fracture risk. The fractures in postmenopausal women are a major cause of disability, mortality and economic burden [1].

In the United States alone, 10 million people have osteoporosis and millions more have low bone mass, placing them at increased risk for more serious bone loss and subsequent fractures. Among them, 80 percent are women [2] and their lifetime risk of osteoporotic hip fractures is greater than breast, cervical and endometrial cancer combined [1,3]. In fact, the risk of dying from the fractures alone (about 20% of all osteoporotic fractures) is the same as that of dying from breast cancer [1,3]. Although several FDA (U.S. Food and Drug Administration) approved medications can help stop or slow bone loss, or help form new bone and reduce the risk of fracture, there is still no cure for osteoporosis [2]. With the aging of people worldwide, the number of people with osteoporotic fractures will increase exponentially [4]. Obviously, there is a great need to further uncover the exact causes of postmenopausal osteoporosis and thereby to develop more effective drugs to combat the disease.

In this review, evidence has been provided to show the possibly causal role of skeletal iron accumulation in the development of postmenopausal osteoporosis. Consequently, a potential therapeutic approach has been outlined for preventing the disease with bone-targeted chelation. The chelation therapy may also have an impact on osteoporosis related to iron overload diseases as well as to aging-iron accumulation in males.

Iron Accumulation and Bone Loss

Postmenopausal osteoporosis has a subtle progression and its causes remain obscure although the etiology is believed to be multifactorial, including genetic, endocrine, exercise, life-style, and aging components [5,6]. Nutrition also plays an important role in the development of osteoporosis [7,8]. Iron is an essential nutrient for virtually all mammalian cells, but it is a double-edged sword. Excessive iron is toxic, which can lead to cellular dysfunction due mainly to being a powerful catalyst for the generation of highly toxic free radicals. These radicals are able to damage all molecular classes including cellular lipids, nucleic acids, proteins and carbohydrates [9].

Indeed, it is recognized that excessive iron in the body increases the risk for a considerable array of diseases such as arthropathy, cardiomyopath, endocrine, infection, neoplasia and neurodegeneration [10,11]. Recent studies have also linked osteoporosis with iron loading conditions by showing that patients with primary and secondary iron overload diseases have a high incidence of osteopenia and osteoporosis [12,13]. It has been found that iron accumulation in the bone microenvironment is toxic to bone remodeling [12]. For example, the deposits of iron are associated with impaired bone formation and increased bone resorption in a secondary iron overload animal model [14]. Additionally, decreases in osteoblast formation and new bone synthesis are observed in iron-loaded animals, in which the iron levels are at the same magnitude as in untreated primary iron overload patients [15]. Clinical investigations have revealed that more than half of HFE-related hemochromatotic (primary iron overload) patients have osteopenia and 34% osteoporosis [16]. Among thalassemic (secondary iron overload) patients with regular transfusions, 41% patients suffer osteoporosis [17]. The rates of osteopenia and osteoporosis are also high in other primary and secondary iron overload patients such as sickle cell anemia and African siderosis [18,19]. Taken together, there is little doubt that the excessive iron plays a key role in bone loss.

It is important to know that because of the lack of a major mechanism of iron excretion in the human body, iron can also accumulate in tissues with aging [20]. Stored body iron as reflected by serum ferritin (SF) concentrations increases rapidly after menopause in women and adolescence in men [21]. The increase continues with age and the iron stores appear to plateau about the sixth decade of life [21]. In postmenopausal women, the average level of stored body iron is about 106 ng/mL, more than twice that in pre-menopausal women at about 43 ng/mL [22]. In adult men, the average concentration of SF is about 121 ng/mL while for males of 5 to 19 years of age it is about 20 to 30 ng/mL [23]. These age-associated iron increases are considered to be moderate compared to the pathological forms of primary and secondary iron overload, with which SF concentrations are more than 300 ng/mL and 200 ng/mL for men and women, respectively [22,23]. However, these increases are still, albeit controversial [24], suggested as risk factors for several chronic diseases such as atherosclerosis [25], cancer [26], diabetes [27], and metabolic disorders associated with the insulin resistance syndrome [28].

Furthermore, our recent studies have found that iron accumulates in severely porous bones of postmenopausal women. Human female bones are examined using an electron paramagnetic resonance (EPR) spectrometer for measurement of free iron [29] followed by Inductively Coupled Plasma-Optical Emission Spectroscopy (ICP-OES) evaluation of total iron [30] (Table 1). The results have shown that both free and total iron contents in bones of three postmenopausal women (one 84 and two 92 years old) with severe bone porosity are significantly higher than that of age-matched bone samples (82, 86 and 90 years old) without severe bone porosity. Also, our studies have revealed that iron concentrations in bones of ovariectomized (OVX) rats increase significantly compared with sham control animals [29,31,32]. The free iron contents in cortical bones of OVX rats measured by EPR are found to be an average of 22.2% (t-test, $p < 0.01$) higher than that of sham controls. These results are consistent with human female bone studies and suggest an association of increased iron content in bones with the development of osteopenia in the OVX model. OVX rats have long been used as a preclinical animal model for investigation of estrogen-deficiency bone loss (postmenopausal osteoporosis) [33].

Osteoporosis is common in postmenopausal women and, in general, iron stores are elevated in this population. However, the relationship between iron accumulation and postmenopausal osteoporosis has rarely been explored. To answer the question of whether the increased iron stores play a causal role in the disease's development or whether this increase is just a consequence of the bone loss, several studies have been conducted. In these studies, a bone-targeted iron chelator has been used to treat OVX animals. The working hypothesis is that if the chelator could deplete iron in the bone of OVX rats and prevent bone loss, iron should be considered as one of culprits for the disease. Importantly, the investigations could lead to a new therapeutic approach to prevent and treat postmenopausal osteoporosis by use of chelation to remove excessive iron from bone.

Table 1. Iron concentrations in human female bones

Samples (number)	Free Iron (a.u.)	Total Iron (ppm)
Bones with severe porosity (3)	510.5 ± 87.2 [a]	25.8 ± 5.6 [a]
Age matched controls (3)	254.7 ± 25.4	6.5 ± 2.3

Mean ± SE. [a] Significantly different from controls, $p < 0.05$.

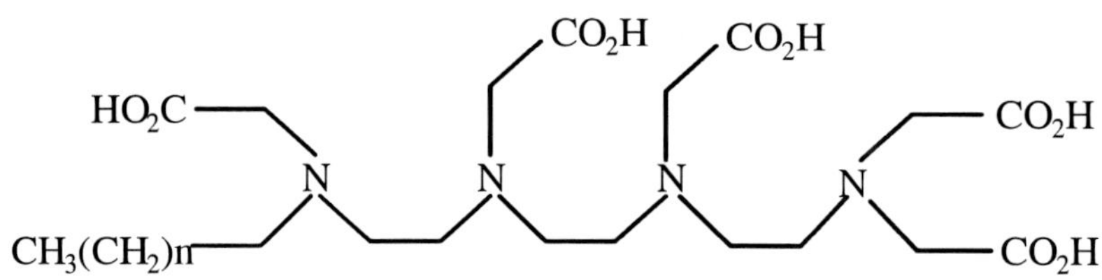

Figure 1. The chemical structure of DoTTPA, an amphiphilic chelator (n = 1920).

Iron Chelation and Bone Protection

1. Bone Targeted Chelator and OVX Rat Model

The chelator used in the studies is 1-N-docosyltriethylenetetraminepentaacetic acid (DoTTPA), an analogue of polyamino polycarboxylic acids (PAPCA) such as disodium ethylenediaminetetraacetic acid (EDTA) and diethylenetriaminepentaacetic acid (DTPA). They are two widely used metal chelation agents for various biomedical applications. The structural difference of DoTTPA from PAPCA is that DoTTPA has a long alkyl chain on the nitrogen atom at position 1 (Figure 1). The addition of the alkyl chain changes the hydrophilic parent chelator, triethylenetetraminehexaacetic acid (TTHA) into an amphiphilic one by assembling together the chelation moiety as a hydrophilic head and fatty chain as a lipophilic tail. Although the alkyl chain shows some hindering effects on metal binding, DoTTPA still retains high metal binding affinity similar to its parent chelator (TTHA) [34]. The chelator has also shown the ability to effectively deplete some metals such as iron, americium and plutonium from skeletal and soft tissues in experimental studies [31,32,35,36]. Interestingly, the chelator possesses oral bioavailability, even though it is highly charged with a molecular weight of 744. A possible explanation is that the chelator may form micelles due to its amphiphilic property, thus increasing intestinal absorption and bone marrow macrophage uptake [35]. The OVX rats have been used to test our hypothesis because they represent themselves as an established preclinical model for postmenopausal bone loss and show the increased iron concentration in bones. Thus, the chelator and OVX rat model provide us with valuable tools to accomplish our studies.

2. Experimental Procedures

Animal treatment: In the studies [31,32], female Sprague-Dawley rats, 3 months of age (Charles River Laboratory, Wilmington, MA, USA) were housed with 12-hour light-dark cycles at constant room temperature (24°C) and humidity. The rats were fed standard rat chow (#8640; Harland Teklad, Madison, WI, USA) and water *ad libitum*. At 6 months of age, the rats were randomly divided into four groups of six rats each. One group was sacrificed as baseline controls at the beginning of the experiment. The remaining groups were sham operated (one group) or bilaterally OVX (two groups) *via* a dorsal approach. Chelation treatment started from the second day after surgery and was given three times a week for 9 weeks. The chelator was dissolved in saline (pH 7.5) and administered through oral gavage (100 µmole/kg). The control groups, including the sham and OVX-operated rats, received the vehicle solution in the same manner. During the chelation treatment, fluorochrome bone markers of calcein (fluorescein-methylene-iminodiacetic acid, 10 mg/kg body weight) and tetracycline-HCl (25 mg/kg body weight) from Sigma Chemical Co., were given by intraperitoneal injections on 10 and 3 days, respectively, prior to necropsy for later evaluation of bone dynamics by histomorphometry. The rats were anesthetized and sacrificed by cardiac puncture and then the humerii and lumbar vertebrae were collected. The experiment was approved by the Institutional Animal Care and Use Committee (University of Utah, Salt Lake City, UT, USA).

Tissue preparation and analyses: After harvest, humeral bone samples were fixed in 70% ethanol for measurements of iron and long-lived organic free radicals (LLOFR) by EPR spectrometer. Lumbar vertebrae were first fixed in 10% phosphate buffered formalin for 24 hours, then dehydrated in ascending concentrations of ethanol and embedded in methyl methacrylate. The blocks were trimmed for peripheral computed tomography (pQCT), micro-computed tomography (Micro-CT) and later prepared for histomorphometric studies.

pQCT densitometry: The third vertebral bodies were examined by pQCT densitometry (Norland Stratec XCT 960A) to determine bone mineral density (BMD) for the part from the middle point to caudal end excluding the primary spongiosa. A scout scan of the vertebra was performed. On the scout view, a reference line was set such that the cross-sectional slices passed through at a distance of 1, 2, 3 and 4 mm from the caudal end of the vertebra body. The voxel size was 196 mm. The contour-mode 2, peel-mode 20, cortical-mode 2 and threshold 570 for cortical bone were chosen for the analysis. The mean BMD for all of the measured slices was then calculated.

Micro-CT measurement: Lumbar vertebrae were scanned using a desktop Micro-CT (µCT-40, Scanco Medical) with a resolution of 10 µm in all three spatial dimensions. The complete third vertebral bodies were scanned with 600 slices, each slice containing 2048 X 2048 pixels. The trabecular and the cortical part of the bodies were separated with semi-automatically drawn contours. The resulting gray-scale images were segmented using a low-pass filter to remove noise, and a fixed threshold to extract the mineralized bone phase. From the binary images, structural indices were assessed with three-dimensional techniques without model-assumptions of the appearance of trabecular bone and were calculated by measuring 3-dimensional distances directly in the trabecular network, and taking the mean over all voxels. The region of interest was trabecular bone in the lumbar vertebral body excluding the primary spongiosa area, 0.5 mm from the growth plate [37].

Histomorphometric measurement: The third vertebral bodies were cut with a precision bone saw (Isomet, Buehler), the sections mounted on plastic slides and ground to about 30 μm in thickness. The sections were left unstained for viewing of the fluorochrome markers. The cancellous bone in one lumbar vertebra from each animal was quantified. The primary histomorphometric indices collected were total bone surface, double-labeled surface, interlabel width and eroded surface. From these, the secondary indices were calculated and included percent of double-labeled surface, corrected mineral apposition rate, bone formation rate and percent of eroded surface. The histomorphometric nomenclature conforms with recommendations [38].

EPR Measurements of iron and LLOFR: The EPR measurement of bone samples was done using modifications of the procedures for alanine and enamel [39,40]. The procedure used a constant rotation goniometer to average out anisotropies, empty EPR tube background subtraction and a manganese standard for accurately aligning the spectra. The spectrometer used was a Bruker 300E (Bruker BioSciences Corp., Billerica, MA, USA). The EPR instrument parameters for iron and LLOFR measurements were 25 mW microwave power, 10 mT magnetic field scan width, 0.5 mT magnetic field modulation amplitude, 10^5 receiver gain, 41 msec. conversion time, 41 msec. time constant, 9.77 GHz microwave frequency and 30 scans. The experimental procedure consisted of taking about 100 mg of bone sample with measurements conducted at room temperature. The EPR signals at $g = 2$ were deconvoluted into their component parts (Figure 2) using the Levenberg-Marquardt method [41,42]. Further details have been described elsewhere [29].

Chelator synthesis: The synthesis of DoTTPA was described previously [34-36]. Briefly, excessive triethylenetetramine reacted with 1-docosyl bromide in order to conjugate a single docosyl group to the triethylenetetramine through a primary amino group (yield about 72%). Then, exhaustive carboxymethylation of the remaining amino groups was conducted using 2-bromoacetic acid (yield about 75%). The pure chelator was obtained after repeated recrystallization with a mixture of acetic acid, methanol and water. The chelator was characterized and its chemical structure confirmed using ^{1}H- and ^{13}C-NMR and mass spectrometry. All chemicals were purchased from Aldrich and used without further purification.

Statistical methods: Results are expressed as the mean ± standard error (SE). Data were analyzed using analysis of variance (ANOVA) followed by a *post hoc* test (Fisher's protected least significant difference, PLSD) or Student's *t* test. A 0.1%, 1.0% or 5.0% significance level was used and differences were considered significant at $p < 0.05$. The Statview Statistical Package (Abacus Concepts, Inc., Berkeley, CA, USA) was used for data analyses.

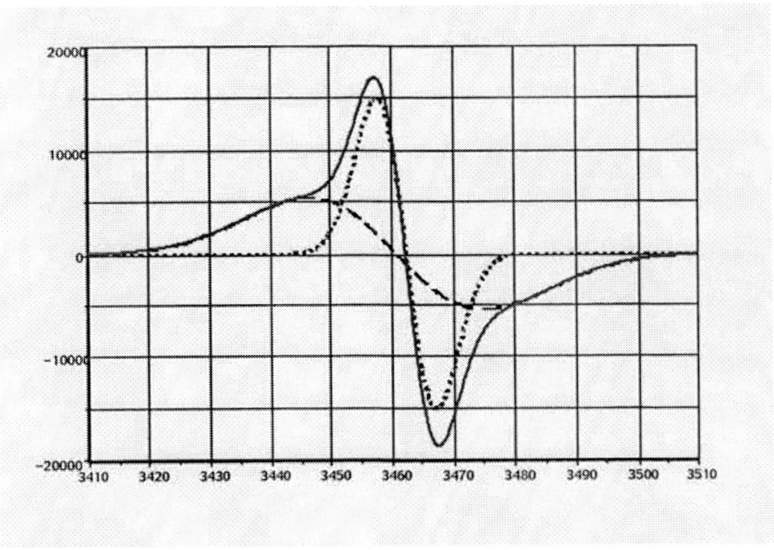

Figure 2. The bone native signal (a solid line) measured by EPR, which is deconvoluted into free iron (dashed line) and LLOFR (dotted line) components. Modification with permission from reference 31.

3. Experimental Results and Discussion

Iron decrease by chelation: As expected, after nine weeks of chelation treatment, the iron content in bones of chelator-treated OVX rats was only 59.8% (t-test, $p < 0.01$) of that of untreated OVX rats, and was 73.0% (t-test, $p < 0.01$) of that of sham controls. These results show that chelation therapy can slow or perhaps even reverse the accumulation of iron in bones of both OVX and normally aging rats. Most significantly, however, the reduction of bone iron in the OVX rats by chelation treatment slowed the development of bone loss. This was demonstrated by measuring BMD with pQCT and bone microstructure with Micro-CT.

BMD protection with iron depletion: Because cancellous bone is more susceptible to osteopenia caused by estrogen deficiency, we have chosen first to measure the BMD in the cancellous bone of the vertebra (Figure 3). The result showed that the average cancellous BMD of chelator-treated OVX rats was significantly greater (12.4%) than that of untreated OVX rats. The average cancellous BMD of untreated OVX rats was 21.6% less than that of sham controls; while the BMD of the chelator-treated OVX rats was just 11.9% less than the sham control. This study suggests that iron chelation treatment slows the loss of cancellous bone mass in estrogen-deficient rats by reducing skeletal iron accumulation.

Bone microstructures protected by chelator: The structure of the cancellous bone was also examined using the Micro-CT and the derived morphological measurements. The ratio of bone volume to tissue volume (BV/TV) in the chelator-treated OVX rats was significantly higher (9.1%) than that of untreated OVX rats, which indicated more trabecular bone mass in the chelator-treated OVX rats (Figure 4A). At the same time, the trabecular separation (Tr. Sp.) was significantly less (10.2%) in the chelator-treated OVX rats compared with the untreated OVX controls (Figure 4B). These results show that iron chelation treatment also slows micro-architectural deterioration of cancellous bone following OVX. The increased trabecular bone volume and decreased trabecular separation are evident in the Micro-CT images (Figure 5) of the chelator-treated OVX rats compared with their untreated controls. These results clearly demonstrate a bone preserving action of iron chelation in a model of estrogen deficiency.

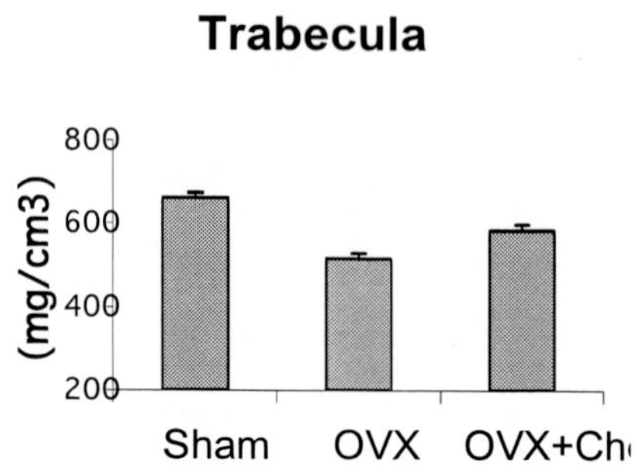

Figure 3. Trabecular BMD of lumbar vertebrae. The BMD of OVX+Chel and Sham groups are significantly higher than that of OVX group with ANOVA ($p < 0.01$) and the BMD of Sham group is also significantly higher than that of OVX+Chel group ($p < 0.01$ by ANOVA). Each group contains 6 rats. All values are expressed as means ± SE. Modification with permission from reference 32.

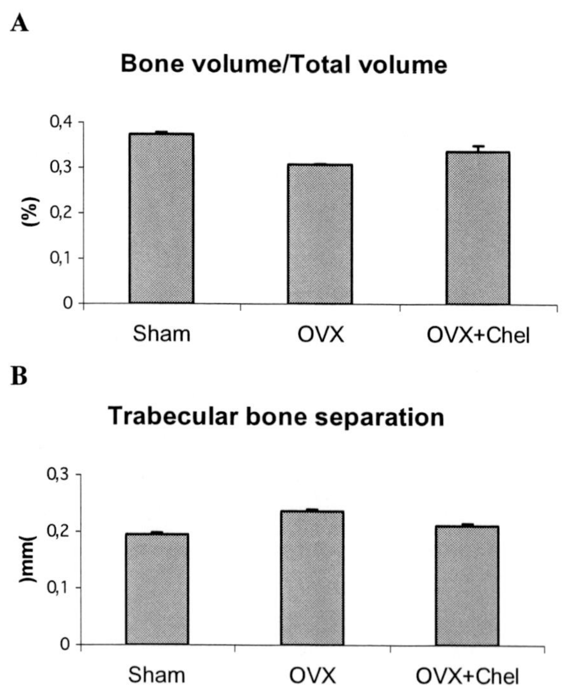

Figure 4. Bone morphological indices of lumbar vertebrae from groups of OVX, OVX+Chel and Sham rats (n = 6 per group). (A) Trabecular bone volume/Total volume measurements are significantly different between the three groups with $p < 0.05$ by ANOVA. (B) Trabecular bone separation measurements are also significantly different between the three groups with $p < 0.01$ by ANOVA. All values are expressed as means ± SE. Modification with permission from reference 32.

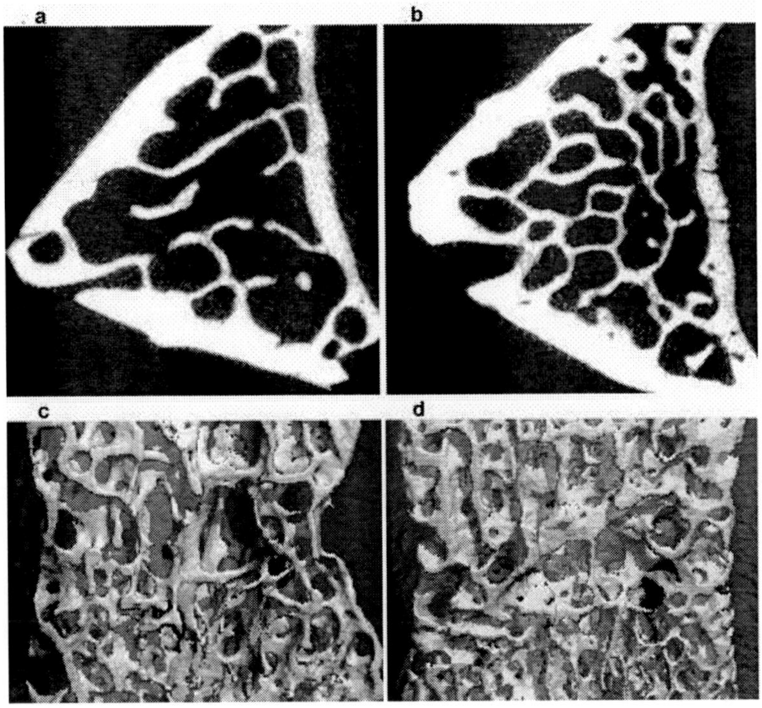

Figure 5. Micro-CT images of lumbar vertebrae from OVX and OVX+Chel rats. Two-dimensional axial slice (a) OVX and (b) OVX+Chel, and three-dimensional reconstruction images (c) OVX and (d) OVX+Chel. The images show the micro-architectural differences between the groups. Permission from reference 32.

Reduced bone resorption and possible bone formation by chelation: As mentioned before, in models of iron overload, iron deposits in the bone microenvironment have been associated with impaired bone formation and increased bone resorption [14]. The suppression of bone formation with the stimulation of bone resorption would result in the development of osteopenia. Thus, it is predictable that iron chelation to prevent or deplete iron accumulation in bone would reverse some of these putative effects of excessive iron on skeletal metabolism. The histomorphometric data showed that the resorption (eroded) surface in the cancellous bone of the chelator-treated OVX rats was about 48% less than that in the untreated OVX rats (Figure 6). There was also a trend ($p > 0.05$ but < 0.1) for a greater cancellous bone formation rate in the chelator-treated animals than in the respective controls. Thus these histomorphometric findings provide a reasonable explanation for the effects of iron reduction on the mitigation of the development of osteopenia in the OVX rat model.

These results indicate that the age-associated iron accumulation in bones of OVX rats plays a significant role in the development of bone loss related to estrogen deficiency. Limiting and/or reducing the free iron concentrations in bone by iron chelation lead to a significant retention of bone mass and a slowing of the deterioration of bone structure. The skeletal protection associated with iron reduction is due to a significant reduction in bone resorption and perhaps maintenance or even an increase in bone formation after ovariectomy.

Additional evidence: Importantly, the effects of chelation on preventing bone loss have also been demonstrated by clinical studies. For example, a clinical investigation examined the effect of EDTA on bone density. Patients with osteoporosis were given EDTA intravenously and bone densitometry reading was measured. The result shows that over the course of EDTA treatment, there is a significant increase in the bone density level from pretest to posttest [43]. With the intravenous EDTA treatment, no adverse effects have been observed [43]. Interestingly, another study has found that women after menopause have higher BMD in population with a habit to drink tea than that of non-tea drinkers [44]. A possible explanation is that (-)-epigallocatechin-3-gallate, a component of the tea is an iron chelator, which has the ability to stimulate mineralization of murine bone marrow mesenchymal cells [44]. Accumulating studies also suggest that lactoferrin, an iron chelation protein for iron scavenging may play an anabolic role in the bone remodeling process by maintaining iron balance [12].

Taken together, these studies provide new insights into pathogenesis of postmenopausal osteoporosis and may lead to novel therapeutic approaches for the disease. However, the possibility that the chelation may also have metabolic effects other than metal chelation should not be excluded.

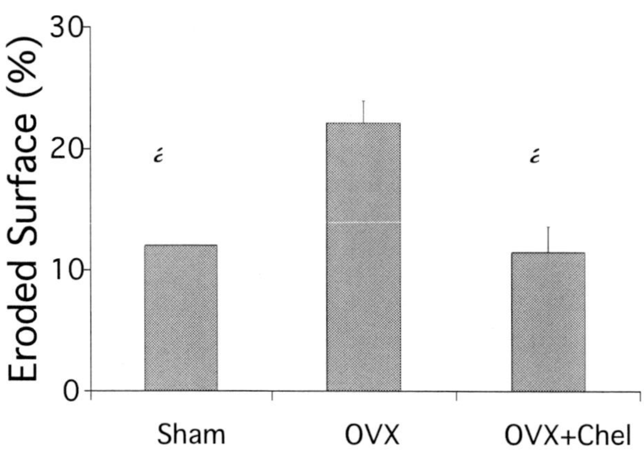

Figure 6. Dynamic bone histomorphometry shows that eroded surfaces (%) of OVX+Chel and Sham groups are significantly lower than that of OVX group with ANOVA (0.1% significance level, $^{a}p <$ 0.0007). There are no significant differences in eroded surface between OVX+Chel and Sham groups. Each group contains 6 animals and all values are expressed as means ± SE. Modification with permission from reference 32.

Iron Associated Oxidation and Osteoporosis

It is believed that an increase in iron content is associated with an increased likelihood of oxidative damage, therefore questions are raised as to whether the iron accumulated in skeletal tissue causes the free radical oxidative damage and consequent bone loss. Indeed, our studies have indicated that there is an increased oxidative level, reflected by LLOFR that is stable in solid matrices [45], in the bones of OVX rats and elderly people with severe bone porosity compared with respective controls [29]. In these bones, iron concentrations are also increased as mentioned above. Additionally, prevention of iron accumulation in the bone of OVX rats by iron chelation treatment has been shown to mitigate osteopenic development

[31,32]. These observations point out a possible link between increased iron content, oxidative damage and bone loss. Here, further evidence is provided to demonstrate the possible mechanism underlying the pathological role of iron associated oxidation in postmenopausal osteoporosis.

To examine the relationship between iron and oxidative damage, and the link of oxidative damage with bone loss, a similar study as aforementioned has been performed using DoTTPA to treatment OVX rats. In the study, EPR technique has been used for measuring both free iron contents and LLOFR levels in the bone.

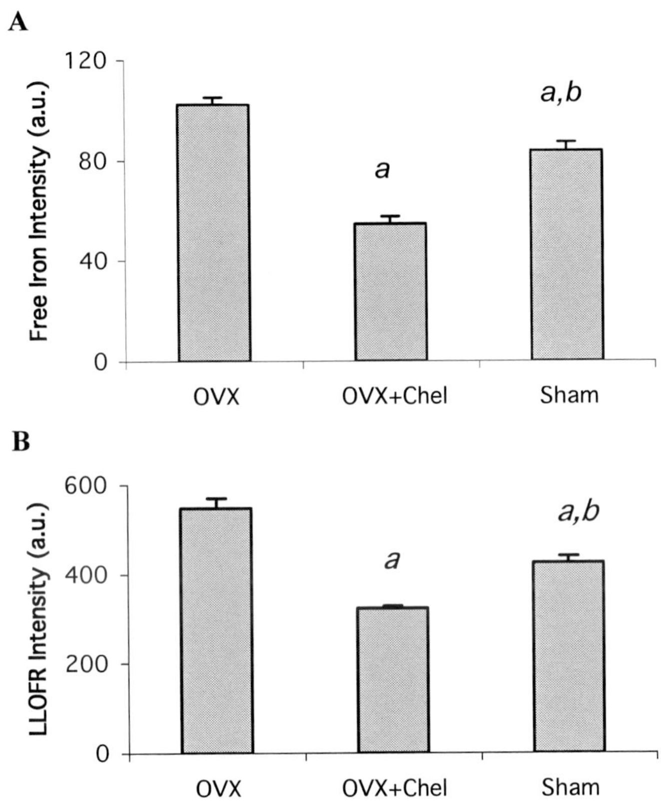

Figure 7. Free iron and LLOFR contents expressed in arbitary units in the bone of OVX, OVX-chelator-treated and Sham-treated rats (n = 6 per group). (A) Iron contents in bone samples. Mean ± SE. [a] Significantly different from OVX, $p < 0.0001$. [b] Significantly different from OVX+Chel, $p < 0.0005$. (B) LLOFR contents in bone samples. Mean ± SE. [a] Significantly different from OVX and Sham, $p < 0.0001$. [b] Significantly different from OVX, $p < 0.001$. Modification with permission from reference 31.

After chelation treatment, the iron and LLOFR contents of the bone have been measured and the results are presented in Figures 7A and B. The mean values for iron and LLOFR levels in the bone of OVX rats are significantly higher (22.1 and 29.2%, respectively) than that of sham controls, indicating that elevated levels of iron and LLOFR follow estrogen deficiency. In contrast, however, chelator-treated OVX rats had significantly less iron and LLOFR contents in the bone than that of untreated OVX rats (46.2% less for iron and 41.0% less for LLOFR), and were 34.3 and 23.8% less, respectively, than that of the sham control. It would appear that increased iron in the bone is associated with the increase of LLOFR and also that iron is a key factor in LLOFR formation because the LLOFR formation can be inhibited by iron chelation. The LLOFR content is positively proportional to iron levels in the bone and the relationship is shown in Figure 8. The decrease in LLOFR in the bones of chelator-treated OVX rats leads to higher BMD and better bone microstructure than that of untreated OVX controls, which are consistent with previous studies.

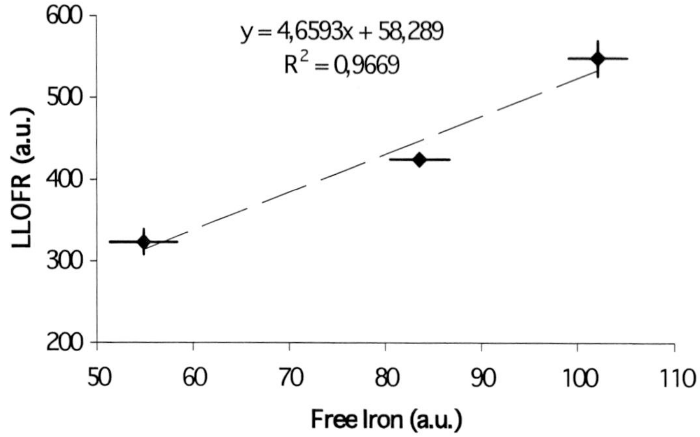

Figure 8. The relationship between free iron and LLOFR in the bone of OVX, OVX-chelator-treated and sham-treated rats (each point represents 6 animals). Modification with permission from reference 31.

It is important to mention that no obvious signs of toxicity associated with the chelation treatment have been found during the experiments. There are no significant differences in the net weight gains between the OVX-chelator-treated and OVX control rats. Also, there are no obvious abnormal changes in organs observed at necropsy. These results show evidence for the safety and tolerability of DoTTPA when administered in a manner that would be used for the chronic treatment of bone loss related to aging or iron overload. Our preliminary studies in vitro are consistent with these results. The toxic profiles of chelators may further be improved by using their zinc salt formulations [46].

Accumulating evidence supports that there is a link between oxidative damage and bone loss. An interesting study shows that lipoxygenase plays a role in bone development and pharmacologic inhibitors of these enzymes improve bone density and strength in animal models of osteoporosis [6]. Lipoxygenases (LOXs) are a family of non-heme iron-containing enzymes that catalyze the dioxygenation of polyunsaturated fatty acids in the biosynthesis of leukotrienes. Leukotrienes have been recognized to be responsible for the effects on an inflammatory response. Besides, the biosynthesis to leukotrienes involves the formation of hydroperoxyl intermediates that can produce highly toxic lipidoxy and lipidperoxy radicals with iron as catalyst [9]. Thus, an inhibition of the lipoxygenases by chelation of its non-heme bound iron [47-50] and/or chelation reduction of iron concentration [31,32,43] merit further investigation as promising therapies for osteoporosis. Evidence also shows that lipids have been found to accumulate in bone of animals and their oxidized products promote bone resorption [51]. Lipids are very susceptible to lipid peroxidation through an autocatalytic chemical chain reaction that can be initiated by iron [52]. Iron appears to be involved with the production of free radicals by tartrate-resistant acid phosphatase (TRAP) that has a redox-active iron center [53]. TRAP is highly expressed in osteoclasts and is an established marker of bone resorption. It is interesting to know that some medications for osteoporosis are strong chelators such as bisphosphonates [54] or antioxidants including estrogen and calcitonin [55,56]. Obviously, chelation, antioxidation or their combination may provide therapeutic effects on osteoporosis.

Although accumulating studies strongly support that chelation is able to prevent bone loss by inhibiting iron associated oxidation in bones, other studies also point out several possible mechanisms underlying the role of natural and synthetic chelation agents in protecting bones. For example, EDTA treatment with osteoporotic patients shows the therapeutic effect by increasing bone density. Although the possible mechanism of EDTA to improve bone structure is controversial, it is suggested that EDTA may stimulate the parathyroid hormone (PTH) secretion by causing transient calcium deficiency because of complexing of EDTA with calcium in blood and then excretion of the complex from kidneys [43]. Therefore, this calcium decrease leads to the increase in PTH, which results in two consequences: releasing calcium from bone (adverse effect: bone resorption) and converting preosteoblasts into osteoblasts (positive effect: bone formation) [43,57]. The total effect in bone should be anabolic because the study shows the increased level of bone density in the patients, which is also demonstrated by our chelation study with OVX rats. It is worth mentioning that PTH increases active reabsorption of calcium from kidneys [58,59] and enhances the absorption of calcium in the intestine by increasing activated vitamin D [60]. In addition, EDTA is a strong chelator for iron [61] and the interaction of EDTA with iron may provide protective effects on bone. Moreover, desferrioxamine (DFO) and (-)-epigallocatechin-3-gallate, two natural iron chelators, have been observed to increase osteogenesis in mesenchymal stem cells possibly due to activating beta-catenin signaling [62] and stimulating mineralization [44], respectively. Lactoferrin has also been found being a possible regulator of bone growth [63], and studies have revealed that lactoferrin has the ability to inhibit bone resorption activity [64,65], to reduce apoptosis and to increase osteoblast proliferation [65,66].

Conclusion

These studies suggest that iron accumulates in the body as it ages and the increased iron levels lead to postmenopausal osteoporosis due probably to iron-mediated free radical damage. Significantly, iron reduction by chelation shows a novel therapeutic opportunity to treat postmenopausal osteoporosis. This approach may also have the potential to treat senile osteoporosis and iron overload bone loss. Our findings may further help raise awareness about iron nutrition, iron supplements and Western diets, which may be associated with excessive iron and less antioxidant intakes, and thereby increase the risks of skeletal disease. Moreover, these studies add further support to the somewhat controversial theory that age-associated iron accumulation and iron-associated oxidative damage in organs increase the risk of diseases. Most importantly, our finding results may lead to new therapeutic approaches to address a number of aging diseases that are or may be related to iron.

ACKNOWLEDGMENT

The authors are very grateful for the financial support from the National Institutes of Health (NIA).

REFERENCES

[1] Cummings, SR; Melton, LJ III. Epidemiology and outcomes of osteoporotic fractures. *Lancet*. 2002 (359). 1761-7.
[2] National Institute of Arthritis and Musculoskeletal and Skin (NIAMS). Osteoporosis. (www.niams.nih.gov/Health_Info/Bone/Osteoporosis/default.asp). Dec. 2007.
[3] Seidman, H; Mushinski, MH; Gelb, SK; Silverberg; E. Probabilities of eventually developing or dying of cancer--United States. *CA Cancer J Clin*. 1985 (35). 36-56.
[4] Cooper, C; Campion, G; Melton, LJ 3rd. Hip fractures in the elderly: a world-wide projection. *Osteoporos Int*. 1992 (2). 285-9.
[5] Raisz, LG; Rodan, GA. Pathogenesis of osteoporosis. *Endocrinol Metab Clin North Am*. 2003 (32). 15-24.
[6] Klein, RF; Allard, J; Avnur, Z; Nikolcheva T, Rotstein D, Carlos AS, Shea M, Waters RV, Belknap JK, Peltz G, Orwoll ES. Regulation of bone mass in mice by the lipoxygenase gene Alox15. *Science*. 2004 (303). 229-32.
[7] Department of Health. Nutrition and bone health: with particular reference to calcium and vitamin D. *Report of the Subgroup on Bone Health, Working Group on the Nutritional Status of the Population of the Committee on Medical Aspects of Food and Nutrition Policy*. The Stationery Office, London. (Report on Health and Social Subjects, No. 49). 1998.
[8] Muhlbauer, RC; Li, F. Effect of vegetables on bone metabolism. *Nature*. 1999 (401) 343-4.
[9] Halliwell, B; Gutteridge, JM. *Free Radicals in Biology and Medicine*. Third ed. Oxford University Press. 1999.
[10] Weinberg, ED. Iron out-of-balance: a risk factor for acute and chronic diseases. *Hemoglobin*. 2008 (32). 117-22.
[11] Weinberg, ED. Therapeutic potential of iron chelators in diseases associated with iron mismanagement. *J Pharm Pharmacol*. 2006 (58). 575-84.
[12] Weinberg, ED. Iron loading: a risk factor for osteoporosis. *Biometals*. 2006 (19). 633-5.
[13] Vogiatzi, MG; Macklin, EA; Fung, EB; Cheung, AM; Vichinsky, E; Olivieri, N; Kirby, M; Kwiatkowski, JL, Cunningham, M; Holm, I; Lane, J; Schneider, R; Fleisher, M; Grady, RW; Peterson, C; Giardina, PJ; for the Thalassemia Clinical Research Network. Bone Disease in Thalassemia: A Frequent and Still Unresolved Problem. *J Bone Miner Res*. 2008 May 27. [Epub ahead of print]2009 (24). 543-57.

[14]Isomura, H; Fujie, K; Shibata, K; Inoue, N; Iizuka, T; Takebe, G; Takahashi, K; Nishihira, J; Izumi, H; Sakamoto, W. Bone metabolism and oxidative stress in postmenopausal rats with iron overload. *Toxicology*. 2004 (197). 93-100.

[15]de Vernejoul, MC; Pointillart, A; Golenzer, CC; Morieux, C; Bielakoff, J; Modrowski, D; Miravet, L. Effects of iron overload on bone remodeling in pigs. *Am J Pathol.* 1984 (116). 377-84.

[16]Guggenbuhl, P; Deugnier, Y; Boisdet, JF; Rolland, Y; Perdriger, A; Pawlotsky, Y; Chalès, G. Bone mineral density in men with genetic hemochromatosis and HFE gene mutation. *Osteoporos Int*. 2005 (16). 1809-14.

[17]Chan, YL; Pang, LM; Chik, KW; Cheng, JC; Li, CK. Patterns of bone diseases in transfusion-dependent homozygous thalassaemia major: predominance of osteoporosis and desferrioxamine-induced bone dysplasia. *Pediatr Radiol*. 2002 (32). 492-7.

[18]Shah, FT; Chatterjee, R; Owusu-Asante, M; Porter, JB. Adult with severe sickle cell anaemia and iron overload have a high incidence of osteopenia and osteoporsis. Blood. 2004 (104). *Annual Meeting American Society for Hematology abstract 1684.*

[19]Schnitzler, CM; Schnaid, E; MacPhail, AP; Mesquita, JM; Robson, HJ. Ascorbic acid deficiency, iron overload and alcohol abuse underlie the severe osteoporosis in black African patients with hip fractures--a bone histomorphometric study. *Calcif Tissue Int.* 2005 (76). 79-89.

[20]McCance, RA; Widdowson, EM. The absorption and excretion of iron following oral and intravenous administration. *J Physiol*. 1938 (94). 148-54.

[21]Howes, PS; Zacharski, LR; Sullivan, J; Chow, B. Role of stored iron in atherosclerosis. *J Vasc Nurs*. 2000 (18). 109-14.

[22]Kato, I; Dnistrian, AM; Schwartz, M; Toniolo P, Koenig K, Shore RE, Zeleniuch-Jacquotte A, Akhmedkhanov A, Riboli E. Risk of iron overload among middle-aged women. *Int J Vitam Nutr Res*. 2000 (70). 119-25.

[23]The British Nutrition Foundation. *Iron: Nutritional and Physiological Significance: the Report of the British Nutrition Foundation's Task Force*. First ed. Chapman & Hall for the British Nutrition Foundation, London, New York. 1995.

[24]Danesh, J; Appleby, P. Coronary heart disease and iron status: meta-analyses of prospective studies. *Circulation*. 1999 (99). 852-4.

[25]Sullivan, JL. Iron and the sex difference in heart disease risk. *Lancet*. 1981 (1). 1293-4.

[26]Stevens, RG; Jones, DY; Micozzi, MS; Taylor, PR. Body iron stores and the risk of cancer. *N Engl J Med*. 1988 (319). 1047-52.

[27]Woo, J; Mak, YT; Law, LK; Swaminathan, R. Plasma ferritin in an elderly population living in the community. *J Med*. 1989 (20). 123-34.

[28]Moirand, R; Mortaji, AM; Loreal, O; Paillard, F; Brissot, P; Deugnier, Y. A new syndrome of liver iron overload with normal transferrin saturation. *Lancet*. 1997 (349). 95-7.

[29]Kenner, GH; Brik, AB; Liu, G; Haskell, EH; Hayes, RB; Knight, JA; Vajda, EG; Miller, SC; Jee, WS; Barrus, JK. Variation of long-lived free radicals responsible for the EPR native signal in bone of aged or diseased human females and ovariectomized adult rats. *Radiation Measurements*. 2005 (39). 255-62.

[30]Harris, DC. *Quantitative Chemical AnalysisThird Edition*. WH Freeman and Company, New York, 1991.

[31]Liu, G; Men, P; Kenner, GH; Miller, SC. Therapeutic effects of an oral chelator targeting skeletal tissue damage in experimental postmenopausal osteoporosis in rats. *Hemoglobin*. 2008 (32).181-90.

[32]Liu, G; Men, P; Kenner, GH; Miller, SC. Age-associated iron accumulation in bone: implications for postmenopausal osteoporosis and a new target for prevention and treatment by chelation. *Biometals*. 2006 (19). 245-51.

[33]Iwaniec, UT; Yuan, D; Power, RA; Wronski, TJ. Strain-dependent variations in the response of cancellous bone to ovariectomy in mice. *J Bone Miner Res*. 2006 (21). 1068-74.

[34]Sonoda, M; Yoshida, I; Murase, I. Synthesis and Determination of Metal Chelate Stabilities of n-Alkyltriethylenetetraaminepentaacetic Acid. *J Coord. Chem*. 2001 (54). 153-65.

[35]Bruenger, FW; Kuswik-Rabiega, G; Miller, SC. Decorporation of aged americium deposits by oral administration of lipophilic polyamino carboxylic acids. *J Med Chem* 1992 (35). 112-8.

[36]Miller, SC; Bruenger, FW; Kuswik-Rabiega, G; Liu, G; Lloyd, RD. Duration and dose related effects of an orally administered, partially lipophilic polyaminocarboxylic acid on the decorporation of plutonium and americium. *J Pharmacol Exp Ther*. 1993 (267). 548-54.

[37]Laib, A; Kumer, JL; Majumdar, S; Lane, NE. The temporal changes of trabecular architecture in ovariectomized rats assessed by MicroCT. *Osteoporos Int*. 2001 (12). 936-41.

[38]Parfitt, AM; Drezner, MK; Glorieux, FH; Kanis, JA; Malluche, H; Meunier, PJ; Ott, SM; Recker, RR. Bone histomorphometry: standardization of nomenclature, symbols, and units. *J Bone Min Res*. 1987 (2). 595-610.

[39]Haskell, EH; Hayes, RB; Kenner, GH. A high sensitivity EPR technique for alanine dosimetry. *Radiat Prot Dosim*. 1998 (77). 43-50.

[40]Hayes, RB; Haskell, EH; Romanyukha, AA; Kenner, GH. Technique for increasing reproducibility in EPR dosimetry of tooth enamel. *Meas Sci Technol*. 1998 (9). 1994-2006.

[41]Press, WH; Teukolsky, SA; Vetterling, WT; Flannery; BP. *Numerical Analysis in C: the Art of Scientific Computing*. 2nd Ed. Cambridge University Press, Cambridge. 1992.

[42]Hayes, RB; Haskell, EH; Kenner, GH. An assessment of the Levenberg-Marquardt fitting algorithm on saturating exponential data sets. *Ancient TL*. 1998 (16). 57-62.

[43]Rudolph, CJ; McDonagh EW; Wussow DG. The Effect of Intravenous Disodium Ethylenediaminetetraacetic Acid (EDTA) upon bone Density Levels. In: Cranton EM, editor. *A Textbook on EDTA Chelation Therapy. Second Edition*. Charlottesville, VA: Hampton Roads Publishing Company, Inc.; 2001; 259-264.

[44]Chen, CH; Ho, ML; Chang, JK; Hung, SH; Wang, GJ. Green tea catechin enhances osteogenesis in a bone marrow mesenchymal stem cell line. *Osteoporos Int*. 2005 (16). 2039-45.

[45]Pearce, RB; Edwards, PP; Green, TL; Anderson, PA; Fisher, BJ; Carpenter, TA; Hall, LD. Immobilized long-live free radicals at the host-pathogen interface in sycamore (Acer pseudoplatanus L.). *Physiol Mol Plant Pathol.* 1997 (50). 371-390.

[46]ORISE: Radiation Emergency Assistance Center/Training Site. Zinc-DTPA Informational Material Package Insert. Nov. 14, 2002 (http://orise.orau.gov/reacts/zinc-dtpa.htm).

[47]Lin, JK; Tsai, SH; Lin-Shiau SY: Antiinflammatory and antitumor effects of flavonoids and flavanoids. *Drugs of the Future.* 2001 (26). 145-157.

[48]Bezáková, L; Muèaji, P; Eisenreichová, E; Haladová, M; Pauliková, I; Obložinský, M. Effect of different compound from *Lilium candidum* L. on lipoxygenase activity. *Acta Facult Pharm Univ Comenianae.* 2004 (51). 45-50.

[49]Prieto, JM; Recio, MC; Giner, RM; Manez, S; Giner-Larza, EM; Rios, JL. Influence of traditional Chinese anti-inflammatory medicinal plants on leukocyte and platelet functions. *J Pharm Pharmacol.* 2003 (55). 1275-1282.

[50]Gutierrez-Lugo, MT; Deschamps, JD; Holman, TR; Suarez, E; Timmermann, BN. Lipoxygenase inhibition by anadanthoflavone, a new flavonoid from the aerial parts of Anadenanthera colubrina. *Planta Med.* 2004 (70). 263-265.

[51]Parhami, F; Garfinkel, A; Demer, LL. Role of lipids in osteoporosis. *Arterioscler Thromb Vasc Biol.* 2000 (20). 2346-8.

[52]Schafer, FQ; Qian, SY; Buettner, GR. Iron and free radical oxidations in cell membranes. *Cell Mol Biol (Noisy-le-grand).* 2000 (46). 657-62.

[53]Halleen, JM; Räisänen, S; Salo, JJ; Reddy, SV; Roodman, GD; Hentunen, TA; Lehenkari, PP; Kaija, H; Vihko, P; Väänänen, HK. Intracellular fragmentation of bone resorption products by reactive oxygen species generated by osteoclastic tartrate-resistant acid phosphatase. *J Biol Chem.* 1999 (274). 22907-10.

[54]Vaisman, DN; McCarthy, AD; Cortizo, AM. Bone-specific alkaline phosphatase activity is inhibited by bisphosphonates: role of divalent cations. *Biol Trace Elem Res.* 2005 (104). 131-40.

[55]Gerschman, R; Gilbert, DL; Nye, SW; Dwyer, P; Fenn, WO. Oxygen poisoning and x-irradiation: a mechanism in common. *Science.* 1954 (119). 623-6.

[56]Berger, CE; Horrocks, BR; Datta, HK. cAMP-dependent inhibition is dominant in regulating superoxide production in the bone-resorbing osteoclasts. *J Endocrinol.* 1998 (158). 311-8.

[57]Rasmussen, H; Bordier, P. *Physiological and cellular bass of metabolic bone disease.* Baltimore: William and Wilkens; 1974, p265.

[58]Parfitt AM. "Parathyroid hormone and periosteal bone expansion." *J. Bone Miner. Res.* 2003 (17). 1741–3.

[59]Martin, TJ. "Does bone resorption inhibition affect the anabolic response to parathyroid hormone?" *Trends Endocrinol. Metab.* 2004 (15). 49–50.

[60]Toromanoff, A; Ammann, P; Mosekilde, L; Thomsen, JS; Riond, JL. Parathyroid hormone increases bone formation and improves mineral balance in vitamin D-deficient female rats. *Endocrinology.* 1997 (138). 2449-57.

[61]Martell, AE; Smith, RM. Critical Stability Constants. Vol. 1: *Amino Acids.* New York: Plenum Press; 1974.

[62]Qu, ZH; Zhang, XL; Tang, TT; Dai, KR. Promotion of osteogenesis through beta-catenin signaling by desferrioxamine. *Biochem Biophys Res Commun*. 2008 (370) 332-7.

[63]Naot, Grey, A ; Reid, IR, Cornish, J. Lactoferrin--a novel bone growth factor. *Clin Med Res*. 2005 (3). 93-101.

[64]Lorget, F; Clough, J; Oliveira, M; Daury, MC; Sabokbar, A; Offord, E. Lactoferrin reduces in vitro osteoclast differentiation and resorbing activity. *Biochem Biophys Res Commun*. 2002 (296). 261-6.

[65]Cornish, J; Callon, KE; Naot, D; Palmano, KP; Banovic, T; Bava; U; Watson, M; Lin, JM; Tong, PC; Chen, Q; Chan, VA; Reid, HE; Fazzalari, N; Baker, HM; Baker, EN; Haggarty, NW; Grey, AB; Reid, IR. Lactoferrin is a potent regulator of bone cell activity and increases bone formation in vivo. *Endocrinology*. 2004 145:4366-74.

[66]Cornish, J; Palmano, K; Callon, KE; Watson, M; Lin, JM; Valenti, P; Naot, D; Grey, AB; Reid, IR. Lactoferrin and bone; structure-activity relationships. *Biochem Cell Biol*. 2006 84 (3). 297-302.

SHORT COMMUNICATIONS

In: Osteoporosis: Etiology, Diagnosis and Treatment
Editors: Bilar E. Mattingly and Albert C. Pillare
ISBN 978-1-60692-397-9

Short Communication A

MECHANISMS OF CORTICOID-INDUCED OSTEOPOROSIS

Eduardo López-Collazo, Alessandra Soares-Schanoski and Pablo Fuentes-Prior

Research Unit, "La Paz" Hospital, Madrid, Spain.

ABSTRACT

Osteoporosis, the most prevalent metabolic bone disease, is characterized by compromised bone strength predisposing to an increased risk of fracture in response to mild trauma. The social and economic burden of osteoporosis is rapidly growing due to the aging of the world population. This disease, therefore, is a severe problem for current public health systems. Postmenopausal women and patients under glucocorticoid treatment are the two main groups of individuals who suffer from osteoporosis. The latter group is of particular relevance, because glucocorticoids are widely used to treat various conditions such as allergic and inflammatory disorders as well as asthma. Currently, physiological actions of glucocorticoids with potential implications in osteoporosis include decreased calcium absorption in the gastrointestinal tract and its increased urinary excretion, thus causing resistance to vitamin D and subsequent loss of bone mineral density. Despite several studies that have focused on the physiological actions of glucocorticoids, we still lack a clear picture of the ultimate molecular mechanism(s) underlying osteoporosis onset and progression in humans.

Osteoclasts are multinucleated cells originated from the fusion of macrophages, which play essential roles in bone development and remodeling. They possess a unique capacity for bone resorption, and are thus important mediators of the bone loss that leads to osteoporosis. Recently, the cellular and molecular bases of osteoclast involvement in osteoporosis have been analyzed in several independent investigations. It has been shown that increases in osteoclast number and/or activity lead to several diseases associated with both general and localized bone loss such as osteoporosis and rheumatoid arthritis, respectively. Here we discuss molecular mechanisms that underlie glucocorticoid-induced osteoporosis, focusing on newly identified regulators of osteoclatogenesis and osteoclast activation such as IRAK-M. Indeed, this pseudokinase not only acts as a negative modulator of innate immune responses mediated by Toll-like receptors (TLRs) and interleukin-1 receptor (IL-1R), but also participates in the control of macrophage differentiation into osteoclasts. IRAK-M knockout mice develop a strong osteoporosis phenotype, suggesting that the down-regulation of this molecule activates osteoclast-mediated bone resorption. Data from human studies indicate that blood monocytes differentiated into osteoclasts express high levels of IRAK-M at both mRNA and protein level. Glucorticoids down-regulate IRAK-M expression, which correlates with an increased activation of bone resorption.

INTRODUCTION

Osteoporosis, the most prevalent metabolic bone disease, is characterized by a progressive decrease of bone strength that predisposes to an increased risk of fracture in response to mild trauma. The social and economic burden of osteoporosis is rapidly growing due to the aging of the world's population. This disease, therefore, is an important challenge to current health systems [1].

The World Health Organization classifies osteoporosis into two classes: primary and secondary [http://bone-muscle.health-cares.net/osteoporosis-types.php]. Primary osteoporosis is the form observed in elder people and post-menopausal women, where bone loss is accelerated due to age (over 70 years) and estrogen loss at menopause, respectively. In contrast, secondary osteoporosis is neither gender- nor age-linked, but is associated with a number of medical disorders (e.g., vitamin D deficiency, gastrointestinal and liver diseases, and alcoholism). Further, exposure to drugs prescribed to treat certain health problems may contribute to trigger or enhance secondary osteoporosis [1]. The most common group of drugs that could affect both quality and quantity of bone are glucocorticoids, and osteoporosis is the most serious complication associated with them. This is of particular medical relevance, since glucocorticoids are widely used to treat several diseases such as allergic and inflammatory disorders as well as asthma [2].

A growing number of reports suggest that the bone loss process is fastest during the first year of glucocorticoid therapy [1-5], with a marked reduction in bone mass being observed three months after therapy start [1-5]. To date, the most accepted hypothesis regarding the implication of glucocorticoids in osteoporosis points to a drug-induced decrease in calcium absorption in the gastrointestinal tract and an increase of its urinary excretion, which causes resistance to vitamin D and subsequently loss of mineral density in bone [3-5].

Despite a number of investigations that describe different aspects of osteoporosis onset and progression, as well as the relevance of glucocorticoids for these processes, we still lack a clear picture of the ultimate molecular mechanism(s) underlying this disease, and in particular of secondary, glucocorticoid-induced osteoporosis. Several studies indicate that these drugs predominantly affect osteoblast proliferation, differentiation and life span [3-6]. Nevertheless, it is conceivable that other cells are also affected, and could directly or indirectly modulate osteoporosis. Osteoclasts are multinucleated cells originated from the fusion of macrophages, and which are specialized in bone removal via bone tissue acidification and proteolytic digestion of collagen and other proteins of the extracellular matrix. In this manner, they counteract osteoblast secretion of osteoid into the resorption cavity [7,8]. Therefore, the balance between osteoblast and osteoclast activity is critical in bone mass regulation.

Because of this essential role in bone development and remodeling, osteoclasts might contribute to the loss of bone observed in patients with glucocorticoid-induced osteoporosis [8,9,10], and this possibility has recently been considered in several studies on the causes of the disease [3-8,10]. In particular, it has been shown that increases in osteoclast number and/or activity lead to several conditions associated with both general and localized bone loss such as osteoporosis and rheumatoid arthritis, respectively [8,9]. Thus, progress in the understanding of osteoclastogenesis and osteoclast activation has notably contributed to advances in osteoporosis research [8,11,12].

The monocyte-macrophage lineage of hematopoietic cells is the precursor of osteoclasts. Their survival and proliferation depends on the presence of functional macrophage colony-stimulating factor (M-CSF) [13,14]. Osteoclast formation requires in addition the presence of receptor activator of NF-κB ligand (RANKL), a member of the tumor necrosis factor (TNF) cytokine family [7,8,14-17]. RANKL, also termed TRANCE (TNF-related activation-induced cytokine), is expressed on the surface of osteoclast-interacting cells (e.g., osteoblasts) and plays a key role in driving the commitment of precursor cells to osteoclasts and their further maturation to multinucleated cells [18]. Both bone marrow-derived monocytes and pre-monocytic lineages could be differentiated into osteoclasts *in vitro* by using M-CSF, RANKL and/or vitamin D [1,8,9,19]. Further, it has been demonstrated that these *in vitro*-produced osteoclasts possess bone resorbing capability [1,8,9,19]. Despite technical difficulties in maintaining these *in vitro* generated osteoclast-like cells in a viable state, this approach allows the establishment of an experimental model to study the molecular mechanisms underlying osteoclastogenesis and osteoporosis.

MOLECULAR MECHANISMS OF OSTEOCLAST DIFFERENTIATION AND ACTIVATION

Studies performed with transgenic mice have clearly demonstrated a critical role for RANK-RANKL signaling in the early phases of osteoclastogenesis [7]. By contrast, the presence of M-CSF is required at later stages of osteclast differentiation, where it activates Akt, c-Fos and ERK pathways that in turn interact with signals downstream of RANK-RANKL interaction [8,9,12,20]. RANK transduces signals by recruiting adaptor molecules, such as the TRAF family of proteins, which leads to NF-κB activation and induction of the ubiquitous transcription factor NFAT (nuclear factor of activated T cells). NFAT cooperates then with other transcriptional partners to activate osteoclast-specific genes such as TRAFs, AP-1, [10,20] and MAPKs signalling pathways [7,8].

Interestingly, it has been reported that some inflammatory cytokines such as IL-1 and TNF also function as osteoclast activators, based on their well known ability to stimulate bone resorption [7,8,12]. They are produced by various cells, such as monocytes/macrophages and mature osteoclasts, in sites of inflammation or around bones, respectively. A growing number of studies currently focus on the IL-1 pathway during osteoclastogenesis and osteoclast activation [7,8,12]. This pathway has also been related to secondary post-menopausal osteoporosis, and our results indicate its implication in glucocorticoid-induced osteoporosis, as we discuss below.

Down-regulation of IRAK-M in Mice Results in Osteoporesis

As mentioned above, it is well established that glucocorticoids induce osteoporosis in humans via a mechanism that is currently not well understood; this represents the most serious drawback of glucocorticoid therapy. In particular, daily glucocorticoid treatment increases the risk of fracture [2,3,21]. A strong correlation between glucocorticoid doses and loss of bone mineral density has been reported [6]. Both *in vitro* and *in vivo* studies have indicated that excess glucocorticoids promote osteoblast apoptosis while extending the life span of pre-existing osteoclasts [3,6]. Several authors suggest that corticosteroid-induced osteoporosis results from direct and indirect actions of these drugs on bone tissue and calcium homeostasis [2,5,22]. Nevertheless, a number of observations suggest that these mechanisms alone do not provide a complete picture of the events that occur during glucocorticoid treatment and their implication for osteoporosis.

It has recently been reported that the pseudokinase IRAK-M plays a critical regulatory role during osteoclast differentiation and activation, and concomitantly in the development of osteoporosis [7,8]. This molecule belongs to a family of kinases termed interleukin-1 receptor-associated kinases (IRAKs). IRAKs are essential for transducing signals downstream of Toll-like receptor (TLR) / interleukin-1 receptor (IL-1R) engagement into a potent inflammatory response. Four members of this family have been identified to date, of which IRAK-1 and IRAK-4 possess intrinsic kinase activity, and are responsible for transducing signals elicited by TLR or IL-1R activation [7,8,23-29]. IRAK-2 and IRAK-M are pseudokinases [8,17-22], and while the former has been recently implicated in a positive feed-back loop [30], IRAK-M acts as a negative regulator of TLR/IL-1R signaling in all systems examined so far. Two mechanisms might explain this negative role of IRAK-M: impaired recruitment of active IRAKs to the initial complex formed between TLR/Il-1R and the critical bipartite adaptor, myeloid differentiation factor 88 (MyD88), or preventing dissociation of IRAK-1 from this membrane-proximal complex bound to TNF receptor associated factor (TRAF)-6 [7,8,23-29].

Unexpectedly, IRAK-M knockout mice were recently shown to present an accelerated osteoclastogenesis, and their osteoclasts possessed increased half-life and hyperactivation of NF-κB and MAKP (mitogen-activated protein-kinases) signaling pathways, via engagement of IL-1R/TLR pathways. Consequently, animals developed severe osteoporosis that started four months after birth [7]. This contrasts with the high levels of IRAK-M that are expressed in osteoclasts from normal mice, which counteract their (hyper)activation [7]. Altogether, IRAK-M emerges as a key regulator of the molecular mechanism(s) underlying bone loss due to osteoclastic bone resorption, at least in mice.

IRAK-M Downregulation in Human and Murine Osteoclasts Boosts Bone Resorbing Activity: A Putative Mechanism for Carticoid-Induced Osteporesis

Osteoclasts from wild-type mice express high basal levels of IRAK-M [7]. It is well established that this pseudokinase plays a crucial role in the regulation of several pro-inflammatory pathways [23-28]. Data obtained from an *in vitro* human model of monocytes-derived osteoclasts indicate that IRAK-M levels increase in a time-dependent manner during the differentiation process, with similar kinetics in both human and murine systems [7,8]. Interestingly, IRAK-M mRNA levels are significantly higher in differentiated osteoclasts derived from both human premonocytic cells THP-1 and isolated human monocytes than in those obtained from RAW cells (about four-fold), thus suggesting a tighter control of osteoclast activation in humans [8] compared to mice [7,8].

Of particular relevance for secondary osteoporosis, we have observed that both mRNA and protein levels of IRAK-M are significantly reduced in the presence of glucocorticoids, in a dose-dependent manner. Furthermore, the bone-resorbing ability is dramatically increased in osteoclast-like cells obtained in the presence of glucocorticoids. These cells exhibit a down-regulation of their IRAK-M expression levels. By contrast, osteoclasts cultivated in the absence of glucocorticoids show a moderate bone-resorbing ability and their levels of IRAK-M are high. In view of the role of IRAK-M as a negative regulator of osteoclast activation, these findings suggest that glucocorticoids induce osteoclast hyperactivation via down-regulation of the pseudokinase. It is important to note that while in macrophages the corticoid up-regulates IRAK-M to control inflammatory responses, in osteoclasts it acts as an inhibitor of IRAK-M expression thus exacerbating bone-resorbing activity.

In summary, clinical data indicate that glucocorticoids have important effects on skeletal turnover, which eventually lead to the development of osteoporosis [3,6,7,22,31,32]. Significant bone loss occurs after the initial exposure to glucocorticoids, and even modest doses of these drugs, frequently considered within the physiological range, increase the risk of fractures [1-7]. A recent report suggests that glucocorticoids act directly on osteoclasts increasing their life span and concomitantly reducing bone density [33]. Other authors have suggested that these drugs have a direct effect on osteoblasts by increasing their expression of RANKL and CSF-1 while down-regulating levels of the inhibitory cytokine, osteoprotegerin [34,35]. Furthermore, glucocorticoids also enhance apoptosis of mature osteoblasts [2-10,34]. Recent findings obtained by us [8] demonstrate that glucocorticoids in addition influence osteoclast activation via down-regulation of IRAK-M. Thus, strategies that counteract this effect might prove beneficial for treatment of osteoporosis in humans.

References

[1] Lane, E.N. Epidemiology, etiology, and diagnosis of osteoporosis. (2006) *Am J Obstet Gynecol. 94*(2 Suppl), 3-11.

[2] Iwamoto, J., Takeda, T., Sato, Y. Prevention and treatment of corticosteroid-induced osteoporosis. (2005). *Yons. Med. J. 46*(4), 456-63.

[3] Canalis, E. (2003) Mechanisms of glucocorticoid-induced osteoporosis. *Curr. Opin. Rheumatol. 15*(4), 454-7.

[4] 4-.Abu EO, Horner A, Kusec V, Triffitt JT, Compston JE. (2007) The localization of the functional glucocorticoid receptor alpha in human bone. 85(2), 883-9.

[5] Leclerc, N., Luppen, C.A., Ho, V.V., Nagpal, S., Hacia, J.G., Smith, E., Frenkel, B. (2004) Gene expression profiling of glucocorticoid-inhibited osteoblasts. *J. Mol. Endocrinol. 33*(1), 175-93.

[6] Sivagurunathan, S., Muir, M.M., Brennan, T.C., Seale, J.P., Mason, R.S. (2005) Influence of Glucocorticoids on Human Osteoclast Generation and Activity. *J. Bone Miner. Res. 20*(3), 390-8.

[7] Li, H., Cuartas, E., Cui, W., Choi, Y., Crawford, T. D., Zhu Ke, H., Kobayashi, K.S., Flavelland, R.A., Vignery, A. (2005) IL-1 receptor–associated kinase M is a central regulator of osteoclast differentiation and activation. *J. Exp. Med. 201*(7), 1169-77.

[8] Soares-Schanoski A, Gómez-Piña V, del Fresno C, Rodríguez-Rojas A, García F, Glaría A, Sánchez M, Vallejo-Cremades MT, Baos R, Fuentes-Prior P, Arnalich F, López-Collazo E. (2007) 6-Methylprednisolone down-regulates IRAK-M in human and murine osteoclasts and boosts bone-resorbing activity: a putative mechanism for corticoid-induced osteoporosis. *J. Leuk. Biol. 82*(3), 700-9.

[9] Sato, K., Takayanagi, H. (2006) Osteoclasts, rheumatoid arthritis, and osteoimmunology. *Curr. Opin. Rheumatol. 18*(4), 419-26.

[10]Kim HJ, Zhao H, Kitaura H, Bhattacharyya S, Brewer JA, Muglia LJ, Ross FP, Teitelbaum SL. (2006) Glucocorticoids suppress bone formation via the osteoclast. *J. Clin. Invest. 116*(8), 2152-60.

[11]Zhang Q, Guo R, Lu Y, Zhao L, Zhou Q, Schwarz EM, Huang J, Chen D, Jin ZG, Boyce BF, Xing L. (2008) *J Biol Chem*. VEGF-C, a lymphatic growth factor, is a RANKL target gene in osteoclasts that enhances osteoclastic bone resorption through an autocrine mechanism. 283(19), 13491-9.

[12]Yao Z, Xing L, Qin C, Schwarz EM, Boyce BF. (2008) Osteoclast precursor interaction with bone matrix induces osteoclast formation directly by an interleukin-1-mediated autocrine mechanism. *J Biol Chem. 283*(15), 9917-24.

[13]Kodama H, Nose M, Niida S, Yamasaki A. (1991) Essential role of macrophage colony-stimulating factor in the osteoclast differentiation supported by stromal cells. *J Exp Med. 173*(5), 1291-4.

[14]Susa, M., Luong-Nguyen, N-H., Capellen, D., Zamurovic, N., Gamse, R. (2004) Human primary osteoclasts: in vitro generation and applications as pharmacological and clinical assay. *J. Trans. Med. 2*(6), 1-12.

[15]Kearns AE, Khosla S, Kostenuik PJ. (2008) Receptor activator of nuclear factor kappaB ligand and osteoprotegerin regulation of bone remodeling in health and disease. *Endocr Rev. 29*(2), 155-92.

[16]Kim Y, Sato K, Asagiri M, Morita I, Soma K, Takayanagi H. Contribution of nuclear factor of activated T cells c1 to the transcriptional control of immunoreceptor osteoclast-associated receptor but not triggering receptor expressed by myeloid cells-2 during osteoclastogenesis. *J Biol Chem. 280*(38), 32905-13.

[17]Fouque-Aubert A, Chapurlat R. (2007) Influence of RANKL inhibition on immune system in the treatment of bone diseases. *Joint Bone Spine.75*(1), 5-10.

[18]Wong BR, Josien R, Choi Y. (1999) TRANCE is a TNF family member that regulates dendritic cell and osteoclast function. *J Leukoc Biol. 65*(6), 715-24.

[19]Avnet, S., Lamolinara, A., Zini, N., Solimando, L., Quacquaruccio, G., Granchi, D., Maraldi, N.M., Giunti, A., Baldini, N. (2006) Effects of antisense mediated inhibition of cathepsin K on human osteoclasts obtained from peripheral blood. *J. Orthop. Res. 24*(8), 1699-708.

[20]Huang, H., Ryu, J., Ha, J., Chang, E-J., Kim, H.J., Kim, H-M., Kitamura, T., Lee, Z.H, Kim, H-H. (2006) Osteoclast differentiation requires TAK1 and MKK6 for NFATc1 induction and NF-κB transactivation by RANKL. *Cell Death Differ. 13*(11), 1879-91.

[21]Van Staa, T.P., Laan, R.F., Barton, I.P., Cohen, S., Reid, D.M., Cooper, C. (2003) Bone density threshold and other predictors of vertebral fracture in patients Receiving oral glucocorticoid therapy. *Arthritis Rheum. 48*(11), 3224-9.

[22]Dempster, D.W., Moonga, B.S., Stein, L.S., Horbert W.R., Antakly, T. (1997) Glucocorticoids inhibit bone resorption by isolated rat osteoclasts by enhancing apoptosis. *J. Endocrinol. 154*(3), 397-406.

[23]del Fresno, C., Otero, k., Gómez-García, L., González-León, M.C., Soler-Ranger, Ll., Fuentes-Prior, P., Escoll, P., Baos, R., Caveda, L., García, F., Arnalich, F., López-Collazo, E. (2005) Tumor cells deactivate human monocytes by up-regulating IL-1 receptor associated kinase-M expression via CD44 and TLR4. *J. Immunol. 174*(5), 3032-40.

[24]del Fresno, C., Gómez-García, L., Caveda, L., Escoll, P., Arnalich, F., Zamora, R., López-Collazo, E. (2004) Nitric oxide activates the expression of IRAK-M via the release of TNF-α in human monocytes. *Nitric Oxide. 10*(4), 213-20.

[25]Escoll, P., del Fresno, C., Gómez-García, L., Vallés, G., Lendínez, M.J., Arnalich, F., López-Collazo, E. (2003) Rapid up-regulation of IRAK-M expression following a second endotoxin challenge in human monocytes and in monocytes isolated from septic patient. *Biochem. Biophys. Res. Commun. 311*(2), 465-72.

[26]Lopez-Collazo, E., Fuentes-Prior, P., Arnalich, F., del Fresno, C. (2006) Pathophysiology of interleukin-1 receptor-associated kinase-M: implications in refractory state. *Curr. Opin. Infect. Dis. 19*(3), 237-44.

[27]González-León, M.C., Soares-Schanoski, A., del Fresno, C., Cimadevila, A., Goméz-Piña, V., Mendoza-Barberá, E., García, F., Marín, E., Arnalich, F., Fuentes-Prior, P., López-Collazo, E. (2006) Nitric oxide induces SOCS-1 expression in human monocytes in a TNF-α dependent manner. *J. Endotoxin Res. 12*(5), 296-306.

[28]del Fresno, C., Soler-Rangel, Ll., Soares-Schanoski, A., González-León, M.C., Gómez-García, L., Gómez-Piña, V., Mendoza-Barberá, E., García, F., Fuentes-Prior, P., Arnalich, F., López-Collazo, E. (2006) Inflammatory responses associated with Acute Coronary Syndrome up-regulate IRAK-M and induce endotoxin tolerance in circulating monocytes. (2007) *J. Endotoxin Res. 13*(1):39-52.

[29]Dauphinee, S.M., Karsan, A. (2006) Lipopolysaccharide signaling in endothelial cells. *Lab. Invest. 86*(1), 9-22.

[30]Kawagoe T, Sato S, Matsushita K, Kato H, Matsui K, Kumagai Y, Saitoh T, Kawai T, Takeuchi O, Akira S. (2008) Sequential control of Toll-like receptor-dependent responses by IRAK1 and IRAK2. 9(6), 684-91..

[31]Chen, T. L. (2004) Inhibition of growth and differentiation of osteoprogenitors in mouse bone marrow stromal cell cultures by increased donor age and glucocorticoid treatment. *Bone 35*(1), 83-95.

[32]van Staa TP. (2006) The pathogenesis, epidemiology and management of glucocorticoid-induced osteoporosis. *Calcif Tissue Int. 79*(3):129-37.

[33]Jia, D., O'Brien, C.A., Stewart, S.A., Manolagas, S.C., Weinstein, R.S. (2006) Glucocorticoids act directly on osteoclasts to increase their life span and reduce bone density. *Endocrinology. 147*(12), 5592-9.

[34]Van Staa, T.P., Leufkens, H.G.M., Cooper, C. (2002) The epidemiology of corticosteroid-induced osteoporosis: a meta-analysis. *Osteoporos. Int. 13*(10), 777-87.

[35]Kondo, N., Tokunaga, K., Arai, K., Amizuka, N., Mingi, L., Kitahara, H., Ito, M., Naito, M., Shu-Ying, J., Odas, K., Murai, T., Tkano, R., Ogose, A., Endo, N. (2006) High dose glucocorticoid hampers bone formation and resorption after bone marrow abaltion in rat. *Microsc. Res. Tech. 69*(10), 839-46.

In: Osteoporosis: Etiology, Diagnosis and Treatment
Editors: Bilar E. Mattingly and Albert C. Pillare
ISBN 978-1-60692-397-9

Short Communication B

PERCUTANEOUS VERTEBROPLASTY AND KYPHOPLASTY IN THE TREATMENT OF OSTEOPOROTIC VERTEBRAL BODY FRACTURES: STATE OF THE ART AND FUTURE DIRECTIONS

S. Masala, F. M. Fucci, M. Mammucari, T. Volpi, F.Massari, A. Ursone and G. Simonetti
University of Rome "Tor Vergata", Rome, Italy.

ABSTRACT

The vertebral fractures are generated when the combination of the axial and rotational charges on the spine exceed the resistance offered by vertebral body.

Reduction in the individual vertebral body strength may result from infiltrative processes created by benign or malignant tumors or, more commonly, from bone mineral loss precipitated by osteoporosis.

Osteoporosis, which may be age-related (primary) or due to steroid use (secondary), is the most common cause of VCF in Europe and United States. The frequency of radiographic evidence of VCF increases from 500/100,000 person years (py) in women aged 50 to 54 years to 2960/100,000 py in women more than 85 years old. Radiographic changes may be present without the patient experiencing pain.

Patients with VCFs may experience severe and prolonged pain that can markedly alter activities of daily living. Complications include progressive kyphosis of the spine and reduction of volumes of the thoracic and abdominal cavities, with consequent reduction of vital capacity (VC) and "forced expiratory volume to 1 second" (FEV1), as well as gastrointestinal dysfunction.

In osteoporotic vertebral collapses a conservative therapy is generally achieved with bed rest, bracing, analgesics, and physical therapy.

Instead for patients with painful bone metastases current conventional treatments are primarily palliative and include localized therapies (fractionated external beam radiation therapy and surgery), systemic therapies (chemotherapy, hormonal therapy, radiopharmaceuticals, and bisphosphonates), and analgesics (opioids and non-steroidal anti-inflammatory drugs).

These conventional therapies with their well known drawbacks and side effects provide reasonable pain relief obtaining variable success rates.

All painful vertebral collapses are adequately treated through percutaneous injection of polymethylmethacrylate (PMMA) bone cement into the vertebral body, described for the first time by Galibert et al. in 1984 as " Vertebroplasty ", and successfully applied to the treatment of C2 aggressive hemangiomas, and subsequently used on VCF secondary to osteoporosis and osteolytic tumors.

Vertebroplasty is a technique utilized in the field of VCF, based on Osteoporosis or neoplasms.

It is extremely useful in the treatment of aggressive vertebral hemangiomas, bone osteolytic metastases and destructive multiple myeloma, which is associated with VCF in 55-70% of the cases.

New tendencies are essentially directed, according to Medline, toward developments of a new generation of injectable bone cements.

Vertebral fractures, defined as a 20% or an at least 4mm height reduction of the vertebral body, occur when the axial and rotational load exceed the resistance offered by the vertebra [1].

Fracture severity is determined by the vertebral height reduction and defined by convention as mild (20 –25%), moderate (25–40%), or severe (40% height loss at any posterior, middle, or anterior point) [1,2,3].

Fractures may also be divided, depending on their morphological characteristics, into:

- *Biconcave* if the height reduction involves only the middle portion of the body with mantained anterior and posterior walls
- *Wedge* if the height reduction involves mainly the anterior wall
- *Crush* in case of a uniform height loss

The most common causes of vertebral fractures are osteoporosis and malignant bone lesions. Primary osteoporosis is responsible of 85% of all vertebral compression fractures (VCF) while secondary osteoporosis and malignant bone lesions are the cause of the remaining 15% [4].

The National Osteoporosis Fundation estimated that over 200 milion individuals are at risk of osteoporosis-induced fractures. The spine is the most frequently affected localization for these fractures: in the U.S., osteoporosis is responsible for 1.5 milion fractures annually, of which 750.000 affect the spine, 250.000 the femur , 250.000 the wrist and the remaining 250.000 other sites [5-8].

Despite their higher incidence, VCF tend to be underdiagnosed, since only 20-25% of radiologically diagnosed fractures are clinically evident. Furthermore, the number of osteoporosis-related fractures is esistimated to increase by four times in the next 50 years due to the demograpchic transition in western countries. Approximately 20-25% of caucasic women above 50 years of age is affected by 1 or more VCF. At the moment, in Europe, 438.750 are diagnosed every year with an incidence of 117 fractures / 100.000 individuals (which means approximately a VCF every 45 seconds) [7].

The estimated risk of being affected by a VCF is 16% for women and 5% for men.

For these reasons, the already high socio-economic expenditures of VCF, are destined to significantly increase. In the European comunity the direct medical cost of VCF has reached €31 bilion and is estimeted to rise over €76 by 2050.

Such high costs are due to the high number of days of hospitalization (an avarage of 10-30 days / patient), to the pharmacological and physical therapy, and to long-term nursing.

Furthermore, indirect costs related to post-fracturative morbidity and to the loss of working days must be considered. Both symptomatic and asymptomatic fractures are associated to a 1,6% increased morbidity and mortality compared to a population of the same age [9,10].

VCF complications maybe divided into acute and chronic. Acute complications are usually represented by transient ileus, by urinary retention and occasionally by back pain [5]. Pain, which is not always present (almost 40% of VCF are aymptomatic) may be due to the irritation of nervous terminations of the periostium and of the articular capsules [11].

Chronic pain is the main long-term complication of VCF and affects almost one third of the patiensts seriously compromising their quality of life. Other chronic effects include insomnia, depression and progressive kyphosis (especially in multilevel wedge VCF) which causes a height reduction of the patient (around 4 cm every 15 degree kyphosis' angle increase), the loss of the physiological lordosis, bulging abdomen but mainly a volumetric reduction of the chest with a consequently reduced pulmonary funtionality [6,12,13]. This latter consists in both a 9% reduction in vital capacity and a decrease of the forced expiratory volume per second for each fractured vertebra [14].

Within the first five years after the fracture, the risk of death incresases proportionally to the number of fractured vertebrae up to 10%; moreover, the subsequent spinal deformity is the cause of biomechanical changes which result in a five times higher risk of fractures of contigous vertebrae; 20% of these latter VCFs occur within the first year [3,14,15]. In case of multiple fractures, the risk of further vertebral collapses is up to 7-9 times higher than in healthy individuals [3].

The first choice treatment options of VCFs include medical therapy associated to rest, eventually to bracing and, in the case of osteoporosis-induced fractures, to specific drugs.

The efficacy of the therapy for osteoporosis, however, requires long-term administration (6 months to 1 year) and, therefore, during this period, patients are exposed to the risk of further fractures which occur in 19% of the cases [15].

In case of persistent pain, interventional radiology techniques , vertebrolpasty and kyphoplasty, may be used. The main indication for percutaneous vertebroplasty are VCFs causing pain which doesn't improve on medical therapy administered either for more than three weeks or at excessively high dosages (causing confusion and sedation) [5,14].

Contraindications may be divided into absolute and relative.

Absolute contraindications are:

- Asymptomatic vertebral body compression fractures
- Patient improving on medical therapy
- Uncorrectable coagulopathy
- Ongoing local or systemic infection
- Unstable fractures with retropulsed bone fragments and spinal compression

- Allergy to bone cement (Polymethilmethacrylate)

Relative contraindications are:

- Radiculopathy in excess of vertebral pain
- Complete vertebral collapses ("vertebra plana", with an height reduction >70%)
- Loss of peduncolar integrity
- Loss of posterior wall integrity
- Prophylaxis in osteoporotic patients with no evidence of vertebral fractures

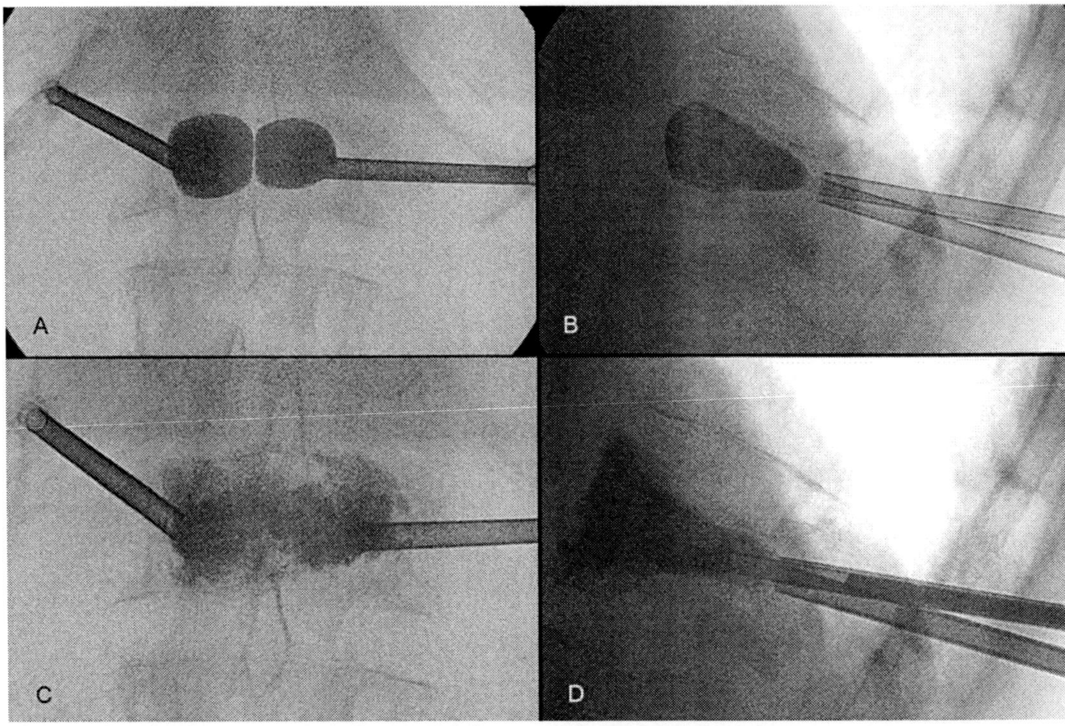

Figure 1. Kyphoplasty treatment. Sequential fluoroscopic images in anterior-posterior and lateral projections: A and B) bilateral inflation of balloon catheters under manometric monitoring; C and D) injection of PMMA into the previously created cavities using filler cannulae.

All eligible patients must undergo an accurate clinical-ananmestic evaluation in order to confirm the role played by the VCF in pain and reduced mobility. As a matter of fact, it is very important to discriminate between pain caused by fractures and all other conditions responsible of spinal pain (radiculopathy, intervertebral disc degeneration, etc.). It is therefore very important to evaluate the characteristics and time of onset of the pain, eventual generating events (traumas), predisposing factors (prolonged corticosteroid therapy), or the presence of previous fractures.

Usually pain caused by a VCF follows low-energy or unnoticed traumas, increases in orthostatism and is improved by lying down [8,16].

Pressing on or laterally mobilizing the spinous process of a fractured vertebra is likely to cause pain.

VCF occurring in the lumbar region are usually characterized by medial pain extended up to 2 levels from the collapsed vertebra; if otherwise, a different cause of pain should be considered.

Furthermore anterior-posterior and lateral radiographs, Computed Tomography (CT), Magnetic Resonance (MR) and bone scintigraphy are performed in each patient for a correct diagnostic evaluation and an accurate procedural planning.

Radiographs show the presence and the localization of the fracture; axial thin slice CT scans with sagittal and coronal reformats are necessary to assess the integrity of the posterior wall and of the pedicles, therefore, reduce the risk of cement leakages, and to exclude the presence of retropulsed bone fragments compromising the spinal canal; through the evaluation of signal alterations within the spinal chord, MR can evidence symptomatic vertebrae eligible for treatment [8,15,17].

Within 30 days from their occurance, acute and subacute osteoporotis induced fractures appear as low signal in T1 weighting and high signal on both T2 weighting and STIR sequences due to the presence of intraspongious edema. The administration of gadolinium causes isointensity of the lesion.

Approximately after a month, the fracture appears isointense in both T1- and T2-weighted sequences. Completely healed fractures show normal bone signal intensity or may appear as low signal in both T1 and T2 weighting due to significant sclerosis. MR is usefull to exclude discal hernia as the cause of pain [16,18]. In case of chronic fractures in which pain doesn't improve, bone scintigraphy should be performed.

A complete evaluation of the patient should include a complete blood test with a study of the leucocytic formula and a complete coagulation test (Prothrombin Time (PT), Partial Thromboplastin Time (PTT), INR) [8]. Subsequently, patients eligible for the procedure undergo cardiological and anaestesiological evaluations, since the intervention is carried out under local anaesthesia. The administration of contrindicated drugs, such as anticoagulants, is temporarily suspended and resumed a few days after the procedure. A few hours prior to the intervention, large spectrum antibiotical coverage (1 2g vial of endovenous Glazidin), gastroprotective drugs (2 20mg vials of endovenous Antra) and corticosteroids (2 20mg vials of endovenous Urbason) are administered for prohylactic purposes. The patient is fasted for eight hours prior to the procedure to allow safe sedation. ECG, saturation and blood pressure are constantly monitorized throughout the entire procedure which is carried out in an angiographic room with the use of a C-Arm fluoroscopy system allowing an accurate view of the spine in multiple planes.

While in case of cervical vertebrae the supine position is preferred, patients undergoing the procedure for the treatment of thoracic or lumbar VCFs are prone positioned; in order to obtain the maximum extension of the spine, three cylinders are placed across the table: one under the patient's thorax, another one under the pelvis and the third one under the ankles [15,17,19,20]. After localizing under fluoroscopy the vertebra to be treated and its pedicles, subcutaneous and periosteal administration of a local anesthetic is performed. A small incision is then followed by the insertion of a 11-13 Gauge bone biopsy needle. The classic either mono- or bilateral transpeduncolar access is preferred in the case of thoracic and lumbar vertebrae due to its major safety, while for upper thoracic vertebrae a costovertebral access is used because of the small sized pedicles.

The correct radiographic profile for the transpeduncolar approach is given by a " En face View " projection view with a 10-20 degree inclination of the C-Arm in which the pedicle appears oval shaped. An important reference point in the anterior-posterior projection is the medial cortical margin of the pedicle which laterally delimits the spinal canal and, therefore, must not be crossed during the progression of the needle which show in an anteromediocaudal direction [15,17,20]. The advance of the needle may eventually be aided by the use of a surgical hammer, and once it is correctly positioned at the anterior third of the vertebral body, PMMA is prepared. PMMA is made up of a powder compound and a liquid catalyst which are mixed inside a sterile container until thick and pasty. The mixture is then loaded into the dedicated filler cannulae and injected under lateral fluoroscopic guidance until the anterior 2/3 of the vertebral body are filled with homogeneous distribution on both sides and between the two endplates. In patients affected by osteoporosis induced collapses 2,5-4 ml of cement allow an optimal obtaining filling both consolidation and pain improvement.

Once the injection is over, pain relief is almost immediate and only in few cases it takes a few hours.

In the first 4 hours after the procedure, patients are kept resting in the supine position to guarantee the complete and uniform consolidation of PMMA inside the vertebral body (cement usually hardens after 20 minutes and reaches 90% of its definitive compactness after an hour); the next day, patients can be dismissed [17].

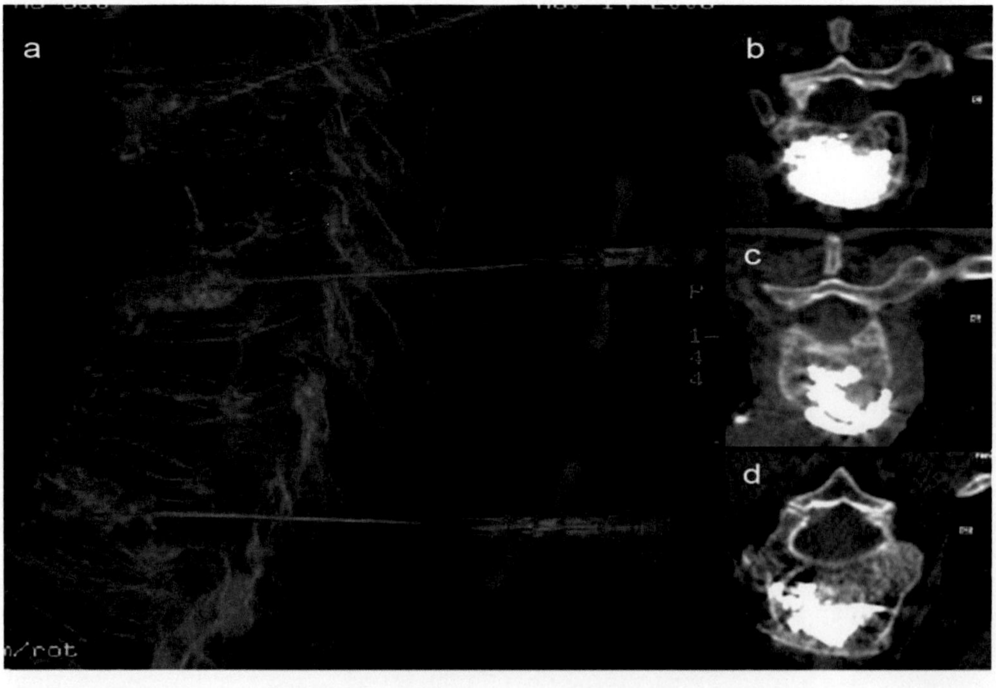

Figure 2. Vertebroplasty treatment of three vertebrae. A) Sagittal reformatted image showing needle placement and cement injection; B,C and D) axial CT scans show the vertebral body after satisfactory application of bone cement.

Vertebroplasty associated complications are:

- cement leakages
- infections
- fractures of the ribs, of the posterior elements or of the pedicles
- the risk of adjacent vertebrae collapses
- allergic reactions
- bleeding of the puncture site

Cement leakages are often asymptomatic;
leakages may involve:

- intervebral disks or paravertebral tissues: these are usually asymptomatic leakages that can however, in severely osteoporotic patients, cause collapses of adjacent vertebral bodies [20].
- the canal or intervertebral foramens: these leakages can cause radiculopathy and paraplegia as the result of the compression of nerve roots and spinal cord respectively. Radiculopathy represents a minor adverse reaction that occurs as a result of the contact of the polimerizing cement with emerging nerve roots and of the heating it produces on these latter. To prevent such complication, a spinal needle should be immediately placed in the involved intervertebral foramen to inject saline solution. Radiculopathy may require the administration of NSAIDs or local analgesics. Spinal compression is instead a major complication that requires immediate neurosurgical decompression in order to avoid permanent neurological sequelae [21,22].
- the paravertebral venous plexus; these leakages can cause pulmonary embolism, which is usually peripheral and asymptomatic ("silent pulmonary microembolism") [14,15].

Furthermore, leakeges may be divided into Minor, Moderate and Major depending on the ratio between their diameter and the nearby structures.

Leakages are considered "minor" if their minor diameter is inferior to that of the closest pedicle, "moderate" if it is greater than that of the pedicle but smaller than the cranio-caudal height of the closest healthy vertebra and "major" if it outmeasures in size the contigous vertebra [22].

Infections, just like fractures of posterior elements or the pedicles occur in less than 1% of the cases. The allergic reaction to PMMA is characterized by hypotension and arrhytmia.

A recent evolution of percutaneous vertebroplasty is percutaneous kyphoplasty which employs balloon catheters inflated with contrast agent to restore the morphology of the collapsed vertebral body and reduce kyphosis before stabilisation with bone cement.

Kyphoplasty can be performed in the thoracic spine on vertebrae T5 to T12 and on all lumbar vertebrae.

The procedure is carried out under general anaesthesia with the patient lying prone on the angiography table.

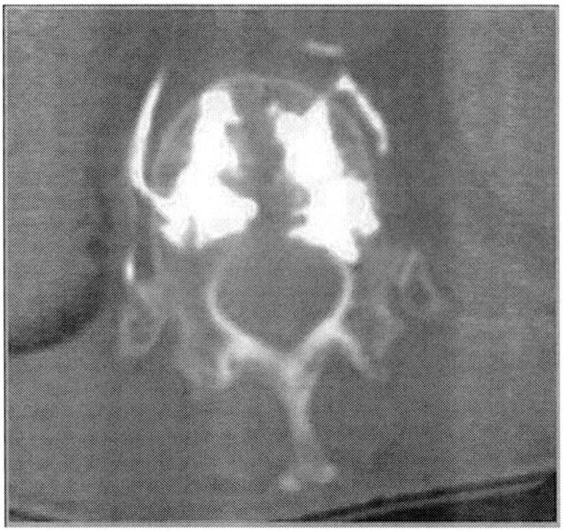

Figure 3. Axial CT scan that shows a paravertebral cement leakage.

There are two possible approaches for the treatment: transpedicular and intercostovertebral. In either case access is bilateral to offer better restoration of vertebral body morphology.

Under fluoroscopic guidance, a C-arm providing adequate visualisation of the spine in the different spatial planes identifies the point of access of the 11G bone-biopsy needle.

After skin incision, the biopsy needle is advanced with the needle tip pointing to 2 or 3 o'clock and to 9 or 10 o'clock on the imaginary clock face traced by the pedicle circumference. The inclination is more horizontal, 3 or 4 o'clock on the right and 8 or 9 o'clock on the left, if the lower somatic endplate shows a depression.

The needle must be advanced in an anteromediocaudal direction. In transpedicular approaches the needle tip must never go beyond the medial cortical margin that delimits the vertebral canal laterally to prevent penetration of the vertebral cavity.

A Kirshner wire is then inserted coaxial to the needle and is used as a guidewire to allow a working cannula to be slid up to 3 mm beyond the posterior wall of the vertebral body.

Subsequently, a bone channel extending distally to a few millimetres from the anterior cortical margin is created with a hand millimetric drill within the spongiosa.

A balloon catheter is inserted into the vertebral body and its exact position checked with lateral fluoroscopy using two radiopaque markers; the balloon is selected on the basis of the morphology of the vertebral body, available sizes being 10,15 and 20 mm with maximum volumes of 4,4 and 6 ml, respectively.

The same procedure is then repeated on the contralateral side.

The balloons in the hemivertebrae are simultaneously inflated with contrast agent under continuous fluoroscopic and manometric control. This generates a radial force that compacts the cancellous bone in the periphery, thereby increasing the strength of the cortical bone and creating a cavity inside the vertebral body. The balloons are inflated until the fracture is set, maximum inflation pressure is achieved, or the balloon is completely distended or encroaching on the cortical margin.

After the balloon catheter has been deflated and removed, the same working cannula is used as an access point to inject PMMA into the newly created cavity.

PMMA is a mixture of a powder compound and a liquid catalyst (methyl-methacrylate monomer in sterile fluid). This compound is mixed until thick and pasty and is then loaded into the dedicated filler cannulae.

The filler cannulae are advanced through the working cannulae, until they reach the anterior third of the bone cavity and the cement is slowly extruded at low pressure through the filler device, under continuous lateral fluoroscopic guidance to check cement distribution.

The number of cannulae required depends on the final volume reached by the inflated balloon catheter and displayed on the inflation system. The cement volume is often 1-2 cubic centimetres more than the final inflation volume to allow the central bolus to mix with the surrounding spongiosa.

The two working cannulae are removed and the skin incisions are sutured under fluoroscopic monitoring in the two orthogonal projections.

Procedure time is approximately 35-45 minutes per level of kyphoplasty. Post-procedure follow-up is performed with conventional radiography and CT.

The patient is kept under observation for fours hours following the procedure and is discharged on the following day [23].

A fundamental role in these minimally invasive procedures is played by bone cement.

There are two main kinds of bone cement: polymer cements and calcium posphate cements.

The role of both is to fill, provide adhesion and stabilize fractures. Polymers are the most used due to their safety and efficacy.

Their use is based on the polymerization of methylmethacrylate (MMA) into polymethylmethacrylate (PMMA), a compound better known as plexiglas while calcium posphate cements take advantage of chemical reactions based on the solubility of reagents and products.

When tricalcium phosphate and calcium phosphate are mixed with water they rapidly precipitate in the form of hydroxyapatite forming a hard compound at body temperature.

Hydroxyapatite is biocompatible material which is believed to form *in vivo* new bone without volume loss.

The disadvantages of this cement consist in the difficulty of injecting it at high pressure inside the vertebral body and the characteristics of its reabsorption which, in osteoporotic patients, may cause bone weakening.

Furthermore, data in literature report that this kind of cement may be less resistant than polymer cements and too fragile to be used in major tratments.

Polimerization may happen in two different ways:

- by the condensation of a funcional group of a monomer with a functional group of the terminal portion of a polymer which grows in length and releases an extra molecule
- by the direct reaction between a polymer chain with a double bond of a monomer without the release of an extra molecule

Polimerization in this latter way begings the very moment in which the monomer becomes unstable reacting with an initiator, a volatile molecule, usually a radical (which contains an unpaired electron).

Commercially available cements are made up of two different compounds:

- a granular powder containing prepolymerized PMMA (or PMMA styrene/copolymer)
- a fluid containing MMA monomers

Benzoyl peroxide (BPO) contained in the powder is the initiator, while the chemical activator is DMTP which is contained in the fluid. In this way polymerization starts only when these two lements are mixed.

To prevent the spontaneous polymerization of the cement, hydroquinone oxide is added to the fluid.

The BPO molecule is split by DMTP and binds the double bond of the MMA monomer.

In this way the polymer grows in length by including PMMA granules into a solid matrix.

Due to the presence of barium sulphate, the resulting cement is radioopaque. However, not all commercially available contain a quantity of barium sulphate and therefore have an adeguate radioopacity.

At the current state, research is oriented towards the developement of an ideal cement which must present all the main discussed characteristics at their highest level (hardness, adhesion force and mechanical strength) without compromising the biomechanics of the spine when used *in vivo*.

References

[1] McKiernan, F; Jensen, R; Faciszewski, T (2003) The dynamic mobility of vertebral compression fractures. *J Bone Miner Res*, *18*(1): 24-9.

[2] Genant, HK et al. (1993) *J Bone Miner Res*, *8*(9) : 1137-1148.

[3] Stallmeyer, MJ; Zoarski, GH; Obuchowski, AM (2003) Optimizing patient selection in percutaneous vertebroplasty. *J Vasc Interv Radiol*, *14*(6): 683-96.

[4] Watts NB (2001) Osteoporotic vertebral fractures. *Neurosurg Focus*, *10*: 1-3.

[5] S.L. Silverman (1992) The Clinical Consequences of Vertebral Compression Fracture. *Bone 13*, S27-S31.

[6] Zoarski, GH; Snow, P; Olan, WJ; Stallmeyer, MJ; Dick, BW; Hebel, JR; De Deyne, M (2002) Percutaneous vertebroplasty for osteoporotic compression fractures: quantitative prospective evaluation of long-term outcomes. *J Vasc Interv Radiol*, *13*(2 Pt 1): 139-48.

[7] Barth, RW; Lane, JM. (1988) Osteoporosis. *Orthop Clin North Am*, *19*: 845-58.

[8] Avery J Evans; Mary E. Jensen; Kevin E. Kip, et al. (2003) Vertebral compression fractures pain reduction and improvement in fuctional mobility after Percutaneous Polymethilmethacrylate Vertebroplasty-Retrospective report of 245 cases. *Radiology* *226*:366-372.

[9] Meunier PJ et al. (1999) *Clin Ther*; *21*(6): 1025-1044.

[10] Ettinger B et al. (1992) *J. Bone Miner Res*, *7*(4):449-456.

[11] Wu SS; Lachmann E; Nagler W (2003) Current medical, rehabilitation and surgical management of vertebral compression fractures. *J Womens Health* (Larchmt), *12*(1): 17-26.

[12] Kaufmann, TJ; Jensen, ME (2001) Age of Fracture and Clinical Outcomes of Pecutaneous Vertebroplasty. *AJNR*, *22*:1860-1863.

[13] Garfin, SR; Yuan HA; Reiley, MA (2001) New technologies in spine: kyphoplasty and vertebroplasty for the treatment of painful osteoporotic compression fractures. *Spine*, *26*(14): 1511-5.

[14] Coumans, JV; Reinhardt, MK; Lieberman, IH (2003) Kyphoplasty for vertebral compression fractures: 1-year clinical outcomes from a prospective study. *J Neurosurg*, *99*(1 Suppl): 44-50.

[15] Higgins, KB; Harten, RD; Langrana, NA; Reiter, MF (2003) Biomechanical effects of unipedicular vertebroplasty on intact vertebrae. *Spine*, *28*(14): 1540-8.

[16] Jang, JS; Kim, DY; Lee, SH (2003) Efficacy of percutaneous vertebroplasty in the treatment of intravertebral pseudarthrosis associated with noninfected avascular necrosis of the vertebral body. *Spine*, *28*(14): 1588-92.

[17] Gangi, A; Tarun, S; Farah, G (2006) Quality Assurance Guidelines for Percutaneous Vertebroplasty. *Cardio Vascolar and Intervetional Radiology 29*:173-178.

[18] Mathis, JM (2002) Vertebroplasty for vertebral fractures with intravertebral clefts. *AJNR Am J Neuroradiol*, *23*(10): 1619-20.

[19] McAllister, A; Spencer, RP; Yannopoulos, AD (2002) Bone densitometry study in a patient with prior kyphoplasty variant of vertebroplasty. *Clin Nucl Med*, *27*(5): 365-6.

[20] Deramond; Cotton, A (1998) Percutaneous Vertebroplasty: State of Art. *Radiographics*, *18*:311-320.

[21] Harrington, KD (2001) Major neurological complications following percutaneous vertebroplasty with polymethylmethacrylate : a case report. *J Bone Joint Surg Am*, *83*-A(7): 1070-3.

[22] Shapiro, S; Abel, T; Purvines, S (2003) Surgical removal of epidural and intradural polymethylmethacrylate extravasation complicating percutaneous vertebroplasty for an osteoporotic lumbar compression fracture. Case report. *J Neurosurg*, *98*(1 Suppl): 90-2.

[23] Masala, S; Massari, F; Simonetti, G (2005) MRI and Bone Scan Imaging in the preoperative evalutation of painful vertebral fractures treated with Vertebroplasty and Kyphoplasty. *In Vivo*, *19*(6):1055-60.

In: Osteoporosis: Etiology, Diagnosis and Treatment
Editors: Bilar E. Mattingly and Albert C. Pillare
ISBN 978-1-60692-397-9

Short Communication C

DETECTING PATIENTS WITH OSTEOPOROSIS PRIOR TO THEM DEVELOPING FRACTURES

Hugh Devlin
School of Dentistry, University of Manchester, Manchester, U.K.

ABSTRACT

Osteoporosis is associated with a considerable degree of mortality and morbidity in elderly patients. Back pain, disfigurement and fractures of the hip and spine are well known consequences of the end stage disease. Hip fracture causes a reduction in life expectancy of almost 6 years in both men and women [1] and often has a devastating effect on the quality of life, with a severe curtailment of independent living. The challenge is to detect fracture-prone patients in the early stages when effective treatment can be instituted.

INTRODUCTION

Recent research has tried to better identify osteoporotic risk factors for fracture. Bone density measurement, by itself, is surprisingly poor at predicting an individual's 10 year risk of hip fracture. This is because of the large numbers of those who have a normal bone density at this site but who subsequently develop hip fractures. The World Health Organization has recently introduced an algorithm which will predict the 10-year probability of an individual having an osteoporotic bone fracture, based on a number of clinical risk factors and bone mineral density (BMD; measured using dual energy X-ray absorptiometry). The clinical risk factors used in this index include body mass index (BMI), a history of fracture, a parental history of hip fracture, consumption of oral glucocorticoids for 3 months or more, rheumatoid arthritis, secondary causes of osteoporosis (such as chronic liver disease), and lifestyle factors such as current smoking, and an alcohol intake of 3 or more units daily [2]. Hip fracture risk is inadequately predicted by measurement of bone mineral density alone, but is considerably improved by using other independent clinical information. Using the algorithm tool for a 65 year-old Caucasian female aged 65 living in the United States (with no additional risk factors, BMD T-score = -2.5, and BMI=24.7), the 10-year probability of hip fracture is 2.8%. The probability of a hip fracture increases to 4.7% in the same individual if the BMD T-score was -3. If an individual's BMD is in the osteoporotic range, treatment is usually indicated because it is cost-effective at any age [3]. However, it is if the patient's BMD is in the osteopenic range (T-score less than -1 but greater than -2.5) that the additional information from clinical risk factors may prove especially helpful in predicting hip fracture probability. For example, if this Caucasian female had an osteopenic BMD T-score of -2, her probability of hip fracture would be 1.6% (with no additional clinical risk factors), but 4.1% if she smoked and consumed 3 or more units of alcohol.

Dawson-Hughes et al [4] used 3% as the threshold probability value which would trigger treatment, but this value will vary according to factors such as a country's ability to afford treatment, the cost of fracture treatment, other health care concerns, the patient's wishes and anxiety, and the availability of cheaper generic drugs. Consideration of additional clinical risk factors in patients with reduced bone density should clarify individual treatment decisions.

Bone Quality

Following the menopause, microarchitectural changes occur in bone which affects its strength independent of the loss of bone mass. As well as the connectedness of bone, the concept of "bone quality" encompasses the microarchitecture, mineralization, and the accumulation of microdamage of bone, but the latter cannot be measured non-invasively in patients. Current radiographic methods of measuring bone quality such as texture and fractal analysis only show moderate correlation with the biomechanical properties of bone. The main determinants of cortical bone strength are its width and porosity, whereas the strength of cancellous bone is dependent on the width and connectivity of individual trabeculae, and at the macroscopic level the geometric shape and anisotropy of the bone. Imaging techniques in development such as in vivo high resolution peripheral quantitative computed tomography (eg XtremeCT, manufactured by Scanco Medical AG) may be useful in examining trabecular bone density, thickness and number and so assist in identifying patients who will develop future fractures. Dual X-ray absorptiometry (DXA) is the current method of choice for determining bone mineral density, due to its accuracy and reproducibility, but only measures areal and not volumetric density.

Determinants of Hip Strength

Low BMD at the femoral neck is a risk factor for a hip fracture. However, only a small proportion of falls result in a fracture, so the nature of the fall must be taken into account. At particular risk of fracture are those individuals who fall sideways and apply high energy loads directly to their hip, perhaps by failing to protect their hip with an outstretched hand or hip protector. Geometric variables of the hip are also important, such as the hip axis length, which are measured from the greater trochanter to the inner pelvic rim, and can be calculated using software packages. Hip axis length may be a significant predictor of hip fracture [5]. Pulkkinen et al [6] found that the assessment of hip fracture risk was considerably improved by combining additional measurements from anterioposterior pelvic roentgenograms with conventional BMD assessment by DXA. Femoral geometric properties, such as neck-shaft angle, cortical thickness and BMD were important. Gregory et al [7] found that the combination of femoral shape, measured using an active shape model, and trabecular structure, measured using a Fourier transform, could almost perfectly classify a small sample of individuals into hip fracture and control groups.

Clinical Risk Factors in Detecting Hip Fractures

It is important to identify strong clinical risk factors for osteoporosis, without overburdening the clinician with lengthy questionnaires. This leads to accurate identification of the true positive osteoporotic proportion in the population, and avoids either failing to detect osteoporotic individuals or providing false positive diagnoses. There are similar parallels to questionnaire design in detecting those who are drinking excessive amounts of alcohol, and providing effective counseling to prevent the social disintegration and self harm which this can bring. There are risk factors, which when identified in a patient's lifestyle, can be used to advise them to avoid future bone fractures. These include tobacco smoking, high alcohol consumption and lack of exercise.

Many hip fractures occur in the very elderly; 41% of hip fractures occurred in the over-80 age group in one study [8]. Large prospective studies are in progress to quantify the contribution of clinical risk factors to hip fracture. Of particular interest to patients are those life-style factors such as smoking, low body weight and alcohol consumption which have been shown to influence hip fracture rate. One in eight hip fractures is attributable to smoking, perhaps through a direct effect on bone [9].

Population screening using DXA is not cost-effective for detecting those most at risk of hip fracture. In addition, there is likely to be a less than adequate provision of DXA facilities needed in the future [10]. Therefore, many studies have explored the possibility of using clinical questionnaires (with or without DXA) to detect groups at particular risk of hip fracture. Dargent-Molina et al [11] used low body weight to select patients for densitometry, and then used clinical risk factors to increase the value of bone mineral density in predicting hip fractures. In their high-risk group, they identified 37% of those women who suffered a hip fracture.

Should this case-finding strategy be implemented there would be a cost saving on densitometric examinations with little reduction in health impact. Other assessment tools such as the FRACTURE index used seven variables (that include age and BMD T-score) which have been shown to predict hip fracture [12].

Other Diseases and Hip Fracture

Rheumatoid Arthritis

Other diseases such as rheumatoid arthritis are associated with an increased risk of osteoporosis, most likely caused by the use of corticosteroids. Less than 14% of those receiving continuous oral glucocorticoids get additional therapy to prevent bone loss, despite the increased risk of fracture [13]. Hip fracture risk is approximately doubled amongst patients with rheumatoid arthritis [14]. Reduced movement, poor nutrition, old age and low body weight may also be significant factors in predicting low bone mass in this disease. The cause of the generalized bone loss in rheumatoid arthritis is controversial, with opinion divided as to whether a reduced bone formation rate or increased resorption rate is the primary etiologic factor. Kr̋ger et al [15] obtained bone biopsies from a group of 119 women with rheumatoid arthritis and found histological evidence of a decreased mineral apposition rate, rather than an increased bone resorption rate. However, osteoporosis is a common complication of patients with rheumatoid arthritis and treatment of these patients with pamidronate (a bisphosphonate which suppresses osteoclastic bone resorption) has been shown in a randomized, double-blind 3-year study, to reduce bone loss and increase bone mass compared with placebo treatment [16].

Bone resorption may be activated by cytokines directly (such as interleukin IL-1) or through them promote the expression of nuclear factor-κB ligand (RANKL), which is necessary for osteoclastic differentiation.

Anorexia Nervosa

A high proportion of those with anorexia nervosa have reduced BMD, as measured by DXA. Winston et al [17] identified osteoporosis in 31% of their sample, with 10% affected at the neck of femur. This is despite the young age of the study group (mean = 26 years, SD=9.9) and a duration of illness of over 12 months. Anorexia especially affects the lumbar spine [18], probably because this is a site with a large proportion of cancellous bone and therefore of more rapid bone turnover. Body mass index [19] and the duration of illness [20] significantly determine the bone mineral density in these patients. Affected women should be counseled about the adverse effects of anorexia on their skeleton, especially as bone loss is not easily reversed and there is an increased rate of non-spine fracture in longitudinal studies [21].

The undernourishment associated with anorexia causes a decrease in serum insulin-like growth factor-I (IGF- I) [22], which when combined with decreased serum estrogen may be responsible for a state of reduced bone formation and increased bone resorption. In anorexia, the serum IGF-1 level may prove to be a useful screening tool as it is related to body mass index and increases during nutritional repletion [23]. Spinal bone density has been shown to increase significantly in anorexic patients in response to recombinant human IGF-I [24]. Doctors need to be aware of the high prevalence of osteoporosis and osteopenia in this group of young individuals (table 1).

Table 1. Some studies show a high prevalence of hip osteoporosis and osteopenia in anorexic individuals

Study	Prevalence of osteoporosis of total hip	Prevalence of osteopenia of total hip
Grinspoon et al [19] (n=130)	16%	47%
Miller et al [25] (n=214)	About 12%	About 42%

Diabetes

In a population of young, middle-aged type I diabetic patients (mean age 38 years) two thirds of the diabetic men and about half of the women had osteopenia of the femoral neck and/or the lumbar spine, as measured by DXA [26]. The hyperglycaemia that is associated with type I diabetes may cause osteopenia and osteoporotic bone fracture through an inhibition of osteoclastic function [27] and osteoblastic mineralization. A deficiency in the insulin-like growth factor system has also been implicated [28]. Bone turnover is therefore affected, with bone formation reduced to a greater extent than bone resorption. Impaired osteoblastic function has been described in diabetic animal studies, where high serum glucose was associated with a decreased mineralization rate [29].

Type II diabetic patients usually have a normal or slightly higher BMD than control subjects, and this may be related to their increased body weight and the active steroids manufactured by adipose tissue.

Conclusion

Recent guidelines recommend that women over the age of 65 years and those aged 60-64 years with clinical risk factors should have their bone density assessed [30]. There is little consensus about which are the best clinical risk factors to use in healthy asymptomatic women; examples in the literature include body mass index [31], age, weight, ethnicity, use of hormone replacement therapy, [32] and a maternal history of fractures [33]. There are some diseases, such as anorexia nervosa and rheumatoid arthritis, and the taking of high doses of glucocorticoid medication for lengthy periods which are generally accepted as being associated with a high risk of osteoporosis. However, other evidence suggests that clinical prediction rules, used alone to screen a healthy community population, will have a high sensitivity but a low specificity, and therefore may not perform well [34]. A low specificity is associated with a large number of normal patients being referred for osteoporotic assessment.

This article is a plea for increased awareness of osteoporosis by doctors in at-risk individuals eg those presenting with low trauma wrist fractures [35] or other risk factors. Some bone densitometry services report receiving requests for investigation in up to 60% of patients with no known risk factors, the “worried well” [36]. Services need to be re-directed to those most in need of osteoporotic investigation.

References

[1] Trombetti A, Herrmann F, Hoffmeyer P, Schurch MA, Bonjour JP, Rizzoli R. Survival and Potential Years of Life Lost After Hip Fracture in Men and Age-matched Women. *Osteoporos Int* 2002; 13:731–737

[2] Kanis JA, Johnell O, Oden A et al. (2008) FRAX™ and the assessment of fracture probability in men and women from the UK. *Osteoporos Int* 2008; 19:385-97.

[3] Kanis JA, Borgstromb F, Zethraeusc N, Johnelld O, Odene A, Jfnssonc B. Intervention thresholds for osteoporosis in the UK. *Bone* 2005; 36:22-32.

[4] Dawson-Hughes B, Tosteson ANA, Melton III LJ, Baim S, Favus MJ, Khosla S, Lindsay RL. Implications of absolute fracture risk assessment for osteoporosis practice guidelines in the USA. *Osteoporos Int*. 2008; 19:449-58.

[5] Faulkner KG, Wacker WK, Barden HS, Simonelli C, Burke PK, Ragi S, Del Rio L. Femur strength index predicts hip fracture independent of bone density and hip axis length. *Osteoporos Int* 2006; 17:593–599.

[6] Pulkkinen P, Partanen J, Jalovaara P, Jämsä T. Combination of bone mineral density and upper femur geometry improves the prediction of hip fracture. *Osteoporos Int*. 2004; 15:274-80.

[7] Gregory JS, Stewart A, Undrill PE, Reid DM, Aspden RM. Bone shape, structure, and density as determinants of osteoporotic hip fracture: a pilot study investigating the combination of risk factors. *Invest Radiol*. 2005; 40:591-7.

[8] Jones G, Nguyen T, Sambrook PN, Kelly PJ, Gilbert C, Eisman JA. Symptomatic fracture incidence in elderly men and women: the Dubbo osteoporosis study (DOES). *Osteopor Int* 1994; 4:277–282.

[9] Law MR, Hackshaw AK. A meta-analysis of cigarette smoking, bone mineral density and risk of hip fracture: recognition of a major effect. *Br Med J* 1997; 315:841–846.

[10] Kanis JA, Johnell O. Requirements for DXA for the management of osteoporosis in Europe. *Osteoporos Int* 2005; 16: 229–238.

[11] Dargent-Molina P, Douchin1 MN, Cormier C, Meunier PJ, Bre´art G, for the EPIDOS study group. Use of Clinical Risk Factors in Elderly Women with Low Bone Mineral Density to Identify Women at Higher Risk of Hip Fracture: The EPIDOS Prospective Study. *Osteoporos Int* 2002; 13:593–599.

[12] Black DM, Steinbuch M, Palermo L, Dargent-Molina P, Lindsay R, Hoseyni MS, Johnell O. An assessment tool for predicting fracture risk in postmenopausal women. *Osteoporos Int*. 2001;12:519-28.

[13] Eastell R, Reid DM, Compston J, Cooper C, Fogelman I, Francis RM, Hosking DJ, Purdie DW, Ralston SH, Reeve J, Russell RG, Stevenson JC, Torgerson DJ. A UK Consensus Group on management of glucocorticoid-induced osteoporosis: an update. *J Intern Med*. 1998; 244:271-92.

[14] Cooper C, Coupland C, Mitchell M. Rheumatoid arthritis, corticosteroid therapy and hip fracture. *Annals of the Rheumatic Diseases*. 1995; 54:49–52.

[15] Krőger H, Arnala I, Alhava EM. Bone Remodeling in Osteoporosis Associated with Rheumatoid Arthritis. *Calcif Tissue Int* 1991; [Suppl] 49:S90.

[16] Eggelmeijer F, Papapoulos SE, van Paassen HC,. Dijkmans BAC, Valkema R, Westedt ML, Landman J-O, Pauwels EKJ, Breedveld FC. Increased bone mass with pamidronate treatment in rheumatoid arthritis. Results of a three-year randomized, double-blind trial. *Arthritis & Rheumatism* 2005; 39:396-402.

[17] Winston AP, Alwazeer AE, Bankart MJ. Screening for osteoporosis in anorexia nervosa: prevalence and predictors of reduced bone mineral density. *Int J Eat Disord.* 2008; 41:284-7.

[18] Misra M, Aggarwal A, Miller KK, Almazon C, Worley M, Soyka LA, Herzog DB, Klibanski A. Effects of anorexia nervosa on clinical, hematologogic, biochemical, and bone density parameters in community-dwelling adolescent girls. *Pediatrics* 2004; 114:1574-1583.

[19] Grinspoon S, Thomas E, Pitts S, Gross E, Mickley D, Miller K, Herzog D, Klibanski A. *Prevalence and predictive factors for regional osteopenia in women with anorexia nervosa.* 2000; 133:790-794.

[20] Legroux-Gérot I, Vignau J, D'Herbomez M, Collier F, Marchandise X, Duquesnoy B, Cortet B. Evaluation of bone loss and its mechanisms in anorexia nervosa. *Calcif Tissue* Int. 2007; 81:174-82.

[21] Rigotti NA, Neer RM, Skates SJ, Herzog DB, Nussbaum SR. The clinical course of osteoporosis in anorexia nervosa. A longitudinal study of cortical bone mass. *JAMA* 1991; 265:1133-1138.

[22] Counts DR, Gwirtsman H, Carlsson LM, Lesem M, Cutler GB Jr. The effect of anorexia nervosa and refeeding on growth hormone-binding protein, the insulin-like growth factors (IGFs), and the IGF-binding proteins *Journal of Clinical Endocrinology & Metabolism* 1992; 75:762-767.

[23] Caregaro L, Favaro A, Santonastaso P, Alberino F, Dipascoli L, Nardi M, Favaro S, Gatta A. Insulin-like growth factor 1 (IGF-1), a nutritional marker in patients with eating disorders. *Clinical Nutrition* 2001; 20: 251- 257.

[24] Grinspoon S, Thomas L, Miller K, Herzog D, Klibanski A. Effects of Recombinant Human IGF-I and Oral Contraceptive Administration on Bone Density in Anorexia Nervosa. *Journal of Clinical Endocrinology & Metabolism* 2002; 87:2883-2891.

[25] Miller KK, Grinspoon SK, Ciampa J, Hier J, Herzog D, Klibanski A. Medical findings in outpatients with anorexia nervosa. *Arch Intern Med.* 2005; 165:561-566.

[26] Kemink SA, Hermus AR, Swinkels LM, Lutterman JA, Smals AG. Osteopenia in insulin-dependent diabetes mellitus; prevalence and aspects of pathophysiology. *J Endocrinol Invest.* 2000;23:295-303.

[27] Wittrant Y, Gorin Y, Woodruff K, Horn D, Abboud HE, Mohan S, Abboud-Werner SL. High d(+)glucose concentration inhibits RANKL-induced osteoclastogenesis. In press. doi:10.1016/j.bone.2008.02.006.

[28] Jehle PM, Jehle DR, Mohan S, Böhm BO. Serum levels of insulin-like growth factor system components and relationship to bone metabolism in Type 1 and Type 2 diabetes mellitus patients. *J Endocrinol.* 1998; 159:297-306.

[29] Shyng YC, Devlin H, Ou KL. Bone formation around immediately placed oral implants in diabetic rats. *Int J Prosthodont.* 2006; 19:513-4.

[30] Nelson HD, Helfand M, Woolf SH, Allan JD. Screening for postmenopausal osteoporosis: a review of the evidence for the U.S. Preventive Services Task Force. *Ann Intern Med.* 2002; 137:529-41.

[31] Meyer HE, Tverdal A, Falch JA. Risk factors for hip fracture in middle-aged Norwegian women and men. *Am J Epidemiol.* 1993;137:1203-11.

[32] Mallmin H, Ljunghall S, Persson I, Bergstro¨m R. Risk factors for fractures of the distal forearm: a population-based case-control study. *Osteoporos Int.* 1994; 4:298-304.

[33] Siris ES, Miller PD, Barrett-Connor E, Faulkner KG, Wehren LE, Abbott TA, et al. Identification and fracture outcomes of undiagnosed low bone mineral density in postmenopausal women: results from the National Osteoporosis Risk Assessment. *JAMA.* 2001; 286:2815-22.

[34] Mauck KF, Cuddihy M-T, Atkinson EJ, Melton JM III. Useof clinical prediction rules in detecting osteoporosis in a population-based sample of postmenopausal women. *Arch Intern Med* 2005; 165:530-536.

[35] Kimber CM, KA Evaluation of current practice: compliance with osteoporosis clinical guidelines in an outpatient fracture clinic. *Aust Health Rev.* 2008; 32:34-43.

[36] Sahota O, Worley A, Hosking DJ. An audit of current clinical practice in the management of osteoporosis in Nottingham. *J Public Health Med.* 2000; 22:466-72.

In: Osteoporosis: Etiology, Diagnosis and Treatment
Editors: Bilar E. Mattingly and Albert C. Pillare
ISBN 978-1-60692-397-9

Short Communication D

DIAGNOSIS AND TREATMENT OF OSTEOPOROTIC PATIENTS IN DENTISTRY

Dubravka Knezović Zlatarić*[1] *and Asja Čelebić

Department of Prosthodontics, School of Dental Medicine, University of Zagreb
Gundulićeva 5, 10000 Zagreb, Croatia

ABSTRACT

Osteoporosis is a multifactorial, age-related metabolic bone disease characterized by low bone mineral density (BMD), deterioration of the microarchitecure of cancellous bone, and changes in the material properties of bone, leading to enhanced bone fragility and to a consequent increase in the risk of fracture.

Those factures do not seem to occur in the jaws. Studies investigating the effect of osteoporosis on the jaws have generally relied on relating changes in bone mass in different skeletal sites to changes in a range of mandibular variables measured in different ways, including height of residual ridge, altered trabecular and cortical pattern, and reduced bone density.

Oral signs of the bone loss in elderly patients are manifested by excessive alveolar ridge resorption and tooth loss. Reduction of the residual alveolar ridges could be described as a resorptive athrophy, a fundamental and physiologic reaction to loss of function and inactivity that presumably is influenced and modulated by individually varying factors, such as condition of the bone, period of edentulousness, denture-wearing habits, and unfavorable loading patterns.

Radiographic intraoral microdensitometry, next to the clinical examination, is definitely one of the most often used bone-mass measuring techniques in assessing the quantity of the mandibular bone loss caused by osteoporosis. It has been developed to increase the precision of bone mass assessment on conventional radiographs, including panoramic radiographs and periapical radiographs. This tool has been proved in several clinical studies to be accurate enough in detecting patients with low bone mineral density.

[1] Corresponging author Assist. Prof. Dubravka Knezović Zlatarić: dkz@email.htnet.hr

In the recent study, determing the relative usefulness of BMD measurements on dental panoramic radiographs in the diagnosis of patients with postmenopausal osteoporosis it was found that the mandibular BMD values, measured on panoramic radiographs, are a significant factor in predicting postmenopausal osteoporosis ($p<0.05$).

Partially and completely edentulous patients, with the diagnosed osteporosis, require special prosthodontic treatment.

Introduction

Osteoporosis is a major public health concern worldwide. The medical, social and psychological consequences can severely impact the health-related quality of life of patients with fractures, and are life-threatening for some patients [1-4].

According to the definition of the World Health Organization (WHO), formulated in 1994, osteoporosis is "a multifactorial, age-related metabolic bone disease characterized by low bone mineral density (BMD), deterioration of the micro-architecture of cancellous bone, and changes in the material properties of bone, leading to enhanced bone fragility and to a consequent increase in the risk of fracture", clearly introducing the association between low bone mass and increased fracture risk, base on bone mineral density [5-7].

Osteoporosis is common among postmenopausal women, but is often asymptomatic [8]. New expert group under the WHO recommended to base the diagnosis of osteoporosis on measurements of BMD in the hip, spine, or lower arm by means of dual X-ray absorptiometry (DXA) [9]. As the annual screening of all postmenopausal women involves high costs, it is suggested that BMD should be measured in subjects with risk factors for osteoporosis, such as low weight or age 65 and over [10,11]. The clinical risk factors for osteoporosis, such as age, height, weight, age at menarche, menopause and its duration, calcium and caffeine intake, alcohol and tobacco use and urinary markers of bone turnover, have been identified and used to develop risk assessment indices [12-16].

However, the results from the National Osteoporosis Risk Assessment showed that large segments of the population of postmenopausal women 50 years old or older with no previous diagnosis of osteoporosis had low skeletal BMD [17].

Osteoporotic Patients in Dentistry

As osteoporosis is a systemic skeletal disease, it also affects bone density and structure of the jaws [18]. Studies investigating the effect of osteoporosis on the jaws have generally relied on relating changes in bone mass in different skeletal sites to changes in a range of mandibular variables measured in different ways, including height of residual ridge, altered trabecular and cortical pattern, and reduced bone density [19-25].

ORAL SIGNS OF THE BONE LOSS

Oral signs of the bone loss in elderly patients are manifested by excessive alveolar ridge resorption and tooth loss. Reduction of the residual alveolar ridges could be described as a resorptive athrophy, a fundamental and physiologic reaction to loss of function and inactivity that presumably is influenced and modulated by individually varying factors, such as condition of the bone, period of edentulousness, denture-wearing habits, and unfavorable loading patterns, as well as bone metabolic diseases. It becomes apparent on a dental panoramic radiograph as thinning of the mandibular cortices and a general radiolucency of the jaws (Figure 1) [26].

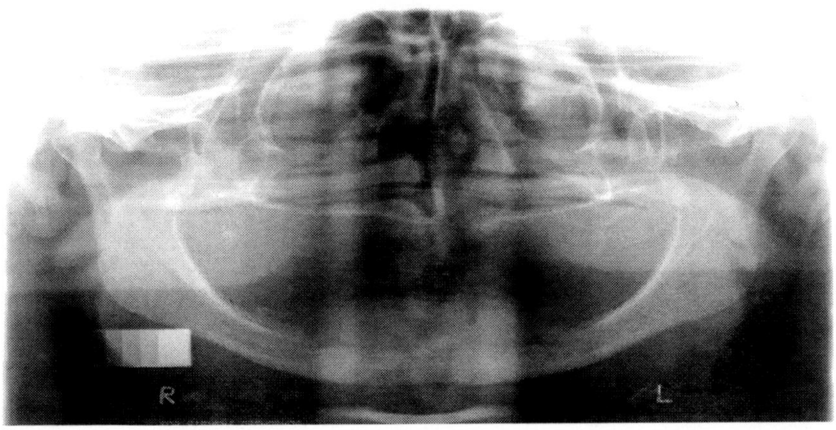

Figure 1. Edentuolous mandible in postmenopausal osteoporotic woman.

DENTAL DIAGNOSTIC TOOLS FOR OSTEOPOROSIS

Recent studies indicate that dental panoramic radiography measures may be useful tools in identifying postmenopausal women with low skeletal BMD [21,27-31], high bone turnover rate [32], or high risk of osteoporotic fractures [33]. Because dental panoramic radiography is frequently performed for the diagnosis of diseases affecting the teeth and jaws in general dental practice, the incidental findings detected on dental panoramic radiographs maybe used to identify women who have no awareness of their low BMD and would benefit from BMD testing [34].

Quantitative linear measurements in form of radiomorphometric indices [23,35], qualitative mandibular cortical index [24,27] or even clinical intraoral bone densitometry [24,36-38] are often used on dental radiographs to assess the bone quality and to find the signs of resorption and osteoporosis.

Ledgerton et al. found that all quantitative indices (mandibular cortical thickness below the mental foramen, at gonion and in region anterior to the gonion) showed a significant, negative correlation with age [35], one of the most important clinical risk factors for osteoporosis.

Knezović Zlatarić et al. also reported that the age-ralated distribution of mandibular cortical index showed an age-related increase in number of individuals with clearly porous lower mandibular cortical line, with significantly higher incidence of women whose mandibular endosteal cortical margins consisted of thick cortical residues in an older age group [24], and significantly lower rates of cortical thicknesses and BMD values among patients of both genders with low body mass indices [23].

Radiographic intraoral microdensitometry, next to the clinical examination, is definitely one of the most often used bone-mass measuring techniques in assessing the quantity of the mandibular bone loss caused by osteoporosis. It has been developed to increase the precision of bone mass assessment on conventional radiographs, including panoramic radiographs and periapical radiographs. This tool has been proved in several clinical studies to be accurate enough in detecting patients with low bone mineral density [18].

In the recent study, determing the relative usefulness of BMD measurements on dental panoramic radiographs in the diagnosis of patients with postmenopausal osteoporosis it was found that the mandibular BMD values, measured on panoramic radiographs, are a significant factor in predicting postmenopausal osteoporosis ($p<0.05$).

Treatment of Osteoporotic Patients in Dentistry

Partially and completely edentulous patients, with the diagnosed osteporosis, require special prosthodontic treatment, due to the resorptive changes of the residual alveolar ridges (Figures 2 and 3).

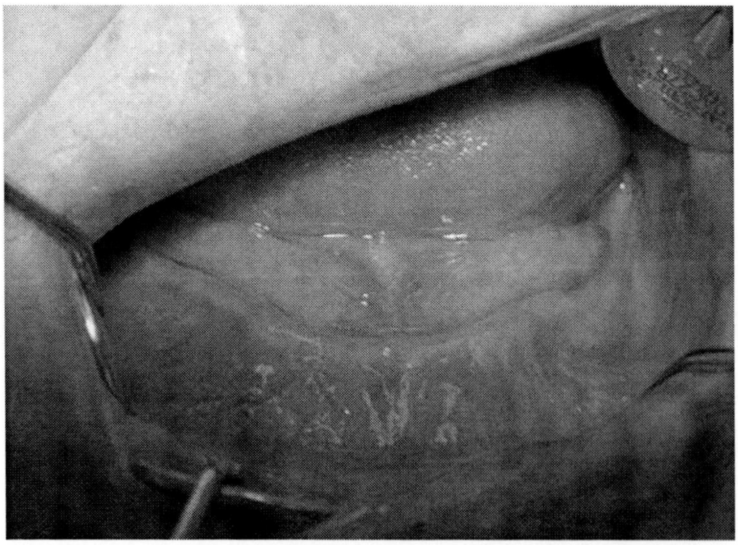

Figure 2. Extremely resorbed edentulous ridge in postmenopausal osteoporotic woman.

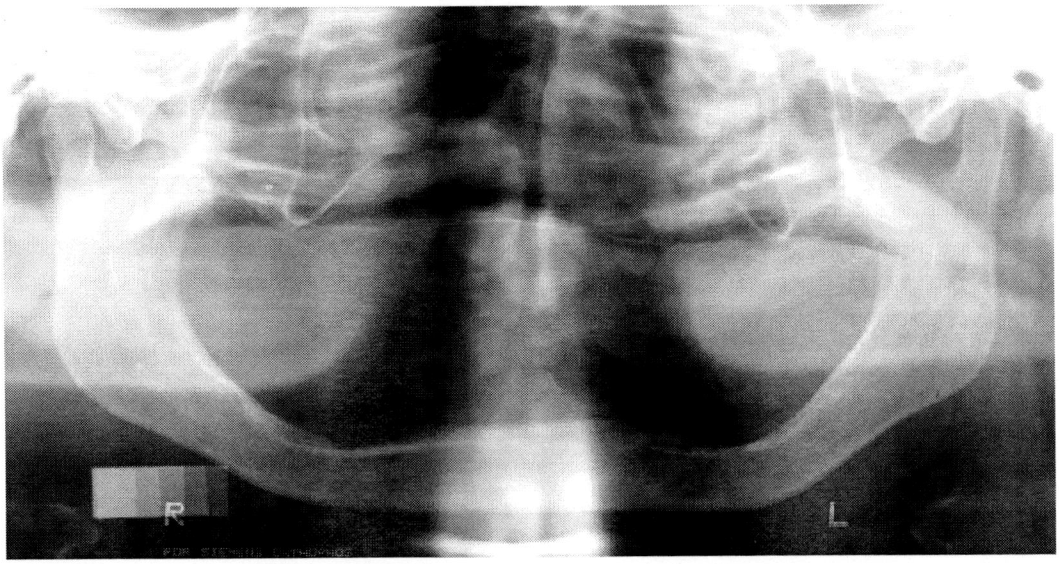

Figure 3. The same alveolar ridge wieved radiographicaly.

Osteoporotic patients can often successfully wear a conventional complete maxillary denture because residual ridge resorption tends to be less dramatic in the maxilla compared to the mandible [42,43], and the most common oral complaint among these patients is a loose conventional mandibular denture.

The relatively frequent experience of advanced mandibular atrophy contributes to denture instability and to a presumed compromise in quality of life [44,45]. Fortunately, this predicament can be remedied routinely by using osseointegrated implants to stabilize a complete mandibular prosthesis.

Oral Bisphosphonate Therapy and Osteonecrosis of the Jaw

Bisphosphonates belong to a group of pyrophosphate compounds that are administered for a constellation of bone disorders. In an oral forme (such as alendronate, risedronate, or etidronate), it is usually prescribed for osteoporosis and osteopenia [43,44].

But, despite these benefits, osteonecrosis of the jaws is a significant complication in a subset of patients receiving these drugs [45]. Since 2003, many cases of osteonecrosis of the jaws have been reported, the vast preponderance associated with the parenteral agents [46-50]. The main reported initiating factor for osteonecrosis of the jaw is dental extraction although periodontal disease and denture trauma have been implicated [51] (Figures 4 and 5).

The risk of developing bisphosphonate osteonecrosis of the jaws in postmenopausal osteoporotic patients treated with oral bisphosponates in still not known, as only a small number of cases have been reported [49,52]. in the review of 368 cases of bisphosphonates related osteonecrosis of the jaws, 18 were associated with oral alendronate, and 13 of these cases occurred in osteoporotic patients without cancer, and almost all of the remaining cases were associated with cancer therapy [52].

It i s important to understand that no casual relationship between bisphosphonate therapy and osteonecrosis of the jaw has been established, only an association has been recognized [47]. There is a need for further research on all aspects of the bisphosphonates, their effec on the jaws and extraction healing, and the relationship between duration of therapy and risks. Inb the meantime however, if the patient is dentally fit before commencement of bisphosphonate therapy and oral health maintained witout extractions, then the risk of osteonecrosis of the jaw should be reduced markedly [53].

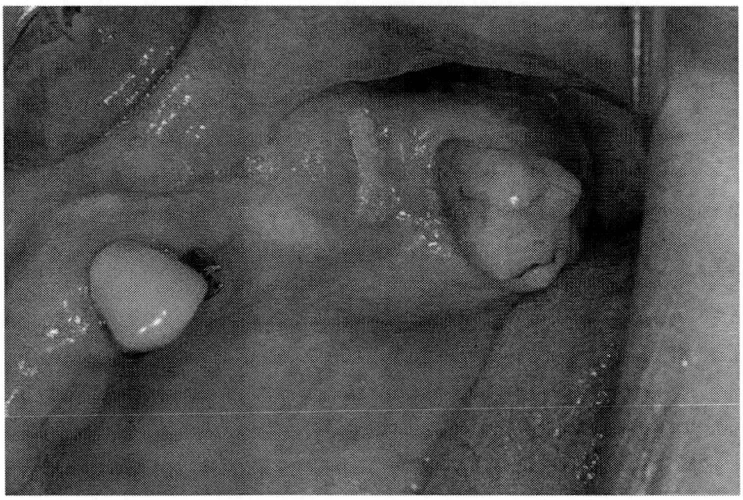

Figure 4. Oral clinical finding of the bisphosphonate osteonecrosis of the jaws.

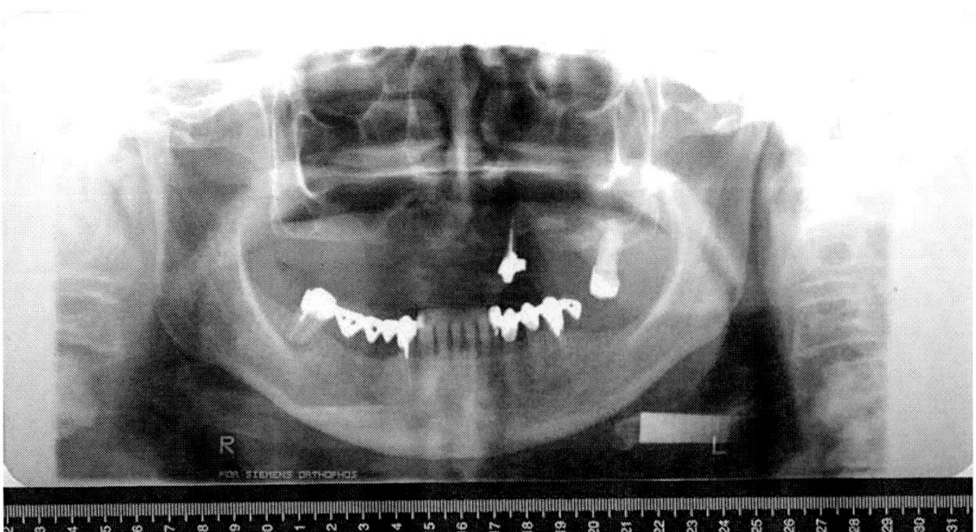

Figure 5. Radiological finding of the bisphosphonate osteonecrosis of the jaws.

REFERENCES

[1] Oleksik A, Lips P, Dawson A, Minshall ME, Shen W, Cooper C, Kanis J. Health-related quality of life in postmenopausal women with low BMD with or without prevalent vertebral fractures. *J Bone Min Res* 2000;15:1384-92.

[2] Oleksik A, Ott SM, Vedi S, Bravenboer N, Compston J, Lips P. Bone structure in patients with low bone mineral density with or without vertebral fractures. *J Bone Miner Res* 2000;15:1368-75.

[3] Randell AG, Nguyen TV, Bhalerao N, Silverman SL, Sambrook PN, Eisman JA. Deterioration in quality of life following hip fracture: a prospective study. *Osteoporos Int* 2000;11:460-6.

[4] Bayles CM, Cochran K, Anderson C. The psychosocial aspects of osteoporosis in women. *Nurs Clin North Am* 2000;35:279-86.

[5] Consensus Development Conference. Prophylaxis and treatment of osteoporosis. *Am J Med* 1991;90:107-10.

[6] Consensus Development Conference. Diagnosis, prophylaxis and treatment of osteoporosis. *Am J Med* 1993;94:646-50.

[7] Consensus Development Conference. Who are candidates for prevention and treatment of osteoporosis? *Osteoporos Int* 1997:7:1-6.

[8] Richy F, Gourlay M, Ross PD, Sen SS, Radican L, De Ceulaer F, Ben Sedrine W, Ethgen O, Bruyere O, Reginster J-y. Validation and comparative evaluation of the osteoporosis self-assessment tool (OST) in a Caucasian populatin from Belgium. *Q J Med* 2004;97:39-46.

[9] WHO scientific group. Prevention and management of Osteoporosis. *WHO Technical Report Series 921*. Geneva. 2003.

[10] Kanis JA, Delmas P, Buchhardt P, Cooper C, Torgerson D. Guidlines for diagnosis and management of osteoporosis: the European Foundation for Osteoporosis and Bone Disease. *Osteoporos Int* 1997;7:390-406.

[11] Physician's Guide to Prevention and Treatment of Osteoporosis. Washington DC, National Osteoporosis Foundation, 1999.

[12] Ribot C, Pouilles JM, Bonneau M, Tremollieres F. Assessment of the risk of post-menopausal osteoporosis using clinical factors. *Clin Endocrinol* 1992;36:225-8.

[13] Lydick E, Cook K, Turpin J, Melton M, Stine R, Byrmes C. Development and validation of a simple questionnaire to facilitate identification of women likely to have low bone density. *Am J Manag cre* 1998;4:37-48.

[14] Cadarette SM, Jaglal SB, Kreiger N, McIsaac WJ, Darlington GA, Tu JV. development and validation of the Osteoporosis Risk Assessment Instrument to facilitate selection of women for bone densitometry. *CMAJ* 2000;162:1289-94.

[15] Gourlay ML, Miller WC, Richy F, Garrett JM, Hanson LC, Reginster JY. Performance of osteoporosis risk assessment tools in postmenopausal women aged 45-64 years. *Osteoporos Int* 2005;16:921-7.

[16] Richy F, Deceulaer F, Ethgen O, Bruyère O, Reginster JY. Development and validation of the ORACLE score to predict risk of osteoporosis. *Mayo Clin Proc* 2004;79:1402-8.

[17] Siris ES, Miller PD, Barrett-Connor E, Faulkner KG, Wehren LE, Abbott TA, Berger ML, Santora AC, Sherwood LM. Identification and fracture outcomes of undiagnosed low bone mineral density in postmenopausal women: results from the National Osteoporosis Risk Assessment. *JAMA*. 2001 Dec 12;286(22):2815-22.

[18] Geraets WGM, Verheij JGC, van der Stelt PF, Horner K, Lindh C, Nicopoulou-Karayianni K, Jacobs R, Harrison EJ, Adams JE, Devlin H. Prediction of bone mineral density with dental radiographs. *Bone* 2007:40:1217-21.

[19] Taguchi A, Ohtsuka M, Tsuda M, Nakamoto T, Kodama I, Inagaki K, Noguchi T, Kudo Y, Suei Y, Tanimoto K. Risk of vertebral osteoporosis in post-menopausal women with alterations of the mandible. *Dentomaxillofac Radiol* 2007;36:143-8.

[20] Arifin AZ, Asano A, Taguchi A, Nakamoto T, Ohtsuka M, Tsuda M, Kudo Y, Tanimoto K. Computer-aided system for measuring the mandibular cortical width on dental panoramic radiographs in identifying postmenopausal women with low bone mineral density. *Osteoporos Int* 2006;17:753-9.

[21] Nakamoto T, Taguchi A, Ohtsuka M, Suei Y, Fujita M, Tanimoto K, Tsuda M, Sanada M, Ohama K, Takahashi J, Rohlin M. Dental panoramic radiograph as a tool to detect postmenopausal women with low bone mineral density: untrained general dental practitioners' diagnostic performance. *Osteoporos Int* 2003;14:659-64.

[22] Taguchi A, Sanada M, Krall E, Nakamoto T, Ohtsuka M, Suei Y, Tanimoto K, Kodama I, Tsuda M, Ohama K. Relationship between dental panoramic radiographic findings and biochemical markers of bone turnover. *J Bone Miner Res* 2003;18:1689-94.

[23] Knezović Zlatarić D, Čelebić A, Kobler P. Relationship between body mass index and local quality of mandibular bone structure in elderly individuals. *J Gerontol A Biol Sci Med Sci* 2002;57A:M588-M593.

[24] Knezović Zlatarić D, Čelebić A. Clinical bone densitometric evaluation of the mandible in removable denture wearers dependent on the morphology of the mandibular cortex. *J Prosthet Dent* 2003;90:86-91.

[25] Knezović Zlatarić D, Čelebić A. Mandibular bone mineral density changes in complete and removable partial denture wearers. A six-month follow-up study. *Int J Prosthodont* 2003;16:661-665.

[26] Devlin CV, Horner K, Devlin H. Variability in measurement of radiomrphometric indices by general dental practitioners. *Dentomaxillofacial radiol* 2001;30:120-5.

[27] Klemetti E, Kolmakov S, Kroger H. Pantomography in assessment of the osteoporosis risk group. *Scand J Dent Res* 1994;102:68-72.

[28] Taguchi A, Suei Y, Ohtsuka M, Otani K, Tanimoto K, Ohtaki M. Usfulness of panoramic radiography in the diagnosis of postmenopausal osteoporosis in women: width and morphology of inferior cortex of the mandible. *Dentomaxillofac Radiol* 1996;25:263-267.

[29] Devlin H, Horner K. Mandibular radiomorphometric indices in the diagnosis of reduced skeletal bone mineral density. *Osteoporos Int* 2002;13:373-378.

[30] Horner K, Devlin H, Harvey L. Detecting patients with low skeletal bone mass. *J Dent* 2002;30:171-175.

[31] Taguchi A, Suei Y, Sanada M, Higashi Y, Ohtsuka M, Nakamoto T, Tsuda M, Ohama K, Tanimoto K. Detection of vascular disease risk in women by panoramic radiography. *J Dent Res* 2003;82:838-43.

[32] Taguchi A, Sanada M, Krall E, Nakamoto T, Ohtsuka M, Suei Y, Tanimoto K, Kodama I, Tsuda M, Ohama K. Relationship between dental panoramic radiographic findings and biochemical markers of bone turnover. *J Bone Miner Res* 2003;18:1689-94.

[33] Bollen AM, Taguchi A, Hujoel PP, Hollender LG. Case-control study on self-reported osteoporotic fractures and mandibular cortical bone. *Oral Surg Oral Med Oral Pathol Oral Radiol Endod* 2000;90:518-24.

[34] Taguchi A, Suei Y, Sanada M, Ohtsuka M, Nakamoto T, Sumida H, Ohama K, Tanimoto K. Validation of dental panoramic radiography measures for identifying postmenopausal women with spinal osteoporosis. *Am J Roentgenol* 2004;183:1755-60.

[35] Ledgerton D, Horner K, Devlin H, Worthington H. radiomorphometric indices of the mandible in a British female population. *Dentomaxillofac Radiol* 1999;28:173-181.

[36] Kribbs PJ, Smith DE, Chestnut CH. Oral findings in osteoporosis. Part I: measurement of mandibular bone density. *J Prosthet Dent* 1983;50, 576-579.

[37] Kribbs PJ, Smith DE, Chestnut CH. Oral findings in osteoporosis. Part II: relationship between residual ridge and alveolar bone resorption and generalized skeletal osteopenia. *J Prosthet Dent* 1983;50, 719-724.

[38] Knezović Zlatarić D, Čelebić A, Milat O. Bone densitometric study of mandibular density using dental panoramic radiographs. *Acta Stomatol Croat* 2002;36, 29-37.

[39] Tallgren A. The contunuing reduction of the residual alveolar ridges in complete denture wearers: A mixed-longitudinal study covering 25 years. *J Prosthet Dent* 1972;27:120-132.

[40] Carlsson GE, Persson G. Morphologic changes of the mandible after extraction and wearing of dentures. A longitudinal, clinical and x-ray celphalometric study covering 5 years. *Odontol Revy* 1967;18:27-54.

[41] Čelebić A, Knezović Zlatarić D. A comparison of patient's satisfaction between complete and partial removable denture wearers. *J Dent.* 2003;31:445-51..

[42] Čelebić A, Knezović Zlatarić D, Papić M, Carek V, Baučić I, Stipetić J. Factors related to patient satisfaction with complete denture therapy. *J Gerontol A Biol Sci Med Sci* 2003;58:M948-M953.

[43] McCarus DC. Fracture prevention in postmenopausal osteoporosis: a review of treatment options. *Obstet Gynecol Surv* 2006;61:39-50.

[44] Sarioglu M, Tazun C, Unlu Z, Tikiz C, Taneli F, Uyanik BS. Comparison of the effects of alendronate and risedronate on bone mineral density and bone turnover markers in postmenopausal osteoporosis. *Rheumatol Int* 2006,26:195-200.

[45] Ruggiero S, Fantasia J, Carlson E. Bisphosphonate-related osteonecrosis of the jaw: background and guidelines for diagnosis, staging and management. *Oral Surg Oral Med Oral Pathol Oral Radiol Endod*. 2006;102:433-41.

[46] Fresco RE, Fernandez NP, Urizar JMA. Bisphosphonates and oral pathology II. Osteonecrosis of the jaws: Review of the literature boefore 2005: *Med Oral Patol Oral Cir Bucal* 2006;11:E456-61.

[47] Koka S, Clarke BL, Amin S, Gertz M, Ruggiero SL. Oral bisphosphonate therapy and osteonecrosis of the jaw: what to tell the concerned patient. *Int J Prosthodont* 2007;20:115-22.

[48] Melo MD, Obeid G. Osteonecrosis of the jaws in patients with a history of receiving bisphosphonate therapy: strategies for prevention and early recognition. *J Am Dent Assoc* 2005;136:1675-81.

[49] Brooks JK, Gilson AJ, Sindler AJ, Ashman SG, Schwartz KG, Nikitakis NG. Osteonecrosis of the jaws associated with use of risedronate: report of 2 new cases. *Oral Surg Oral Med Oral Pathol Oral Radiol Endod* 2007;103:780-6.

[50] Dimitrakopoulos I, Magopoulos C, Karakasis D. Bisphosphonate-induced avascular osteonecrosis of the jaws: a clinical report of 11 cases. *Int J Oral Maxillofac Surg* 2006;35:588-93.

[51] Marx RE. Pamicronate (Aredia) and zolendronate (Zometa) induced avascular necrosis of the jaws: A growing epidemic. *J Oral Maxillofac Surg* 2003;61:1115-1117.

[52] Woo SB, Hellstein JW, Kalmar JR. Systemic (narrative) review: Bisphosphonates and osteonecrosis of the jaws. *Ann Intern Med* 2006;144:753-761.

[53] Sambrook P, Olver I, Goss AN. Bisphosphonates and osteonecrosis of the jaw: Position statement on behalf of the Australian and New Zealand Bone and Mineraal Society, Osteoporosis Australia, Medical Oncology Group of Australia na the Australian Dental Association. *Aust Fam Physician* 2006;35:801-803.

In: Osteoporosis: Etiology, Diagnosis and Treatment
Editors: Bilar E. Mattingly and Albert C. Pillare
ISBN 978-1-60692-397-9

Short Communication E

Nordic Walking - Is it Suitable for Patients with Fractured Vertebra?

J. Wendlová *

University Derer's Hospital and Policlinic, Osteological Centre, Bratislava, Slovakia.

Abstract

This article brings the biomechanical analysis of sport – Nordic walking – for patients with osteoporotic fractured vertebrae and shows that it is suitable for them.

Based on the biomechanical model of skeletal load we have developed a method of walking movement for patients, different from the method of walking movement for healthy people. And so came into being the "first sport"for patients with osteoporotic fractures. They can go for regular walks in easy terrains outdoors with friends and family, and so be liberated from social isolation. It requires only one-off financial costs of buying the poles and special footwear.

Keywords: osteoporosis – fractured vertebra – biomechanics – exercise - Nordic walking.

Introduction

Patients with Fractured Vertebra and Sport?

I have put the question mark deliberately, as it could seem absurd to some people without it. However, I know from my clinical experience that most of these patients strive to defy the heavy odds and want to overcome their handicap by physical activity. Many patients are aware that inactivity will aggravate their health, their muscles will slacken and their

* Correspondence concerning this article should be addressed to: Ass Prof Jaroslava Wendlová MD, PhD Krížna 30, 811 07 Bratislava. jwendlova@mail.t-com.sk.

efficiency will diminish, and the back pain will get worse. The patients will have to rely on the help of other people or a care service, which they often cannot afford for financial reasons. This is the reason why there is a growing interest in regular motion activities. I often hear in my surgery statements like "*Could you advise me some group exercise for people with the same handicap I have?"* The best exercise for patients with osteoporotic vertebra fractures is a regular group exercise lead by an experienced physiotherapist as well as exercise in a swimming pool (excluding swimming).

Unfortunately, there are not many towns and villages where the patients have the opportunity to participate in regular and long-term exercise organised by experienced physiotherapists. Other sport activities are not suitable for patients with osteoporotic vertebra fractures, either for the increased risk of injury or for increased strain on weakened skeleton.

When we pondered over the questions asked by my patients and considered what easy sport would be suitable for them, we have chosen – Nordic Walking. This assumption was confirmed by a biomechanical analysis. Based on the biomechanical model of skeletal load we have developed a method of walking movement for patients, different from the method of walking movement for healthy people. And so came into being the "first sport" suitable for patients with osteoporotic fractures. They can go for regular walks in easy terrains outdoors with friends and family, and so be liberated from social isolation. It requires only one-off financial costs of buying the poles and special footwear.

Nordic Walking – Walking with Supporting Poles

Nordic Walking is a dynamic fitness walking outdoors in different terrains, using a pair of special telescopic poles with exchangeable tips for different surfaces. When walking on less concrete surfaces, such as grass or dirt, the poles with classical spike tips are used, on hard surfaces, such as asphalt, the poles with rubber tips are used. The stride rhythm is given by swinging opposite arms and legs alternately forward and backward.

The correct pole length should represent about 70 – 72% of the body height and to calculate it there is a simple formula using one's own height multiplied by 0.66. The walker's elbow should be at approximately a 90° angle when holding the pole by the grip with the tip on the ground. We have chosen the Nordic Walking as a suitable sport for patients with osteoporosis, especially for patients with osteoporotic vertebra fractures. This conclusion was reached on the basis of biomechanical analysis of vertebra load. Firstly, we simulated the vertebra load as a patient with kyphosis walked with outstretched arms without supporting poles, to demonstrate the lever arms and components of the force of gravity of the upper part of the body acting upon the vertebra. Consequently, we unloaded the upper part of the body by poles held in arms extended forward during walking.

Biomechanical Analysis

Calculation of Static Load of Vertebra during mild Trunk Bending without the Support of the Poles [1–8]

Model example No.1

We are interested in static load, e.g., of the Th12 vertebra (12th thoracic vertebra) by the force of gravity of the upper part of the body above the mentioned vertebra, if both elbows of upper limbs are held at a 90° angle (i.e., without being supported by poles).

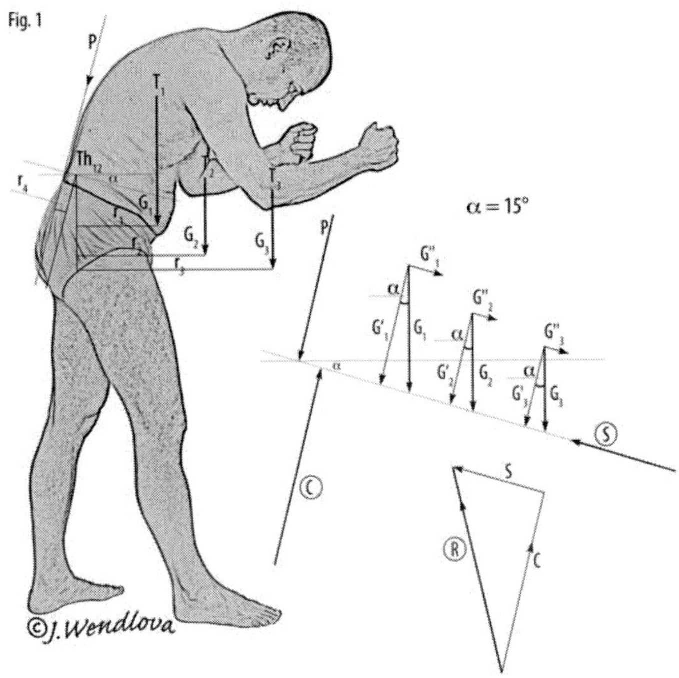

Figure[#] 1. Static load of vertebra Th12 during mild trunk bending without the support of the poles.

Mathematical definitions:

mass: $m = \dfrac{G}{g}$ (kg)

force of gravity: G = m x g ($kgms^{-2}$)

acceleration due to gravity $g = 9.80665ms^{-2}$

gravity force moment M = G x r

r – arm, to which the force is applied

Solution

Static load will be calculated for the Th12 vertebra.

[#] Figures are created by author. Figurant in figures: Martin Petrik.

Patient's weight is m = 70 kg, his force of gravity is $G = m \times g \approx 700$ N

Bending forward, the spine is bent at a 15° angle.

When bending forward, there are four forces (G_1, G_2, G_3, P) acting upon the Th 12 vertebra:

1. G_1 - resultant gravity force of the upper part of the torso and head G_1 (over the Th12 vertebra), producing approx. 50% of the body mass (Table 1). G_1 = 350N, is applied in the gravity centre of the upper torso T_1.
2. G_2 ,G_3 - resultant gravity forces of both upper limbs stretched forward with elbows held at a 90° angle, producing 5.6% x 2 = 11.2% of body mass. G_2 = 39.20 N acting upon the gravity centre of the left upper limb (UL) T_2.
3. G_3 = 39.20 N acting upon the gravity centre of the right UL T_3. P - is force produced by the contraction of erector spinae muscles (consisting of muscles: • m. iliocostalis thoracis, • m. spinalis thoracis, • m. longissimus thoracis). The magnitude of the P force is unknown; we know only its direction and the point of application (it is an imaginary point in erector spinae muscles above the Th12 vertebra body).

Table1. The Mass Ratio of Different Body Parts to the Whole Body in Percentage (Body mass = 100%) [13]

Body Part	The Ratio of the Body Part Mass to the Whole Body in % (according to Fischer)	The Ratio of the Body Part Mass to the Whole Body in % (according to Dempster)
Head	8.8	8.1
Torso	45.2	49.7
Thigh	11.0	9.9
Crus	4.5	4.6
Leg	2.1	a.4
Arm	2.8	2.8
Forearm	2.0	1.6
Hand	0.8.	0.6

Calculation of the P Force Magnitude

All four forces, namely G_1, G_2 , G_3, P, are acting upon arms of different length (r_1, r_2, r_3, r_4) related to the imaginary point in Th12, producing four bending moments for this point.

Arms, on which the forces are applied, are real distances measured on the patient

r_1 = 0,25 m, r_2 =0,30 m, r_3 =0,40 m , r_4 =0,05 m

Explanatory note to symbols used in equations

The clockwise acting force moment is called a positive moment, marked by the symbol (+), the counter clockwise acting force moment is called a negative moment and marked by the symbol (-).

Forces of gravity G_1, G_2 and G_3 produce positive bending moments.

$M_1 = G_1 \times r_1$

$M_2 = G_2 \times r_2$

$M_3 = G_3 \times r_3$

The contraction force P in m. erector spinae produces a negative bending moment

$-M_4 = P \times r_4$

Bending moment M_4 is the counterbalancing moment to bending moments M_1, M_2, M_3.
The P force magnitude is calculated from the first condition of equilibrium:
The sum of the moments in the plane acting upon a given point is equal to zero.

$$\sum_{i=1}^{4} M_i = 0$$

$$M_1 + M_2 + M_3 + (-M_4) = 0$$

$$G_1 \times r_1 + G_2 \times r_2 + G_3 \times r_3 = P \times r_4$$

$$P = \frac{(G_1 \times r_1) + (G_2 \times r_2) + (G_3 \times r_3)}{r_4} = \frac{(350 \times 0.25) + (39.20 \times 0.30) + (39.20 \times 0.40)}{0.05} = 2298.80N$$

P = 2298.80 N

Forces of gravity G_1, G_2 and G_3 are resolved in a polygon of forces into compressive forces G_1' G'_2 G_3' and shearing forces G_1'', G_2'', G_3''. By both these forces the gravity forces G_1 G_2 and G_3 are acting upon Th12 vertebra at a 15° angle of bent back..

Calculation of Reactive Compressive Force C in Th12 Vertebra

Component compressive forces G_1', G'_2 , G_3' and the contraction force of muscles P, acting upon Th12 vertebra, condition the rise of the reactive compressive force C in the vertebra, which is in equilibrium with the forces G_1' ,G'_2 , G_3' and P (the equilibrium is upset in case of vertebra fracture).

The magnitude of the resultant reactive compressive force C in vertebra is unknown; we know only its direction and point of application. Its direction is opposite to the direction of G_1' G'_2 G_3' and P forces, and its point of application is in Th 12 vertebra.

The C force is calculated from the second condition of equilibrium.

The sum of parallel forces in the plane is equal to zero.

$$\sum forces = 0$$

Magnitudes of component compressive forces G_1', G'_2, G_3' are calculated from right-angled triangles by trigonometrical function for cosine:

$$\alpha = 15^0$$

$$\cos\alpha = \frac{G_1'}{G_1} \qquad G_1' = \cos 15° \times G_1 = 0.966 \times 350 = 338.10\ \text{N}$$

$$\cos\alpha = \frac{G_2'}{G_2} \qquad G_2' = \cos 15° \times G_2 = 0.966 \times 39.20 = 37.87\ \text{N}$$

$$\cos\alpha = \frac{G_3'}{G_3} \qquad G_3' = \cos 15° \times G_3 = 0.966 \times 39.20 = 37.87\ \text{N}$$

$$(\cos 15° \times G_1) + (\cos 15° \times G_2) + (\cos 15° \times G_3) + P + (- C) = 0$$

$C = (\cos 15° \times G_1) + (\cos 15° \times G_2) + (\cos 15° \times G_3) + P = 338.10 + 37.87 + 37.87\text{N} + 2298.80 = 2712.64$ N

C = 2712.64 N

Calculation of Reactive Shearing Force S in Th12 Vertebra

Component gravity forces G_1'' G_2'' G_3'' are shearing forces acting upon the vertebra, where the reactive shearing force S comes into being, in equilibrium with the forces G_1'' G_2'' G_3'' (the equilibrium is upset in case of vertebra fracture). The magnitude of the reactive shearing force S in the vertebra is unknown; we know only its direction and a point of application. It acts in the opposite direction than forces G_1'' G_2'' G_3'' and its point of application is in Th12 vertebra.

Magnitudes of component shearing forces G_1'' G_2'' G_3'' are calculated from right-angled triangles by trigonometrical function for sine:

$$\alpha = 15^0$$

$$\sin\alpha = \frac{G_1''}{G_1} \qquad G_1'' = \sin 15° \times G_1 = 0.259 \times 350\text{N} = 90.65\ \text{N}$$

$$\sin\alpha = \frac{G_2''}{G_2} \qquad G_2'' = \sin 15° \times G_2 = 0.259 \times 39.20 = 10.15\ \text{N}$$

$\sin\alpha = \frac{G_3^{''}}{G_3}$ $G_3^{''} = \sin 15° \times G_3 = 0.259 \times 39.20 = 19.15$ N

The S force is calculated from the second condition of equilibrium.

The sum of parallel forces in the plane is equal to zero.

$$\sum forces = 0$$

$G_1'' + G_2'' + G_3'' + (-S) = 0$

$S = G_1'' + G_2'' + G_3'' = 90.65 + 10.15 + 10.15 = 110.95$ N

S = 110.95 N

We calculated the magnitudes of reactions (reactive forces) C and S in the vertebra to compressive and shearing components of gravity forces G_1 G_2 G_3.

Calculation of Resultant Reactive Force R

As the forces C and S act perpendicularly upon each other, we can calculate the magnitude of their resultant R from the Pythagorean Theorem:

$$R = \sqrt{C^2 + S^2} = \sqrt{2712.64^2 + 110.95^2} = 864.94N$$

R = 864.94 N

R is a resultant reactive force, produced in Th12 vertebra due to static load by the upper part of the body during bending the back at a 15° angle with upper limbs extended forward and elbows held at 90 ° angles. The direction of the action of the resultant force R is determined graphically by the composition of forces S and C.

The procedure for the calculation of static load for other dorsal vertebra is identical. The angle of action of component forces upon the vertebra changes as well as the magnitude of component forces depending upon the magnitude of resultant gravity force of the body part above the given vertebra. Less gravity force of the body acts upon proximally placed vertebra (upper vertebra) than upon distally placed vertebra (lower vertebra).

Forces transferred into poles during Nordic Walking [3, 4, 8–12]

Model example No. 2

We start from the identical position of the trainee as in the example No. 1 – the spine is at a 15° angle during trunk bending (identical picture).

The force of gravity of the upper part of the torso and the head G_1 (the point of application is in the centre T_1) and forces of gravity of both upper limbs G_2 , G_3 (acting upon the centres T_2 , T_3) are transferred into poles during walking with the poles held in extended arms. We consider two independent solutions – the trainee supported with one vertical pole and the trainee supported with one deflected pole.

Solution A

Transfer of forces into the right-hand vertical pole.

Solution B

Transfer of forces into the left-hand pole, deflected from the vertical at an acute angle.

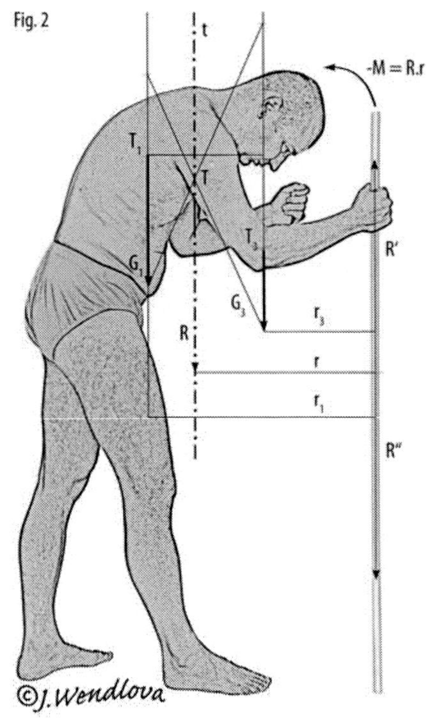

Figure 2. Solution A.

Solution A (Figure 2)

Transfer of Forces into the Right-hand Vertical Pole

To find out how the forces are transferred into the pole, at first we have to determine the magnitude, direction and the point of application of the resultant gravity force R and then add a couple of forces in the pole to the force R. These two forces are formed by two equally large forces acting in the same beam and point of application; they are of an opposite direction, while it applies that:

$$R = R' = R''$$

The equilibrium status of forces is not changed, as the effects of both added forces are cancelled mutually. Vertical distances of centres T_1 and T_3 from the pole are arms r_1, r_3, upon which act the gravity forces G_1, G_3. We calculated them in the Model example No. 1. We find out the magnitude of the arm r, upon which acts the resultant of gravity forces R. The resultant of vertical gravity forces equals their sum.

$G_1 = 350$ N $\quad G_3 = 29.20$ N $\quad r_1 = 0.52$ m $\quad r_3 = 0.30$ m

$R = G_1 + G_3 = 350 + 29.20 = 379.20$ N

R = 379.20 N

From the condition of equality of moments we calculate the arm, upon which acts the resultant R: The moment of the resultant set of forces in the plane to a given point equals the sum of moments of individual forces for this point

$G_1 \times r_1 + G_3 \times r_3 = R \times r$

$$r = \frac{G_1 \times r_1 + G_3 \times r_3}{R} = \frac{(350 \times 0.52) + (29.20 \times 0.30)}{379.20} = 0.503m$$

r = 0.503 m

We know now the resultant R, arm r, upon which acts the R and its direction (in the picture we determined its direction graphically), but we do not know its point of application – the centre T. The centre of the resultant R can be determined graphically or by calculation. This mathematical process is not the target of this analysis, because for physicians it is important to explain in a simple way the principle of the transfer of forces into poles, and the position of the centre T affects neither the magnitude of moments of gravity forces, nor the magnitude of the compressive force R´´ transferred into the pole.

The resultant moment M is produced by the gravity force R, acting upon the arm r.

- M = R x r = 379.20 x 0.503 = *190.74 Nm*

In the course of walking with a pole in an outstretched hand, the total resultant of gravity forces R of the upper part of the body is transferred as the compressive force R´´ (379.20 N). To provide stability, a couple of forces R, R´ (negative bending moment, - M = 190.74 Nm) are acting from the pole towards the upper part of the body against the forward inclination of the walker. Taking into consideration two vertical poles, while the distance of the centres of upper limbs from the poles is the same, a half of compressive force R´´ of the resultant gravity force R is transferred into each pole.

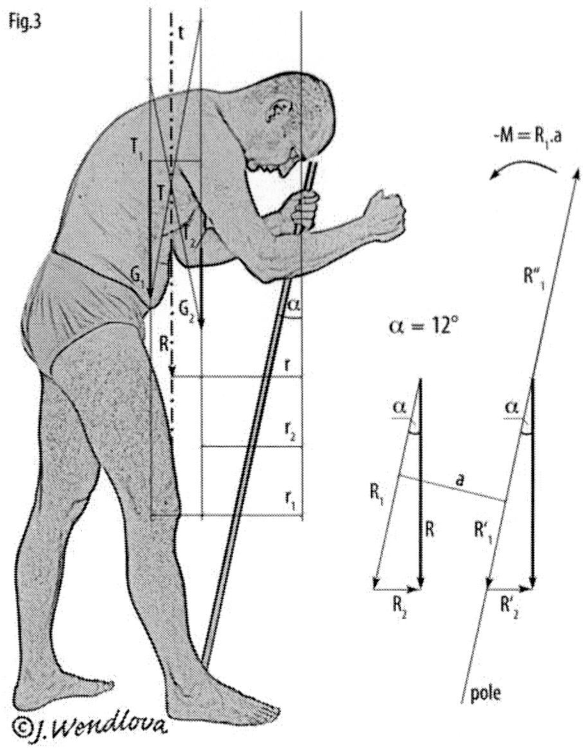

Figure 3. Solution B.

Solution B (Figure 3)

Transfer of forces into the left-hand pole, deflected from the vertical at an acute angle.

The magnitude of the resultant force R of the upper part of the body is calculated in the same way as in Solution A, i.e., for an imaginary vertical left-hand pole.

$G_1 = 350$ N $\quad G_2 = 29.20$ N $\quad r_1 = 0.43$ m $\quad r_2 = 0.30$ m

$R = G_1 + G_2 = 350 + 29.20 = 379.20$ N

$R = 379.20\ N$

$G_1 \text{ x } r_1 + G_2 \text{ x } r_2 = R \text{ x } r$

$$r = \frac{G_1 \times r_1 + G_2 \times r_2}{R} = \frac{(350 \times 0.43) + (29.20 \times 0.30)}{379.20} = 0.42m$$

$r = 0.42\ m$

Equally as in the Solution A, we do not calculate the point of application of the force T, to make the analysis simpler. We know its magnitude, the arm, upon it acts and direction (determined graphically in the picture), which is sufficient for the explanation of application of forces.

The resultant force R is divided into two component forces R_1 a R_2.

The magnitude of component forces R_1 a R_2 is calculated from trigonometrical functions for sine and cosine of the angle:

$$\alpha = 12^0$$

$$\cos\alpha = \frac{R_1}{R_2} \qquad R_1 = \cos 12° \text{ x } R = 0.978 \text{ x } 379.20 = 370.858 \text{ N}$$

$$\sin\alpha = \frac{R_2}{R} \qquad R_2 = \sin 12° \text{ x } R = 0.208 \text{ x } 379.20 = 78.874 \text{ N}$$

$$R_1 = R_1' = R_1'' \qquad a = r = 0.42 \text{ m}$$

$$- M = R_1 \text{ x } a = 370.858 \text{ x } 0.42 = 155.760 \text{ Nm}$$

The resultant force R, passing the axis of the gravity centre t, is transferred by its component R_1 at an 12° angle into the pole deflected from the vertical by 12°. We add to the component force R_1 of the resultant gravity force R two forces in the axis of the deflected pole, both of equal magnitude, acting in one beam but in the opposite direction. The equilibrium of forces does not change, because the effects of both added forces are mutually cancelled. The distance *a* is the distance of component force R_1 from the axis of the pole and simultaneously it creates the lever arm for two forces R_1 and R_1''. To provide stability, a couple of forces R_1 and R_1'' (negative bending moment, - M = 155.760 Nm) are acting from the pole towards the upper part of the body against the forward inclination of the walker. The remaining force R_1' (370.858 N) is the compressive component force R_1 of the resultant gravity force R transferred into the pole. The horizontal component force R'_2 (78.874 N) of the resultant gravity force R prevents the sliding of the pole. If the two poles are deflected at the same angle and the axes of gravity force of upper limbs are at the same distance from the poles, then a half of the compressive component force R_1 of resultant gravity force R is transferred into each pole.

THE CONCLUSION OF BIOMECHANICAL SOLUTION OF FORCE TRANSFER INTO THE POLES

In the model example the Th12 vertebra of the trainee, bent in the spine at a 15° angle and stretching out the arms (without the poles) with elbows at a 90° angle, is loaded by a force of *864.94 N*.

If in the same position we put vertical poles in the trainee's hands, then *379.20 N* of the force of gravity of the upper part of the body is transferred into the poles; to provide stability two forces R and R′ (negative bending moment) are acting from each pole towards the upper part of the body against the forward inclination of the walker. Using two vertical poles, the static load of the Th12 vertebra is reduced by 379.20 N and the vertebra is loaded by *485.74 N* force.

If we put into the trainee's hands two poles, deflected from the vertical at a 12° angle, then *370.858 N* of the force of gravity of the upper part of the body is transferred into the poles; to provide stability the two forces R_1 and R_1'' (negative bending moment) are acting from each pole against the forward inclination of the walker. Horizontal component forces of the resultant gravity force R, transferred into the poles, prevent their sliding. Using two poles, deflected from the vertical, the static load of the Th12 vertebra is reduced by 370.858 N and the vertebra is loaded by *494.08N* force.

EFFECTS OF NORDIC WALKING

Positive effects for osteoporotic patients with fractured vertebra:

- strengthening the muscles of shoulders, arms, breast, abdomen, spine, and upper and lower limbs
- stretching the muscles of the neck, shoulders and trunk
- enlargement of the support area and improvement of stability while walking (Figure 5)
- partial relief of vertebra from the gravity force of the head and trunk
- reduction of tensile forces in spinal muscles by osteoporotic kyphosis
- improvement of motion coordination → prevention of falls
- improvement of muscle performance → improvement of mobility
- sparing the knee and hip joints while walking
- even longer walks do not worsen the back pain

Overall effects upon the organism:

- up to a 20 to 50% increase in energy consumption compared with ordinary walking without poles
- 30% less load on the locomotory system compared with slow running combined with walking (jogging)
- strengthening the cardiac muscle

Differences in the Walking Methods between Healthy Persons and Patients with Osteoporotic Vertebra Fractures

Healthy Person (Figure 4)

The motion rhythm is given by alternate diagonal walking. The right upper limb is forward, the left lower limb is extended backwards, the left upper limb is stretched backwards, the right lower limb is extended forward and in the next step the positions of the limbs alternate. There is a rotation of the axis of the left (right) shoulder joint against the axis of the left (right) hip joint.

Patient with Osteporotic Vertebra Fractures (Figure 5)

We suggest the same motion rhythm, given by alternate diagonal walking; however, the upper limbs are bent in the elbows and stay outstretched during walking to reduce partially the gravity force of the head and trunk upon the spine. The right upper limb is forward, left lower limb is extended backwards, the left upper limb is forward, but with the pole closer to the body as the right upper limb, the right lower limb is stretched forward. In the next step the positions of the limbs alternate. There is no counter-rotation of the axes of shoulder and hip joints and so the osteporotic spine is spared the stress of the torsion forces.

Fig. 4

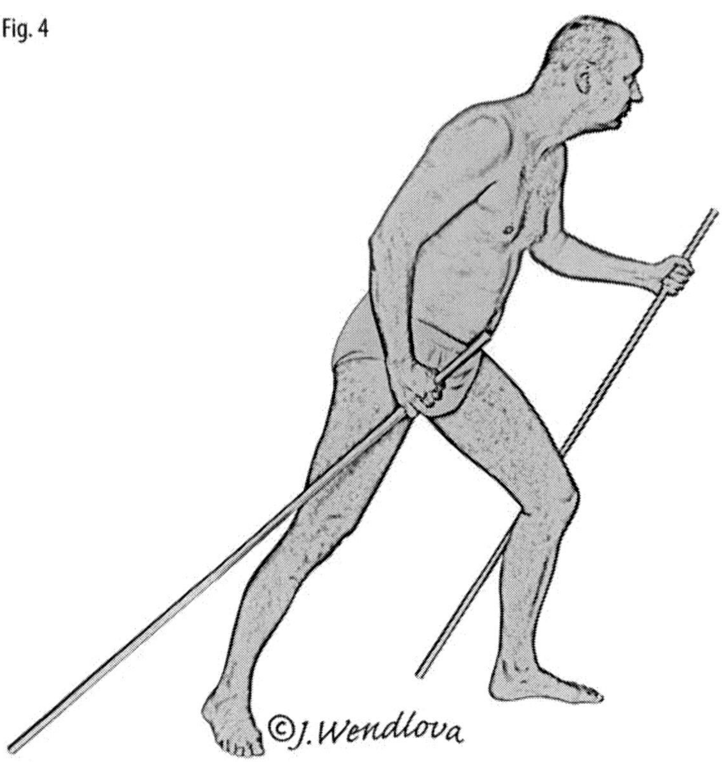

Figure 4.

Fig. 5

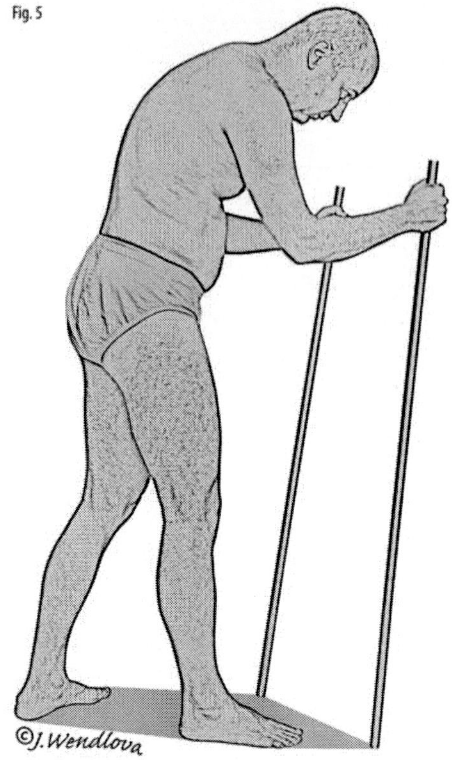

Figure 5.

Conclusion

Based on the biomechanical analysis we recommend Nordic Walking as a suitable sport for patients with osteoporotic fractures, under the conditions of the change of the method of motion rhythm, as suggested in the article.

Regular motion activities stimulate new bone formation. The bone mineral density (BMD) and also the periosteal apposition of bone increase. The periosteal apposition brings the bone mineral further away from the central axis, the cross – sectional area (CSA) of bone and following the cross - sectional moment of inertia (CSMI) enlarge. Increasing in BMD and in CSMI improve the bone strength. Less than 1 mm increase in outer diameter can compensate for 10% loss in BMD [14].

References

[1] Wendlová J: Biomechanika chrbtice a jej význam v pohybovej liečbe pri osteoporóze. (Biomechanics of spine and its signification in exercise therapy for osteoporotic patients) *Eurorehab* 1999, vol.2, č. 3 – 4, 174 – 177.

[2] Wendlová J: Odľaženie chrbtice o hmotnosť horných končatín v štádiu hojenia akútnej fraktúry stavca (Unloading the spine by the weight of upper extremities during healing of acute fracture of vertebra) *Rehabil fyz lék* 2004 vol.11, č. 2, 95 – 101.

[3] Obetková V, Mamrillová A, Košinárová A: *Teoretická mechanika. Vydavateľstvo technickej a ekonomickej literatúry ALFA*, Bratislava, 1990, 30 – 94.

[4] Adamča LF, Marton P, Pavlík M, Trávníček F: *Teoretická mechanika. Vydavateľstvo technickej a ekonomickej literatúry ALFA*, Bratislava, 1992, 27 – 37.

[5] Homminga J. Van-Rietbergen B. Lochmuller EM. Weinans H. Eckstein F. Huiskes R: The osteoporotic vertebral structure is well adapted to the loads of daily life, but not to infrequent "error" loads. *Bone* 2004, 34, 510-516.

[6] Bono CM, Einhorn TA: Overview of osteoporosis: Pathophysiology and determinants of bone strength. [Review] *Europ Spine J* 2003, 12, 90-96.

[7] Lohfeld S, Barron V, Mc Hugh PE: Biomodels of bone: A review An of *Biomed Engineering* 2005, 10, 145 – 150.

[8] Burr DB: Biomechanics *Clin Reviews in Bone and Miner Metab*, 2006, 3, 112 – 117.

[9] Bouxein ML: Biomechanics of osteoporotic fractures. *Clin Reviews in Bone and Miner Metab*, 2006, 3, 118 – 126.

[10] Ferguson JS, Steffen T: Biomechanics of the aging spine. *Europ Spinal J*, 2003, Suppl 2, 167 – 169.

[11] Özkaya N, Nordin M: *Fundamentals of biomechanics: Equilibrium, motion and deformation*, 2nd ed, Springer – Verlag, New York, 1999, 45 – 51.

[12] Fernandez JW, Mithraratne P, Thrupp SF, Tawhai MH, Hunter PJ: Anatomically based geometric modeling of the musculo – sceletal system and other organs. *Biomech and Model in Mechanobiology*, 2004, 3, 444 – 450.

[13] Koniar M, Leško M: *Biomechanika Slovenské pedagogické nakladateľstvo*, Bratislava, 1992, 37.

[14] Faulkner KG, Wacker WK, Barden HS, Simonelli C, Burke PK, Ragi S, Del Rio L: Femur strength index predicts hip fracture independent of bone density and hip axis length. *Osteoporos Int*, 2006, 4, 593 – 599.

In: Osteoporosis: Etiology, Diagnosis and Treatment
Editors: Bilar E. Mattingly and Albert C. Pillare
ISBN 978-1-60692-397-9

Short Communication F

T - Plus Z – Score in the Assessment of Relative Fracture Risk

J. Wendlová*

University Derer´s Hospital and Policlinic, Osteological Centre, Bratislava, Slovakia.

Abstract

Patients and methods. We analysed 498 (n = 498) densitometric findings from the area of proximal femur: Neck (ROI_1), Ward ´s area (ROI_2), great trochanter (ROI_3) (DXA - dual energy X–ray absorptiometry, from the population of Bratislava women of the average age of 59.71 years ⟨58.63; 60.80⟩. Measured values of T and Z– score were categorized as follows: 1 – increased fracture risk (T – score < - 2.5 SD/ T = 1, Z–score ≤ - 1.0 SD/ Z = 1), 0 – without increased fracture risk (T – score > - 2.5 SD/ T = 0, Z – score > - 1.0 SD / Z = 0).

The objective of the study. We aimed to prove that the relative risk of fractures (RR) is higher in women whose T and Z–score values come under the category of increased risk than in the women whose T–score only falls within the category of increased risk.

Statistical analysis: 1. Contingency tables, measurement of the intensity of the association of categorized variables 2. Determination of probability (P) and relative risk (RR)

Results: RR for development of fracture was higher for all measurement sites (ROI_1 – 29.87; ROI_2 – 15.3; ROI_3 – 5.5) for women having T – score < - 2.5 SD and simultaneously Z – score ≤ - 1.0 SD than for the women having T – score < - 2.5 SD and simultaneously Z – score > - 1.0 SD. When the women were divided according to age into two groups: a) women< 65 years, b) women ≥ 65 years, it was found that the RR of fracture for women < 65 years having T – score < - 2.5 SD and also Z – score ≤ - 1.0 SD is very high (RR = ∞), old women (≥ 65 years) had the RR for ROI_1 – 32.61, for ROI_2 – 7.72, and for ROI_3 – 6.9. Probability (P) of the presence of women with T – score values < - 2.5 SD and Z – score ≤ - 1.0 SD in the group under 65 years is for ROI_1 – 12.5%;

* Correspondence concerning this article should be addressed to: Ass Prof. Jaroslava Wendlová, MD, PhD Krížna 30, 811 07 Bratislava. jwendlova@mail.t-com.sk.

ROI_2 – 34.4%; ROI_3 – 20.5%, and the probability for women ≥ 65 years is for ROI_1 – 75%; ROI_2 – 98%; and ROI_3 – 100%.

Conclusions: The study's contribution lies in the finding that the relative fracture risk in proximal femur in women increases, if T-core < - 2.5 SD and, simultaneously, Z-score ≤ - 1.0 SD, and this risk is especially high for women under the age of 65.

In assessing the individual fracture risk by questionnaires in female patients we recommend to add also Z – score values in the measured area to T –score values and to other anamnestic and biochemical risk factors.

Keywords: total hip - osteoporosis – female – T- score – Z - score.

Introduction

The assessment of individual fracture risk has been constantly improved and made more accurate. The assessment of individual fracture risk by applying only the T – score values does not take into consideration other risk factors, and is, therefore, distorted. For example, in the past the same fracture risk was assessed for T – score - 2.6 SD in a woman of 45 as well as a woman of 65, without considering the age factor [1,2,3]. This was the reason why other risk factors began to be added to T – score values, as age, sustained fracture after the age of 50, femur neck fracture in mother, increased biochemical markers of osteoresorbtion, smoking, body mass under 56 kg, and the like. These risk factors in the individual assessment of fracture risk are evaluated together with T – score from the area of proximal femur (total hip) using various questionnaires with good sensitivity and specificity, contributing to the objectification of the risk assessment [4].

Z – score determination is a part of all densitometric measurements and it is given in all densitometric findings. Its significance in the assessment of individual fracture risk is defined as a risk increase with the decrease of standard deviation (SD) by every

-1.0 SD. However, in practice it is not used for individual fracture assessment at all. An important finding is that in postmenopausal women with reduced Z-score values it is necessary to consider the presence of secondary osteoporosis.

We have set up the hypotheses in the study in order to objectively prove the significance of Z– score values in the individual fracture risk assessment and to introduce it into the medical practice.

The Objective of the Study:

1. To establish how many times the relative fracture risk is higher in the group of women with T-score < - 2.5 SD and, simultaneously, with Z-score ≤ - 1.0 SD, in comparison with women with T-score < - 2.5 SD and Z-score > - 1.0 SD.
2. To divide the cohort of women into two groups according to age:
   2.1. age ≥ 65 years (old age)
   2.2. age < 65 years

To establish how many times the relative fracture risk is higher for women ≥ 65 years with T-score < - 2.5 SD and, simultaneously, with Z-score ≤ - 1.0 SD, in comparison with women ≥ 65 years with T-score < - 2.5 SD and Z-score > - 1.0 SD.

To establish how many times the relative fracture risk is higher for women < 65 years with T-score values< - 2.5 SD and, simultaneously, with Z-score ≤ - 1.0 SD, in comparison with women < 65 years with T-score < - 2.5 SD and Z –score > - 1.0 SD.

Characteristics of the Sample of Examined Female Patients and Methods Applied

We analysed 498 (n = 498) densitometric findings from the area of proximal femur in the sample of population of Bratislava women of the average age of 59.71 ⟨58. 63, 60. 80⟩.

In the group of women from different Bratislava districts there were patients with osteoporosis and osteopenia who underwent control BMD measurement, as well as women with osteoporosis risk factors who undergo densitometric examination at the first time. The women with osteoporosis risk factors were selected in accordance with the indication list of the International Society for Clinical Densitometry (Official Positions 2004) [5]. Within the group of risk women, new patients were diagnosed with osteoporosis and osteopenia. All women were examined with the same densitometer DXA (dual energy X–ray absorptiometry) Bone mineral density (BMD) was determined in standard regions of interest for DXA (ROI - region of interest) – Neck (ROI_1), Ward's area (ROI_2), great trochanter (ROI_3). BMD values were given in absolute numbers in g of Ca- hydroxyapathite crystals for cm^2 (g/cm^2), as well as in relative numbers as T-score (the number of standard deviations from the reference group of young healthy women) and Z-score (the number of standard deviations from the relevant age group of healthy women). Osteoporosis was diagnosed in accordance with the WHO criteria:

Classification of bone density	**T- score:**
Normal	> – 1,0 SD
Osteopenia	⟨–1,0; - 2,5) SD
Osteoporosis	≤ – 2,5 SD

Statistical Analysis [6,7,8, 20]

We have used the statistical program systems Statgraphics plus version 3 and SPSS version 6 for the analysis of the female group data.

1) Test for normality of distribution of T – score and Z - score values in ROI_1, ROI_2, ROI_3 (χ^2 – goodness-of-fit statistic, Kolmogorov – Smirnov statistics)
2) Contingency tables (association)

We have the T and Z – scores categorized as:

a) *Presence of higher fracture risk* (designation of category 1)

for T – score < - 2.5 SD and for Z – score ≤ - 1.0 SD
(categorized T = 1, Z = 1)

b) *Absence of higher fracture risk* (designation of category 0)

for T – score > - 2.5 SD and for Z – score > - 1.0 SD.
(categorized T = 0, Z = 0)

3) Verification of association and measurement of the intensity of association between categorized variables T and Z – score in contingency tables:
   a) Phi coefficient
   b) Cramer's V coefficient
   c) Pearson's contingency coefficient
4) Assessment of relative fracture risk in the sample (6) according to T - score with regard to Z – score values

Because the incidence of osteoporosis in Slovakia is less than 10% according the EVOS study [EVOS, 9], we can in retrospective study use RR instead of the OR [10]. RR is more better to interpret.

RESULTS

Measured values of T – score in ROI_1 , ROI_2 have normal distribution (Graph 1, 2), lognormal distribution of frequency is in ROI_3 (Graph 3). Z– score values in ROI_1, ROI_2, ROI_3 are normally distributed.

Probability (P) and Relative Risk (RR) for ROI

ROI_1 (Tables 1a,b)

$$P_1 = \frac{a}{a+b} = \frac{15}{20} = 0.25 = 25\%$$

$$P_2 = \frac{c}{c+d} = \frac{4}{478} = 0.00836 = 0.8\%$$

$$RR = \frac{0{,}25}{0.00836} = 29.875$$

ROI_2 (Tables 2a,b)

$$P_1 = \frac{a}{a+b} = \frac{70}{111} = 0.631 = 63.1\%$$

$$P_2 = \frac{c}{c+d} = \frac{16}{378} = 0.0413 = 4.13\%$$

$$RR = \frac{0.631}{0.0413} = 15.3$$

Table 1a

	T – score (SD) ROI$_1$		Total count in row
Z – score (SD) ROI$_1$	> - 2,5 (count)	≤ - 2,.5 (count)	
> - 1,0	474 d	4 c	478
≤ - 1,0	15 b	5 a	20
Total count in column	489	9	498

a, b, c, d, - frequencies.

Table 1b

Coeficient of assotiation	Intensity of assotiation	Approximate significance
Phi	0,35613	*
Cramer´s V	0,35613	*
Pearson´s	0,33549	*

$\alpha = 0{,}05$; $p > 0{,}05$; * statistical significance.

Table 2 a

	T – score (SD) ROI$_2$		Total count in row
Z – score (SD) ROI$_2$ (count)	> - 2,5 (count)	≤ - 2,.5 (count)	
> - 1,0	371 d	16 c	387
≤ - 1,0	41 b	70 a	111
Total count in column	412	86	498

Table 2b

Coeficient of assotiation	Intensity of assotiation	Approximate significance
Phi	0,64885	*
Cramer´s V	0,64885	*
Pearson´s	0,54431	*

$\alpha = 0{,}05$; $p > 0{,}05$.

Table 3a

	T – score (SD) ROI$_3$		Total count in row
Z – score (SD) **ROI$_3$** (count)	> - 2,5 (count)	≤ - 2,.5 (count)	
> - 1,0	430 d	25 c	455
≤ - 1,0	31 b	12 a	43
Total count in column	461	37	498

Table 3b

Coeficient of assotiation	Intensity of assotiation	Approximate significance
Phi	0,24004	*
Cramer´s V	0,24004	*
Pearson´s	0,23341	*

$\alpha = 0,05$; $p > 0,05$.

ROI$_3$ (Tables 3a,b)

$$P_1 = \frac{a}{a+b} = \frac{12}{43} = 0.279 = 27.9\%$$

$$P_2 = \frac{c}{c+d} = \frac{25}{455} = 0.055 = 5.5\%$$

$$RR = \frac{0.279}{0.055} = 5.07$$

Probability (P_1) that women in selected group have T – score < - 2.5 SD, if they have simultaneously Z – score ≤ - 1.0 SD, is for:

1) ROI$_1$ - 25%
2) ROI$_2$ – 63.1%
3) ROI$_3$ – 27.9%

Probability (P_2) that women in selected group have T – score < - 2.5 SD, if they have simultaneously Z – score > - 1.0 SD, is for:

1) ROI$_1$ - 0.8%
2) ROI$_2$ – 4.13%
3) ROI$_3$ – 5.5%

We define RR for sustaining fracture according to T – score with regard to Z – score in ROI$_1$, ROI$_2$, ROI$_3$ as follows:

$$RR = \frac{P(T = 1 / Z = 1)}{P(T = 1 / Z = 0)}$$

Relative risk (RR) for sustaining fracture *in the sample* is for:

1) ROI$_1$ - 29.875 times

2) ROI_2 – 15.300 times
3) ROI_3 – 5.070 times

higher for women having T – score < - 2.5 SD and simultaneously Z – score ≤ - 1.0 SD than for the women having T – score < - 2.5 SD and simultaneously Z – score > - 1.0 SD.

In the population the RR is with probability 95% from the interval:

1) ⟨13.86; 64.39⟩ for ROI_1
2) ⟨11.22; 20.75⟩ for ROI_2
3) ⟨2.85; 9.04⟩ for ROI_3

There was a statistical significance of association intensity (Tables 1b, 2b, 3b) for dichotomous variables in contingency tables (Tables 1a, 2a, 3a) for all ROIs. The closest association was found for the contingency table Table 2a (ROI_2), r = 0.648 (Table 2b).

Probability (P) and Relative Risk (RR) for Women< 65 Years

ROI_1

$$P_1 = \frac{a}{a+b} = \frac{2}{16} = 0.125 = 12.5\%$$

$$P_2 = \frac{c}{c+d} = \frac{0}{306} = 0.0 = 0.0\%$$

$$RR = \frac{0.125}{0.0} = \infty$$

ROI_2

$$P_1 = \frac{a}{a+b} = \frac{21}{61} = 0.344 = 34.4\%$$

$$P_2 = \frac{c}{c+d} = \frac{0}{261} = 0.0 = 0.0\%$$

$$RR = \frac{0.344}{0.0} = \infty$$

ROI_3

$$P_1 = \frac{a}{a+b} = \frac{8}{39} = 0.205 = 20.5\%$$

$$P_2 = \frac{c}{c+d} = \frac{0}{283} = 0.0 = 0.0\%$$

$$RR = \frac{0.205}{0.0} = \infty$$

Probability (P_1) that women in selected group aged < 65 years
have T – score < - 2.5 SD, if they have simultaneously Z – score ≤ - 1.0 SD is for:

1) ROI_1 - 12.5%
2) ROI_2 – 34.4%
3) ROI_3 – 20.5%

Probability (P_2) that women in selected group aged < 65 years have T – score < - 2.5 SD, if they have simultaneously Z – score > - 1.0 SD, is for:

1) ROI_1 - 0%
2) ROI_2 – 0%
3) ROI_3 – 0%

No woman was found in the female group aged < 65 years for measurements in all ROIs, who would have T - score *<- 2.5 SD and, simultaneously, Z – score >- 1.0 SD.*

Therefore the RR for fracture risk *in the sample* equals infinity, what means that the RR for women with T – score < - 2.5 SD and, simultaneously, Z – score ≤ - 1,0, is infinite times higher than for women with T – score < - 2.5 SD and, simultaneously, Z – score > - 1.0 SD.

RR *in the population* cannot be calculated, because RR in the sample equals ∞.

Table 4a

Age < 65 years			
Z – score (SD) ROI_1 (count)	**T – score (SD) ROI_1** (count)		Total count in row
	> - 2,5	≤ - 2,.5	
> - 1,0	306 d	0 c	306
≤ - 1,0	14 b	2 a	16
Total count in column	320	2	322
Age ≥ 65 years			
> - 1,0	168 d	4 c	172
≤ - 1,0	1 b	3 a	4
Total count in column	169	7	176

Table 4b

Age < 65 years		
Coeficient of assotiation	Intensity of assotiation	Approximate significance
Phi	0,34573	*
Cramer´s V	0,34573	*
Age ≥ 65 years		
Phi	0,55422	*
Cramer´s V	0,55422	*

$\alpha = 0{,}05$; $p > 0{,}05$.

There was a statistical significance of association intensity (Tables 4b, 5b, 6b) for dichotomous variables in contingency tables (Tables 4a, 5a, 6a) for all ROIs. The closest association was found for the contingency table Table 5a (ROI_2), r = 0.546 (Table 5b).

Table 5a

Age < 65 years			
Z – score (SD) ROI_2 (count)	**T – score (SD) ROI_2** (count)		Total count in row
	T- score > - 2,5	≤ - 2,.5	
Z - score > - 1,0	261 d	0 c	261
≤ - 1,0	40 b	**21** a	61
Total count in column	301	21	322
Age ≥ 65 years			
> - 1,0	110 d	16 c	126
≤ - 1,0	1 b	**49** a	50
Total count in column	111	65	176

Table 5b

Age < 65 years		
Coeficient of assotiation	Intensity of assotiation	Approximate significance
Phi	0,54636	*
Cramer´s V	0,54636	*
Age ≥ 65 years		
Phi	0,79709	*
Cramer´s V	0,79709	*

$\alpha = 0{,}05$; $p > 0{,}05$.

Table 6a

Age < 65 years			
Z – score (SD) ROI₃ (count)	**T – score (SD) ROI₃** (count)		Total count in row
	T- score > - 2,5	≤ - 2,.5	
Z - skóre > - 1,0	283 d	0 c	283
≤ - 1,0	31 b	8 a	39
Total count in column	314	8	322

Age ≥ 65 years			
> - 1,0	147 d	25 c	172
≤ - 1,0	0 b	4 a	4
Total count in column	147	29	176

Table 6b

Age < 65 years		
Coeficient of assotiation	Intensity of assotiation	Approximate significance
Phi	0,42997	*
Cramer´s V	0,42997	*
Age ≥ 65 years		
Phi	0,34334	*
Cramer´s V	0,34334	*

$\alpha = 0{,}05$; $p > 0{,}05$.

Probability (P) and Relative Risk (RR) for Women ≥ 65 Years

ROI₁

$$P_1 = \frac{a}{a+b} = \frac{3}{4} = 0.75 = 75\%$$

$$P_2 = \frac{c}{c+d} = \frac{4}{172} = 0.023 = 2.3\%$$

$$RR = \frac{0.75}{0.023} = 32.61$$

ROI₂

$$P_1 = \frac{a}{a+b} = \frac{49}{50} = 0.98 = 98\%$$

$$P_2 = \frac{c}{c+d} = \frac{16}{126} = 0.127 = 12.7\%$$

$$RR = \frac{0.98}{0.127} = 7.72$$

ROI₃

$$P_1 = \frac{a}{a+b} = \frac{4}{4} = 1.0 = 100\%$$

$$P_2 = \frac{c}{c+d} = \frac{25}{172} = 0.145 = 14.5\%$$

$$RR = \frac{1.0}{0.145} = 6.9$$

Probability (P_1) that women in selected group aged ≥ 65 years have T – score < - 2.5 SD, if they have simultaneously Z – score ≤ - 1.0 SD, is for:

1) ROI_1 - 75%
2) ROI_2 – 98%
3) ROI_3 – 100%
4)

Probability (P_2) that women in selected group aged ≥ 65 years have T – score < - 2.5 SD, if they have simultaneously Z – score > - 1,0 SD, is for:

4) ROI_1 - 2.3%
5) ROI_2 – 12.7%
6) ROI_3 – 14.5%
7)

Relative risk (RR) for sustaining fracture *in the sample* is for:

1) ROI_1 - 32.61 times
2) ROI_2 – 7.72 times
3) ROI_3 – 6.90 times
4)

higher for women aged ≥ 65 years, having T – score < - 2.5 SD and, simultaneously, Z – score ≤ - 1,0 SD, than for the women having T – score < - 2.5 SD and, simultaneously, Z – score > - 1.0 SD.

In the population the RR is with probability 95% from the interval:

1) for ROI_1 – big scatter in the interval, because there are small counts for a, b, c, so the result is not valid
2) ⟨1.09; 54.58⟩ for ROI_2
3) for ROI_3 the RR cannot be calculated, because b equals 0 in the contingency table

There was a statistical significance of association intensity (Tables 4b, 5b, 6b) for categorized variables in contingency tables (Tables 4a, 5a, 6a) for all ROIs. The closest association was found for the contingency table Table 5a (ROI_2), $r = 0.797$ (Table 5b)

Discussion

T and Z – score values are different in measurements by DXA densitometer in various skeleton sites not only in the same osteoporotic patient, but also in a healthy individual. This is conditional on the uneven bone mass loss in the skeleton.

In measurement sites with fast bone mass loss (DXA - vertebrae in lateral projection, DXA - Ward's area) the WHO criterion for T-score overestimates pathologies of BMD, and, conversely, in sites with a slow bone mass loss (DXA - total hip, DXA - trochanter) it underestimates pathologies of BMD [11,12]. Intermediate bone mass loss is found when DXA is used at the distal forearm, at the vertebrae in AP projection and at the femoral neck area.

Therefore, the WHO set the BMD measurement by DXA instruments in the proximal femur area (total hip) as a gold standard for osteoporosis diagnosis. According to the WHO criteria, the osteoporotic fracture risk increases for both T - and Z - scores for every –1.0 standard deviation, and the increased fracture risk for the patient is imminent when the measurement results for T-score < - 2.5 SD and for Z-score ≤ - 1.0 SD. We used these criteria in statistical categorisation of both T- and Z - scores as the presence of increased fracture risk and the absence of increased risk.

In the study we determined how many times the fracture risk in women having both T and Z-score values within the increased risk category differs from the risk in women having only the T-score values within the increased fracture risk category. The study confirmed that women having both T and Z-scores within the increased fracture risk category face statistically significant higher fracture risk for all measured regions of interest in proximal femur area in comparison with women having only the T-score in the increased risk category. The highest RR of fracture for the whole sample of women according to T plus Z-score values was found in ROI_1 (Neck). When the sample was divided into the old-age women (≥ 65 years) and the women aged < 65 years, we found out that in the latter group there was no woman having T-score < - 2.5 SD and, simultaneously, Z – score ≤ - 1.0 SD for measurements in all three ROIs. In the group of women under the age of 65 the RR of fracture equals infinity, there is an infinitely more times higher RR for women having T-score < - 2.5 SD and simultaneously, Z-score ≤ - 1.0 SD, than for women having T-score < - 2.5 SD and simultaneously, Z-score > - 1.0. This result is of high statistical significance, demonstrating that it is very important in the fracture risk assessment in postmenopausal women under the age of 65 to evaluate also the decrease of the number of standard deviations for Z-score. In the old age group there was a very high probability that if a woman had T-score < - 2.5 SD, she had also Z-score v ≤ - 1.0 SD. For ROI_3 (total hip) it reached even 100%! It means that for ROI_3 all women had Z-score ≤ - 1.0 SD, if they had T-score < - 2.5 SD. The fracture risk in old women (> 65 year) was the highest one for ROI_1, as in the whole cohort, if both T - and Z- scores were within the increased fracture risk category.

The intensity of association of categorized T- and Z - scores was statistically significant for all selected relations. The highest intensity of association was found for the values measured in ROI_2 in the whole cohort, in the group of women under the age of 65 and also in the old women group (> 65 years), where it reached the value of 0.797. This highest intensity of association is conditional on the measurement of greater fraction of trabecular bone in the Ward's area in comparison with ROI_1 and ROI_3, and so measurement errors resulting from osteoarthrotic changes in Ward´s area are less significant. As Ward's area has a quicker bone loss than other measurement sites, it is not used for osteoporosis diagnosis with DXA instruments.

We have not come across a similar solution of the problem in the available literature, and, therefore, we do not have the possibility to compare our results with other authors. However, there are many studies comparing the sensitivity and specificity of T - and Z - scores for differentiating osteoporotic women from healthy ones by different measurement techniques and different measurement sites [13–18]. In these studies Z-score demonstrates a very good sensitivity and specificity. For example, in the study by Bergot C. et al., the authors proved that Z-score for QCT measurement had the highest sensitivity in differentiating osteoporotic women from the normal ones in comparison with T-score for QCT and with T - and Z - scores for DXA [19]. The precise BMD classification according to Z-score for osteoporosis diagnosis is not yet determined.

CONCLUSION

The study's contribution lies in the finding that the relative fracture risk in proximal femur area in women increases, if T-score < - 2.5 SD and, simultaneously, Z-score ≤ - 1.0 SD, and this risk is especially high for women under the age of 65.

In assessing the individual fracture risk in female osteoporotic patients (by questionnaires) we recommend to add also Z – score values from the measured area to T – score values from proximal femur area and to other anamnestic risk factors (age, sustained fracture after the age of 50, femur neck fracture in mother, increased biochemical markers of osteoresorbtion, smoking, body mass index lower than 19, and the like).

REFERENCES

[1] Kanis JA, Johnell O, Oden A, Jonsson B, Dawson A, Dere W: Risk of hip fracture derived from relative risk: An analysis applied to the population of Sweden. *Osteoporosis Int* 2000, 11, 120 – 127.

[2] Kanis JA, Johnell O, Oden A, Oglesby AK, De Laet C, Jonsson B: Ten year probabilities of osteoporotic fracture according to BMD and diagnostic thresholds, *J Bone Miner Res* 2001, 16 (Suppl 1), 194.

[3] Leslie WD, Metge C, Ward L: Contribution of clinical risk factors to bone density – based absolute fracture risk assessment in postmenopausal women. *Osteoporos Int*, 2003, 14, 334 – 338.

[4] Black DM, Steinbuch L, Palermo L, Dargent – Molina P, Lindsay R, Hoseyni MS, Johnell O: An assessment tool for predicting fracture risk in postmenopausal women. *Osteoporosis Int* 2001, 12, 519 – 528.

[5] Leib ES, Lewiecki EM, Binkley N, Hamdy RC: Official positions of the international society for clinical densitometry. *J Clin Densitom* 2004, 7, 1 – 6.

[6] Hilgers RD, Bauer P, Scheber V: *Einfuhrung in die medizinische Statistik*, Springer Verlag Berlin Heidelberg, 1. Ausgabe, 2003, 217 – 220.

[7] Pacakova V: *Štatistika pre ekonómov (Sstatistics for economist)*, IURA EDITION, Bratislava, 1. vydanie, 2003, 193 – 234.

[8] Schumacher M, Schulgen Gabi: *Methodik klinischer Studien* Verlag Berlin Heidelberg, 1. Ausgabe, 2002, 89 – 104.

[9] Matthis C, Weber T, O 'Neil W, Raspe H: Health impact associated with vertebral deformities: Results from the European Vertebral Osteoporosis Study (EVOS). *Osteoporos Int* 1998, 8, 364 – 372.

[10] Zhang J, Yu KF: What is relative risk? A method of correcting the odds ratio in cohort studies of common outcomes. *JAMA* 1998, 280, 1690 – 1691.

[11] Fualkner KG, von Stetten E, Steiger P, Miller P: Discrepancies in osteoporosis prevalence at different sceletal sites: impact on the WHO criteria. *Bone* 1998, 23 (Suppl), 194.

[12] Mazess RB: T – score differ among skeletal sites. Calcif Tissue Int 1999, 64, 104.

[13] Molyvda – Athanasopoulou E, Sioundas A, Kaltziioannou K: Dual X – ray absorptiometry reference data for Greek. *Europ J Radiol* 2000, 36, 36 – 40.

[14] Henry MJ, Pasco JR, Pocock NA et al: Refence ranges for bone densitometers adopted Australia – wide: Geelong osteoporosis study. *Austral Radiol* 2004, 48, 473 -. 475.

[15] McMahon K, Nightingale J, Pocock N: Discordance in DXA male reference ranges. *J Clin Densitom*, 2004, 7, 121 – 126.

[16] Wendlova J: Differences in distribution of T – scores and Z – scores among bone densitometry tests in postmenopusal women (a comparative study). *Wien Med Wschr* 2002, 152, 591 – 595.

[17] Blake GM, Knapp KM, Fogelman I: Absolute fracture risk varies with bone densitometry technique used. A theoretical and in vivo study of fracture cases. *J Clin Densitom* 2002, 5, 109 – 116.

[18] Newton LJ, Kenny RA, Frearson R, Francis MR: A prospective evalution of bone mineral density measurement in females who have fallen. *Age Ageing* 2003, 32, 497 – 502.

[19] Bergot C, Laval – Jeantet AM, Hutchinson K et al: A comparison of spinal quantitative computed tomograpfy with dual energy X - ray absorbtiometry in European women with vertebral and nonvertebral fractures. *Calcif Tissue Int* 2001, 68, 74 – 82.

[20] Labudová V: Analýza sociálnej situácie domácnosti Slovenskej republiky na báze údajov , EU SILC 2006 , Slovenská štatistika a demografia, 2008, 18, 108-137

In: Osteoporosis: Etiology, Diagnosis and Treatment
Editors: Bilar E. Mattingly and Albert C. Pillare
ISBN 978-1-60692-397-9

Short Communication G

WHICH STATISTICAL TESTS FOR ESTIMATING OSTEOPOROTIC FRACTURE RISK?

J. Wendlová *

University Derer's Hospital and Policlinic, Osteological Centre, Bratislava, Slovakia.

ABSTRACT

The article presents an analysis of statistical methods used for estimating fracture risk in patients with osteoporosis. Mathematical relations of different methods are explained (risk – R, risk ratio - RR, RD – risk difference, odds - O, odds ratio - OR, Yule's Q, Yule's Y, logistic model). What is important to keep in mind is that: 1) relative risk and odds ratio are statistics that only describe an association, not causation; 2) relative risk and odds ratio refer to a population, not to an individual patient; 3) the studies of small groups are more likely to find an association that might actually just be due to chance, the larger the groups, the less likely the association between a risk factor and an outcome (fracture); 4) when the incidence of an outcome of interest in the study population is low (< 10%), the OR is close to the RR, the more frequent the outcome becomes, the more the OR will overestimate the RR when it is more than 1 or underestimate the RR when it is less than 1.

Sophisticated statistical packages are available which can calculate many of the tests of association but the problem is that the investigator must know which the desirable is. The incorrect option of statistical analysis, the incorrect interpretation of risk ratio or odds ratio and overestimation of the importance of a risk factor may lead to unintentional errors in the economic analysis of potential programs or treatments in osteoporosis. This article could be a contribution for investigators, who are concerned with assessment of fracture risk.

Keywords: relative risk - odds ratio – Yule's Q, Yule's Y – fracture risk – osteoporosis.

INTRODUCTION

There increase the costs of the complex care of patients with osteoporotic fractures from year to year. The detection and adequate treatment of patients with a higher fracture risk is of great interest. The criteria for the evaluation of a fracture risk have constantly been reassessed and updated with one goal – to maximise the validity and accuracy of the applied methods.

The aim of the article is to present the statistical methods enabling the analysis of fracture risk estimation in patients with osteoporosis in an investigated population. Mathematical relations of different methods are explained. At present there are two priorities in the centre of interest in the research of osteoporotic patients:

1. observation of the influence of risk factors on the bone mineral density (BMD) values and on the onset of fractures (observational studies)
2. observation of the influence of antiosteoresorptive, bone formation stimulating or dual acting drugs on BMD values and the reduction of fracture risk (interventional studies – trials)

ANALYSIS

The evaluation of the fracture risk for patients with osteoporosis can be realized in both observational and interventional studies by retrospective (case – control) or prospective (cohort, incidence) studies. A retrospective study determines: How did the exposure to risk factors influence the fracture? How did the antiosteoresorptive, bone formation stimulating or dual acting drugs decrease the incidence of fractures? A prospective study determines: Will the exposure to risk factors condition the incidence of a fracture in the future? Will the antiosteoresorptive or bone formation stimulating drugs prevent the patient from the fracture in the future? [1,2,3]

It is preferred to use the odds ratio in retrospective studies and the relative risk or relative risk corrected to odds ratio in prospective studies (see eq. 2, 3 and 7). In the observation of the influence of fracture risk factors, or the influence of drugs on the reduction of fracture incidence we are working with dichotomous variables. Dichotomous variables characterise the quality of the observed parameter and we classify them by "yes" or "no", and in the statistical evaluation by the values of 0 and 1.

Association among dichotomous variables can be judged by contingency tables 2x2 and can be measured by several statistical methods:

- risk (R)
- risk ratio (RR)
- odds (O)
- odds ratio (OR)

* Correspondence concerning this article should be addressed to: Ass Prof Jaroslava Wendlová, MD, PhD Krížna 30, 811 07 Bratislava. jwendlova@mail.t-com.sk.

- approximation (correction) of OR to RR (RR_{cor})
- Yule's Q and Yule's Y ratio (Q, Y)

As an illustration we present a simple 2x2 contingency table with dichotomous variables in the article (Table 1).

- risk factor – present, absent (+, -)
- fracture – present, absent (+, -)

Table 1. Contingency table 2x2

Risk factor	*Fracture*	
	+	–
+	**a**	**b**
–	**c**	**d**

a, b, c, d – fequencies.

Risk (R) [4,5,6]

Risk R_1 -- yields the risk for the fracture in patients with the risk factor
Risk R_2 -- yields the risk for the fracture in patients without the risk factor

$$R_1 = \frac{a}{a+b} \quad \text{(eq. 1a)}$$

$$R_2 = \frac{c}{c+d} \quad \text{(eq. 1b)}$$

$$R = probability(p) = \frac{x}{n} \quad \text{(eq. 1c)}$$

$$R(\%) = probability(p) = \frac{x}{n} \cdot 100\% \quad \text{(eq. 1d)}$$

$$R\langle 0,1 \rangle$$

The risk R_1 is a ratio of the number of patients with fractures exposed to risk factor (a) to the total number of observed patients exposed to risk factor ($a + b$). The risk R_2 is a ratio of the number of patients with fractures without exposure to risk factor (c) to the total number of patients not exposed to risk factor ($c + d$) (Table 1). From the statistical point of view it is actually the risk expressed as a probability (p) – the number of positive or negative cases (x) (event rates) to the total number of observed cases (n).

Risk values vary within the interval $\langle 0,1 \rangle$

Relative Risk = Risk Ratio (RR) [4,5,6,7,8,9]

RR – is the ratio of the risk for the fracture in patients with the risk factor, to the risk for the fracture in patients without the risk factor. In the equation 2a, the RR is expressed also by means of the probabilities ratio.

$$RR = \frac{R_1}{R_2} = \frac{\frac{a}{a+b}}{\frac{c}{c+d}} \quad \text{(eq. 2)}$$

$$RR = \frac{p_1}{p_2} = \frac{\frac{x_1}{n_1}}{\frac{x_2}{n_2}} \quad \text{(eq. 2a)}$$

The RR takes on values between zero (0) and infinity (∞). One (RR = 1) is the neutral value and means that there is no difference between the groups compared, close to zero (RR ≈ 0) or infinity (RR $\approx \infty$) means a large difference between the two groups on the variable concerned. A risk ratio larger than one (RR > 1) means that group one has a larger proportion than group two, if the opposite is true the risk ratio will be smaller than one (RR < 1). The RR multiplicated by 100% gives the percentage proportion in classification between one and group two. It needs to be calculated for each value of RR the 95% confidence interval (C.I.).

Risk difference (RD)

$$RD = R_1 - R_2 \quad \text{(eq. 2b)}$$

RD gives difference between risk R_1 for the fracture in patients with the risk factor, to the risk R_2 for the fracture in patients without the risk factor.

Example No 1:

We can compare two groups with different risks (R_1, R_2) for hip fracture from data in prospective epidemiological study. For example we have investigated that, the risk (R_1) for patients suffering from hip fracture with BMD T – score = -1. 4 SD is 0. 05 (5 %) (group A), while the risk (R_2) in the group B with BMD T – score = - 2,6 SD is 0.20 (20%). The RR equals 0, 25 ($R1/R_2$ = 0.05 / 0.20).

The difference from neutral value 1 is 0. 75 (1 – 0. 25 = 0. 75 .100 = 75%).

75% fewer patients in group A are in the relative risk to suffer hip fracture.

We chose for T - score in the example No 1 only the categorical level without the C.I. for simple interpretation.

Odds (O) [8 - 14]

O – is given as a probability (p) that the fracture will happen, divided by the probability that the fracture will not happen.

$$O = \frac{p}{1-p} \qquad \text{(eq. 3)}$$

In the eq. 3 the probability (p) can be substituted by the risk (R)

$$O = \frac{R}{1-R} \qquad \text{(eq. 4)}$$

INTERPRETATION OF ODDS RESULTS

Odds values (O) vary within the interval $\langle 0, \infty)$. If the value O > 1, there are higher odds that the fracture will occur in the observed group. If the value O < 1, there are higher odds that the fracture will not occur. The odds that the fracture will definitely occur equal infinity (O $= \infty$), and the odds that the fracture will not occur at all equal zero (O = 0).

The ratio of two odds values is expressed as odds ratio.

Odds Ratio (OR) [8 - 14]

OR – is the ratio of the odds of the fracture for patients with the risk factor, to the odds of the fracture for patients without the risk factor.

$$OR = \frac{O_1}{O_2} = \frac{\dfrac{p_1}{1-p_1}}{\dfrac{p_2}{1-p_2}} = \frac{\dfrac{\frac{a}{a+b}}{1-\left(\frac{a}{a+b}\right)}}{\dfrac{\frac{c}{c+d}}{1-\left(\frac{c}{c+d}\right)}} = \frac{\frac{a}{b}}{\frac{c}{d}} = \frac{a.d}{b.c} \qquad \text{(eq. 5)}$$

The OR takes values between zero (0) and infinity (∞). One (OR = 1) is the neutral value and means that there is no difference between the groups compared, close to zero (OR $\approx$ 0) or infinity (OR $\approx \infty$) means a large difference. An OR larger than one (OR > 1) means that group one has a larger proportion than group two (positive association), if the opposite is true the OR will be smaller than one (OR < 1) (negative association).

Example No 2:

If 10 % of patients in group A1 having BMD T- score = -1. 4 SD suffer from hip fracture, than the odds (O_1) for suffering from hip fracture is 0.11 (0.10 / 0.90) (eq. 3). The patients in group A1 have 0.11 times higher chance of getting fracture than of not getting fracture.

If 15% of patients in group B1 with BMD T – score = - 2. 6 SD suffer from hip fracture, than the odds (O_2) for suffering from hip fracture is 0.176 (0.15 / 0.85) (eq. 3).

The patients in group B1 have 0.176 times higher chance of getting fracture than of not getting fracture. The odds ratio (OR) equals 0.625 (O_1/O_2 = 0.11 / 0.176). The patients in group A1 have 0.625 times higher chance of getting fracture than in group B1. The inverse of the odds ratio (O_2/O_1 = 1/OR) equals 1.6 (0.176 / 0.11). The patients in group B1 have 1.6 times higher chance of getting fracture than patients in group A1.

OR indicates how much the odds of the fracture for patients with the risk factor is higher than the odds of the fracture for patients without the risk factor.

$$OR = \frac{\frac{a}{b}}{\frac{c}{d}} = \frac{\frac{a}{c}}{\frac{b}{d}} = \frac{\frac{d}{b}}{\frac{c}{a}} = \frac{\frac{d}{c}}{\frac{b}{a}} = \frac{a.d}{b.c} \qquad \text{(eq. 6)}$$

In equation (eq. 6) we see that the OR can be interpreted in various ways. We can compare the patient groups *a, b, c, d*, in the contingency table (Table 1) in a horizontal or vertical direction, but not in cross direction, regardless of whether one is concerned with risk or without risk, or whether one has a fracture or has not – the outcome is the same. If an observation is higher in value as another observation on both the horizontal and the vertical marginals, the pair of observations is called concordant; if this is not the case the pair is discordant.

Some research papers present an incorrect opinion that OR and RR are identical statistical methods [15]. The eq. 2 and eq. 5 in our analysis indicate the opposite. Relative risk is not the same as odds ratio.

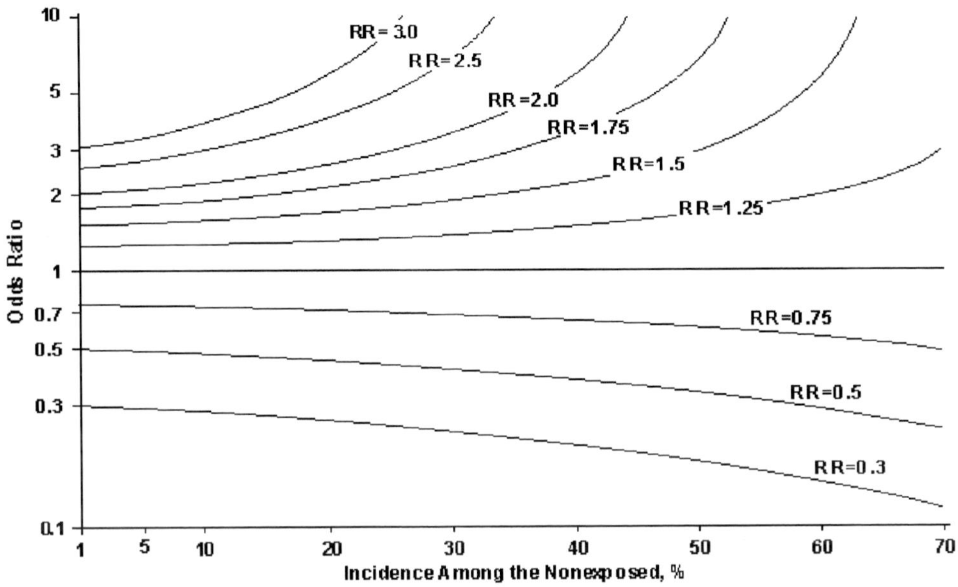

Graph 1. The relationship between risk ratio (RR) and odds ratio (OR) by variable incidence of the outcome (Zhang J, Kai F : What is the relative risk? *JAMA*, 1998, 280, 19, 1690 – 91).

The graph 1 shows that when the incidence of an outcome of interest in the study population is low (< 10%), the OR is close to the RR. The more frequent the outcome becomes, the more the OR will overestimate the RR when it is more than 1 or underestimate the RR when it is less than 1.

The RR is easier to interpret than the OR. However, in practice the odds ratio is used more often. This has to do with the fact that the OR is more closely related to frequently used statistical techniques such as logistic regression. Also, the OR has the attractive property that, however is turned the table (Table 1), it will always take on the same value (eq. 6).

There must be calculated the 95% confidence interval (C.I.) for each value of OR and RR (for example in SAS^R system).

WHEN TO USE RR AND OR IN THE EVALUATION OF THE ASSOCIATION OF DICHOTOMOUS VARIABLES? (TABLE 2)

The relevant literature states that OR is more appropriate for the evaluation of retrospective studies and RR or RR_{cor} (eq. 7) is better for prospective studies [13,14,16].

Table 2. Types of studies frequently used to determine the fracture risk and recommended statistical analysis

Studies	Recommended statistical analysis
case – control studies (retrospective)	**OR** **Yule's Q, Yule's Y**
cohort studies (prospective, incidence)	**RR, RR$_{cor}$**

Corrected RR (RR$_{cor}$) [5]

In a cohort study, if the incidence of outcome is more than 10% (Graph 1) and the OR is more than 2.5 or less than 0.5, a correction of the OR may be desirable to more appropriately interpret the magnitude of an association.

$$RR_{cor} = \frac{OR}{(1-p_0)+(p_0 \cdot OR)} \qquad \text{(eq. 7)}$$

p_0 – indicates the incidence of the outcome of interest in the not exposed group, it is the ratio of patients without a risk in a group to the total in the group.

Yule's Q, Yule's Y (Q, Y) [13]

If we want to compare the influence of two risk factors separately on the fracture onset as a comparison of two OR (two contingency tables: 2 x 2 and 2 x 2), we have to evaluate which risk factor has higher OR to condition the fracture onset (which drug has higher OR to reduce the risk of a fracture) by using two mathematical and statistical methods – Yule's Q and Yule's Y.

$$Q = \frac{OR-1}{OR+1} \qquad \text{(eq. 8)}$$

$$Y = \frac{\sqrt{OR}-1}{\sqrt{OR}+1} \qquad \text{(eq. 9)}$$

Both methods compare two OR. The Q and Y transform the odds to the range $\langle +1,-1 \rangle$ with Q (Y) = 0 when OR = 1, Q (Y) = - 1 when OR = 0 and Q (Y) approaches 1 as OR approaches infinity, Q and Y are the gamma statistic.

Yule's Q and Y are based on the OR and a symmetric measure taking on values between -1, and +1. One (1) implies perfect negative or positive association, zero (0) no association. By Yule's Y the measure tends to estimate association more conservatively than Yule's Q and has little substantive or theoretical meaning.

Transformation of the result of the ration of two OR from the original interval $\langle 0, \infty \rangle$ into the interval $\langle +1, -1 \rangle$ makes its interpretation more clear.

MORE THAN TWO RISK FACTORS

Logistic Model [8,9,16]

When observing *k* risk factors ($R_1, R_2, \ldots R_k$) and their influence upon the fracture onset at once, we can use *k* contingency tables (type $n_i \times 2$), where n_i is the number of levels of risk factors R_i ($i = 1, 2, 3, \ldots\ldots k$).

For more than two risk factors these possibilities are to calculate:

- OR for all pairs separately in each group one risk factor (present, absent) and one dichotomous outcome (fracture, no fracture) → simple analysis
- logistic regression analysis

Logistic regression uses the explanatory variables, which can be categorical or continuous, to predict the probability that the outcome or response variable takes on a given value. In other words, logistic regression is designed to describe probabilities associated with the values of the outcome variable. Probabilities are bounded by 0 and 1, so a linear model cannot be used because linear functions are inherently unbounded. The solution to this problem is to transform the probabilities to *logits,* which are unbounded, so that a linear regression model can be used because the logits are linear in the parameters.

The logistic regression model describes the relationship between a categorical outcome (response) variable *Y* and a set of explanatory variables (X_i). It models the conditional probability of a successful outcome, which is denoted $p = P(Y = 1/X = x)$. The relationship between probability *p* and a set of explanatory variables (X_i) is not linear

$$p = \frac{\exp(\beta_0 + \beta_1 X_1 + \beta_2 X_2 + \ldots + \beta_k X_k)}{1 + \exp(\beta_0 + \beta_1 X_1 + \beta_2 X_2 + \ldots + \beta_k X_k)}$$

The relationship between *logit* and a set of explanatory variables (X_i) is linear:

$$Logit = \ln(odds) = \ln \frac{p}{1-p} = \beta_0 + \beta_1 X_1 + \beta_2 X_2 + \ldots + \beta_k X_k$$

Unlike linear regression, the categorical response is not normally distributed and the variances are not the same. Also, logistic regression usually requires a more complex iterative estimation method called maximum likelihood to estimate the parameters than linear regression. This method finds the parameter estimates that are most likely to occur given the data. It accomplishes this by maximizing the likelihood function that expresses the probability of the observed data as a function of the unknown parameters.

Individual (Absolute) Risk of Fracture

Individual risk of the fracture in a patient has been determined in the last few years through a popular form of various questionnaires, where, besides the bone mineral density values in the total hip area, the points are given for the answers concerning the presence of a risk factor in the anamnesis – e.g., age, weight, a fracture sustained after the age of 50, hip fracture in mother after the age of 50, biochemical markers of osteoresorption, smoking, and the like [17]. Each questionnaire after its completion has to be tested for sensitivity, specificity, positive predictive value, and negative predictive value – the most proper statistical test methods include the $\chi 2$ - square test and the ADALINE programme [18,19].

WHO Fracture Assessment Tool (FRAX) – Probability of racture [20].

The FRAX tool has been developed by WHO to calculate fracture risk of patients. It is based on individual patient models that integrate the risks associated with clinical risks factors as well as bone mineral density (BMD) at the femoral neck. The FRAX models have been developed from studying population – based cohorts from Europe, North America, Asia and Australia in their most sophisticated form. The FRAX tool is computer - driven and is available on link www.iofbonehealth.org.

The FRAX algotithms give the 10 – year probability of fracture. The output is a 10 – year probability of hip fracture and the 10 – year probability of a major osteoporotic fracture (clinical spine, forearm, hip or shoulder fracture).

The series of meta – analyses identified several clinical risk factors that might be used for assessing fracture risk. These included body mass index as a continous variable, as well as dichotomous variables comprising a parental history of hip fracture, a prior fragility fracture, current smoking, exposure to oral glucocorticouds, theumatoid arthritis and the consumption of more than two units of alcohol daily. Each of the risk factors was examined for interactions with sex, age, BMD and the variable itself.

Conclusion

In this article we have reviewed the methods used to analyse associations between variables – risk factor and fracture in 2 x 2 contingency tables. What is important to keep in mind is that:

1. relative risk and odds ratio are statistics that only describe an association, not causation
2. relative risk and odds ratio refer to a population, not to an individual patient
3. when the incidence of an outcome of interest in the study population is low (<10%), the OR is close to the RR, the more frequent the outcome becomes, the more the OR will overestimate the RR when it is more than 1 or underestimaye the RR when it is less than 1.

It is important that before starting a research, its annotation should be seriously prepared with a clear intention and selection of a proper method for statistical evaluation. Sophisticated statistical packages are available which can calculate many of the tests of association but problem is that the investigator must know which is the desirable one. The incorrect option of statistical analysis, the incorrect interpretation of risk ratio or odds ratio and overestimation of the importance of risk factor may lead to unintentional errors in the economic analysis of potential intervention programmes or treatments in osteoporosis.

REFERENCES

[1] Kanis JA, Johnell O, Oden A, Jonsson B, Dawson A, Dere W : Risk of hip fracture derived from relative risk: An analysis applied to the population of Sweden. *Osteoporosis Int* 2000, 11, 120 – 127.

[2] Kanis JA, Johnell O, Oden A, Oglesby AK, De Laet C, Jonsson B: Ten year probabilities of osteoporotic fracture according to BMD and diagnostic thresholds, *J Bone Miner Res* 2001, 16 (Suppl 1), 194.

[3] Mc Nutt LA, Wu CH, Xue X, Hafner JP: Estimating the relative risk in cohort studies and clinical trials of common outcomes. *Am J Epidemiol* 2003,157, 940 – 943.

[4] Sinclair JC, Bracken MB: Clinically useful measures of treatment effect in binary analyses of randomized trials. *J Clin Epidemiol* 1994, 47, 881 – 889.

[5] Zhang J, Yu KF: What is relative risk? A method of correcting the odds ratio in cohort studies of common outcomes. *JAMA* 1998, 280, 1690 – 1691.

[6] Greenland S: Model – based estimation of relative risks and other epidemiologic measures in studies of common outcomes and in case – control studies. *Am J Epidemiol* 2004, 160 (4), 301 – 305.

[7] Melton JL III, Atkinson E, O'Connor MK, O'Fallon WM, Riggs BL: Bone density and fracture risk in men. *J Bone Miner Res*1998, 13, 1915 – 1917.

[8] Hilgers RD, Bauer P, Scheber V: *Einfuhrung in die medizinische Statistik* Springer Verlag Berlin Heidelberg, 1. Ausgabe, 2003, 217 – 220.

[9] Kleinbaum DG, Klein M : *Logistic regression. Statistics for Biology and Health*, Springer, 2nd edition 2002, corr. 4th printing 2005, 2 – 45.

[10] Lee J: Odds ratio or relative risk for cross – sectional data? *Int J Epidemiol* 1994, 23, 201 – 203.

[11] Bland JM, Altman DG: The odss ratio. *Brit Med J* 2000, 320, 1468.

[12] Davies HTO, Crombie IK, Tavakoli M: When can odds ratios mislead? *BMJ* 1998, 316, 989 – 991.

[13] Last JM : *A dictionary of epidemiology*, 4 th ed, RA Spasoff, SS Harris and MC Thuriaux eds. Oxford, Oxford University Press, 2001, 45 – 82.

[14] Jaeschke, Guyatt G, Shannon H, Walter S, Cook D, Heddle N: Assessing the effects of treatment: measures of association. *CMAJ* 1995, 152, 351 – 357.

[15] Mikulecky M: Association of nominal variables – contingency tables. *Euro Rehab* 2003, 9, 88 – 96.

[16] Egger M, Davey Smith G, Philips AN: Meta analyses principles and procedures. *BMJ* 1997, 315, 1533 – 1537.

[17] Black DM, Steinbuch L, Palermo L, Dargent – Molina P, Lindsay R, Hoseyni MS, Johnell O: An assessment tool for predicting fracture risk in postmenopausal women. *Osteoporosis Int* 2001, 12, 519 – 528.

[18] Widrow B, Smith FW Pattern recognizing control systems. In: Tou JT., Wilcox RH. *Computer and Information science. Collected papers on learning adaptation and control in information systems*. 2nd ed, Washington, Sparten Books, 1964, 40 – 47.

[19] Mikulecky M, Komornik J, Ondrejka P Automatizacia matematicko – statistickych odhadov a testov na zaklade binomickeho rozdelenia. PC software, Comtel, 1997.

[20] Kanis JA, Johnell O, Oden A, Johansson H, McCloskey E:

[21] FRAX™ and the assessment of fracture probability in men and women from UK.

[22] Osteoporos Int 2008, 19, 385 – 397

In: Osteoporosis: Etiology, Diagnosis and Treatment
Editors: Bilar E. Mattingly and Albert C. Pillare
ISBN 978-1-60692-397-9

Short Communication H

Determination of the Centre of Gravity in the Methodology of Kinesitherapy for Osteoporotic Patients

J. Wendlová*

University Derer´s Hospital and Policlinic, Osteological Centre, Bratislava, Slovakia.

Abstract

The article brings a biomechanical analysis of the determination of the position of gravity centre of a trainee in the plane, both graphically and by calculation.

The importance of determining the position of the gravity centre in different postures of a trainee should not be underestimated, as it belongs to the basic principles in the development of methodology of kinesitherapy for both healthy and ill people.

An erudite methodology of kinesitherapy for osteoporotic patients can be developed only on the basis of biomechanical analysis of each exercise element, i.e., the knowledge of the position of the gravity centre, the knowledge of the support area and the distance of the gravity centre projection from the stability limit, the knowledge of the magnitude of the stability angle, and the knowledge of the regularity of mechanical stress of weakened osteoporotic vertebrae. A correctly chosen methodology of kinesitherapy for osteoporotic patients prevents the development of microfractures in the vertebrae, prevents patient's fall during the exercise, and stimulates the bone neoformation with increasing the bone mineral density and periosteal apposition of bone, followed by the enlargement of the bone cross sectional area as well as of the cross sectional moment of inertia.. The resulting effect is an improvement of the bone quality and its mechanical resistance.

Keywords: biomechanics –determination of centre of gravity – osteoporosis – methodology of kinesitherapy.

* Correspondence concerning this article should be addressed to: Ass Prof. Jaroslava Wendlová MD, PhD Krížna 30, 811 07 Bratislava. jwendlova@mail.t-com.sk.

INTRODUCTION

The knowledge of mechanical conditions of the static and dynamic balance of the skeleton is an important factor in the development of the methodology of kinesitherapy, especially for osteoporotic patients. Incorrectly chosen methodology of kinesitherapy with improperly stressed osteoporotic skeleton may result in the development of microfractures in the vertebrae and infractions in the ribs. Ignorance of the regularity of shifting the point of gravity centre of the body during the changes in the body's positions may lead to the development of exercises that have a reduced stability in individual postures and represent for an osteoporotic patient a risk of falling during the exercise and, consequently, a risk of a fracture with low energy injury.

BIOMECHANICAL CONDITIONS OF THE STATIC AND DYNAMIC BALANCE OF THE SKELETON

In the performance of everyday movements during physical work and exercise, the gravity force (G) acts upon each material point of human body. To maintain a balance while standing or moving, it is necessary that the effects of all forces acting upon a man are mutually cancelled, i. e., they have to equal zero.

Definitions [1 - 4]

Mass (m) is a feature of a material body, manifested in a gravitational field by force effects, i.e., the gravity.

The body mass in the biomechanics is represented by a specific amount of mass and is determined by weighting. It is marked by the letter m and measured values are given in kg according to the international units. It is directly proportional to the gravity force (G) and inversely proportional to the gravitational acceleration (g).

The force of gravity (***G***) is the force with which the Earth acts upon the body mass and its magnitude depends upon a distance of the body from the Earth's centre. It is directly proportional to the body mass and gravitational acceleration.

The force of gravity is determined by the place of its action, magnitude, direction, and sense.

Mathematical definitions

mass: $m = \frac{G}{g}$ (kg)

gravity force: $G = m \times g$ (kg.ms^{-2})

gravitational acceleration: $g = 9.80665 ms^{-2}$

From the mechanical point of view the **balance constancy** in any posture of a man is determined by:

- the magnitude of the **support area**
- the position of the body's **gravity centre** in relation to the support area
- the distance of the body's median (the **gravity centre projection**) from the edge of the support area
- the magnitude of the **stability angle**

The **support area** of a man is represented by the area limited by the outer limit of the body's contact point with the ground. The outer limit of this support area is called the **edge of the support area** or the **stability limit**. The **gravity centre** (*T*) of the body is represented by a material point, concentrating the whole force of the body's gravity (the body mass). It is called also the mass centre. The body mass is equally distributed from this point to all sides. The **median** (*t*) is a vertical line passing through the gravity centre. The **gravity centre projection** (*PT*) is the point in the support area, crossed by the median (Figure 1).

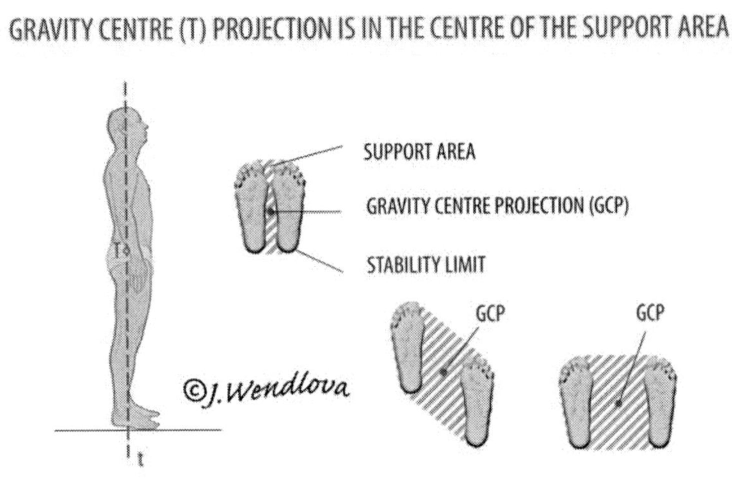

Figure 1. Healthy Skeleton. Support Area and the Gravity Centre Projection into the Support Area.

When the gravity centre projection in different exercise positions gets over the edge of the support area, i.e., beyond the stability limit, the trainee is in an unbalanced position a falls down to the ground. In patients with osteoporotic fractures of vertebrae the projection of the gravity centre into the support area gets close to the stability limit of the support area in the upright position, and so these patients are prone to falls when leaning forward or to sides (Figure 2).

The gravity centre position depends upon

- the mass
- the form } of the individual body parts
- the length

The **stability angle** is the angle formed by the median and the line passing through the gravity centre and the edge of the body's support area (Figure 3).

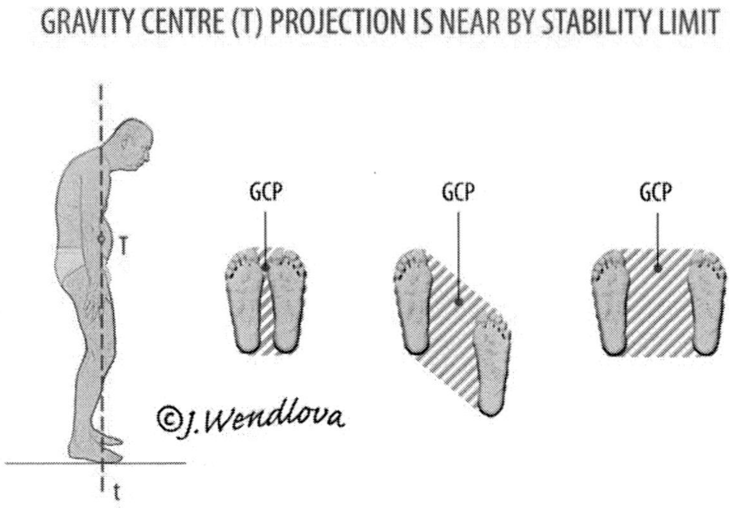

Figure 2. Osteoporotic Skeleton with Fractured Vertebrae Support Area and the Gravity Centre Projection into the Support Area.

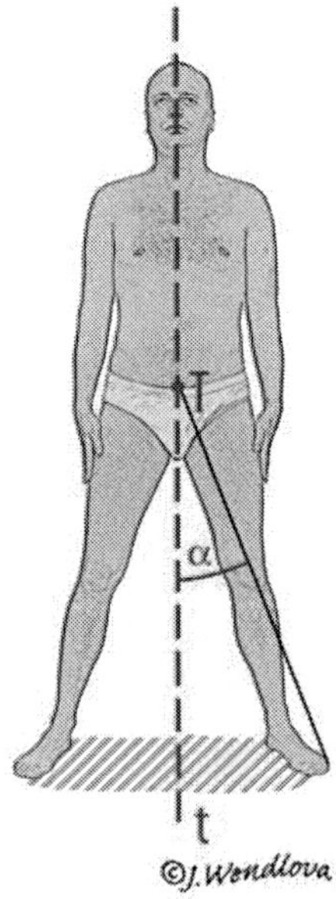

Figure 3. Stability Angle

The **stability of the skeleton** is increased by

- the enlargement of the support area
- the approximation of the gravity centre to the support area

- the approximation of the median (gravity centre projection) to the centre of the support area
- the enlargement of the stability angle
-

The gravity centre of different parts of the limbs lies upon the join of the joint centres of a given limb part (the gravity centre divides the join into two parts in the ratio of 4:5 in the direction from the proximal towards the distal joint). The position of the gravity centre is determined by the distance from the proximal joint and is given in cm or in percentage from the overall length of the limb part.

The gravity centre of the head and the torso lies in the saggital plane (in the vertical axis of the body) and is determined by the distance from the proximal part of the head and the torso, and is given in cm or percentage from the overall length of the torso and the head.

The gravity centre position of the individual body parts is determined, e.g., according to Donskoy, on the basis of the percentage expression from the overall length of the body part (Table 1).

Table 1. The gravity centre positions of individual body parts expressed in % of the overall length of a given body part (Donskoy) [2]

Body parts	The gravity centre position to the proximal end of the body part (%)
upper arm	0.47
forearm	0.42
thigh	0.44
lower leg	0.42
foot	0.44
torso	0.44
head	0.44

The body's gravity centre position when standing upright is situated about five centimetres over the articulation coxae (hip joint) in the saggital plane (the plane of body's symmetry) in the pelvis behind the symphysis pubis (pubic bone). The gravity centre point is at the 52% of the overall length of the person calculated from the support area (Figure 4). The body's gravity centre position depends upon many factors, primarily upon the body mass, its shape, the ratio of the mass of individual body parts to their length. The gravity centre position in women is about 0.5 to 2% lower than in men.

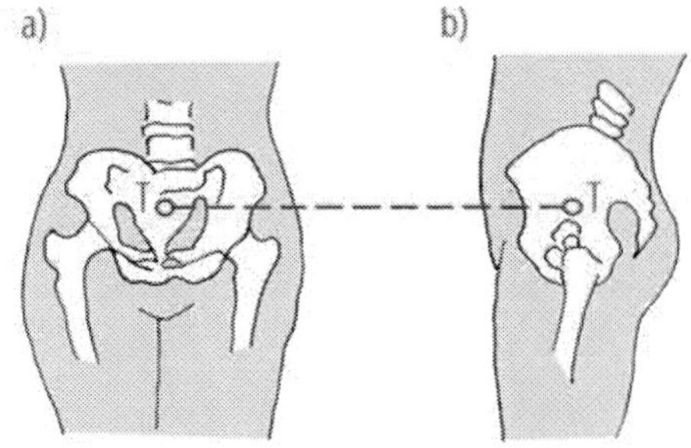

Figure 4. The Body's Gravity Centre Position in Healthy Skeleton.

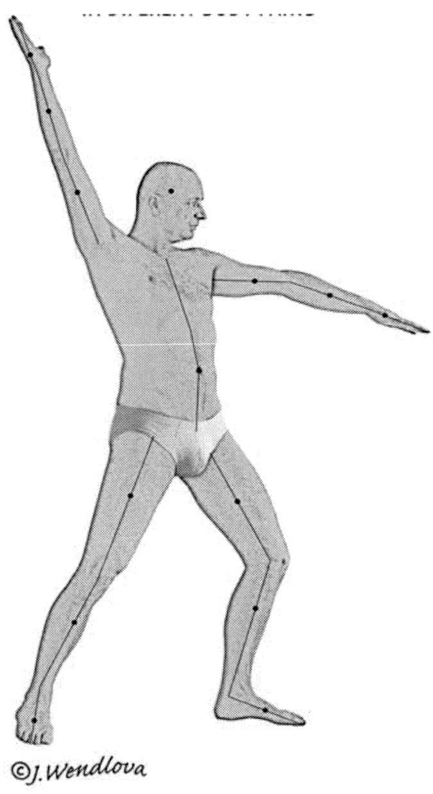

Figure 5. The Gravity Centre Position in Different Body Parts.

Approximate determination of the gravity centre position in different body parts (Figure 5)

- gravity centre of the head – situated inside the head behind sella turcica (Turk' saddle)
- gravity centre of the torso – situated at the frontal area of the first lumbar vertebra
- gravity centre of the torso with head – situated at the frontal side of the 11th thoracic vertebra
- gravity centre of the whole upper limb – situated at the elbow joint

- gravity centre of the upper arm – situated over the half of its length closer to the shoulder joint
- gravity centre of the forearm – situated over the half of its length closer to the elbow joint
- gravity centre of the hand – situated at the lower protuberance of the second wristbone
- gravity centre of the whole lower limb – situated at the rear side of the thighbone about 8 cm over the knee
- gravity centre of the thigh – situated at the frontal side of the thighbone between the upper and the middle third
- gravity centre of the lower leg – situated at the rear side of the shinbone between the upper and middle third
- gravity centre of the foot – situated at the navicular bone.

The importance of determining the position of the gravity centre in different postures of a trainee should not be underestimated, as it belongs to the basic principles in the development of methodology of kinesitherapy for both healthy and ill people.

Therefore, we demonstrate the method of the body's gravity centre calculation on a model example.

Determination of the Body's Gravity Centre Position of a Trainee in the Plane

The body's gravity centre in the plane can be determined in two ways:

1. graphically
2. by calculation

1. Graphical Determination of the Gravity Centre Position (Figure 6) [5,6]

The principal force acting upon each material point in the body of the trainee is the force of gravity G.

According to Table 1, in the trainee's photograph we determine the gravity centres of different body parts in his exercise posture (the photograph with gravity forces is called *the main diagram*). The following resultants of the gravity forces will be applied in the individual body parts T_1 to T_6: The head – G_1, the right UL* – G_2, the left UL – G_3, the torso – G_4, the right LL** – G_5, the left LL – G_6, through which we draw the rays of the gravity forces.

UL* – upper limb

LL** –lower limb

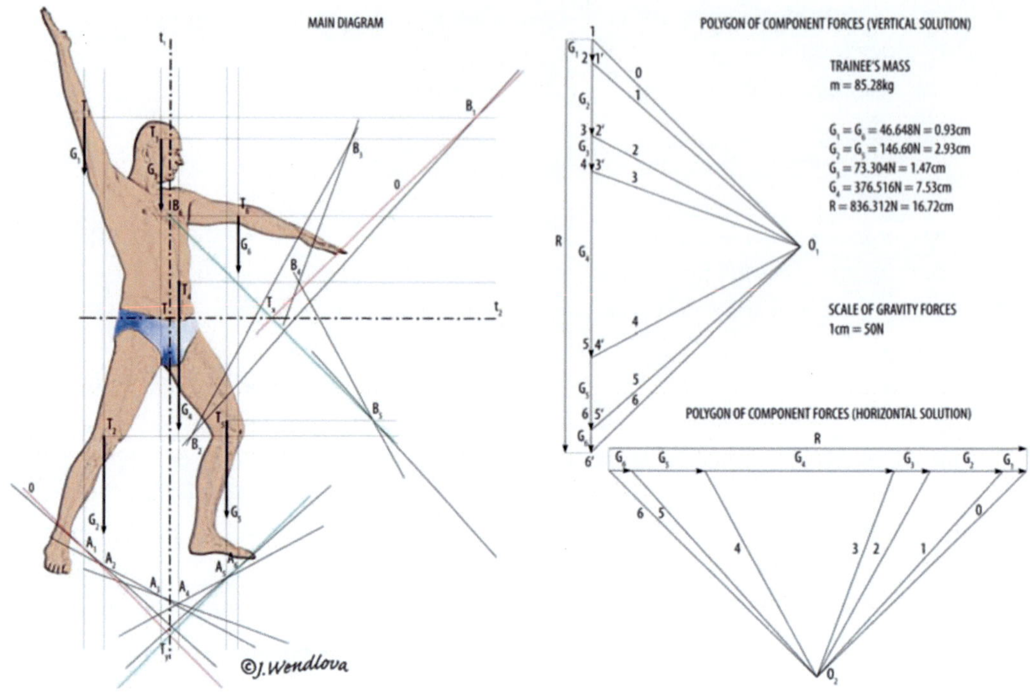

Figure 6. Graphical Determination of the Gravity Centre Position.

Model Example 1

Task assignment

According to Table 2 (Fischer) we calculate the masses of individual body parts, multiply them by the gravitational acceleration (g) and the results are the gravity forces of the body parts.

Table 2. The ratio of the mass of different body parts to the whole body in percentage (Body mass = 100%) [2]

Body part	The ratio of the mass of a body part to the whole body in % (according to Fischer)	The ratio of the mass of a body part to the whole body in % (according to Dempster)
head	8.8	8.1.
torso	45.2	49.7
thigh	11.0	9.9
lower leg	4.5	4.6
foot	2.1	1.4
upper arm	2.8	2.8
forearm	2.0	1.6
hand	0.8	0.6

The trainee's mass is m = 85.28 kg, G = 836.332 N
Head ....73.304 N
Torso...............376,516 N
Thigh..................91.36 N
Lower leg............37.485 N
Foot....................17.493 N
LL = thigh + lower leg + foot = 146.608 N
Upper arm...........23.324 N
Forearm..............16.66 N
Hand....................6.664 N
UL = upper arm + forearm + hand = 46.648 N

To transfer the gravity forces into a *polygon of component forces* we select a scale, for instance:

1 cm = 50 N

The aim of the solution

To determine the gravity centre position of the trainee in a chosen posture in a graphical way.

The solution of the example

As all forces are acting vertically and in the same direction, we can compose them into one vertical line, called the resultant of the forces of gravity R. In the composition of forces of gravity each force is marked by its determination segment. The magnitude of the force G_1 is given by the determination segment 1; 1', G_2 – 2; 2', G_3 – 3; 3', G_4 – 4; 4', G_5 – 5; 5', G_6 – 6; 6'.

Polygon of Component Forces (Vertical Solution)

We select a pole O_1 at a random distance from the resultant R and we draw from it polar rays (marked 0 to 6). The ray 0 is drawn towards the beginning of the determination segment of the gravity force G_1 and the rest of rays towards the ends of individual determination segments. The picture with composed gravity forces and polar rays is called a *polygon of component forces.* We draw parallels with individual polar rays from the *polygon of component forces* into the *main diagram.* The parallel with the polar ray 0 crosses the vertical ray of the gravity force G_1 in the point A_1 . From the point A_1 we draw a parallel with the ray 1 from the component picture until it crosses the vertical ray of the gravity force G_2 in the *main diagram*. This forms the point A_2. From the point A_2 we draw a parallel with the vertical ray 2 from the *polygon of component forces* until it crosses the vertical ray of the gravity force G_3 and so we get the point A_3 . We continue in the same way until the formation of the point A_6. The intersection of the ray 0 passing through the point A_1 with the ray 6 passing through the point A_6 forms the point T_y , through which passes the median (t_1), parallel with the gravity forces G_1 up to G_6.

Polygon of Component Forces (Horizontal Solution)

We rotate the polygon of forces in the clockwise direction in the plane by 90° and we let the gravity forces act upon the same gravity centres but in the horizontal direction, i.e., in the perpendicular direction to the vertical gravity forces.

In the *main diagram* we produce parallels with individual polar rays from the *polygon of component forces*. The parallel with the ray 0 crosses the horizontal ray of the gravity force G_1 in the point B_1. From the point B_1 we draw a parallel with the ray 1 from the *polygon of component forces* until it crosses the horizontal ray of the gravity force G_2 in the *main diagram*. Thus we get the point B_2. From the point B_2 we draw a parallel with the ray 2 from the *polygon of component forces* until it crosses the horizontal ray of the gravity force G_3 and produces so the point B_3. We continue in the same way until the production of the point B_6. The point T_x , produced by the intersection of the ray 0 with the ray 6, is passed through by the median (t_2), parallel with the horizontal rays of gravity forces G_1 to G_6 .

The gravity centre T of the trainee is situated in the intersection of both medians t_1 and t_2

2. Determination of the Gravity Centre Position by Calculation (Figure 7) [5 - 8]

Let us situate the picture of the trainee, used in the example 1, with marked gravity centres and gravity forces of individual body parts, into a coordinates system of two, mutually perpendicular axes x,y.

Model Example 2

Task assignment

The mass of the trainee is 85.28 kg (m = 85.28 kg), the resultant gravity force is G = 836.332 N

The gravity forces of individual body parts are calculated as in the model example 1.

UL............$G_1 = G_6 = 46.648$ N
LL............$G_2 = G_5 = 146.608$ N
Head......... $G_3 = 73.304$ N
Torso.........$G_4 = 376.516$ N

The aim of the solution

To determine the gravity centre position of the trainee in a chosen posture by calculation.

The solution of the example

We draw parallel rays with the axis y through the gravity centres T_1 to T_6 and gravity forces G_1 to G_6. We turn these forces by 90° and we draw parallel rays with the axis x through the gravity centres T_1 to T_6.

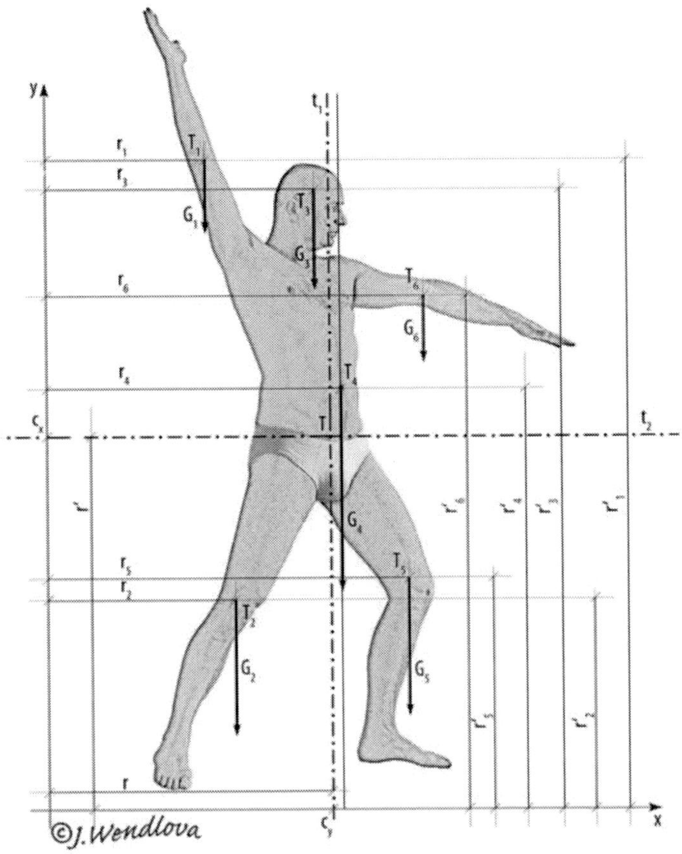

Figure 7. Determination of the Gravity Centre Position by Calculation

The calculation of the gravity centre position of the trainee is based upon two moment conditions:

1. The moment of the resultant gravity forces to the axis ***y*** (M_y) equals the sum of the moments of individual gravity forces to the axis ***y***.
2. The moment of the resultant gravity forces to the axis ***x*** (M_x) equals the sum of the moments of individual gravity forces to the axis ***x***.

The moment of the gravity force is given by the product of the gravity force and the arm (perpendicular distance to the axis *x* or *y*) upon which the gravity force is acting

M = G x r

Perpendicular distances of partial gravity centres T_1 to T_6 from the axis y are arms of the forces r_1 to r_6 upon which the individual gravity forces G_1 to G_6 are acting.

The arms of the forces r_1 to r_6 can be measured from the picture (in cm)

$r_1 = 4.67$ cm, $r_2 = 5.46$ cm, $r_3 = 7.80$ cm, $r_4 = 8.53$ cm, $r_5 = 10.45$ cm, $r_6 = 10.91$ cm

According to the 1st Moment Condition it is Valid that:

The moment of the resultant of forces to the axis *y* (M_y) equals:

$M_Y = G_1 \text{ x } r_1 + G_2 \text{ x } r_2 + G_3 \text{ x } r_3 + G_4 \text{ x } r_4 + G_5 \text{ x } r_5 + G_6 \text{ x } r_6 = 46.648 \text{ x } 4.67 + 146.608 \text{ x } 5.46 + 73.304 \text{ x } 7.80 + 376.516 \text{ x } 8.53 + 146.608 \text{ x } 10.45 + 46.648 \text{ x } 10.91 = \mathit{6842.759\ N}$

$G = 836.332$ N

$M_Y = 6842.759$ N

$M_Y = G \text{ x } r$

$$r = \frac{M_Y}{G} = \frac{6842.759Ncm}{836.332N} = 8.18cm$$

The length of the arm to the axis y, upon which the resultant gravity force *G* acts, is 8.18 cm. We apply the length of the arm $r = 8.18$ cm on the axis *x* and so produce the point C_y. We draw a parallel with the axis y through the point C_y and call it the median t_1.

Perpendicular distances of partial gravity centres T_1 to T_6 from the axis *x* are the arms of the forces r'_1 to r'_6 upon which the individual gravity forces G_1 to G_6 would act in case we turn the picture of the trainee by 90°.

The arms of the forces r'_1 to r'_6 can be measured again from the picture (in cm)

$r'_1 = 19.07$ cm, $r'_2 = 6.16$ cm, $r'_3 = 18.16$ cm, $r'_4 = 12.32$ cm, $r'_5 = 6.8$ cm, $r'_6 = 15.06$ cm

According to the 2nd Moment Condition it is Valid that:

The moment of the resultant of forces to the axis *x* (*Mx*) equals:

$M_X = G_1 \text{ x } r'_1 + G_2 \text{ x } r'_2 + G_3 \text{ x } r'_3 + G_4 \text{ x } r'_4 + G_5 \text{ x } r'_5 + G_6 \text{ x } r'_6 = 46.648 \text{ x } 19.07 + 146.608 \text{ x } 6.16 + 73.304 \text{ x } 18.16 + 376.516 \text{ x } 12.32 + 146.608 \text{ x } 6.8 + 46.648 \text{ x } 15.06 = \mathit{9462.013\ Ncm}$

$M_X = G \text{ x } r'$

$$r' = \frac{M_X}{G} = \frac{9462.013}{836.332N} = 11.313cm$$

The length of the arm to the axis x, upon which the resultant gravity force *G* acts, is 11.31 cm. We apply the length of the arm r' = 11.31 cm on the axis *y* and so produce the point C_x. We draw a parallel with the axis *x* through the point C_y and call it the median t_2.

The trainee's gravity centre *T* is situated in the intersection of both medians t_1 and t_2.

CONCLUSION

Determination of the gravity centre position of the trainee during a sports performance is made by means of a film camera and special computer software, using biomechanical method of determination of the gravity centre position especially by calculation. It serves to educate sportsmen, because the watching of the film record and the analysis of the gravity centre positions enable them to rectify their faults in further performances and facilitate the drill of correct technique of movement and maintaining stability during performances of different sport events. The analysis of the gravity centre position is also used in the methodology of developing new exercises in gymnastics, figure skating, aerobics, etc.; it also ensures the stability of a trainee in any exercise position.

The analytical method of determination of the gravity centre position starts to be used also in the development of the methodology of kinesitherapy for patients with osteoporosis and other diseases of musculoskeletal system [9 – 10].

An erudite methodology of kinesitherapy for osteoporotic patients can be developed only on the basis of biomechanical analysis of each exercise element (the knowledge of the position of the gravity centre, the knowledge of the magnitude of support area and the distance of the gravity centre projection from the stability limit, the knowledge of the magnitude of the stability angle, the knowledge of the regularity of mechanical stress of weakened osteoporotic vertebrae). A correctly chosen methodology of kinesitherapy for osteoporotic patients prevents the development of microfractures in the vertebrae, prevents patient's fall during the exercise, and stimulates the bone neoformation with increasing the bone mineral density and periosteal apposition of bone, followed by the enlargement of the bone cross sectional area as well as of the cross sectional moment of inertia. The resulting effect is an improvement of the bone quality and its mechanical resistance [11].

REFERENCES

[1] Wendlová J : Biomechanika chrbtice a jej význam v pohybovej liečbe pri osteoporóze. (Biomechanics of the spine and its importance in kinesitherapy for osteoporotic patients). *Eurorehab*, 1999, vol.2, No. 3 – 4, pp. 174 – 177.

[2] Koniar M, Leško M: Biomechanika (Biomechanics). *Slovenské pedagogické nakladateľstvo* (Slovak Pedagogical Publishing House), Bratislava, 1992, 37.

[3] Burr DB : Biomechanics. *Clin Reviews in Bone and Miner Metab*, 2006, 3, 112 – 117.

[4] Özkaya N, Nordin M: *Fundamentals of biomechanics: Equilibrium, motion and deformation*. 2nd ed., Springer – Verlag, New York, 1999, 45 – 51.

[5] Obetková V, Mamrillová A, Košinárová A: *Teoretická mechanika*.(Theoretical Mechanics). Vydavateľstvo technickej a ekonomickej literatúry (Publishing House of Technical and Economic Literature) ALFA, Bratislava, 1990, 30 – 94.

[6] Adamča LF, Marton P, Pavlík M, Trávníček F: *Teoretická mechanika*. (Theoretical Mechanics). Vydavateľstvo technickej a ekonomickej literatúry (Publishing House of Technical and Economic Literature) ALFA, Bratislava, 1992, 27 – 37.

[7] Bono CM, Einhorn TA : Overview of osteoporosis: Pathophysiology and determinants of bone strength. [Review] *Europ Spine J*, 2003, 12, 90-96.

[8] Bouxein ML: Biomechanics of osteoporotic fractures. *Clin Reviews in Bone and Miner Metab*, 2006, 3, 118 – 126.

[9] Fernandez JW, Mithraratne P, Thrupp SF, Tawhai MH, Hunter PJ: Anatomically based geometric modeling of the musculosceletal system and other organs. *Biomech and Model in Mechanobiology*, 2004, 3, 444 – 450.

[10] Ferguson J. S., Steffen T: Biomechanics of the aging spine. *Europ Spinal J*, 2003, Suppl 2, 167 – 169.

[11] Wendlová J.: Didaktika a metodika liečebného telocviku pre pacientov s osteoporózou. (Didactics and methodology of kinesitherapy for patients with osteoporosis). *Osteolog Bull*, 1997, vol. 2, č. 2, 49 – 51.

In: Osteoporosis: Etiology, Diagnosis and Treatment
Editors: Bilar E. Mattingly and Albert C. Pillare
ISBN 978-1-60692-397-9

Short Communication I

WHY IS SO IMPORTANT TO BALANCE THE MUSCULAR DYSBALANCE IN MM. COXAE AREA IN OSTEOPOROTIC PATIENTS? (BIOMECHANICAL ANALYSIS, CLINICAL APPLICATION)

J. Wendlová *

University Derer´s Hospital and Policlinic, Osteological Centre, Bratislava, Slovakia.

ABSTRACT

The article presents a biomechanical model of articulatio and mm. coxae with the characteristics of the vectors of reaction forces generated in flexors and extensors 1) in muscular balance; 2) in muscular dysbalance; 2a) with permanent load of the model of a hip by the body weight; 2b) with simulated live load during a fall or an impact. In case of muscular dysbalance the application of action force on a hip during a fall results in a sharp increase of the reaction compressive force in flexors and the tensile force in extensors. Muscular dysbalance of external (extensors) and internal (flexors) muscles of mm. coxae facilitates in this way complicated splintered fractures in the collum femoris area, and in the pertrochanteric and subtrochanteric areas.

Muscular balance achieved by balancing exercises and mechanical protection of the joint reduce the risk of splintered and complicated fractures in the described area.

Keywords: Osteoporosis - muscular dysbalance - mm. coxae - biomechanics – hip fracture - therapeutic exercise.

* Correspondence concerning this article should be addressed to: Ass. Prof. Jaroslava Wendlová MD, PhD Krížna 30, 811 07 Bratislava. jwendlova@mail.t-com.sk.

INTRODUCTION

The collum femoris fracture is one of the most frequent complications of osteoporosis. The incidence of fractures in the femoral area increases exponentially with age and it is higher in women. In women it increases after the onset of menopause, in men after the age of 70 [1,2].

Increased incidence of fractures in the area of collum femoris, pertrochanter and subtrochanter acquires a world-wide importance, as it brings about an increase of the number of days in hospital beds as well as of costs for treatment of these patients. That is the reason why the prevention of osteoporotic fractures comes to the forefront of attention.

This article describes muscular dysbalance in mm. coxae area (Table 1, Figure 1), which until now has been a less discussed factor contributing to splintered fractures of coli femoris, pertrochanter and subtrochanter. Human musculoskeletal system is demonstrated as a biomechanical construction transfering external load evenly from one part of the system to another. Basic knowledge of technical mechanics is applied in the study, namely the laws of statics. We simulate the magnitude and orientation of vectors of action and reaction forces in the biomechanical model of articulatio and mm. coxae. We use the method of composition and resolution of concurrent forces acting to a point in a plane, while the resultant of the forces is represented by a diagonal of a parallelogram, the so-called polygon of forces [3,4].

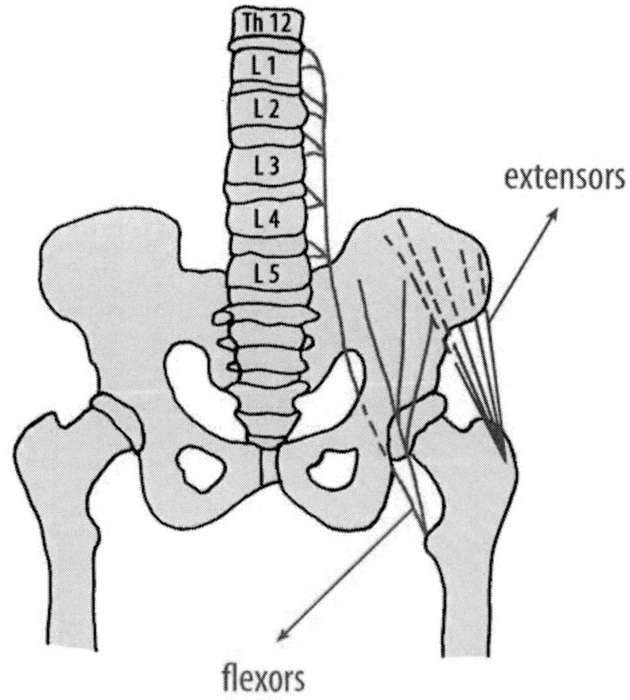

Figure 1. Anatomical scheme of mm. coxae (flexors, extensors).

Table 1.

Muscles with tendency towards reduction of length

A. Flexors
m. iliopsoas: - m. psoas major - m. iliacus - m. psoas minor

Muscles with tendency towards weakening

B. Extensors
- m. gluteus maximus - m. gluteus medius - m. gluteus minimus

Biomechanical Model of Articulatio and MM. Coxae [5,6,7].

We simplified articulatio and mm.coxae schematically to a biomechanical construction, which we used to simulate the application of individual forces and their assumed effects. We divided the loads applied to the biomechanical construction as follows:

1) internal permanent load - the weight of the construction itself (muscles, skeleton)
2) external permanent load - body weight minus the weight of muscles and skeleton
3) external live load - physical work, exercise, fall, impact, blow - applied to the construction only for limited time.

All external forces influencing the musculoskeletal construction are called action forces. These forces induce internal forces of the same quantity in the musculoskeletal system, which function against original action forces and we call them reactions, reaction forces. The stability of any construction, including a biological one, is preserved when the action and reaction forces are in balance. In our diagram of a biomechanical model articulatio and mm. coxae the force vector F_1 simulates a reaction compressive force in flexors and the vector F_2 in extensors in permanent load of the weight of the upper part of the body (Q) over articulatio coxae (Figure 2). In the paper we do not give concrete values of Q and F forces in Newtons ($N = m.kg.s^{-2}$), but only their vectors, as the main purpose of the paper is to demonstrate clearly the changes in the magnitude and orientation of individual vectors a) in muscular balance, b) muscular dysbalance , c) in simulation of external live load (a fall) and their influence on the risk of fractures in the area of proximal femur. For the concrete values of Q and P forces it is possible with the help of polygons of forces [a scale is to be selected: *x (cm)* = *y (N)*] to calculate corresponding values of forces F_1, F_1', F_1'' and F_2, F_2', F_2'', which are discussed in the paper.

In case of regular motoric activity the reaction forces F_1 and F_2 (i.e. their tonus) are of the same magnitude ($F_1 = F_2$). It means that there is a balance between muscular groups of agonists and antagonists. Reaction forces F_1 and F_2 are also in balance with permanent load Q ($F_1 + F_2 = Q$), while the sum of F forces is to be considered in the sense of the sum of vectors (the method of composition and resolution of concurrent forces) (Figure 2).

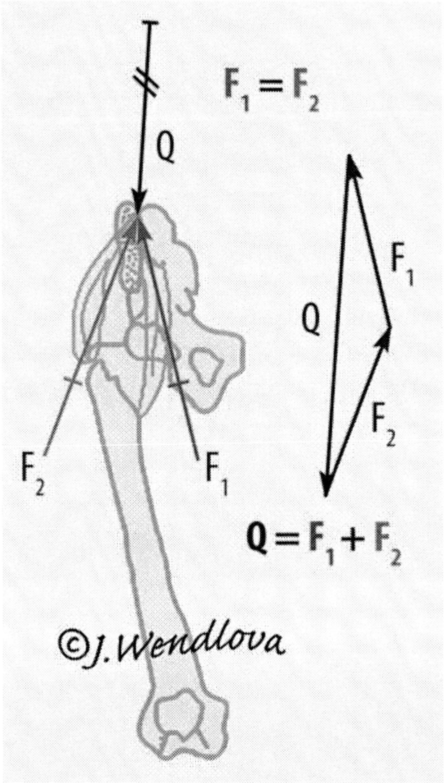

Figure 2. Biomechanical scheme of force resolution in muscular balance. Q - the force vector, which simulate the action of the weight of the upper part of the body on articulatio and mm. coxae. Force Q resolutes into force F_1 acting on flexors and F_2 acting on extensors. F_1 - the force vector transferred into flexors; F_2 - the force vector transferred into extensors.

Sedentary life style of today's civilised society results almost in general dysbalance between muscular groups of agonists and antagonists. Also flexors of mm. coxae are shortened and their neutral tonus is growing. The vector of reaction compressive force F_1 is gradually increasing to the vector of F_1' force ($F_1 < F_1'$). External muscles of mm. coxae become flabby and have a tendency to elongation. Their neutral tonus decreases. The magnitude of the vector of compressive reaction force F_2 is diminished to the vector F_2' ($F_2 > F_2'$). Muscular dysbalance is the result, demonstrated by a change of force effect on the site of muscle tendons attached to a corresponding bone (Figure 3).

Even in muscular dysbalance the balance status is preserved between reaction forces F_1', F_2' and permanent load Q, however, the flexors are overburdened by a growing compressive reaction force F_1' ($F_1' > F_2'$, $F_1' + F_2' = Q$).

Muscular dysbalance in patients with osteoporosis becomes clinically significant:

1) in case of the increase of permanent load Q (weight gain)
2) in case of the increase of live load
   a) physical work, exercise
   b) fall, impact
3) in case of reduction of bone mass.
4)

In these cases there is a distortion of balance status between reaction forces of external load (body weight, physical work, fall, impact) and reaction forces in muscles and bones.

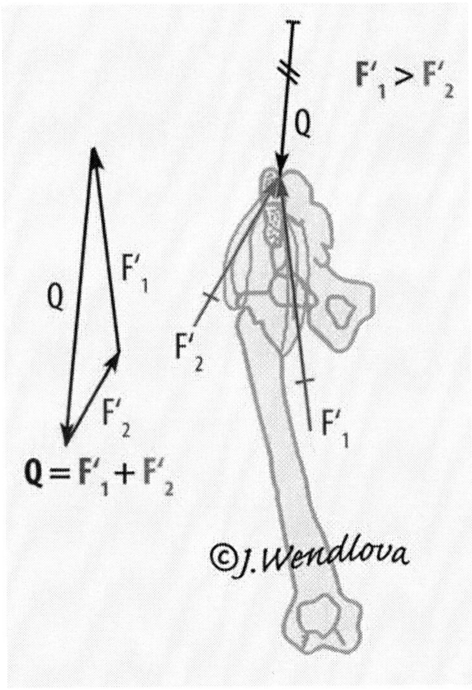

Figure 3. Biomechanical scheme of force resolution in muscular dysbalance. Tonus of flexors is greater than that of extensors. F_1' - the force vector transferred into flexors; F_2' - the force vector transferred into extensors.

In the biomechanical model of mm.coxae we simulated the influence of live load in the form of a vector of P force (blow, impact, fall). In case of low energy of the injury and normal density of bone mass the P value is submaximal, so there is a balance between action and reaction forces ($P + Q = F_1 + F_2$) and, therefore, muscle fibres are not damaged and the bone is not broken. The magnitude of impact force P, which does not cause a fracture in healthy bone, increases the risk of fractures in osteoporotic patients just with the disruption of the balance of forces. In Figure 4 we simulated a different direction of application of impact forces P, having a vector of the same magnitude ($P_1 = P_2 = P_3$). In Figure 5 it can be seen how the vector of impact force P changes the magnitude and direction of force vectors in flexors (F_1'') and extensors (F_2'') in muscular dysbalance. Uniting the effects of vectors of impact force P and permanent load Q gives their resultant R. The influence of R resultant vector on mm.coxae (resolution of force effects of the R vector) results in the increase of reaction compressive force in flexors F_1'' and, at the same time, there occurs an important phenomenon, when the compressive force in extensors is changed into tensile force F_2'', because the vector of this force is oriented in opposite direction from the resultant R. Growing force F_2'' in traction is transferred to muscle tendons in the trochanter major area.

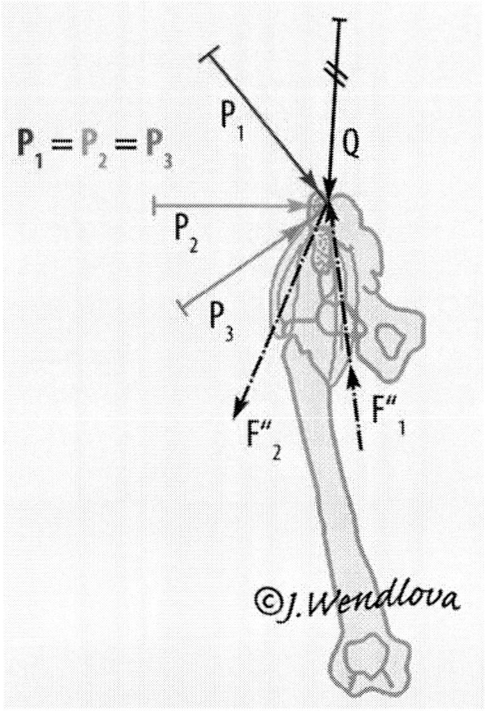

Figure 4. The different directions of application of impact forces P_1, P_2 and P_3 on the hip. Q – the force vector of the upper part of the body, P_1, P_2 , P_3 – the force vectors of live loads (blow, impact, fall), F_1''- the force vector in flexors; F_2''- the force vector in extensors.

The most unfavourable direction of the vector of the P force is the one with a perpendicular action upon the hip, as not only the reaction compressive force increases in F_2'' flexors, but also tensile force in F_2'' extensors. From the mechanical aspect there is a risk of the increase of just the tensile force in extensors weakened by muscular dysbalance, because there is a possibility of disrupting the integrity of muscular fibres as well as of complicated splintered hip fractures by a transfer of tensile force to trochanter major.

To prevent a sharp increase of tensile force F_2'' which contributes to complicated fractures in the collum femoris area by a fall, it is necessary to remove muscular dysbalance of mm. coxae by balancing exercises. Balancing the muscular dysbalance puts to normal the tonus of extensors, thus improving the muscle quality as a tenacious material and increasing the value of yield stress and tensile strength - the resistance of the muscle against the effects of tensile force is growing. Muscular dysbalance can be diagnosed by tests, evaluating the length of internal muscles (the motion range of flexors) and the power of external muscles (extensors).

To remove muscular dysbalance in the mm. coxae area it is recommended to use the following techniques in balancing exercises for osteoporotic patients [8]:

1. for shortened muscles (flexors) we set up a programme of statical stretching exercises on the principle of post-isometric relaxation (tension - relaxation - stretching)
2. for weakened muscles (extensors) we set up a programme of muscle conditioning exercises (slow statical submaximum isometric exercises and slow dynamic conditioning exercises).

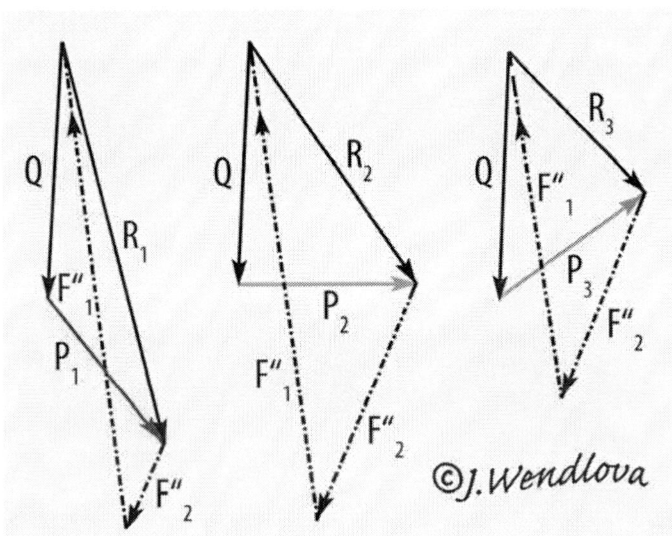

Figure 5. Polygon of forces shows how can the vector of impact forces $P_1 - P_3$ change the magnitude and direction of force vectors in flectors (F_1'') and extensors (F_2'') in muscular dysbalance. R_1, R_2, R_3 – the resultant forces of a vector of Q and P_1, P_2, P_3 forces.

CONCLUSION

An asset of this paper is the new knowledge that muscular dysbalance between flexors and extensors of mm.coxae could contribute during a fall or an impact upon the hip to complicated splintered fractures. In addition to well-known preventive measures against fractures in the collum femoris area as

1. early diagnosis and therapy of osteoporosis
2. rational nutrition
3. regular motoric activity
4. mechanical protection of hip in risk patients

we would recommend also a *targeted therapeutic exercise to balance the muscular dysbalance of mm.coxae.*

An important role in providing regular long-term therapeutic exercise for osteoporotic patients is played by trained instructors of therapeutic exercise who manage in a professional way self-helping groups of patients associated in patient's organisations. Therapeutic exercise should become a very important part of complex care of outdoor osteoporotic patients.

Clinical Application of the Biomechanical Analysisi

Suggested Compensatory Exercises program To Remove Muscular Dysbalance in the Mm. Coxae Area

In compensatory exercises we have chosen stretching for shortened muscles and strengthening exercises for weakened muscles [9].

Stretching the Flexors of MM. Coxae

M. Iliopsoas

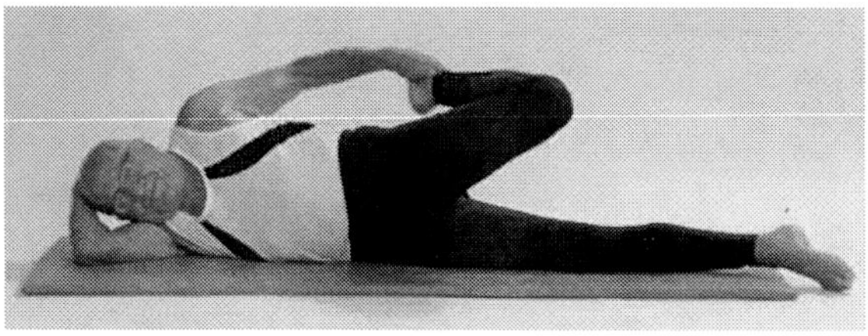

Photo 1.

The patient lies down on his/her right side and puts his head on his/her right UL (upper limb). He/she bends his/her left LL (lower limb) in the knee and by his/her left hand grips the end of hi/her bended leg. He/she pulls his/her leg backwards. He/she alternates the limbs in the given position.

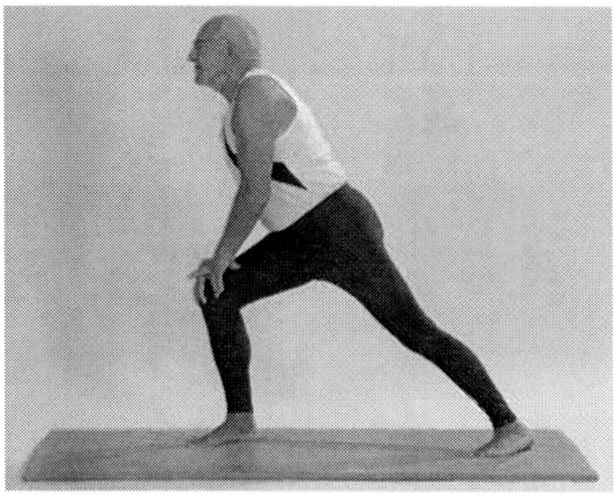

Photo 2.

Squatting on the left leg with outstretched right leg the patient transfers the weight to the front to his/her right LL until feeling in the bent LL the traction of muscles in the frontal part of the thigh. In this exercise it is not allowed to increase the bending in the lumbo-sacral area (LS).

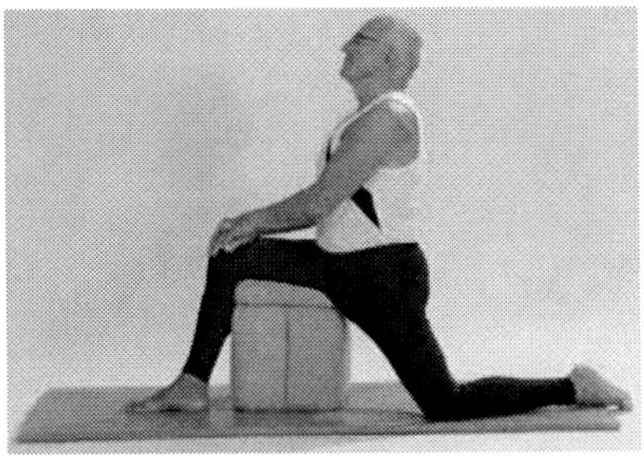

Photo 3.

The patient sits astride on a square shape stool and moves his/her leg backwards until feeling the traction in the frontal part of the thigh of that lower limb. The trunk is held straight, the pelvis must not be turned to a side.

Strengthening of MM. Coxae Abductors

M. Gluteus Maximus

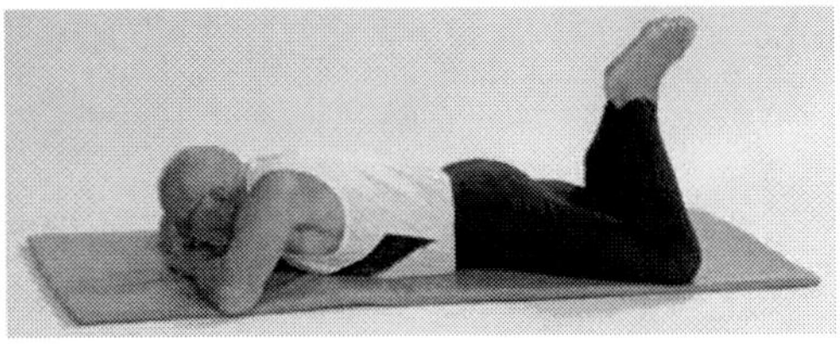

Photo 4.

In a prone position the patient bends the lower limbs in the knees and for a few seconds pushes the soles of his/her feet together, alternating tension and relaxation several times.

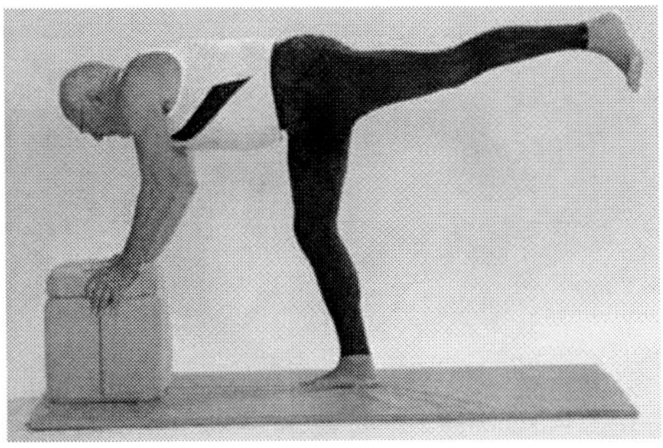

Photo 5.

The patient leans with his/her hands on the stool, stretches one LL backwards in a horizontal plane. The sole of the stretched LL is relaxed; the point of his/her foot is turned downwards.

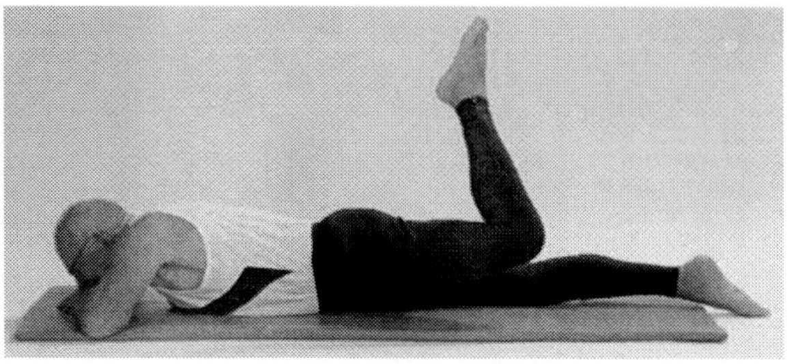

Photo 6.

In a prone position the patient bends one LL and lifts it slightly above the pad. He/she must not bend in the LS area. The patient alternates the limbs in given positions.

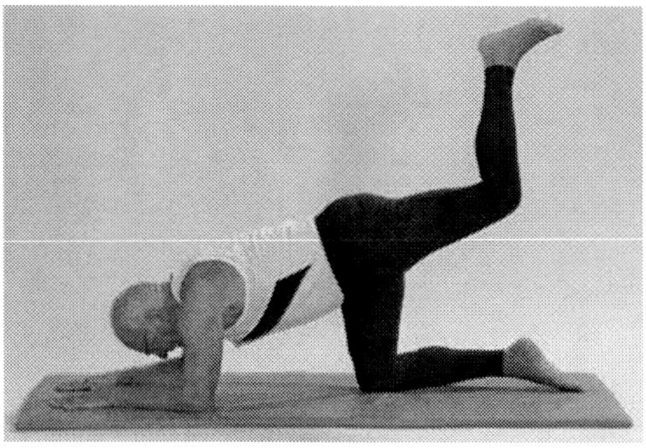

Photo 7.

In a kneeling position, leaning on his/her hands, the patient stretches backwards one bent LL, pulling it upwards, the thigh and the spine is in one line, the point of the bent LL is not tense. The positions of limbs are alternated.

M. Gluteus Medius and Minimus

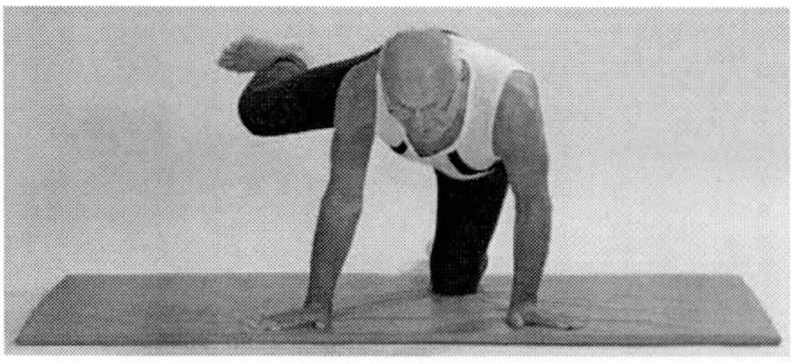

Photo 8a. (frontal view).

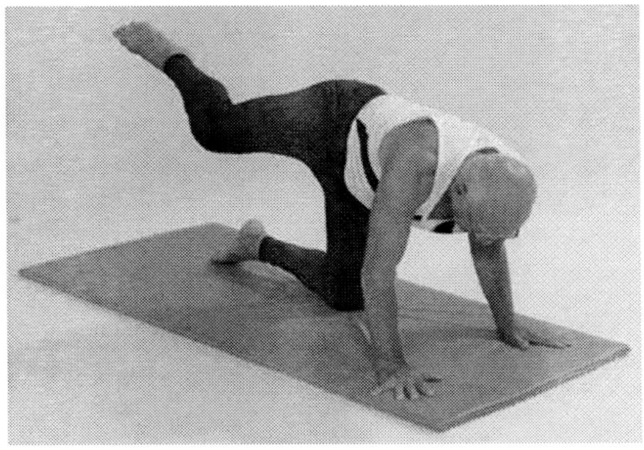

Photo 8b. (side view).

In a kneeling position, leaning on his/her hands, the patient puts one leg to the side and bends it, not turning the pelvis and keeping the whole trunk in one plane. The patient pushes him/herself away from the floor with the hands not to allow the chest to protrude between the shoulders. The knee of the bent LL should be positioned higher than the sole. He/she maintains this position for about 5 to 10 minutes.

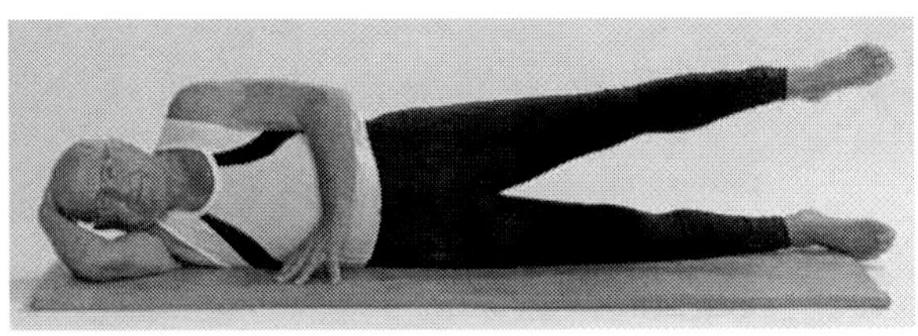

Photo. 9a.

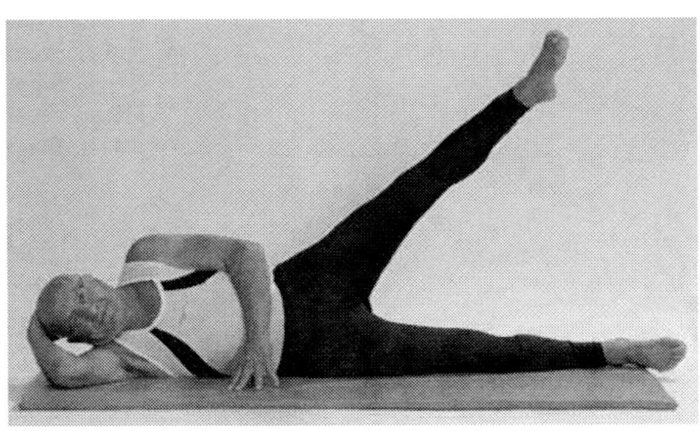

Photo. 9b.

The patient lies on his/her side. With one outstretched LL he/she slightly swings up and down without entirely putting the legs together. The patient alternates the position of the LL.

Caution

Patients with advanced osteoporosis with wedge-shaped deformations of vertebrae do not perform exercises in Figures 1, 3, 4, 6, 7 and 8.

REFERENCES

[1] Ringe JD, Meunier P: *Senile Osteoporose. Prevention von Schenkelhalsfrakturen.* Georg Thieme Verlag, Stuttgart – New York 1996, 2 – 3.

[2] Lu – Jao GL, Baron JA, Barret JA, Fisher ES: Treatment and survival among elderly Americans with hip fractures: A population based study. *AMJ Public Healths*, 1994, 84, 1287 – 1291.

[3] Obetková V, Mamrilová A, Košinárová A: *Theoretical mechanics*. Publishing House of technical and economic literature ALFA, Bratislava, 1990, 30 – 94.

[4] Adamča LF, Marton P, Pavlík M, Trávníček F: *Theoretical mechanics*. Publishing House of technical and economic literature ALFA, Bratislava, 1992, 27 – 37.

[5] Koniar M, Leško M: *Biomechanics* Slovak pedagogic publishing house, Bratislava, 1995, 30 – 33.

[6] Burr DB: Biomechanics *Clin Reviews in Bone and Miner Metab*, 2006, 3, 112 – 117.

[7] Bouxein ML: Biomechanics of osteoporotic fractures *Clin Reviews in Bone and Miner Metab*, 2006, 3, 118 – 126.

[8] Wendlová J, Wendl J: Didactics and method of therapeutic exercise in patients with osteoporosis. *Osteological bulletin*, 1997, 2, 49 – 51.

[9] Lewit K: *Manipulační léčba v rámci léčebné rehabilitace*, 1. vydání, Vydavatelství NADAS, Praha 1990, 258 – 269.

In: Osteoporosis: Etiology, Diagnosis and Treatment
Editors: Bilar E. Mattingly and Albert C. Pillare
ISBN 978-1-60692-397-9

Short Communication J

WHY DOES DEPRESSION DEVELOP IN COMPLICATED OSTEOPOROSIS? (CLINICAL STUDY)

J. Wendlová[*]

University Derer´s Hospital and Policlinic, Osteological Centre, Bratislava, Slovakia.

ABSTRACT

Patients and methods: In a prospective study we observed which female patients developed depression following an acute and painful vertebral fracture. On the day of diagnosing the vertebral fracture the patients filled the questionnaires 1 and 2. The depression developed in some patients was diagnosed by means of the DSM – IV questionnaire. For the statistical evaluation of questionnaires we chose randomly 32 patients with depression (out of 33 patients) aged 51-73, and 32 patients without depression (out of 44 patients) aged 52-70.

The aim of the study: To verify the hypothesis that the patients with more traumatic experience in the anamnesis (Questionnaire No. 1) are more depression prone following the osteoporotic vertebrae fractures and their character features are typical for subjects with higher emotional vulnerability (Questionnaire No. 2).

Statistical analysis: 1. Questionnaires 1 and 2 were evaluated by two statistical methods:

a) automatization of mathematical and statistical estimates and tests based on binomial distribution;
b) ADALINE Programme. 2. Assessment of relative risk for developing depression.

[*] Correspondence concerning this article should be addressed to: Ass. Prof. Jaroslava Wendlová MD, PhD Krížna 30, 811 07 Bratislava. jwendlova@mail.t-com.sk.

Results: 1. Questionnaire No. 1 completed by depressed patients contained statistically significant higher number of positive answers to questions defining experienced stress situations (differences in values of weights of questionnaire parameters expressed in percentages within linear combination of the whole group). 2. Questionnaire No. 2 completed by depressed patients contained statistically significant higher number of positive answers by more depression prone subjects in comparison with non-depressed patients (differences in values of weights of questionnaire parameters. 3. Patients lapsed into depression most often on the 32nd day following the vertebra fracture. 4. Proposed questionnaires are according to validity criteria (sensitivity, specificity, prediction value of positive test, prediction values of negative test, test effectiveness) indicated for identification of persons risking the onset of depression following the osteoporotic fracture of vertebrae. 5. Relative risk (RR) for developing depression in patients with osteoporotic fracture, which answered in Questionnaire No. 1 eight and more questions positive is *7,0 time* higher than in patiens with osteoporotic fracture, which answered in Questionnaire No. 1 less than eight guestions positive. For Questionnaire No. 2 it is *8,5 time* higher.

Conclusion: We recommend to use questionnaires No. 1 and 2 in female patients with acute painful vertebrae fractures to select patients with the risk of depression development. These patients should be followed more frequently as outpatients and in case of first clinical symptoms of depression should be recommended for special psychiatric care. Early therapy of depression enables to accelerate the mobilisation, rehabilitation and resocialisation of patients, to improve the quality of their lives and to reduce the costs of analgetic treatment of pain, sedatives and rehabilitation.

Keywords: Aetiology – depression – osteoporosis – post menopause – vertebrae fracture.

INTRODUCTION

Fractures as complications of osteoporosis represent an important social and economic problem, because they increase the costs of treatment and complex care of patients. Risk factors for osteoporotic fractures are: female sex, premature menopause, age, primary or secondary amenorrhoea, primary and secondary hypogonadism in man, Asian or white ethnic origin, previous fragility fracture, low bone mineral density, glucocorticoid therapy, high bone turnover, family history of hip fracture, low bodyweight, neuromuscular disorders, smoking, excessive alcohol consumption, long-term immobilisation, low dietary calcium intake, vitamin D deficiency [1]. According to Cummings et al. cohort study [2] a 50-year-old Caucasian woman has a 32% chance of a vertebral fracture occurring in her remaining lifetime. Even more striking, women with prevalent vertebral deformities have a risk of sustaining a subsequent vertebral fracture that is five times that of women without prevalent vertebral deformities [3,4].

Vertebral fractures lead to deformations of the chest – kyphosis, conditioning biomechanical changes in the musculoskeletal system with subsequent clinical symptomatology:

- discopathies, pseudoradicular or radicular syndrome, muscular dysbalance of the trunk musculature (chronic backache)

- ileocostal-friction syndrome (friction of costal arches with ala ossis ilii during the trunk movement)
- increase of intraabdominal pressure (loss of appetite, dyspeptic problems, diffused pain in the abdomen and under the right costal arch, obstipation)
- growth of pressure forces on pulmonary parenchyma (the disposition to infection of upper respiratory tract and lungs, the reduction of maximal breathing capacity, and the decrease of right ventricular systolic ejection fraction in combination with the increased diastolic content of the right ventricle represent a risk for the development of cor pulmonale chronicum)
- disposition to falls mainly in leaning forward (deviating the body's centre of gravity from its normal position, disruption of skeletal statics)

Osteoporotic fracture represents for a patient a long-term stress situation, as it brings about a lifestyle change with the limitation of everyday activities and the loss of total independence. The success of the vertebral fracture therapy is often complicated by the development of depression, which is frequently diagnosed late or not at all; sometimes it is treated by sedatives as a neurasthenic syndrome, without the effect of such a treatment.

In the osteological department we were able to observe in some patients with osteoporotic vertebral fractures a very slow and unsuccessful mobilisation, rehabilitation and reconvalescence in comparison with other patients whose mobilisation was relatively quick, and they could return to their original lifestyle with some limitations. In the group of unsuccessfully mobilised patients persisted a marked vertebrogenic algic syndrome, aversion to cooperation with the physician and physiotherapist, and inability to live a normal life. These patients were prevailingly diagnosed as depressive.

The above-mentioned clinical experience brought us to the annotation of a prospective study to answer this question: Why did some women, following the clinical vertebral fracture, despite a standard therapy, develop depression and some women did not.

The Aim of the Study:

1. To find out the confidence interval (C.I.) and median ($\widetilde{x}$) for time interval of the onset of clinical symptoms of depression from the onset of osteoporotic fracture of vertebra.
2. To set up Questionnaire No.1 focused on the anamnesis of experienced mental stress situations.
3. To compare anamnestic data (positive or negative answer) focused on experienced mental traumas, obtained by means of *Questionnaire No. 1* in the group of depressed female patients with osteoporotic vertebrae fractures, with the group of female patients with osteoporotic vertebrae fractures, but without depression.
4. To compare the differences in positive and negative answers in completed *Questionnaire No. 2* (characteristics of depression prone personality - according F.Flach) between the groups of depressed and non-depressed patients.
5. To evaluate validity criteria for Questionnaires No. 1 and 2:

- sensitivity
- specificity
- prediction values of the positive test
- prediction value of the negative test
- test effectiveness
-

6. To calculate the relative risk (RR) for developing depression in patients with osteoporotic fracture.

Questionnaire No. 1.

For every life situation you experienced in the past insert the plus sign (+), or the minus sign (-) if such an event did not happen to you during your lifetime		
	D	**NonD**
1. Wrong lifestyle – disorganised lifestyle		
1.1. Long-term lack of sleep	**18**	**6**
1.2. Repeated overwork and exhaustion by excessive work	**26**	**14**
1.3. Lack of regular exercise	**29**	**30**
2. Previous diseases, long-term care of gravely ill person close to you		
2.1. Post-natal depression	**6**	**2**
2.2. Operations (give number, e.g.: 3)	**12**	**7**
2.3. Personal experience of serious illness	**25**	**12**
2.4. Long-term care of gravely ill close person who died	**16**	**4**
3. Experience of failure or sin feeling		
3.1. I failed in a serious situation and I still blame myself for it	**15**	**10**
3.2. I have a feeling that I sinned and I cannot come to terms with it	**16**	**9**
4. Difficult life trials		
I experienced:		
4.1. Death of a family member (give number)	**28**	**29**
4.2. Divorce	**10**	**7**
4.3. Disintegration of the family	**11**	**3**
4.4. Job loss	**5**	**6**
4.5. Serious financial difficulties	**21**	**24**
4.6. Loneliness, desertedness	**26**	**7**
4.7. Repeated failures in activities I felt very strongly about	**23**	**7**
4.8. Long-term conflict relations in the workplace	**22**	**4**
4.9. Nursing of physically or mentally handicapped child	**1**	**0**
4.10. I experienced an alcohol addiction	**0**	**0**

Characteristics of the Cohort of Examined Female Patients and Methods Applied

During the period of six years the study gradually included patients with one newly sustained (painful) clinical vertebral fracture, who in the past had none or at most two vertebral fractures. The patients were diagnosed with a primary or secondary osteoporosis (condition after a hysterectomy and bilateral adnexectomy, malabsorption syndrome – asymptomatic coeliacia, chronical atrophic gastritis with achlorhydria, M. Crohn). The study did not include patients with osteoporosis, induced by glucocorticoids. On the very day when the acute vertebral fracture was diagnosed, each patient filled a questionnaire No. 1 and 2.

Questionnaire No. 2.

Depression Prone Personality Profile **If you identify with a feature fitting you in the past, insert the plus sign (+), if not, insert the minus sign (-).**		
	D	**NonD**
1. I took things very seriously, I had a feeling of a high moral responsibility for everything I did	29	14
2. I was very ambitious, I always tried to perform well	19	10
3. I was definitely a competitive person	27	22
4. I always had a feeling of having a lot of energy, that I am indefatigable, that I can work myself "into the ground"	27	4
5. I always cared too much how other people feel	18	4
6. I never wanted to hurt other people's feelings	17	5
7. I was always too much dependent on people I loved	27	19
8. I reacted too emotionally to anything that could even in a smallest way possible reduce the feeling of my self-esteem	29	13
9. Any tactlessness from other people hurt me too deeply (every humiliation or insult)	18	2
10. I was at a loss what to do in confrontation with a hostile attitude of other people, I was often helpless against attacks by other people	22	3
11. If I was verbally attacked I had troubles to pull myself together and defend myself – even in case when the defence was really justified	23	6

Questionnaire 1 was set up to include the most frequent model situations of stress and mental trauma in people' s lives. Questionnaire 2 was set up according to Frederic Flach [5], including character features of persons inclined to develop depression following stressful life situations.

All patients, both in acute and chronical stage of vertebral fracture, received a standard treatment by analgesics, nonsteroid antirheumatics, myorelaxants and physical therapy:

1) in the acute stage: local application of cold, electrotherapy, tender relaxing back massage;

2) in the chronical stage: kinesitherapy directed at the removal of muscular dysbalance in the area of trunk muscles.

The choice of analgesic drug and its dosage were on individual basis, aimed at removing or minimising backache.

Depression in patients was diagnosed by means of the DSM-IV questionnaire [6].

Depressive patients were adequately treated by antidepressants. For the final evaluation of comparison of questionnaires we chose at random 32 (D) depressive patients (from the overall number of 33) and 32 (nonD) nondepressive patients (from the overall number of 44). We chose the same number of patients in both groups (observation and control) to meet the criteria for proper evaluation of qualitative features by means of questionnaires. In the depressive patients group (D) there were four patients who had already sustained one clinical vertebral fracture in the past. In the non-depressive patients group (nonD) there were four patients who had overcome a vertebral fracture and one patient had overcome two vertebral fractures. From all patients with vertebral fractures (n = 64) 5 were treated with bisphosphonates (1 – 3 years), 4 with calcitonin (2 – 3 years), 6 with selective estrogen receptor modulators (1 – 2 years). In 49 patients were established the diagnosis of osteoporosis, when they suffered from osteoporotic vertebral fracture. These patients were not treated in the past. The age of patients in the D group ranged from 51 to 73 years, in the nonD group from 52 to 70 years.

Statistical Analysis

1. Time for developing depression following osteoporotic fracture

We calculated the confidence interval (95% C.I.) and median ($\widetilde{x}$) for time interval (given as the number of days from the onset of vertebra fracture) characteristic for the onset of clinical signs of depression.

2. Evaluation of Questionnaires

In the completed questionnaires we compared:

a) presence or absence in the anamnesis of experienced stress situation,
b) presence or absence of character feature for a depression prone personality (DPP),

in the cohort of depressed and non-depressed female patients with osteoporotic vertebrae fractures.

In statistical evaluation we used two methods for the comparison of qualitative signs:

2.1. Automatization of Mathematical and Statistical Estimates and Tests based on Binomial Distribution [7,8]

According to this statistical method the number of positive answers (x) to all questions (n) in Questionnaires No. 1 and 2 is given as a percentage of positive answers (P) from the total number of questioned patients in the D or NonD groups (n = 32).

$$P = \frac{x}{n} \cdot 100\%$$

Differences between percentage values of positive answers in Questionnaires No 1 and 2 for D and NonD groups were evaluated by χ^2 (chi – square test) Statistically significant difference between answers was achieved when the following condition was met:

$$\chi^2 > 3.841$$

2.2. ADALINE, PC Software [9]

Using ADALINE program we calculated absolute values of parameter weights in Questionnaires No 1 and 2 and their percentage expression within linear combination of the whole group. Absolute values of weights of individual parameters are given in bar diagrams. We evaluated also validity parameters of the questionnaires (sensitivity, specificity, prediction value of positive test, prediction value of negative test, effectiveness). The ADALINE program includes also the production of a recognition patterns matrix.

Recognition Patterns

Every questionnaire item has a binary character (positive or negative answer). Positive answer (the presence of experience in the anamnesis, presence of DPP character feature) was indicated by the plus sign (y = +1), negative answer by the minus sign (y = - 1). Recognition patterns in the form of a matrix show graphically the differences in answers to every question by every investigated patient.

3. Calculation of Relative Risk (RR)

We calculated relative risk [10,11] for developing depression in patients with acute vertebrae fractures by means of binary association – contingency tables (Tables: K1, K2).

Table K1. Contingency table for Questionaire No.1

	Depression	
Questionaire No. 1	Yes	No
Positive	28 (a)	4 (b)
Negative	4 (c)	28 (d)

Table K2. Contingency table for Questionaire No.2

	Depression	
Questionaire No. 2	Yes	No
Positive	29 (a)	5 (b)
Negative	3 (c)	27 (d)

a, b, c, d – frequencies.

The risk (R_1) is a ratio of the number of patients with depression exposed to risk factors (a) to the total number of observed patients exposed to risk factors (a + b). The risk (R_2) is a ratio of the number of patients with depression without exposure to risk factors to the total number of patients not exposed to risk factors. Relative risk (RR) is the ratio of the risk for depression by patients with the risk factors to the risk for depression by patients without the risk factors.

$$R_1 = \frac{a}{a+b}$$

$$R_2 = \frac{c}{c+d}$$

$$RR = \frac{R_1}{R_2} = \frac{\frac{a}{a+b}}{\frac{c}{c+d}}$$

RESULTS

Median for developing depression was the 32nd day following the onset of the osteoporotic vertebra fracture. Patients developed depression at the least after 7 days, at the most after 52 days.

$\tilde{x}$ (median) for 95% C.I = 32nd day
95% C.I.: - upper limit 38th day
- lower limit 24th day

Table 1. Percentage representation of parameters weights of Questionnaire No.1 within linear combination of the whole group ($\alpha = 0,05$)

Question No.	Weights of parameters of questionnaire (in %)	
	D	NonD
1.1.	1,93	- 4,73
1.2.	6,22	- 0,42
1.3.	5,81	8,24
2.1.	- 4,99	- 8,35
2.2.	- 5,39	- 4,98
2.3.	4,29	- 3,60
2.4.	1,71	- 3,15
3.1.	- 1,97	- 3,38
3.2.	0,28	- 2,36
4.1.	10,57	5,90
4.2.	- 3,65	- 5,29
4.3.	- 1,78	- 6,08
4.4.	- 10,07	- 5,30
4.5.	0,31	2,82
4.6.	5,54	- 2,85
4.7.	5,56	- 6,47
4.8.	1,88	- 5,15
4.9.	- 12,73	- 10,42
4.0.	- 15,33	- 10,42

Evaluation of Questionnaire No.1

Questionnaires completed by depressed patients included statistically significant higher number of positive answers to questions defining experienced stress situation in life (Table 1).

Differences in weights values of questionnaire parameters expressed in percentages within linear combination of the whole group are given in Table 2 (questions are numbered). Table 2 contains those questions, statistically significant for diagnosing risk patients, where the weights of answers reached positive numbers (in % or in absolute numbers) in the D group and negative numbers in the NonD group. The number of questions meeting these criteria is, at the same time, a minimum number of questions to which the patient has to give a positive answer to be included into the depression development risk group. For Questionnaire No. 1 it is a minimum of eight positive answers.

Table 2. Comparison of the number of positive answers (expressed in percentage % from the overall number of questioned patients n = 32) in Questionnaire No. 1 for every question in the group of depressed patients (D) and non-depressed patients (NonD) by means of χ^2 ($\alpha = 0,05$)

Question No.	D n = 32 (%)	NonD n = 32 (%)	χ^2 (chi – square test)
1.1.	56	19	10,252
1.2.	84	44	12,485
1.3.	88	94	0,756
2.1.	22	6	3,505
2.2.	38	22	1, 01
2.3.	78	38	11,562
2.4.	50	16	9,194
3.1.	44	31	1,074
3.2.	50	28	3,281
4.1.	88	88	0,000
4.2.	34	23	1,086
4.3.	34	9	6,363
4.4.	16	19	0,075
4.5.	66	75	0,677
4.6.	78	22	22,841
4.7.	72	22	17,647
4.8.	72	13	27,077
4.9.	3	0	0,178
4.10.	0	0	0,000

According to validity criteria (Table 3) we consider Questionnaire No 1 indicated for the recognition of depression development risk patients following an acute painful vertebra fracture.

Table 3. Validity criteria of Questionnaire No. 1. ($\alpha = 0,05$)

	Validity criteria (in %)								
group	**TN**	**FP**	**FN**	**TP**	**sensitivity**	**specificity**	**Prediction values of the positive test**	**Prediction values of the negative test**	**Test effectivness**
D	25	7	1	31	96,88	78,13	81,58	96,15	87,50
NonD	31	1	7	25	78,13	96,88	96,15	81,58	87,50

TP – true positives;
TN – true negatives;
FP – false positives;
FN – false negatives.

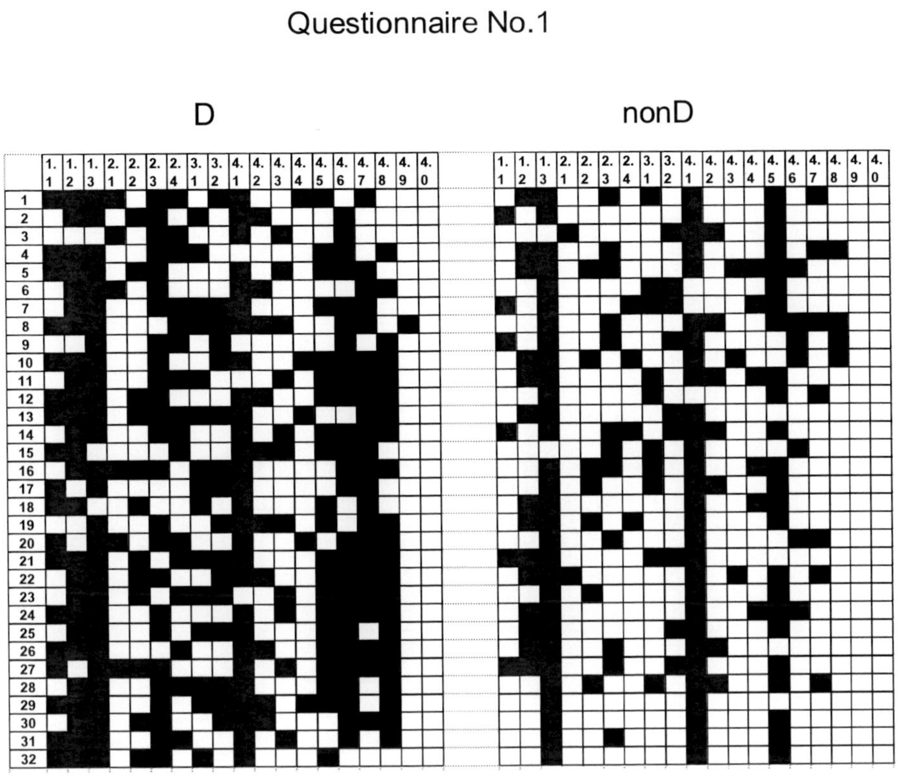

Figure 1. Discrimination analysis of recognition patters for Questionnaire No. 1. (Columns are numbered by questions numbers in Questionnaire No. 1, the lines are numbered by serial numbers of individual patients n = 32, positive answer – black field, negative answer – white field).

Evaluation of Questionnaire No. 2

Questionnaires completed by depressed patients included statistically significant higher number of positive answers for character features of depression prone persons in comparison with non-depressed patients (Table 4).

Table 4. Percentage representation of parameters weights in Questionnaire No. 2 within linear combination of the whole group ($\alpha = 0{,}05$)

Question No.	Weights of parameters of questionnaire (in %)	
	D	NonD
1	12,48	6,85
2	5,17	- 13,64
3	19,26	4,53
4	11,08	- 10,86
5	0,35	- 9,45

Table 4. (Continued)

Question No.	Weights of parameters of questionnaire (in %)	
	D	NonD
6	- 0,55	- 7,98
7	18,80	8,75
8	19,00	3,83
9	1,51	- 13,44
10	4,81	- 16,65
11	7,00	- 4,00

Table 5. Comparison of the number of positive answers (expressed in percentage % from the overall number of questioned patients n = 32) in Questionnaire No. 2 for every question in the group of depressed patients (D) and non-depressed patients (NonD) by means of χ^2 (α = 0,05)

Question No.	D n = 32(%)	NonD n = 32 (%)	χ^2 (chi square – test)
1.	91	44	18,447
2.	59	31	5,254
3.	84	69	2,234
4.	84	13	41,273
5.	56	13	15,160
6.	53	16	10,774
7.	84	59	5,188
8.	91	41	20,686
9.	56	6	22,687
10.	69	9	28,423
11.	72	19	20,356

Differences in weights values of questionnaire parameters expressed in percentages within linear combination of the whole group are given in Table 5.

Table 5 contains the questions, statistically significant for diagnosing risk patients, where the weights of answers reached positive numbers (in % or in absolute numbers) in the D group and negative numbers in the NonD group. The number of questions meeting these criteria is, at the same time, a minimum number of questions to which the patient has to give a positive answer to be included into the depression prone person risk group. For Questionnaire No. 2 it is a minimum of six positive answers.

According to validity criteria we consider Questionnaire No. 2 indicated for diagnosing depression prone persons (Table 6).

Table 6. Validity criteria of Questionnaire No. 2 for evaluation of character features of depression prone persons (DPP) (α = 0,05)

	Validity criteria (in %)								
group	TN	FP	FN	TP	senzitivity	specificity	Prediction values of the positive test	Prediction values of the negative test	Test effectiveness
D	30	2	4	28	87,50	93,75	93,33	88,24	90,63
NonD	28	4	2	30	93,75	87,50	88,24	93,33	90,63

Figure 2 brings differences in character features of depressed and non-depressed patients by means of recognition patterns (positive answer – black field, negative answer – white field).

Calculation of Relative Risk for Questionnaire No. 1 (Table K1)

$$RR = \frac{R_1}{R_2} = \frac{\frac{a}{a+b}}{\frac{c}{c+d}} = \frac{\frac{28}{28+4}}{\frac{4}{4+28}} = \frac{0{,}875}{0{,}125} = 7.0 \qquad 95\%\ \text{CI for RR}\ (6.\ 4;\ 8.\ 1)$$

RR for developing depression in patients with osteoporotic vertebrae fractures is 7,0 time higher for patients, which answered in Questionnaire No. 1 eight and more questions positive then in patients with osteoporotic fractures, which answered in Questionnaire No. 1 less than eight questions positive

Calculation of Relative Risk for Questionnaire No. 2 (Table K2)

$$RR = \frac{R_1}{R_2} = \frac{\frac{a}{a+b}}{\frac{c}{c+d}} = \frac{\frac{29}{29+5}}{\frac{3}{3+27}} = \frac{0{,}8529}{0{,}1000} = 8.529 \qquad 95\%\ \text{CI for RR}\ (7.6;\ 9.2)$$

RR for developing depression in patients with osteoporotic vertebrae fractures is 8,5 time higher for patients, which answered in Questionnaire No. 2 six and more questions positive, then in patients with osteoporotic fractures, which answered in Questionnaire No. 2 less than six questions positive.

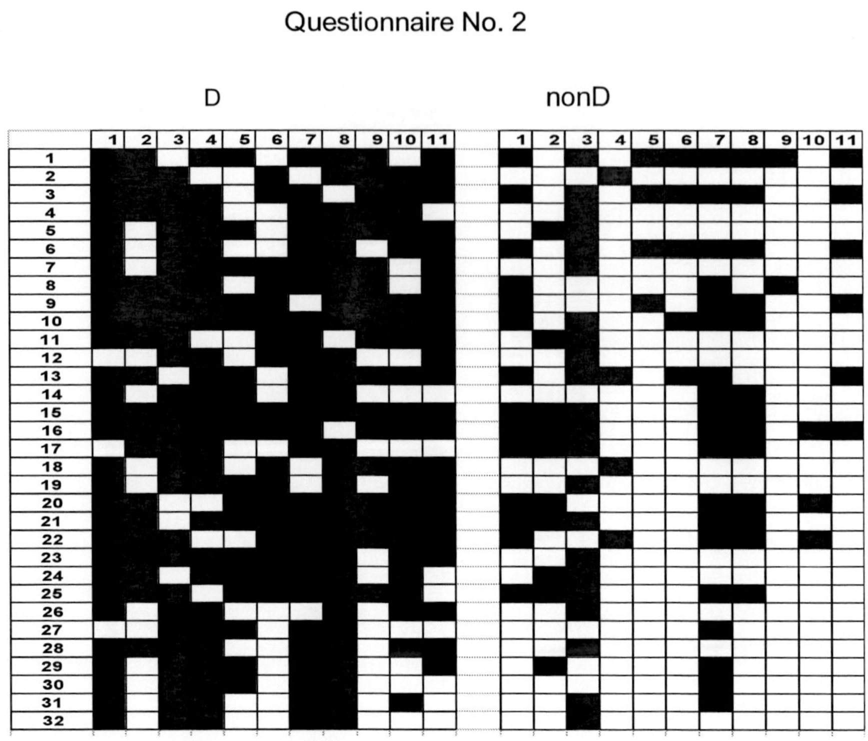

Figure 2. Discrimination analysis of recognition patters for Questionnaire No. 2. (Columns are numbered by numbers of questions about character features of depression prone persons in Questionnaire No. 2, the lines are numbered by serial numbers of individual patients n = 32, positive answer – black field, negative answer – white field).

Discussion

We have not met a similar study in literature to compare our results with. Several studies, whose authors investigated clinical symptomatology accompanying osteoporotic vertebrae fractures, present also the reactive depression as one of the symptoms [12-17], but do not examine its reasons.

In our study we have been dealing with the reasons of the development of reactive depression in female patients in acute or chronically stage of painful osteoporotic vertebra fractures. We found out that those patients developed depression who had in their anamnesis more frequent incidence of traumatic experiences and a long-term overexertion on the job or at home. The onset of osteoporotic vertebra fracture with following vertebrogenic pain syndrome, disruption of sleep regime, limited mobility, loss of physical performance and independence represented for the patients a long-term stress situation. The median for developing depression was the 32nd day after the osteoporotic vertebra fracture. In this study we did not point out only that female patients with osteoporotic vertebrae fractures in acute or chronically stage of the illness may develop reactive depression, but we tried to answer the question: Why do only some female patients develop depression? We see the contribution of our study in the finding that depression is developed more frequently in those women who have in their anamnesis a number of traumatic experiences and their character features are typical for depression prone persons (DPP).

Conclusion

Based on the result of our study we recommend the use of Questionnaires No. 1 and 2 in patients with acute painful vertebrae fractures for detecting risk patients for depression development. These patients should be followed more frequently within ambulatory care and in case of first clinical symptoms of depression should be recommended for special psychiatric care. Early anti-depression treatment by antidepressants of the 3rd and 4th generation (selective serotonine reuptake inhibitors - SSRI, serotonine and noradrenaline reuptake inhibitors – SNRI, noradrenergic, specific serotonergic antidepressants – NaSSA, etc.) could accelerates the mobilisation, rehabilitation and resocialisation of patients, could improves quality of their lives and reduces the costs of analgetic pain treatment, sedatives and rehabilitation. It has to be investigated in future studies.

References

[1] Kanis JA: Diagnosis of osteoporosis and assessment of fracture risk. *Lancet* 2002, 359, 1929 – 1936.

[2] Cummings SR, Black DM, Rubin SM: Lifetime risks of hip, Colle´s, or vertebral fractures nad coronary heart disease among Caucasian postmenopausal women. *Arch Intern Med* 1989, 148, 2445 – 2448.

[3] Black DM, Arden NK, PalermoI, Pearson J, Cummings SR : Prevalent veretebral deformities predict hip fractures and new vertebral deformities but not wrist fracture: Study of osteoporotic fractures research group. *J Bone Miner Res* 1999, 14, 821 – 828.

[4] Klotzbuecher CM, Ross PD, Lansman PB, Abbot TA, Berger M : Patients with prior fracture have an increased risk of future fractures: a summary of the literature and statistical synthesis. *J Bone Miner Res* 2000, 15, 721 – 739.

[5] Flach FF: *The secret strength of depression.* 2nd ed, Philadelphia, Lippincott, 1974 26 – 28.

[6] American Psychiatric Association. *Diagnostic and Statistical Manual of Mental Disorders*, 1994 , 4 th ed., Washington DC, American Psychiatric Association.

[7] Mikulecky M, Komornik J, Ondrejka P: A*utomatizacia matematicko – statistickych odhadov a testov na zaklade binomickeho rozdelenia*. PC software, Comtel, 1997.

[8] Labudová V: Analýza sociálnej situácie domácnosti Slovenskej republiky na báze údajov EU SILC 2006 , Slovenská štatistika a demografia, 2008, 18, 108-137

[9] Widrow B, Smith FW Pattern recognizing control systems. In: Tou JT., Wilcox RH.: *Computer and Information science*. Collected papers on learning adaptation and control in information systems. 2nd ed, Washington, 1964 Sparten Books, 40 – 47.

[10] Pacaková V: Statistics for economists, Publishing Hose: IURA EDITION, Bratislava, 1st ed, 2003, 193 – 234.

[11] Mc Nutt LA, Wu CH, Xue X, Hafner JP: Estimating the relative risk in cohort studies and clinical trials of common outcomes. *Am J Epidemiol* 2003, 157, 940 – 943.

[12] Cizza G, Ravn P, Chrousos GP, Golg PW: Depression a major unrecognised risk factor for osteoporosis ? *Trends Endocrinol Metab* 2001, 12, 198 – 203.

[13] Papaioannon A, Watts NB, Kendler DL, Yuen ChK et al.: Diagnosis and management of vertebral fractures in elderly adults. *Am J Med* 2002, 113, 220 – 228.

[14] Greendale GA, Barret – Connor E, Ingles S, Haile R: Late physical and functional effects of osteoporosis fracture in women. The Rancho Bernardo study. *J Am Geriatr Soc* 1995, 48, 546 – 549

[15] Greendale GA, De Amicis TA, Bucur A et al.: A prospective study of the effect of fracture on measured physical performance : results from the Mac Arthur Study – MAC. *J Am Geriatr Soc* 2000, 43, 955 – 961.

[16] Cook DJ, Guyatt GH, Adachi JD et al.: Quality of life issues in women with vertebral fractures due to osteoporosis. *Arthritis Rheum* 1993, 36, 750 – 756.

[17] Rapado A: General management of vertebral fractures. *Bone* 1996, 18, 191 – 196.

In: Osteoporosis: Etiology, Diagnosis and Treatment
Editors: Bilar E. Mattingly and Albert C. Pillare
ISBN 978-1-60692-397-9

Short Communication K

OSTEOPOROSIS IN A FEMALE POPULATION FROM BRATISLAVA - AGE-RELATED BMD CHANGES

J. Wendlová[1,*] and V. Pacáková[2]

[1]University Derer´s Hospital and Policlinic, Osteological Centre, Bratislava, Slovakia;
[2]Economy University, Department of Statistics, Bratislava, Slovakia.

ABSTRACT

Patients and methods. We analysed 498 women (n = 498) in Bratislava (BA) population aged 21 to 90. We measured bone mineral density (BMD) in the area of proximal femur with one densitometric instrument DXA (dual energy X–ray absorptiometry), applying BMD and T-score values in three standard regions of interest: Neck (ROI_1), Ward ´s area (ROI_2), great trochanter (ROI_3).

Statistical analysis: 1. Chi-square goodness-of-fit statistics (χ^2 - test). 2. Analysis of variance (ANOVA).

Results: Measured values of T–score in ROI_1 , ROI_2 have normal distribution and a lognormal distribution of frequency in ROI_3. Using χ^2 - test (chi-square goodness-of-fit statistics), we determined the distribution of frequency of T-score values and the percentage of osteoporosis incidence in Bratislava female population. The osteoporosis incidence in Bratislava female population, according to T-score values measured in ROI_1 is 2.40%, in ROI_2 16.34% and in ROI_3 3.83% . Following the division of women into ten-year intervals, the statistically significant sample averages of T-score values were decreasing in relation to age only for ROI_2. The osteoporosis incidence in age intervals was rising with age for ROI_2, for ROI_1 the number of osteoporotic patients in the 61 to 70-year interval was lower than in the 41 to 50-year interval, and for ROI_3 the number of osteoporotic patients in the 51 to 60-year interval was lower than in the 41 to 50-year interval. Expect of the above mentioned intervals, T-score values decreased in relation to

* Correspondence concerning this article should be addressed to: Ass Prof Jaroslava Wendlová MD, PhD Krížna 30, 811 07 Bratislava. jwendlova@mail.t-com.sk.

age also in ROI_1 and ROI_3 . According to the analysis of variance, the age category explains 9.6% of the overall variability of T-score values for ROI_1, 24.7% for ROI_2 and 11.70% for ROI_3.

Conclusion: As in ROI_2 (Ward's area) greater fraction of the trabecular bone is measured in comparison with ROI_1 and ROI_3, the ROI_2 reflects best the age-related BMD changes. It is due to the fact that the trabecular bone is eight times more active metabolically than the cortical bone, and so it is more sensitive than the cortical bone for the determination of BMD changes. In ROI_1 and ROI_3 the relation was distorted by a greater fraction of cortical bone in comparison with ROI_2 and by an accidental selection of a higher number of osteoarthrotic patients in the 61 to 70-year interval for ROI_1 , and in the 51 to 60-year interval for ROI_3 . The age of patients is a significant risk factor. Bone mass decreases with age independently of the period of other risk factors activities, and also independently of the fact whether the patient suffers from primary or secondary osteoporosis (osteopenia). The development and application of densitometric methods measuring separately the trabecular and cortical bone excludes the distorting factor of osteoarthrosis and should be preferred in densitometric examination methods for a continuous observation of BMD changes.

Keywords: bone mineral density – proximal femur – osteoporosis – women – epidemiological study.

Introduction

Skeletal osteoporosis [1] is the reason for 90% of vertebrae and femoral neck fractures, 70% fractures in the distal forearm area, and about one third of Caucasian women over 50 sustain a fracture in one of these skeletal sites. Therefore, two priorities are preferred in osteology: 1) active screening of patients with risk factors, who undergo densitometric examination; 2) reduction of individual fracture risk by complex treatment of osteopenia and osteoporosis [3].

The objective of densitometric measurement is the diagnosis of osteoporotic patients and in combination with anamnestic data and biochemical markers of osteoresorbtion, the determination of individual fracture risk. According to the WHO, a gold standard for osteoporosis diagnosis and the fracture risk assessment is DXA (dual-energy X-ray absorptiometry) in the proximal femur area (total hip). The problem of the DXA densitometry lies in the discrepancy of results given by densitometers from different manufacturers, in the discrepancy of BMD in measurements in various skeleton sites, differences in selected reference groups of healthy young adults, osteoarthrotic changes in the measured site, sclerotic plates in the aorta, scoliosis and obesity in patients [4,5].

Objective of the Study:

1. To determine the percentage of osteopenia and osteoporosis incidence in Bratislava female population.

2. To divide the sample group into ten-year intervals and to determine the number of osteoporosis cases (in %) in each age interval according to T-score values in the Neck (ROI_1), Ward's area (ROI_2) and great trochanter (ROI_3).
3. To determine which ROI detects best the age-related BMD changes.
4. To determine, using the analysis of variance, the percentage of age participation in the overall variability of T-score values for ROI_1, ROI_2 and ROI_3.

Characteristics of the Examined Patients Group and Methods Applied

General practitioners as well as specialists from different Bratislava districts were sending female patients with primary or secondary osteoporosis and osteopenia and patients with risk factors who did not undergo previous densitometric examination, to one densitometric centre. Women with risk factors were selected for densitometric examination in accordance with the indication list of the International Society for Clinical Densitometry (Official Positions 2004) [6].

So we had a random selection of patients with osteoporosis and osteopenia from Bratislava districts, and simultaneously, in the random selection of risk patients we diagnosed new patients with osteoporosis or osteopenia.

In the Bratislava population sample group there were 498 (n= 498) women of the average age of 59.71 ⟨58. 63; 60. 80⟩.

All women were examined with the same densitometer DXA (dual energy X–ray absorptiometry). Bone mineral density (BMD) was determined in standard regions of interest for DXA (ROI - region of interest) – Neck (ROI_1), Ward's area (ROI_2), great trochanter (ROI_3). BMD values were given in absolute numbers in *g* of Ca-hydroxyapathite crystals for cm^2 (g/cm^2), as well as in relative numbers as T-score (the number of standard deviations from the reference group of young healthy women) and Z-score (the number of standard deviations from the relevant age group of healthy women). Osteoporosis was diagnosed in accordance with the WHO criteria:

Classification of bone density	**T- score:**
Normal	> -1.0 SD
Osteopenia	⟨–1.0; - 2.5) SD
Osteoporosis	≤ -2.5 SD

Statistical Analysis [7,8]

We have used the statistical program systems Statgraphics plus version 3 and SPSS version 6 for the analysis of the female group data.

5) Test for normality of distribution of T – score and Z - score values in ROI_1, ROI_2, ROI_3 (χ^2 – goodness-of-fit statistic, Kolmogorov – Smirnov statistics)

6) Division of the female cohort into 10–year age groups and determination of osteoporosis incidence percentage in each age group for T – score in ROI_1, ROI_2, ROI_3
7) Analysis of variance for comparison of mean T-score values for ROI_1, ROI_2, ROI_3 in age groups divided in ten-year intervals
8) Spearman rank correlation between variables of age and T-score for ROI_1, ROI_2, and ROI3.

RESULTS

Measured values of T – score in ROI_1 and ROI_2 have normal distribution (Graph 1, 2), lognormal distribution of probabilities is in ROI_3 (Graph 3).

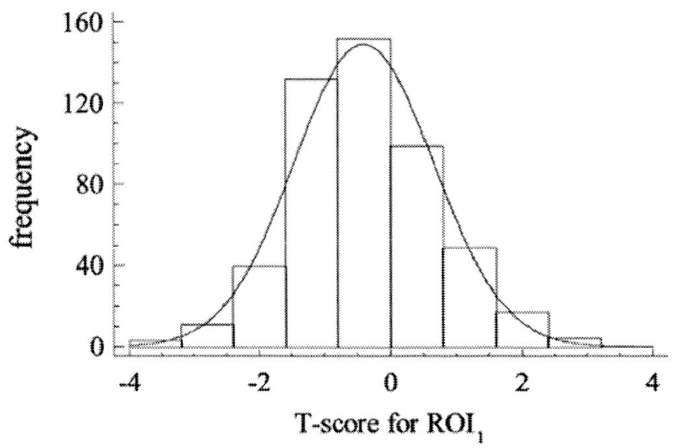

Graph 1.

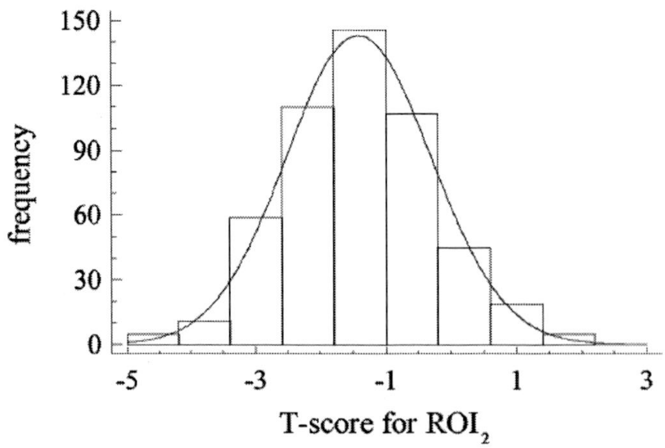

Graph 2.

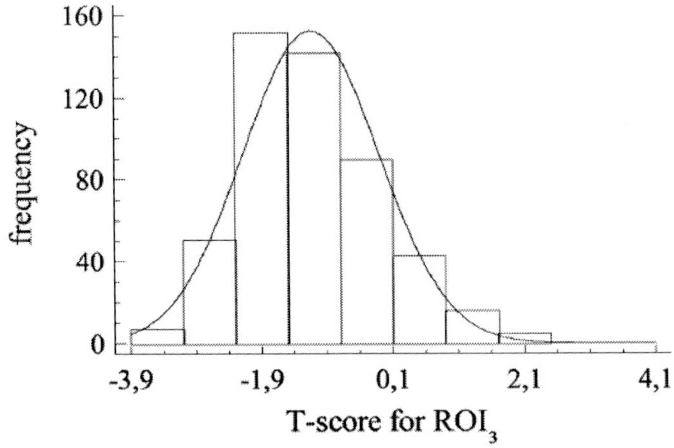

Graph 3.

Table 1. Frequency in observed group and in expected group by means of Chi – square goodness – of – fit statistic. Expected count of female osteoprotic patients in population from Bratislava in %

T – score (SD)	Observed frequency (count)	Expected frequency (count)	Expected frequency in %
ROI_1			
⟨ - 2,5; - ∞)	9	12	**2,46**
(- 2,5; - 1,0⟩	143	131	26,23
(- 1,0; 0,0⟩	181	179	35,88
(0,0;+ ∞)	165	176	35,43
ROI_2			
⟨ - 2,5; - ∞)	86	81	**16,34**
(- 2,5; - 1,0⟩	240	239	47,98
(- 1,0; 0,0⟩	123	127	25,39
(0,0;+ ∞)	49	51	10,29
ROI_3			
⟨ - 2,5; - ∞)	37	19	**3,83**
(- 2,5; - 1,0⟩	264	296	59,47
(- 1,0; 0,0⟩	130	120	23,99
(0,0;+ ∞)	67	63	12,71

$\alpha = 0{,}05$; $p > 0{,}05$;
χ^2 – square test for $ROI_1 = 9{,}338$ with 4 d.f. p - value = 0,053;
χ^2 – square test for $ROI_2 = 2{,}878$ with 6 d.f. p – value = 0,824;
χ^2– square test for $ROI_3 = 13{,}609$ with 7 d.f. p – value = 0,058.

We determined the character of probability distribution by χ^2 – goodness-of-fit test for the comparison of empiric frequency distribution of T-score values found in the sample group with expected frequencies in the Bratislava female population at the significance level α = 0.05 (table 1). The percentage of expected number of women with osteoporosis and osteopenia in the Bratislava population is given in Table 1.

The percentage of osteoporotic patients in ten-year age intervals is given in Table 2.

Table 2. Count of female osteoporotic patients (in %) in 10 – year age groups for ROI_1, ROI_2, ROI_3

Age group	ROI_1		ROI_2		ROI_3	
	T score > - 2,5 SD n_1 n_2 (%)	T - score < - 2,5 SD n_1 n_2(%)	T score > - 2,5 SD n_1 n_2(%)	T - score < - 2,5 SD n_1 n_2(%)	T score > - 2,5 SD n_1 n_2(%)	T - score < - 2,5 SD n_1 n_2(%)
21 – 30	16 100,0	0 0	16 100,0	0 0	16 100,0	0 0
31 - 40	11 100,0	0 0	11 100,0	0 0	11 100,0	0 0
41 – 50	75 100,0	0 0	72 96,0	3 **4,0**	72 96,0	3 4,0
51 - 60	158 98,7	2 1,3	153 95.6	7 **4.4**	157 98,1	3 **1,9**
61 – 70	136 99,3	1 **0,7**	108 78.8	29 **21,2**	129 94,2	8 5,8
71 – 80	78 95,1	4 4,9	44 53,7	38 **46,3**	65 79,3	17 20,7
81 - 91	15 88,2	2 11,8	8 47,1	9 **52,9**	11 64,7	6 35,3

n_1 – count of female patients in age group;
n_2 - % of female osteoporotic (or nonosteoporotic) patients in age group.

Osteoporosis incidence in age intervals according to T-score values in measured ROIs:

1) ROI_1 – the percentage of osteoporotic patients is higher in the 51 to 60 age interval than in the 61 to 70 interval, otherwise the osteoporosis incidence percentage rises with age;
2) ROI_2 – osteoporosis incidence percentage rises with age in all age intervals;
3) ROI_3 – the percentage of osteoporotic patients is higher in the 41 to 50 age interval than in the 51 to 60 interval, otherwise the osteoporosis incidence percentage rises with age in all intervals.

Sample averages of T-score values in ROI_1, ROI_2, ROI_3 and their confidence intervals (C.I.) for set age groups are illustrated in Graphs 4, 5 and 6. They show that the values of sample intervals are decreasing with age. Statistically significant differences among compared T-score values from all set ten-year age intervals can be found only in ROI_2 (Graph 5).

In the variance analysis (ANOVA) the age category explains 9.6% of the overall variability of T-score values for ROI_1, 24.7% for ROI_2, and 11.7% for ROI_3 (Table 3).

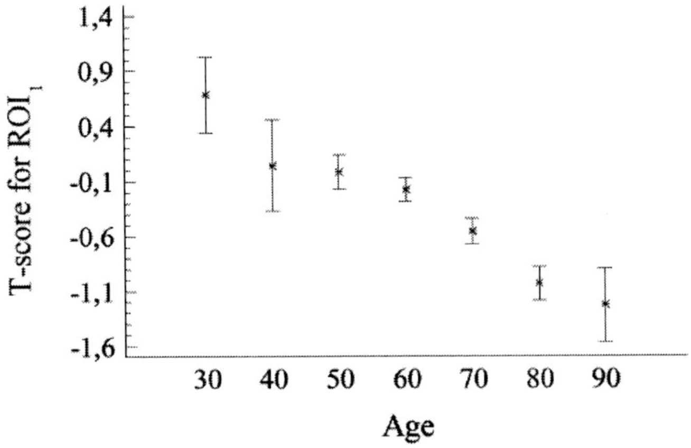

Graph 4.

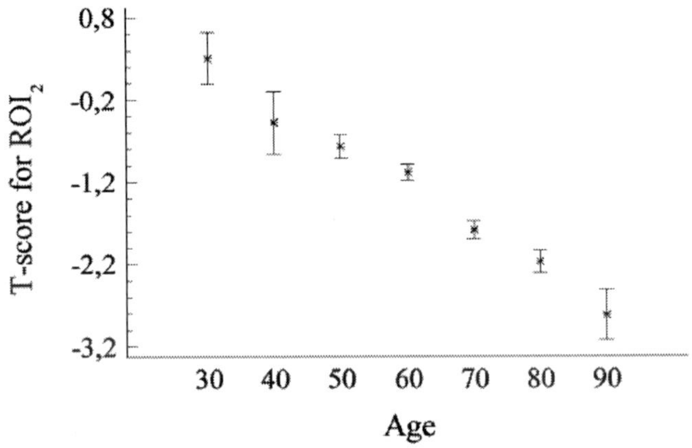

Graph 5.

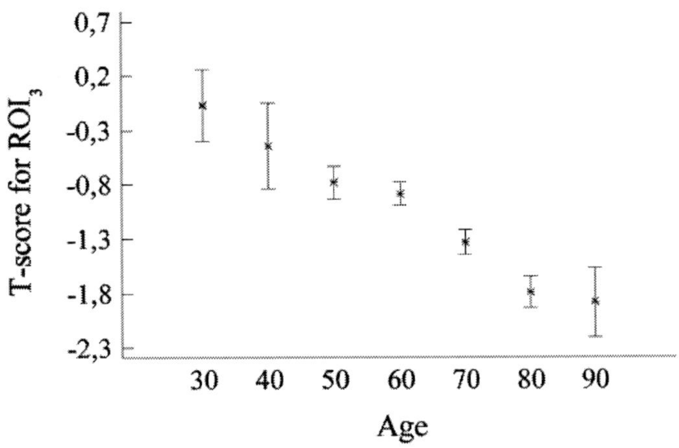

Graph 6.

Fisher's test (F–test) at the significance level of $\alpha = 0.05$ confirmed the significance of the age factor.

Statistically most significant negative correlation between age and T-score was determined for ROI_2 ($r = -0.5785$).

Table 3. ANOVA analysis for age and T – score in ROI_1, ROI_2, ROI_3. P - value < 0,05 - alternative hypothesis H_1 is accepted

ROI_1	Sum of squares	F – ratio	p - value	Variance determined with age in %
Variance between groups	54,285			
Variance within groups	512,912	8,66	0,001	9,6
Total variance	567,197			
ROI_2				
Variance between groups	151,989			
Variance within groups	463,761	26,82	0,001	24,7
Total variance	615,75			
ROI_3				
Variance between groups	63, 227			
Variance within groups	477,092	10,85	0,001	11,7
Total variance	540,319			

F – ratio (Fisher – ratio).

Discussion

Osteoporosis incidence in Bratislava female population, according to T-score values measured in ROI_1 is 2.40%, in ROI_2 16.34% and in ROI3 is 3.83%. In comparison with the results of the European Vertebral Osteoporosis Study (EVOS) [9], which found the osteoporosis incidence in European women to be 12% according to BMD in vertebrae, the osteoporosis incidence in Bratislava female population is, according to measurements in proximal femur for ROI_1 and ROI_3 lower and for ROI_2 higher than European average values in EVOS study. Women aged 50 to 79 from 19 European countries were randomly selected for the EVOS study and were divided into groups according to 5-year age intervals. The age was the only criterion for the inclusion of women in the study [10]. The incidence of osteoporosis according to BMD values in vertebrae is higher than that according to BMD in neck or total hip in postmenopausal women [11–13]. In dividing the cohort of examined women into ten-year age intervals we found that the osteoporosis incidence percentage rises in each consequent age group for T-score values only in ROI_2 (Ward's) as well as the ROI is not acceptable for diagnosis of osteoporosis. As in ROI_1 and ROI_3 greater fraction of the cortical bone is measured in comparison with the ROI_2, the higher incidence of osteoporotic patients in the lower age interval than in the higher age interval is conditional on random selection of higher number of patients with arthrotic changes in measurement sited ROI_1 and ROI_3. Through random selection a higher number of patients with osteoarthrosis in measured

ROI_1 site got into the 61 to 70 age interval as well as in the 51 to 60 age interval for ROI_3. Measurement in ROI_2 area, independently of osteoarthrosis, detects well the bone mass loss, even though the bone mass loss is faster in this area than in other parts of proximal femur [14,15]; therefore, it is not used for osteoporosis diagnosis. Important finding is that Fisher's test confirmed the significance of age risk factor. Bone mass was decreasing with age, independently of other risk factors and time of their activities (which we have no evaluated), as well as independently of whether the patient had primary or secondary osteoporosis (osteopenia). The age-related decrease of BMD was reflected best in Ward's area. T-score values in this area showed the closest negative correlation with age ($r = 0.5785$). The trabecular bone is eight times more active metabolically than the cortical bone and, therefore, the methods measuring changes in the trabecular bone BMD are the most sensitive [5].

Exclusion of distorting factor of osteoarthrosis is supported by the development and application of quantitative computer tomography (QCT) densitometric method. QCT method measures separately the cortical and trabecular bones in the area of the vertebrae and proximal femur and gives the number of Ca-hydroxyapathite crystals in cubic measure units (g/cm^3), in contrast to DXA, which gives the number of Ca-hydroxyapathite crystals in square measure units (g/cm^2), and measures the cortical and trabecular bones together [5].

It follows from this that DXA and QCT do not provide identical information on BMD of measured bones. QCT measurements values are age-related, but independent of arthrotic calcification in the vertebrae and proximal femur areas, sclerotic plates in aorta, and patient's scoliosis. Therefore, the QCT examination is suitable for all age and weight categories [16]. Several authors [16–18] compared the sensitivity of DXA and QCT in differentiating a normal from an osteoporotic population. Higher sensitivity was found in QCT measurements, using t-test, logistic regression analysis, odds ration, ROC (receiver operator characteristics), and Wilcoxon's pair test. Highest sensitivity of differentiation of osteoporotic patients from healthy individuals was achieved by Z-score for QCT, in comparison: a) with T-score for QCT b) with T-score for DXA c) with Z-score for DXA. The introduction of a localiser into a scanner for QCT methods, as well as the determination of *mAs* dose for patients according to their height and weight, reduce the radiation load by 50% and more, and QCT methods acquire an important position in densitometry [19,20].

Standard application of QCT methods requires a whole range of prospective clinical studies determining a relative fracture risk in a time interval in treated and non-treated postmenopausal women. The WHO criteria for BMD classification by means of T-score for DXA may not provide the best predictive ability to detect individuals with the greatest risk for fracture. They are novel approaches in DXA and QCT measurement methods, with the possibility to calculate the geometric values of proximal femur. These geometric values of proximal femur combined with BMD of proximal femur provide valuable clinical information, which is more sensitive for QCT, because here is the possibility to win 3D scan and to measure separately the cortical and trabecular bones in the selected area of the vertebrae and proximal femur.

Conclusions

Summary:

1. Osteoporosis incidence in Bratislava female population, according to T-score values measured in ROI_1 is 2.40%, in ROI_2 16.34% and in ROI_3 3.83%.
2. Patient's age is a significant risk factor for osteoporosis. Bone mass decreases with age, independently of the period of other risk factors activities, and also independently of the fact whether the patient suffers from primary or secondary osteoporosis (osteopenia).
3. Age category provides for the highest percentage in the variability of T-score values (24.7%) for measurements in ROI_2.
4. In all three measured ROIs, the statistically most significant negative correlation can be found between age and T-score measured in the trabecular bone in ROI_2 (Ward's area).
5. Separately measurement of the trabecular bone, which is eight times more active metabolically than the cortical bone, should be preferred in densitometric examination methods for a continuous observation of BMD changes.

References

[1] Melton LJ, Thamer M, Ray NF et al: Fractures attributable to osteoporosis: Report from the National Osteoporosis Foundation. *J Bone Miner Res* 1997, 12, 16 – 23.

[2] Melton LJ, Chrisschilles EA, Cooper C et al: How many women have osteoporosis? *J Bone Miner Res* 1992, 7, 1005 – 1110.

[3] Blake GM, Knapp KM, Fogelman I: Absolute fracture risk varies with bone density techniques used. A theoretical and in vivo study of fractures cases. *J Clin Densitom* 2002, 5, 109 – 116.

[4] McMahon K, Nightingale J, Pocock : Discordance in DXA male reference ranges. *J Clin Densitom* 2004, 7, 121 – 126.

[5] Liu G, Peacock M, Eliam O, et. al: Effect of osteoarthritis in the lumbar spine and hip on bone mineral density and diagnosis of osteoporosis in elderly men and women. *Osteoporos Int* 1997, 7, 564 – 569.

[6] Leib ES, Lewiecki EM, Binkley N, Hamdy RC: Official positions of the international society for clinical densitometry. *J Clin Densitom* 2004, 7, 1 – 6.

[7] Hilgers RD, Bauer P, Scheber V: *Einfuhrung in die medizinische Statistik* Springer Verlag Berlin Heidelberg, 1. Ausgabe, 2003, 217 – 220.

[8] Pacakova V: *Štatistika pre ekonómov (Statistics for economists)*, IURA EDITION, Bratislava, 1st edition, 2003, 193 – 234.

[9] Matthis C, Weber T, O ´Neil W, Raspe H: Health impact associated with vertebral deformities: Results from the European Vertebral Osteoporosis Study (EVOS). *Osteoporos Int* 1998, 8, 364 – 372.

[10] Bartl R, Bartl Ch: *Osteoporose – Manual. Diagnostik, Prävention und Therapie*, Springer Verlag Berlin, 1. Ausgabe, 2004, 201.

[11] Kanis JA, Gluer CC: An update on the diagnosis an assessment of osteoporosis with densitometry. *Osteopor Int* 2000, 11. 192 – 202.

[12] Oden A, Dawson A, Dere W et al: Lifetime risk of hip fractures is underestimated. *Osteoporos In* 1998, 8, 599 – 603.

[13] Kanis JA, Melton LJ, Christiansen C et al: The diagnosis of osteoporosis. *J Bone Miner Res* 1994, 9, 1137 – 1141.

[14] Faulkner KG, von Stetten E, Steiger P, MIller P: Discrepancies in osteoporosis prevalence at different skeletal sites: impact on the WHO criteria. *Bone* 1998, 23, (Suppl), 194.

[15] Mazess RB: T – score differ among skeletal sites. *Calcif Tissue Int* 1999, 64, 104.

[16] Bergot C, Laval – Jeantet AM, Hutchinson K et al: A comparison of spinal quantitative computed tomography with dual energy X-ray absorptiometry in European women with vertebral and nonvertebral fractures. *Calcif Tissue Int* 2001, 68, 74 – 82.

[17] Yu W, Gluer CC, Grampp S, Jergas M et al: Estimates of volumetric bone density from projectional measurements improve the discriminatory capability of dual X–ray absorbptiometry. *J Bone Miner Res* 1995, 10, 1101 – 1110.

[18] Lafferty FW, Rowland DY: Correlation of dual energy X–ray absorptiometry, quantitative computed tomography and single photon absorptiometry with spinal and non–spinal fractures. *Osteoporos Int* 1996, 6, 407 – 415.

[19] Kalender WA: Effective dose values in bone mineral measurements by photon absorptiometry and computed tomography. *Osteoporos Int* 1992, 2, 82 – 87.

[20] Weigert JM: QCT, the most accurate method of measuring bone mineral density? *J Bone Miner Res*, 1997, 12, 1954 – 1955.

In: Osteoporosis: Etiology, Diagnosis and Treatment
Editors: Bilar E. Mattingly and Albert C. Pillare
ISBN 978-1-60692-397-9

Short Communication L

Determination of NTx in Second Morning Urine (Draft Standardisation of Morning Urine Collection)

J. Wendlová[1,*] and M. Mikulecký[2]

[1]University Derer´s Hospital and Policlinic, Osteological Centre, Bratislava, Slovakia;
[2]Institute of Preventive and Clinical Medicine, Bratislava, Slovakia.

Abstract

According to the instruction manual of the producer of kits for determining the levels of aminoterminal telopeptide of type I collagen of organic bone matrix (NTx), the time of the collection of second morning urine is arbitrary, i.e., that a patient can urinate anytime within the period from about 6 to 8.30 a.m. This time interval is within the period of the change in circadian rhythm of the NTx excretion (maximum excretion with the transition into the fast decrease of excretion). That is the reason why we considered appropriate to standardise conditions for the collection of second morning urine and we suggested to apply the so-called two-hour morning diuresis NTx2 (from 6 to 8.00 a.m. after an overnight fast). We examined 48 women patients aged 33-65 with a primary or secondary osteopenia or osteoporosis (all patients had normal renal functions). In these patients we determined NTx (Osteomark, OSTEX, USA) in a standardly used 24-hour diuresis (NTx24) and in the suggested two-hour morning diuresis (NTx2).

Aim of the study: To find a mathematical character of the dependence of values of dependent variable NTx2 from an independent variable NTx24 and to evaluate the statistic significance of this dependence. To compare the ratio of the widths of 95% confidence intervals (C.I.) for NTx2 and NTx24 in patients (index: IO) with the ratio of the widths of reference limits for NTx in arbitrary second morning urine ($NTx2_{ostex}$) and

* Correspondence concerning this article should be addressed to: Ass Prof Jaroslava Wendlová MD, PhD Krížna 30, 811 07 Bratislava. jwendlova@mail.t-com.sk.

in 24-hour diuresis ($NTx24_{ostex}$) in healthy women (index: IR). To evaluate the suggested two-hour diuresis for the determination of NTx.

Statistical analysis: Stochastic and deterministic linear regressive analysis. Index of 95% C.I., index of reference limits.

Results: Statistically significant ($p < 0.01$) regressive dependence ($r^2 = 0.781$) was found between the values of NTx24 and NTx2. The index of the widths of reference limits (IR) is 1.5 times bigger that the index for osteopenic and osteoporotic patients (IO), meaning that the scatter of the $NTx2_{ostex}$ values is bigger than NTx2 in the suggested two-hour diuresis.

Conclusion: Based on statistically significant linear regressive dependence between NTx24 and NTx2 values it is possible to use the suggested two-hour morning diuresis to determine the NTx levels in women. The introduction of two-hour morning diuresis NTx2 will decrease the fluctuation range of NTx values in its repeated examination and will make the conclusiveness of its values more accurate in comparison with the determination of $NTx2_{ostex}$ in any second morning urine in compliance with the instructions of the producer of kits OSTEX, USA.

Keywords: NTx - osteoresorption - dueresis - osteoporosis.

INTRODUCTION

Aminoterminal telopeptide of type I collagen of organic bone matrix (NTx) urine parameter is one of sensitive markers of laboratory diagnostics of bone resorption.

Indications for NTx determination are detection of the character of bone turnover (osteoresorption) during peri- and postmenopause, identification of risk patients for the development of osteoporosis, monitoring the effectiveness of antiosteoresorption therapy (bisphosphonates, hormonal replacement therapy, calcitonine, selective modulators of oestrogen receptors), diagnostics and therapy effectiveness control in Paget's disease [1,2].

The NTx value decrease by 30% and more reflects significant changes in bone resorption [3]. Selecting a proper drug and doses, in 4 to 8 weeks following the beginning of the therapy the urine NTx level should drop by 30% compared to the initial level prior to therapy. If this does not happen, the therapy is probably unsuccessful [4,5,6].

The producer of the kits for determining NTx (Osteomark, OSTEX, USA) recommends in its instruction manual two different methods of urine collection for determining NTx:

1. 24-hour urine collection ($NTx24_{ostex}$)
2. any second morning urine ($NTx2_{ostex}$)

While the 24-hour urine collection ($NTx24_{ostex}$) is precisely defined, there are no standard conditions for the urine collection given for the second morning urine ($NTx2_{ostex}$). According to observation by different authors [7,8,9], NTx levels are subject to circadian variations. Maximum NTx excretion in urine in healthy as well as patients with osteoporosis is between 3 and 7 a.m. and minimum excretion between 3 and 7 p.m. Roughly defined second morning urine collection can be made, e.g., between 6.30 and 7 a.m., this period overlapping with the time period of maximum NTx excretion, or between 7 and 8.30 a.m. when the excretion of NTx levels decreases. As the time interval of roughly defined second morning urine collection (between 6.30 and 8.30 a.m.) is within the time of the change in circadian rhythm (maximum excretion with transition to fast decrease of excretion), it can be assumed that the NTx values will markedly fluctuate just in this second morning urine, especially in repeated control urine collections.

Therefore we consider it proper to standardise conditions for the collection of second morning urine and suggest the so-called two-hour morning diuresis NTx2 (6 to 8 a.m.)

THE AIM OF THE STUDY

To find a mathematical character of the dependence of values of TNx2 in the suggested two – hour morning diuresis from values of NTx24 in a standardly used 24 – hour diuresis and based on the character of the statistical significance to evaluate the suggested two – hour diuresis for the determination of TNx.

SUBJECTS AND METHODS

We examined 48 women with primary or secondary osteoporosis aged 33-65 (all examined patients had normal renal functions). The NTx was determined in those patients in 24- and 2-hour diuresis after an overnight fast. Seven days prior to the examination the patients did not use any medications. One day prior to the examination, at 6 a.m. they urinated into the toilet, then they were collecting the urine into a glass vessel. At 6 a.m. on the second day they urinated to the collection vessel for the last time and so finished the 24-hour urine collection. Following the 24-hour urine collection they did not urinate at home any more, they also did not eat and drink and came to the surgery with the whole volume of urine. At 8 a.m. they urinated again and this sample was taken in separately. In this way standard conditions were ensured for the second morning diuresis, which we called two-hour morning diuresis (6 to 8 a.m.).

METHODS

Densitometry

The women enrolled in he study were assigned as osteopenic or osteoporotic according to the WHO classification based on measurement with DXA in the proximal femur (DXA, Hologic, USA).

Laboratory Methods

1) NTx in urine, Osteomark™, OSTEX, USA.
Assay principles.

The Osteomark™ assay is a competitive – inhibition enzyme – linked immunosorbent assay (ELISA). Quantitation of the NTx concentration in the specimen is determined spectrophotometrically and calculated from a standard calibration curve, Assay values are corrected for urinary dilution by urinary creatinine analysis and expressed in nanomoles NTx per liter per millimole creatinine per liter.

Total assay precision: 7-10 %

Urine specimen storage:

The urine samples have been storaged by – 20° C or below for 5 – 7 weeks. They did not undergo thaw cycles.

The samples handling were strictly standardized to keep the components stable and to provide reproducible conditions for their measurement.

2) Creatinine in urine, Biotrol creatinine H.P., Biotrol Diagnostic, France

Biotrol creatinine H.P. is based on modifications of the Jaffe procedure.

The intensity of formation of the red coloured complex measured at 510 nm is directly proportional to the amount of creatinine present in the sample.

$$\text{Creatinine} + \text{picric acid} \xrightarrow[\text{pH}]{\text{ALKALINE}} \text{red complex}$$

3) Calculation the ratio: NTx (nmol/l) : Creatinine in urine (mmol/l)

– in 24 – hour and 2 – hour urine collection

Statistical Analysis

D'Agostino's test for $n > 30$ was used to test the normality of the distribution of statistical signs [10].

One-way dependence of the dependent variable **y (NTx2)** from independent variable **x (NTx24)** was expressed using stochastic and deterministic linear regression $(y = a + bx)$, where a, b are regressive coefficients [11,17].

To compare the scatter of the NTx2 and $NTx2_{ostex}$ we used the following indices [17 - 18]:

1) Index (IO) of the widths 95% C.I. for NTx2 and NTx24 in female patients
2) index (IR) of the widths 95% C.I. of reference limits for $NTx2_{ostex}$ and $NTx24_{ostex}$ in healthy women (equations in Table 3).

RESULTS

Measurement sets of variable values NTx2 and NTx24 were characterised by a median ($\tilde{x}$) and 95% C.I. because they did not show normal distribution (non-parametric distribution) Table 1.

Using linear regressive analysis to determine the character of mutual dependence between NTx values in the suggested two-hour morning diuresis (NTx2) and NTx values in standard 24-hour diuresis (NTx24) in osteopenic and osteoporotic women.

(NTx2 = a + b. NTx24) it was found out that the dependence of the dependent variable NTx2 from independent variable NTx24 is statistically significant (r^2 = 0.78). According to the determination coefficient (r^2) 78% of values of dependent variable NTx2 is linear dependent upon the values of independent variable NTx24, and only 22% of NTx2 values are not subject to this dependence (Table 2).

The main message of the graphic depiction of the regression (Grapf1) is a fair congruence between confidence corridor and the line of identity *(y = x, a = 0, b = 1)*. In the little square demarked with the 95% confidence intervals for either variable NTx2, NTx24 (dotted and dashed straight lines) is better shown this fair congruence between line of means (middle full line of 95% confidence corridors) and line of identity.

Table 1. The point and interval estimates of NTx (nmol/mmol creat.) urine output for the present data as well as for those given in instruction manual for OSTEX

Gender	Variable	Mean	Median	95% C.I.	Reference intervals OSTEX
female	NTx24	---	37.4	27.9 ; 43.0	---
n = 48	NTx2	---	39.3	29.8 ; 48.9	---
female	NTx24	28.0	---	---	14 ; 42
OSTEX	NTx2	32.0	---	---	6 ; 58

Table 2. The point estimates and their 95% confidence intervals (C.I.) for the regression coefficients a, b of the linear function (NTx2 = a + b.NTx24), with corresponding coefficients of determination (r^2)

Gender	a		b		r^2
	mean	95% C.I.	mean	95% C.I.	
	NTx2 / creat.		*P* = *NTx2/ creat.* / NTx24/ creat.		
Females	11,2 *	4,7 ; 17,7	0,84 *	0,70 ; 0,97	0,781

*significantly (α = 0.01) different from zero.

P – proportion

Table 3 contains equations used for calculating the index for reference values of NTx $_{ostex}$ (IR) and the index for measured values of NTx (IO).

Table 3. Index of widths of 95% C. I. for osteoporosis (IO), index of widths of 95% C. I. for reference ranges given by OSTEX (IR) and index (I) of IR to IO

Gender	Index for osteoporosis (IO)	Index for reference ranges, OSTEX (IR)	$I = \frac{IR}{IO}$
females	1.26	1.86	1.5

$$IO = \frac{\text{width of 95\% C. I. for NTx2}}{\text{width of 95\% C. I. for NTx24}}$$

$$IR = \frac{\text{width of reference ranges for NTx2 OSTEX}}{\text{width of reference ranges for NTx24 OSTEX}}$$

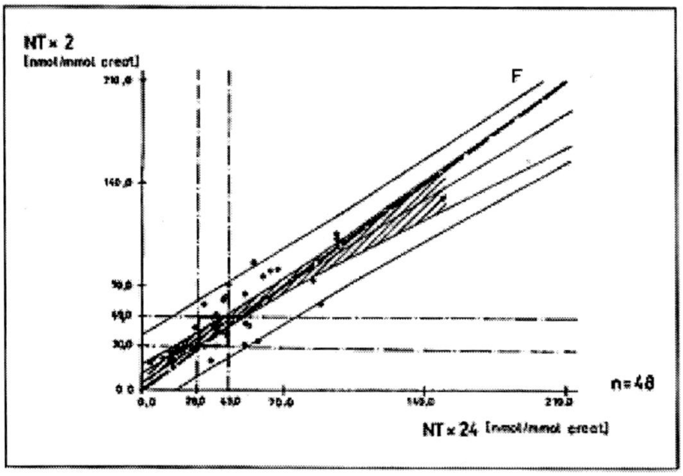

Graph 1. The NTx2 values in 48 female patients with osteoporosis plotted versus their NTx24 values. The data (dots) were approximated with the aid of the linear regression function (l.r.f.) NTx2 = a + b.NTx24. The point estimate of the l.r.f. is accompanied by the 95% confidence (shadowed) and 95% tolerance (wider) corridors. The theoretical line of identity is shown by heavy dashed straight line.

Ratio for reference ranges given by OSTEX ($NTx2_{ostex}/NTx24_{ostex}$) is 1.5 times higher than for osteoporosis (NTx2/NTx24) in the present study, i.e., the scatter of $NTx2_{ostex}$ data is higher than of NTx2.

In the graph 2 the line of identity (LI) is nearer to the diagonal of the little guadrangular (F) as to the bigger one (f). There is a better congruity of both NTx24 and NTx2 values with the line of identity in the present data as the reference data for $NTx2_{ostex}$ and $NTx24_{ostex}$.

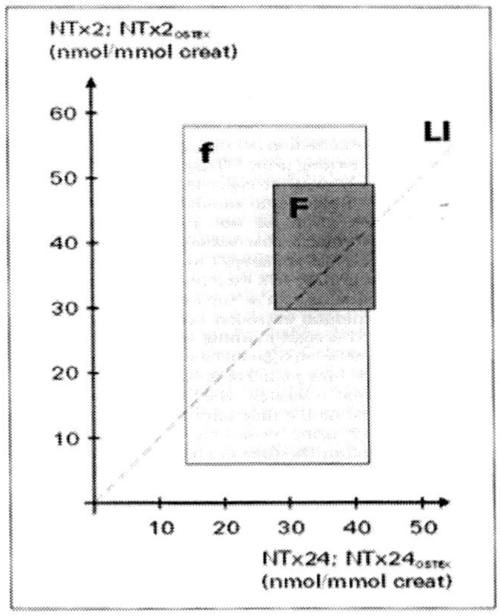

Graph 2. Quadrangular area delimited by univariate 95% confidence intervals for NTx24 and NTx2 (F = female patients). For comparison, analogical areas are shown for the reference intervals given by OSTEX for $NTx24_{OSTEX}$ and $NTx2_{OSTEX}$ (f = females). The theoretical line of identity (LI) is given too.

Discussion

In general intra – individual variability expressed as coefficient of variation (CV % = SD/ x .100 %) is lower for serum bone formation markers than for urinary resorption markers although urinary NTx (U - NTx) is the most sensitive marker for prediction of bone loss and for monitoring therapy effect. The intra – patient CV is around 14,2% for U – NTx and only 7,2% for serum NTx [12].

Sources of biological variability can be divided into two categories: (1) uncontrollable factors such as age, gender, renal function, ethnicity, pregnancy, lactation, some drugs, certain diseases, recent fractures, menopausal status, oral contraception, immobility and (2) controllable factors such as circadian rhythms, menstrual cycle, seasonal variation, exercise, diet, reference ranges [13].

The preanalytical controllable factors that influence variability of U – NTx are in the first place circadian rhythms, choice of reference group and exercise.

Circadian variability has more impact on markers of bone turnover than most other sources of variability [7]. According to the Committee of Scientific Advisors of the International Osteoporosis Foundation each laboratory should establish own reference ranges separately for men, premenopausal and postmenopausal women. Standardized time and conditions for sample collection must also be defined for each reference range [13]. Persistent and acute exercises affect the variability of bone markers. In most studies the acute effect of exercise is to increase markers of collagen degradation by 10 – 15%. The patients have to refrain from exercise for at least 24 h before samples are collected [14]. Other preanalytical controllable factors such as menstrual cycle, seasonal variation and diet have a small impact on variability of U – NTx so that the effect may be regarded as insignificant. From preanalytical uncontrollable factors is the most important renal function and immobility. Care should be taken in the interpretation of U – NTx when the creatinine clearance decreases below 30-ml/min [15].Bed rest results in a very rapid increase in markers of bone resorption [16].

The significance of circadian variability for our study can be discused as follows.

As the second morning diuresis just falls within the time interval of the change in circadian rhythm of NTx excretion, we consider necessarily the introduction of standard conditions for urine collection. In our study we presented the two-hour morning diuresis we use in osteological surgery.

Statistically significant regressive dependence between NTx24 and NTx2 values in female patients with osteopenia or osteoporosis indicates that both urine collections can be used for the measurement of NTx levels.

Because of economic reasons we did not examine NTx2 and NTx24 levels in a healthy control group. In accordance with the rules of statistical data processing it is not admissible to compare measured values with reference values and that was the reason why we chose the method of comparing relative values - indices.

There is a linear dependence between measured NTx2 and NTx24 values as well as between $NTx2_{ostex}$ and $NTx24_{ostex}$ reference values, i.e., the increase of NTx24 ($NTx24_{ostex}$) value is accompanied also by the increase of NTx2 ($NTx2_{ostex}$) value, while the mutual ratio NTx2/NTx24 ($NTx2_{ostex}$ /$NTx24_{ostex}$) is a constant one, and exactly this constant ratio of linearly growing values was the basis for the calculation of indices. The comparison of the index of reference values with the index of values of female patients is possible in this case, because the ratio of NTx values in the second morning urine and in 24-hour diuresis in both patients and healthy women is a constant one, regardless whether the values are increasing or decreasing, pathological or normal.

The index of reference limits of the OSTEX Co. ($NTx2_{ostex}$ /$NTx24_{ostex}$) which is higher than the index of the widths 95% C.I. (NTx2/NTx24) of measured values in our study points out that there is a bigger scatter of $NTx2_{ostex}$ values than of NTx2 values in the suggested diuresis.

The two-hour diuresis was chosen on practical grounds, so that the patients did not have to transport the urine from their homes to the surgery and, at the same time, so that the collection of second morning urine was standardised. In conclusion, statistically significant positive regressive dependence was found out between NTx24 and NTx2 values. Suggested two-hour morning diuresis can be used to determine the NTx levels in women. $NTx2_{ostex}$ values present bigger scatter than NTx2 values. The introduction of two-hour diuresis for determining NTx levels instead of presently used any second morning urine will reduce the scope of fluctuation of NTx values in repeated examinations and will make the conclusiveness of NTx values in morning diuresis more accurate.

To reduce the effect of circadian rhythms on the clinical interpretation of markers of bone turnover it is essential that the timing of sample collection be standardized.

References

[1] Hanson D.A, Weis M.A., Bollen A., Maslan S.L., Singer F.R., Eyre D.R.: A specific immunoassay for monitoring human bone resorption: quantification of type I. collagen cross-linked N-telopeptide in urine. *J Bone Miner Res*, 1992, 11, 125-130.

[2] Calvo MS, Eyre D.R., Gundberg C.M.: Molecular Basis and clinical application of biological markers of bone turnover. *Endocrinol Rev*, 1996, 4, 333-367.

[3] Schneider DL, Barrett - Connor - EL: Urinary N - telopeptide levels discriminate normal, osteopenic, and osteoporotic bone mineral density. *Arch Intern Med* 1997, 157, 1241 – 1245.

[4] Ravn P, Hosking D, Thompson D., Cizza G., Wasnich R.D., McClung M., Yates A.J., Bjarnason N.H., Christiansen C.: Monitoring of alendronate treatment and prediction of effects on bone mass by biochemical markers in the early postmenopausal intervention cohort study. *J Clin Endocrinol Metab* 1999, 7, 2363 – 68.

[5] Braga de Castro Machado A, Hannon R, Eastell R: Monitoring alendronate therapy for osteoporosis. *J Bone Miner Res*, 1999, 4, 602 – 608.

[6] Eastell R., Calvo MS, Burritt MF, Offord KP, Russell RG, Riggs BL: Abnormalities in circadian patterns of bone resorption and renal calcium conservation in type I. osteoporosis. *J Clin Endocrinol Metab* 1992, 74, 487 – 494.

[7] Blumsohn A, Herrington K, Hannon A, Shao P, Eyre DR, Eastell R: The effect of calcium supplementation on the circadian rhythm of bone resorption. *J Clin Endocrinol Metab* 1994, 3, 730 – 735.

[8] Greenspan SL, Dresner - Pollak R, Rarker RA, London D, Ferguson L: Diurnal variation of bone mineral turnover in elderly men and women. *Calcif Tissue Int* 1997, 60, 419 – 23.

[9] Ju HS, Leung S, Brown B, Stringer M.A., Leigh S., Scherrer C., Shepard K., Jenkins D., Knudsen J., Cannon R.: Comparison of analytical performance and biological variability of three bone resorption assays. *Clin Chem* 1997, 43, 1570 – 1576.

[10] Procházka B: *Biostastics for doctors. Principles of basic methods and their interpretation*. Charles University Prague, Publishing House Carolinum, Prague, 1999, 65 – 72.

[11] Pacakova V: *Štatistika pre ekonómov (Statistics for economists)*, IURA EDITION, Bratislava, 1st edition, 2003, 193 – 234.

[12] Eastell R., Mallinak N., Weiss S., Ettinger M., Pettinger M., Cain D., Flessland K., Chesnut III. C: Biological variability of serum and urinary N – telopeptides of type I. collagen in postmenopausal women. *J Bone Miner Res* 2000, 15, 594 – 598.

[13] Delmas P.D., Eastell R., Garnero P., Seibel M.J., Stepan J.: The use of biochemical markers of bone turnover in osteoporosis. *Osteoporos Int* 2000, Suppl.6, 2 – 17.

[14] Thorsen K., Kristofferson A., Lorenztzon R.: The effect of brisk walking on markers of bone and calcium metabolism in postmenopausal women. *Calcif Tissue Int* 1996, 58, 221 – 225.

[15] Watts N.B: Clinical utility of biochemical markers of bone remodelling. *Clin Chem* 1999, 45, 1359 – 1368.

[16] Zerwekh J.E., Ruml L.A., Gottschalk F., Pak C.Y.: The effects of twelve weeks of bed rest on bone histology, biochemical markers of bone turnover and calcium homeostasis in eleven normal subjects. *J Bone Miner Res* 1998, 13, 1594 – 1601.

[17] Varga S.: Robust Estimations in Classical Regression Models versus Robust Estimations in Fuzzy Regression Models. *Kybernetika* 2007, vol. 43, č. 4, 503-508.

[18] Stankovičová I, Vojtková M: Multi – dimensional statistical methods with applications.

[19] Publishing house: *Iura Edition, Bratislava*, 2007, 202-241, ISBN 978-80-8078-152-1

INDEX

A

C

D

E

F

G

H

I

J

K

L

M

N

O

P

S

T

U

V

W

X

Y

Z